PHYSICAL THERAPY CASE FILES® Orthopedics

Second Edition

Jason Brumitt, PT, PhD, ATC, CSCS, CSPS
Associate Professor of Physical Therapy
School of Physical Therapy
George Fox University
Newberg, Oregon
Adjunct Faculty
Rocky Mountain University of Health Professions
Provo, Utah

Erin E. Jobst, PT, PhD
Clinical Associate Professor of Physical Therapy
Doctor of Physical Therapy Program
Oregon State University—Cascades
Bend, Oregon

New York   Chicago   San Francisco   Athens   London   Madrid   Mexico City
Milan   New Delhi   Singapore   Sydney   Toronto

Physical Therapy Case Files®: Orthopedics, Second Edition

1 2 3 4 5 6 7 8 9   LCR   28 27 26 25 24 23

ISBN 978-1-264-28600-3
MHID 1-264-28600-7

Notice

Medicine is an ever-changing science. As new research and clinical experience broaden our knowledge, changes in treatment and drug therapy are required. The authors and the publisher of this work have checked with sources believed to be reliable in their efforts to provide information that is complete and generally in accord with the standard accepted at the time of publication. However, in view of the possibility of human error or changes in medical sciences, neither the editors nor the publisher nor any other party who has been involved in the preparation or publication of this work warrants that the information contained herein is in every respect accurate or complete, and they disclaim all responsibility for any errors or omissions or for the results obtained from use of the information contained in this work. Readers are encouraged to confirm the information contained herein with other sources. For example and in particular, readers are advised to check the product information sheet included in the package of each drug they plan to administer to be certain that the information contained in this work is accurate and that changes have not been made in the recommended dose or in the contraindications for administration. This recommendation is of particular importance in connection with new or infrequently used drugs.

This book was set in Adobe Jenson Pro by KnowledgeWorks Global Ltd.
The editors were Sydney Keen Vitale and Christina M. Thomas.
The production supervisor was Catherine H. Saggese.
Project management was provided by Nitesh Sharma of KnowledgeWorks Global Ltd.

Library of Congress Cataloging-in-Publication Data

Names: Brumitt, Jason, editor.
Title: Physical therapy case files. Orthopedics / [edited by] Jason
    Brumitt.
Other titles: Physical therapy case files. Orthopaedics. | Orthopedics
Description: Second edition. | New York : McGraw Hill, [2024] | Preceded by
    Physical therapy case files. Orthopaedics / [edited by] Jason Brumitt.
    c2013. | Includes bibliographical references and index. | Summary: "This
    second edition of Physical Therapy Case Files - Orthopedics contains 33
    cases on common musculoskeletal conditions: 7 on the upper extremity, 8
    on the spine, and 18 on the lower extremity. Twenty-six cases from the
    1st edition have been updated to incorporate new practices and evidence
    over the past decade. Examples include the use of diagnostic ultrasound
    to confirm the diagnosis of patellar tendinopathy (Case 22) and the use
    of dry needling as an adjunctive treatment for plantar heel pain (Case
    33). Six new cases reflect exciting advancements in physical therapy
    practice, including blood flow restriction training in the treatment of
    patellofemoral pain (Case 21) and the utilization of physical therapists
    in the primary care setting (Case 15). We hope this new edition will
    inspire continued learning, inform practice, and help improve the lives
    of your patients"—Provided by publisher.
Identifiers: LCCN 2023007787 (print) | LCCN 2023007788 (ebook) | ISBN
    9781264286003 (paperback) | ISBN 9781264286010 (ebook)
Subjects: MESH: Physical Therapy Modalities | Musculoskeletal
    Diseases—therapy | Orthopedic Procedures—methods | Needs Assessment |
    Case Reports
Classification: LCC RM725 (print) | LCC RM725 (ebook) | NLM WB 460 | DDC
    615.8/2—dc23/eng/20230620
LC record available at https://lccn.loc.gov/2023007787
LC ebook record available at https://lccn.loc.gov/2023007788

CONTENTS

Lane Bailey, PT, DPT, PhD, CSCS
Director of Sports Medicine and Research
Memorial Hermann Health System
Houston, Texas

David S. Bailie, MD
Orthopedic surgeon
Arizona Institute of Sports Knees and Shoulders (AZISKS)
Scottsdale, Arizona

Jolene Bennett, PT, OCS, Cert MDT
Physical therapist
Spectrum Health Rehabilitation Services
Grand Rapids, Michigan

Jake Bleacher, PT, MSPT, OCS, FAAOMPT, MTC, CSCS
Co-coordinator of the Orthopedic Manual Physical Therapy
  Fellowship Program
The Ohio State Medical Center Sports Medicine at Care Point in
  Gahanna
Ohio State's Wexner Medical Center
Gahanna, Ohio

Jason Brumitt, PT, PhD, ATC, CSCS, CSPS
Associate Professor of Physical Therapy
School of Physical Therapy
George Fox University
Newberg, Oregon
Adjunct Faculty
Rocky Mountain University of Health Professions
Provo, Utah

Michael R. Conway, PT, DPT
Sports Physical Therapist
Gundersen Health System
Onalaska, Wisconsin

Tyler Cuddeford, PT, PhD
Professor of Physical Therapy
School of Physical Therapy
George Fox University
Newberg, Oregon

Barry Dale, PhD, PT, OCS, SCS, CSCS, ATC (Ret.)
Professor and Chair
Department of Physical Therapy
University of Tennessee Health Science Center
Memphis, Tennessee

George J. Davies, DPT, MEd, PT, SCS, ATC, LAT, CSCS, PES, CSMS, FAPTA
Professor
Georgia Southern University
Savannah, Georgia
Assistant Director
Georgia Southern University Biodynamics & Human
  Performance Center
Savannah, Georgia
Sports Physical Therapist
Coastal Therapy & Sports Rehab
Savannah, Georgia
Sports Physical Therapist
Gundersen Health System
Onalaska, Wisconsin

Carl DeRosa, PT, PhD, FAPTA
Professor and Director
Physical Therapy Program
Rasmussen University
Eagan, Minnesota

Todd S. Ellenbecker, DPT, MS, CSCS, FAPTA
Board Certified in Orthopaedic Physical Therapy
Director of Shoulder Rehabilitation and Clinical Research
Rehab Plus Sports Therapy Scottsdale
Vice President Medical Services, ATP Tour
Scottsdale, Arizona

Charles Greene, PhD, PT, MS, ATC
Physical Therapist
Rocky Mountain University of Health Professions
Provo, Utah

Laurie Griffin, PT, DPT, OCS
Physical Therapist
Howard Head Sport Medicine
Vail, Colorado

Barbara J. Hoogenboom, PT, EdD, SCS, ATC
Professor and Associate Chair, Physical Therapy Department
Grand Valley State University
Grand Rapids, Michigan

Jeff Houck, PT, PhD
Program Director
School of Physical Therapy
George Fox University
Newberg, Oregon

Daniel Jenkins, PT, DPT
Physical Therapist & Assistant Department Manager
Lebanon Community Hospital
Lebanon, Oregon

Daniel Kang, PT, DPT
Dean, Interprofessional Education
Interim Dean, College of Allied Health
Associate Professor, School of Physical Therapy
George Fox University
Newberg, Oregon

Kristi Greene Kelch, PT, OCS, FAAOMPT
Physical Therapist
Agile Physical Therapy
Palo Alto, California

Marcey Keefer Hutchison, DPT, SCS, ATC, CMP
Clinical Associate Professor of Physical Therapy
Doctor of Physical Therapy Program
Oregon State University—Cascades
Bend, Oregon

Douglas Lauchlan, MCSP, MSc Physiotherapy
Senior Lecturer in Physiotherapy
Glasgow Caledonian University
Glasgow, Scotland, United Kingdom

Brianne Lewis, PTA
Physical Therapist Assistant
Rehab Plus Sports Therapy Scottsdale
Scottsdale, Arizona

Janice K. Loudon, PT, PhD, SCS, ATC, CSCS
Professor
Department of Physical Therapy Education
Rockhurst University
Kansas City, Missouri

Robert C. Manske, PT, SCS
Professor of Physical Therapy
Department of Physical Therapy
Wichita State University
Wichita, Kansas

Danny J. McMillian, PT, DSc, OCS
Clinical Professor
School of Physical Therapy
University of Puget Sound
Tacoma, Washington

Erik P. Meira, PT, DPT
Board Certified in Sports Physical Therapy
Director
PTSC Group, Inc.
Happy Valley, Oregon

Matt Mymern, PT, DPT, SCS, MHA, CSCS
Physical Therapist
Howard Head Sport Medicine
Vail, Colorado

Nathan R. Neff, PT, DPT, SCS, MTC, CSCS
Physical Therapist
Howard Head Sports Medicine
Vail, Colorado

Luke T. O'Brien, PT, M.Phty (Sports), SCS
Head of Physical Therapy
Milwaukee Bucks
Milwaukee, Wisconsin

Thomas J. Olson, PT, DPT, SCS
Physical Therapist
Vail, Colorado

Johnny Owens, MPT
Physical Therapist
Owens Recovery Science, INC
San Antonio, Texas

Mark V. Paterno, PT, PhD, MBA, SCS, ATC
Scientific Director
Division of Occupational Therapy and Physical Therapy
Cincinnati Children's Hospital Medical Center
Cincinnati, Ohio
Professor
Department of Pediatrics
University of Cincinnati
Cincinnati, Ohio

Li-Zandre Philbrook, PT, DPT
Assistant Professor of Physical Therapy
School of Physical Therapy
George Fox University
Newberg, Oregon

Laura S. Pietrosimone, DPT, PhD
Assistant Professor
Doctor of Physical Therapy Division
Department of Orthopedic Surgery
School of Medicine
Duke University
Durham, North Carolina

Paul Reuteman, PT, DPT, ATC
Board Certified Clinical Specialist in Orthopedic Physical Therapy
Clinical Professor
Program of Physical Therapy
University of Wisconsin–La Crosse
La Crosse, Wisconsin

Michael D. Rosenthal, PT, DSc, ATC
Associate Professor of Physical Therapy
College of Allied Health Professions
University of Nebraska Medical Center
Omaha, Nebraska

Michael D. Ross, PT, DHSc, OCS, FAAOMPT
Associate Professor
Daemen University
Amherst, New York

Ellen Shanley, PhD, PT, OCS
Sr. Director Care Delivery Optimization
  Research Scientist—ATI Physical Therapy
Director, Athletic Injury Research, Prevention, and Education
SC Center for Effectiveness Research in Orthopedics
Greenville, South Carolina

Lyndsay Stutzenberger, PT, DPT, PhD
Assistant Professor of Physical Therapy
School of Physical Therapy
George Fox University
Newberg, Oregon

Christy Sweeney, PT
Senior Physical Therapist
Beacon Orthopaedics and Sports Medicine
Cincinnati, Ohio

Casey A. Unverzagt, PT, DPT, DSc
Board Certified in Orthopaedic & Sports Physical Therapy
Fellow, American Academy of Orthopaedic Manual Physical Therapists
Clinical Associate Professor
Academic Coordinator for Baylor Scott & White—Baylor University
  Orthopaedic Residency
Baylor University Doctor of Physical Therapy ProgramWaco, Texas

Charles Nathan Vannatta, PT, DPT, SCS
Sports Physical Therapist
Gundersen Health System
Onalaska, Wisconsin
Associate Program Director for Sports Physical Therapy Residency
  Program
Gundersen Medical Foundation
Onalaska, Wisconsin
Adjunct Graduate Faculty
La Crosse Institute of Movement Science
University of Wisconsin–La Crosse
La Crosse, Wisconsin

Shane A. Vath, PT, DSc, SCS
Physical Therapist
Physical Therapy Department
Naval Medical Clinic Annapolis
Annapolis, Maryland

Paul E. Westgard, PT, DPT, OCS, SCS, CSCS
Physical Therapist
Howard Head Sports Medicine
Vail, Colorado

Tyler Whited, PT, DPT
Assistant Professor of Kinesiology
Kinesiology Program
George Fox University
Newberg, Oregon

Brett Windsor, PT, MPA, PhD
Associate Professor of Physical Therapy
Physical Therapy Program
Rasmussen University
Eagan, Minnesota

Pedro Zavala, PT, DPT
Sports Physical Therapist
Twin Cities Orthopedics
Woodbury, Minnesota

Sadie J. Zebell, PT, DPT, ATC
Sports Physical Therapist
Gundersen Health System
Onalaska, Wisconsin

ACKNOWLEDGMENTS

We would like to thank each of the authors who contributed cases for the second edition of this book. Your participation in this project has helped us to create what we believe will be an invaluable book for students, new clinicians, and seasoned professionals. We were fortunate to have leading clinical and academic physical therapists share their expertise.

Jason Brumitt and Erin E. Jobst

It is especially an honor for me that this book includes cases from George Davies, Todd Ellenbecker, Rob Manske, and Erik Meira. These therapists have informed my clinical practice and inspired my research. I am also excited to include cases from my friends and colleagues at George Fox University.

Next, I would like to thank my friend and project partner Erin Jobst, PT, PhD. Erin is the Series Editor for the *Physical Therapy Case Files* books. Her editing and project oversight has elevated the quality of each case presented in this book.

I would also like to thank my wife Renee and children Rex, Halsey, and Stone for their love and support. Finally, I would like to thank Tom Petty and the Heartbreakers, Pearl Jam, Slash featuring Myles Kennedy and the Conspirators, Miles Davis, and Buddy Guy. Their music played non-stop in the background during the writing and editing process.

Jason Brumitt, PT, PhD, ATC, CSCS

Thank you to all my students—past and present—that keep me engaged and eager to continue learning. Without your questions and attention, there would be no reason for writing any textbook. And, always, thank you dear Ken for always providing me encouragement and endless love and support.

Erin E. Jobst, PT, PhD

As the physical therapy profession continues to evolve as a doctoring profession, so does the rigor of entry-level physical therapist education. Students must master foundational courses while integrating an understanding of new research in all areas of physical therapy. Evidence-based practice is clinical decision-making that incorporates current best evidence with the expertise of the clinician and the values and circumstances of the patient. Evidence-based practice is emphasized in physical therapy education. However, the most challenging task for students is making the transition from didactic classroom-based knowledge to its application in developing a physical therapy diagnosis and implementing appropriate interventions. Ideally, instructors who are experienced and knowledgeable in every diagnosis and treatment approach would guide students at the "bedside" and students would supplement this training by independent reading. While there is certainly no substitute for clinical education, clinical rotations cannot cover the scope of each physical therapy setting. In addition, it is not always possible for clinical instructors to be able to take the time necessary to guide students through the application of evidence-based tests and measures and interventions. Perhaps an effective approach includes teaching with structured case studies. At the time of writing the *Physical Therapy Case Files* series, there were no physical therapy textbooks containing case studies that reference current literature to support an illustrated examination or treatment. In my own teaching to physical therapy students, I have designed case scenarios based on my personal patient care experiences, those experiences shared by my colleagues, and searches through textbooks, journals, and websites to find a case study illustrating a particular concept. There are two problems with this approach. First, neither my own nor my colleagues' experiences cover the diversity of patient diagnoses, examinations, and interventions. Second, designing a case scenario that is not based on personal patient care experience or expertise takes an overwhelming amount of time. In my experience, detailed case studies that incorporate application of the best evidence are difficult to design "on the fly" in the classroom. The twofold goal of the *Physical Therapy Case Files* series is to provide resources that contain multiple real-life case studies within an individual physical therapy practice area that will minimize the need for physical therapy educators to create their own scenarios and maximize the students' ability to implement evidence into the care of individual patients.

The cases within each book in the *Physical Therapy Case Files* series are organized for the reader to either read the book from "front to back" or to select scenarios based on specific interest. A list of cases by case number and by health condition is included in Section II. Each case follows an organized format using language from both the World Health Organization's International Classification of Functioning, Disability, and Health (ICF) framework[1] and the American Physical Therapy Association's *Guide to Physical Therapist Practice*.[2] Section titles within each case were chosen to guide the reader through each step of patient/client management.

The front page of each case begins with a patient encounter followed by a series of open-ended questions. The discussion following the case is organized into *seven* sections:

1. **Key Definitions** provide terminology pertinent to the reader's understanding of the case. **Objectives** list the instructional and/or terminal behavioral objectives that summarize the knowledge, skills, or attitudes the reader should be able to demonstrate after reading the case. *PT considerations* provides a summary of the physical therapy plan of care, goals, interventions, precautions, and potential complications for physical therapy management of the individual presented in the case.

2. **Understanding the Health Condition** presents an abbreviated explanation of the medical diagnosis. The intent of this section is *not* to be comprehensive. The etiology, risk factors, epidemiology, and medical management of the condition are presented in enough detail to provide background and context for the reader.

3. **Physical Therapy Patient/Client Management** provides a summary of the role of the physical therapist in the patient's care. This section may elaborate on how the physical therapist's role augments and/or overlaps with those of other healthcare practitioners involved in the patient's care, as well as any referrals to additional healthcare practitioners that the physical therapist should provide.

4. **Examination, Evaluation, and Diagnosis** guides the reader how to organize and interpret information gathered from the chart review (in inpatient cases), appreciate adverse drug reactions that may affect patient presentation, and structure the subjective evaluation and physical examination. Not every assessment tool and special test that could possibly be done with the patient is included. For each outcome measure or special test presented, available reliability, validity, sensitivity, and specificity are discussed. When available, a minimal clinically important difference (MCID) for an outcome measure is presented to help the clinician to determine the "the minimal level of change required in response to an intervention before the outcome would be considered worthwhile in terms of a patient/client's function or quality of life."[3]

5. **Plan of Care and Interventions** elaborates on a few physical therapy interventions for the patient's condition. The advantage of this section and the previous section is that each case does *not* exhaustively present every outcome measure, special test, or therapeutic intervention that *could be* performed. Rather, only selected outcome measures or examination techniques and interventions are discussed. This is done to simulate real-life patient interaction in which the physical therapist uses clinical reasoning to determine the most appropriate tests and interventions to use with *that* patient during *that* episode of care. For each intervention, evidence to support its use with individuals with the same diagnosis (or similar diagnosis, if no evidence exists to support its use in that particular patient population) is presented.

6. **Evidence-Based Clinical Recommendations** includes a minimum of three clinical recommendations for diagnostic tools and/or treatment interventions for the patient's condition. Each recommendation is graded using the Strength of

Recommendation Taxonomy (SORT),[4] which has been used by several medical journals including *American Family Physician, Journal of the American Board of Family Practice, Journal of Family Practice*, and *Sports Health*. The SORT system has been chosen because it is simple and its rankings are based on patient-oriented outcomes. The SORT system has only three levels of evidence: A, B, and C. Grade A recommendations are based on consistent, good-quality patient-oriented evidence (*e.g.*, systematic reviews, meta-analysis of high-quality studies, high-quality randomized controlled trials, high-quality diagnostic cohort studies). Grade B recommendations are based on inconsistent or limited-quality patient-oriented evidence (*e.g.*, systematic review or meta-analysis of lower-quality studies or studies with inconsistent findings). Grade C recommendations are based on consensus, disease-oriented evidence, usual practice, expert opinion, or case series (*e.g.*, consensus guidelines, disease-oriented evidence using only intermediate or physiologic outcomes). Contributing authors provided a grade based on the SORT guidelines. The grade for each statement was then reviewed and sometimes altered by the editors. Key phrases from each clinical SORT recommendation are bolded within the case to enable the reader to easily locate where the cited evidence was presented.

7. **Comprehension Questions and Answers** include 2 to 4 multiple-choice questions that reinforce the content or elaborate on related concepts to the patient's case. When appropriate, detailed explanations about why alternative choices would *not* be the best choice are also provided.

My hope is that these real-life case studies will be a useful resource to help incorporate evidence into everyday practice. With the persistent push for evidence-based healthcare to promote quality and effectiveness as well as the advent of evidence-based reimbursement guidelines, case studies with evidence-based recommendations will be an added benefit as physical therapists continue to face decreased reimbursement rates and need to demonstrate evidence supporting their services. I hope physical therapy educators, physical therapy students, physical therapists, and professionals preparing for Board Certification in clinical specialty areas will find these books helpful to translate classroom-based knowledge to evidence-based assessments and interventions.

Erin E. Jobst, PT, PhD

December 28, 2022

1. World Health Organization. International Classification of Functioning, Disability and Health (ICF). Available at: https://www.who.int/standards/classifications/international-classification-of-functioning-disability-and-health. Accessed December 28, 2022.

2. American Physical Therapy Association. *Guide to Physical Therapist Practice*. Available at: https://store.apta.org/guide-to-physical-therapist-practice-3-0.html. Accessed December 28, 2022.

3. Jewell DV. *Guide to Evidence-Based Physical Therapy Practice*. Sudbury, MA: Jones and Barlett; 2008.

4. Ebell MH, Siwek J, Weiss BD, et al. Strength of Recommendation Taxonomy (SORT): a patient-centered approach to grading evidence in the medical literature. *Am Fam Physician*. 2004;69:548-556.

Introduction

This second edition of *Physical Therapy Case Files – Orthopedics* contains 33 cases on common musculoskeletal conditions: 7 on the upper extremity, 8 on the spine, and 18 on the lower extremity. Twenty-six cases from the 1st edition have been updated to incorporate new practices and evidence over the past decade. Examples include the use of diagnostic ultrasound to confirm the diagnosis of patellar tendinopathy (Case 22) and the use of dry needling as an adjunctive treatment for plantar heel pain (Case 33). Six new cases reflect exciting advancements in physical therapy practice, including blood flow restriction training in the treatment of patellofemoral pain (Case 21) and the utilization of physical therapists in the primary care setting (Case 15). We hope this new edition will inspire continued learning, inform practice, and help improve the lives of your patients.

Listing of Cases

Listing by Case Number

Listing by Health Condition (Alphabetical)

Listing by Health Condition (Alphabetical)

Thirty-Three Case Scenarios

Subacromial Impingement

Christy Sweeney

An 18-year-old right-hand dominant male presents to an outpatient clinic with a physical therapy prescription from an orthopedic physician to evaluate and treat right shoulder subacromial impingement. The patient states he started to experience shoulder pain approximately 4 weeks ago. He attributes the cause to playing tennis 3 times during the past week after not playing at all over the winter. His right shoulder pain increases with reaching forward or behind his back, lifting any type of weight with his right arm, and playing tennis. He also reports not being able to reach behind his back to loop his belt or tuck his shirt in, activities he could previously do without difficulty. The only position that relieves his shoulder pain is keeping his arm at his side. His physician started him on a course of nonsteroidal anti-inflammatory drugs, which has helped decrease the pain intensity. X-rays (performed in the physician's office) of the acromioclavicular and glenohumeral joints were negative for any bony abnormalities or structural defects. The patient's medical history is otherwise unremarkable.

▶ Based on the patient's diagnosis, what do you anticipate may be the contributing factors to his condition?
▶ What examination signs may be associated with this diagnosis?
▶ What are the most appropriate physical therapy interventions?
▶ What possible complications may limit the effectiveness of physical therapy?

KEY DEFINITIONS

SCAPULAR DYSKINESIS: Visible alterations in scapular position and movement patterns

SUBACROMIAL IMPINGEMENT SYNDROME: Compression, entrapment, or mechanical irritation of the rotator cuff tendons beneath the coracoacromial arch

Objectives

1. Describe subacromial impingement syndrome (SAIS).

2. Identify possible causes of subacromial impingement.

3. Discuss signs and symptoms of subacromial impingement based on examination findings.

4. Select appropriate joint range of motion and/or flexibility exercises for an individual with SAIS.

5. Select appropriate resistance exercises for a person with SAIS.

Physical Therapy Considerations

Physical therapy considerations during management of the individual with a diagnosis of SAIS:

▶ **General physical therapy plan of care/goals:** Decrease pain; increase glenohumeral joint range of motion; increase flexibility; increase rotator cuff and scapular muscle strength; improve function with activities of daily living

▶ **Physical therapy interventions:** Patient education regarding shoulder anatomy and pathomechanics of the diagnosis; modalities as needed to decrease pain; manual therapy to decrease pain and improve joint and muscular flexibility; range of motion and flexibility exercises; resistance exercises to increase muscular strength and endurance; proprioceptive exercises to promote joint and muscular control

▶ **Precautions during physical therapy:** Monitor vital signs; address precautions or contraindications for exercise based on patient's pre-existing condition(s)

▶ **Complications interfering with physical therapy:** Lack of adherence with exercise program

Understanding the Health Condition

Shoulder pain affects one in five adults, and SAIS accounts for half of all conditions causing shoulder pain.[1-3] An impingement syndrome involves degeneration and/or mechanical compression of soft tissue structures.[4] In the case of SAIS, the rotator cuff, the long head of the biceps, and the subacromial bursa are compressed between the acromion, the coracoacromial ligament, and the humeral head.[4-6]

The **etiology of SAIS is multifactorial**—caused by extrinsic and/or intrinsic mechanisms. Extrinsic mechanisms of compression include anatomical factors, biomechanical factors, or a combination of both.[7] Anatomical variations that can narrow the subacromial space include variations in the shape of the acromion,[7-11] orientation of the slope or angle of the acromion,[7,12-15] and osseous changes to the acromioclavicular (AC) joint or coracoacromial ligament.[7,11,16,17] Subacromial and AC joint spurs are other anatomical factors that can contribute to rotator cuff impingement.[7] Biomechanical factors leading to subacromial impingement include abnormal scapular and humeral kinematics (specifically anterior-superior translation of the humeral head over the glenoid fossa[18,19] and scapular anterior tilt[5,20,21]), postural abnormalities, rotator cuff and scapular muscle weakness, and decreased flexibility of the pectoralis minor or posterior shoulder tissues.[7] Intrinsic mechanisms of rotator cuff tendinopathy that may lead to SAIS result from tendon degradation due to the natural aging process,[7,22-25] poor vascularity,[7,26-30] altered biology,[7,22,31-33] and mechanical properties that result in damage with tensile or shear loads.[7,34-37] Rotator cuff tendons in individuals with tendinopathy have decreased total collagen content, increased proportion of type III collagen fibers, and greater cell death compared to normal tendons.[7,33,38,39] These factors can contribute to thinning and weakening of the rotator cuff tendons, which can lead to impingement.[7,40,41]

Nonsurgical treatment options for SAIS include physical therapy and oral and injected medications. Some studies have demonstrated decreased pain and increased function with nonsurgical rehabilitation programs for individuals with SAIS.[42] If nonsurgical interventions fail to resolve symptoms, a surgical decompression of the subacromial space is indicated.[4]

Physical Therapy Patient/Client Management

There are multiple physical therapy interventions for SAIS based on the patient's presentation. Interventions may include modalities, manual therapy, therapeutic exercise (stretching and resistance training), postural education, and patient education on how to prevent recurring problems.[4,7,42] In some cases, patients may not benefit from physical therapy interventions and will need to be referred to an orthopedic physician for a surgical consultation. Standard practice is to provide physical therapy for 3 to 6 weeks (~6-12 visits) before considering a surgical consultation.[4]

Examination, Evaluation, and Diagnosis

When evaluating an individual with SAIS, it is important to start with a thorough subjective evaluation. The patient's history often contains a description of repetitive overhead work or athletic activity involving overhead movements that aggravate the patient's shoulder pain.[4] A patient may complain of pain in the anterior aspect of the shoulder with movements that decrease the size of the subacromial space, causing impingement of the subacromial bursa, long head of the biceps, or rotator cuff tendons. The patient's functional limitations should be discussed since these are usually the primary reasons for which the patient has sought treatment. In addition to changes in objective measurements, improvements in functional tasks (*e.g.*, being able to loop a belt or tuck in a shirt behind the back) can be used to document progress in physical therapy. Questions should also be asked about previous medical history, current medications, and any diagnostic imaging that has been performed.

A comprehensive objective evaluation begins with screening the cervical spine to rule out referred symptoms from the neck as the etiology of the shoulder pain. Unrestricted cervical active range of motion and a clear neurologic screen of the upper quadrant (testing of dermatomes, myotomes, and deep tendon reflexes from C5-C8) help rule out cervical spine involvement.[4,43] A summary of the objective examination for the patient with suspected SAIS is presented in Table 1-1.

Table 1-1 SUMMARY OF OBJECTIVE EXAMINATION FOR PATIENT WITH SUSPECTED SAIS

Test	Patient Position and Movement	Positive Findings
Posture observation	Standing posterior view	Posterior view: atrophy of infraspinatus and supraspinatus; winging of scapula
	Standing lateral view	Lateral view: thoracic kyphosis, shoulder protraction
Active range of motion	Standing: 1. Shoulder flexion 2. Shoulder abduction 3. Shoulder external rotation (ER) with elbow at 90° 4. Shoulder internal rotation (IR): ask patient to place hand behind back; measure level of thumb to highest spinous process	Painful arc of motion (60°-120°) with shoulder flexion Pain at end range of shoulder flexion and/or shoulder abduction Decreased IR on affected side, as demonstrated by inability to reach spinous process equal to that of unaffected shoulder
Passive range of motion	Supine: 1. Shoulder flexion 2. Shoulder abduction 3. Shoulder ER at 90° abduction 4. Shoulder IR at 90° abduction	Decreased IR on affected side
Manual muscle testing: 1. Teres minor and infraspinatus 2. Subscapularis 3. Supraspinatus 4. Serratus anterior 5. Middle trapezius 6. Lower trapezius	Therapist applies force in direction opposite of muscle action. 1. Standing ER with arm at side and elbow at 90° 2. Standing IR with arm at side and elbow at 90° 3. Standing shoulder horizontal abduction at 40° anterior to frontal plane 4. Seated with shoulder at 120° of flexion 5. Prone with shoulder at 90° horizontal abduction with ER 6. Prone with arm parallel to body and shoulder at 145° horizontal abduction	All muscles tested have the potential to be graded as weak, but the most common weaknesses are found in the supraspinatus (mostly due to pain) and scapular muscles (serratus anterior, middle trapezius, and lower trapezius).

The physical therapist carefully observes the patient's standing posture from posterior and lateral views. From the posterior view, note any atrophy of the rotator cuff muscles in the infraspinatus and supraspinatus fossae. Compare the heights of the shoulders and look for the presence of scapular winging with the patient's arms by his side. Due to increased upper trapezius activity and decreased serratus anterior strength, the patient's involved shoulder may be elevated and scapular winging present.[44] From the lateral view, evaluate for the presence of excessive thoracic kyphosis and shoulder protraction.[45] Patients with SAIS often have increased thoracic kyphosis and decreased thoracic mobility that contribute to altered movement patterns.[44,46] The shoulder affected by SAIS is often in a protracted position due to the increased thoracic kyphosis and a tight pectoralis minor muscle.[21] Both of these postural abnormalities contribute to a decreased subacromial space and impingement of the underlying tissues.[7,21]

During an active range of motion movement screen of the shoulder, **patients with SAIS may demonstrate scapular dyskinesis.** Scapular dyskinesis refers to visible alterations in scapular position and movement patterns.[47] Dyskinesis may be caused by adaptive shortening of the pectoralis minor muscle,[44,45,48,49] posterior shoulder tightness,[7,50] decreased scapular and rotator cuff strength,[7,21] and increased thoracic kyphosis.[7,44,46,51] Generally, the affected shoulder demonstrates decreased scapular posterior tilting, decreased upward rotation, and increased internal rotation of the scapula.[7,44] This positioning results in failure of the anterior aspect of the acromion to move away from the humeral head during shoulder flexion, contributing to a reduction in subacromial space and rotator cuff impingement.[7,44] A method for identifying scapular dyskinesis is the scapula dyskinesis test (SDT, Fig. 1-1).[47] The patient performs 5 repetitions of bilateral and weighted shoulder flexion followed by bilateral and weighted shoulder abduction while the physical therapist observes

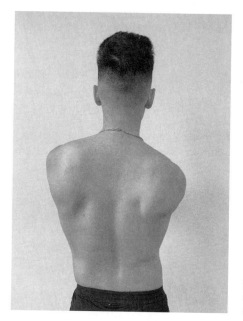

Figure 1-1. Note the obvious scapular winging on the right as the patient performs the scapula dyskinesis test.

from the posterior and superior views.[47] The shoulder of a patient with a positive SDT demonstrates scapular winging, dysrhythmia, or both.[4,47,52]

Evaluating muscle strength helps to further refine the contributing factors to SAIS. Weakness of the serratus anterior, lower trapezius, and middle trapezius muscles can lead to altered scapular kinematics in patients with SAIS.[4,7,44,53] The serratus and trapezius muscles stabilize the scapula and produce scapular upward rotation, external rotation, and/or posterior tilting of the scapula to allow the humeral head to clear the acromion with elevation.[7,54] Patients with SAIS often complain of increased pain and decreased strength with shoulder flexion. This is due to scapular weakness and altered kinematics on the affected side, which leads to rotator cuff impingement in the subacromial space. In a study performed by Tate et al.,[55] manually repositioning the scapula (using the scapula reposition test) resulted in less pain during impingement testing and increased strength in athletes that had a positive impingement test. The scapula reposition test involves manually posterior tilting, externally rotating, and retracting the scapula to permit the normal scapular mechanics to occur with shoulder elevation and thus prevent impingement of the rotator cuff (Fig. 1-2). In addition to strength testing of the scapular stabilizers, manual muscle tests of the supraspinatus, teres minor, infraspinatus, and subscapularis muscles should also be performed. These muscles frequently demonstrate weakness, and strength testing may cause increased pain in patients with SAIS.[4]

Special tests for the shoulder (Table 1-2)[56] are performed at the end of the musculoskeletal examination. Impingement tests that may help confirm the diagnosis of SAIS are the Neer test, Hawkins test, and empty can test. Tate et al.[4] reported that patients with SAIS demonstrate the following: (1) a positive Neer, Hawkins, or empty can test, (2) a painful shoulder arc of motion, and (3) pain or weakness with resisted shoulder external rotation with the arm at the side. Kelly et al.[57] found the

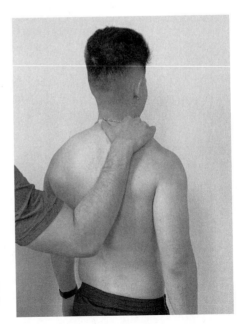

Figure 1-2. Scapula reposition test. Physical therapist manually repositioning the scapula prior to the patient elevating the right arm.

Table 1-2 SPECIAL TESTS ASSOCIATED WITH IMPINGEMENT SYNDROME[60]

Special Test	Patient Position	Findings
Neer impingement test	With the patient seated or standing, the physical therapist passively flexes the shoulder while stabilizing the scapula with the other hand	Positive test: pain with full forced flexion is a positive sign of supraspinatus impingement
Hawkins impingement test	With the patient seated or standing, the physical therapist passively flexes the shoulder to 90° and internally rotates the shoulder with elbow flexed to 90°	Positive test: pain is a positive sign of supraspinatus tendonitis/impingement
Empty can test	With patient seated or standing, the patient flexes the shoulder to 90° in the scapular plane with full internal rotation (thumb down) and resists downward pressure placed at the wrist by the physical therapist	Positive test: pain and/or muscle weakness is a positive sign of supraspinatus tendonitis/impingement
Scapula dyskinesis test	Standing, the patient performs 5 repetitions of shoulder flexion with weight in hand (2.3 kg for patients weighing >68.0 kg and 1.4 kg for patients weighing <68.0 kg)[3]	Patients are rated as having normal scapular motion, subtle abnormalities, or obvious abnormalities. Abnormalities are defined as winging or dysrhythmia.[3]
Scapula reposition test	With the patient standing, the physical therapist applies a moderate force to the patient's scapula to encourage posterior tilting and external rotation of the scapula.	Manually repositioning the scapula reduces pain and increases shoulder elevation strength in patients with impingement.

Hawkins test to be the most accurate for diagnosing any degree of SAIS. Calis et al.[58] confirmed that the Hawkins test was the most sensitive for diagnosing shoulder impingement, followed by the Neer impingement test. Additional special tests should be performed to rule out labral tears, shoulder instability, and rotator cuff tears.

Plan of Care and Interventions

Physical therapy interventions for patients with SAIS must address deficits and limitations found in the objective examination. **Therapeutic exercise has a positive effect in retraining muscle imbalances and restoring normal movement patterns.**[4,20,42,59,60] Manual therapy techniques help decrease pain, improve range of motion, and increase function in these patients.[4]

Several studies have evaluated the effectiveness of therapeutic exercise programs for SAIS. Tate et al.[4] evaluated a 6- to 8-week three-phase intervention for patients with SAIS. Table 1-3 details the interventions used by Tate et al., which included progressive strengthening (Fig. 1-3), manual stretching, thrust and non-thrust manipulations to the shoulder and spine, patient education, activity modification, and a daily

Table 1-3 EXAMPLE SAIS TREATMENT PROGRAM

Treatment Technique	Treatment Specifics
Motor control/ strengthening	Phase 1: rotator cuff strengthening with humerus in neutral position
	Phase 2: add shoulder flexion exercises, focus on more aggressive strengthening of serratus anterior (Fig. 1-3) and trapezius
	Phase 3: higher-level strengthening and endurance training at multiple levels of shoulder flexion; incorporate trunk strengthening
Manual therapy	Manual stretching techniques focusing on improving flexibility of the posterior shoulder and inferior glenohumeral capsule
	Thrust and non-thrust manipulation techniques directed at the thoracic spine to improve thoracic extension
Self-stretches	Stretches performed independently by the patient to increase mobility of the glenohumeral capsule and flexibility of the pectoral and thoracic spinal muscles
Home exercise program	Selective combination of strengthening exercises and self-stretches to be performed once daily at home, using same repetitions and resistance as was performed in the clinic

home exercise program of stretching and strengthening. Eight of the ten subjects reported successful outcomes based on symptomatic and functional improvement after completion of the treatment program. The outcome measures used to define success included: the three pain subscale questions of the Penn Shoulder Scale, the Disabilities of the Arm, Shoulder and Hand (DASH) questionnaire, and the Global

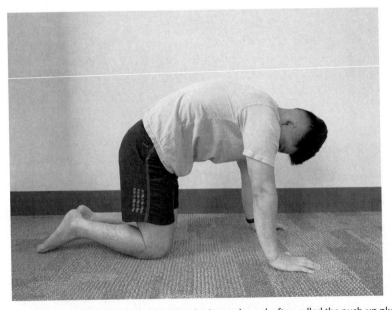

Figure 1-3. Serratus anterior strengthening exercise in quadruped, often called the push-up plus exercise. Patient moves from quadruped position to pictured push-up plus position.

Rating of Change (GRC) question that allowed subjects to rate the perceived change in their shoulder condition since starting the strengthening program.[4]

Bernhardsson et al.[59] demonstrated that a **12-week eccentric strengthening program decreased pain and improved function in patients with SAIS.** The exercise regimen targeted the supraspinatus and infraspinatus muscles, emphasizing the eccentric phase of strengthening for these two muscles, along with scapular stabilizing exercises to promote correct movement patterns.

Turgut et al.[20] evaluated the effects of 6-week stretching program in subjects with SAIS. Exercises targeting the pectoralis minor (Fig. 1-4), posterior capsule (Fig. 1-5), levator scapulae (Fig. 1-6), and latissimus dorsi muscles (Fig. 1-7) were performed for 3 sets of 5 repetitions daily with each stretch held for 30 seconds.[20] After the 6-week program, the subjects experienced increased flexibility and decreased pain and disability.[20] Increased flexibility of the pectoralis minor muscle and of the posterior shoulder capsule in particular improves posture, helps align the scapula, and optimizes glenohumeral arthrokinematics during dynamic upper extremity movements—all of which decrease subacromial impingement.

The studies by Tate et al.[4], Bernhardsson et al.[59], and Turgut et al.[20] focused on specific exercise programs and types of exercises for the treatment of SAIS. In a systematic review, Pieters et al.[60] appraised 16 studies to determine the effectiveness of exercise, manual therapy, electrotherapy, and multimodal approaches in the treatment of SAIS.[60] Multimodal therapy included combined nonsurgical treatments such as passive physical modalities, exercise, manual therapy, taping, glucocorticoids, and electrotherapy. While the authors concluded that stronger evidence supporting exercise as a primary intervention for SAIS is accumulating, the *specific* exercises as well as the *dosing* are still unclear.[60] The authors' appraisal also strongly supported the use

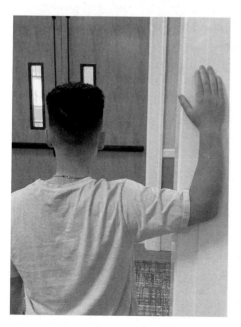

Figure 1-4. Static stretch for the pectoralis minor, often called the one-arm doorway stretch.

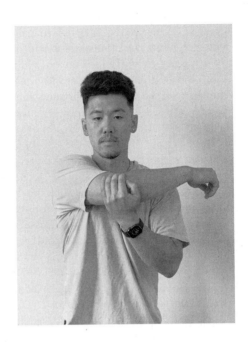

Figure 1-5. Posterior capsule stretch, often called the shoulder cross-arm stretch.

of manual therapy in the form of shoulder girdle and cervical spine mobilizations or manipulations, soft tissue techniques, neurodynamic mobilizations, and mobilizations with movement of the shoulder girdle or spine in conjunction with exercises.

It is worth mentioning that Roddy et al.[1] found physiotherapist-led exercise led to greater improvements in pain and function than simply providing an exercise

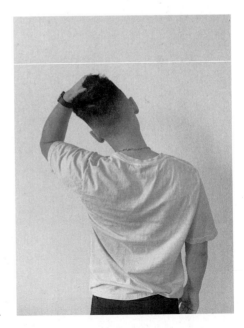

Figure 1-6. Right levator scapulae stretch.

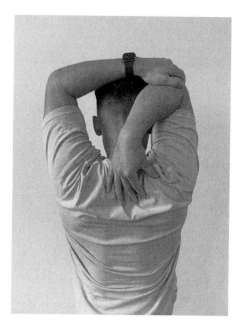

Figure 1-7. Right latissimus dorsi stretch.

handout to patients with subacromial pain. Thus, as with any diagnosis, a plan of care that focuses on improving the patient's specific objective and functional deficits may be more effective. For the patient with SAIS in this case study, after 2 weeks of treatment, the physical therapist should reassess his pain intensity with reaching in various directions and lifting objects, and his progress toward being able to loop his belt and tuck a shirt in behind his back. If his symptoms remain unchanged, the treatment strategy and focus of exercises may need to be altered.

Evidence-Based Clinical Recommendations

SORT: Strength of Recommendation Taxonomy

A: Consistent, good-quality patient-oriented evidence
B: Inconsistent or limited-quality patient-oriented evidence
C: Consensus, disease-oriented evidence, usual practice, expert opinion, or case series

1. Intrinsic and extrinsic factors contribute to the development of SAIS. **Grade A**

2. Patients with SAIS demonstrate scapular dyskinesis. **Grade B**

3. Therapeutic exercise helps retrain muscle imbalances, restore normal movement patterns, and decrease pain in individuals with SAIS. **Grade B**

COMPREHENSION QUESTIONS

1.1 An outpatient physical therapist evaluates a patient suffering from right shoulder subacromial impingement syndrome (SAIS). While observing the patient's active range of motion, the therapist notes altered right scapular movement. Weakness in which muscles is *most* likely to be responsible for this scapular dyskinesis?

A. Supraspinatus, infraspinatus, teres minor

B. Supraspinatus, serratus anterior, lower trapezius

C. Serratus anterior, lower trapezius, middle trapezius

D. Middle trapezius, pectoralis minor, biceps brachii

1.2 SAIS involves degradation and/or mechanical compression of which of the following soft tissue structures?

A. Rotator cuff

B. Long head of the biceps

C. Subacromial bursa

D. All of the above

1.3 Scapular dyskinesis can be caused by:

A. Adaptive shortening of the pectoralis minor muscle and posterior shoulder tightness

B. Decreased scapular and rotator cuff strength

C. Thoracic kyphosis

D. All of the above

ANSWERS

1.1 **C.** Weakness of the serratus anterior, lower trapezius, and middle trapezius muscles can lead to altered scapular kinematics in patients with SAIS.[23,24,25,40,44] The serratus anterior and trapezius muscles stabilize the scapula and cause scapular upward rotation, external rotation, and/or posterior tilting of the scapula to allow the humeral head to clear the acromion with shoulder elevation.[29,40]

1.2 **D.** Impingement syndrome involves degeneration and/or mechanical compression of soft tissue structures.[44] In the case of SAIS, the rotator cuff, long head of the biceps, and the subacromial bursa are compressed between the acromion, the coracoacromial ligament, and the humeral head.[27,31,44]

1.3 **D.** Scapular dyskinesis may be caused by adaptive shortening of the pectoralis minor muscle,[44,45,48,49] posterior shoulder tightness,[7,50] decreased scapular and rotator cuff strength,[7,21] and increased thoracic kyphosis.[7,44,46,51]

REFERENCES

1. Roddy E, Ogollah RO, Oppong R, et al. Optimising outcomes of exercise and corticosteroid injection in patients with subacromial pain. *Br J Sports Med.* 2021;55:262-271.

2. Luime JJ, Koes BW, Hendriksen IJM, et al. Prevalence and incidence of shoulder pain in the general population; a systematic review. *Scand J Rheumatol.* 2004;33:73-81.

3. van der Windt DA, Koes BW, de Jong BA, Bouter LM. Shoulder disorders in general practice: incidence, patient characteristics, and management. *Ann Rheum Dis.* 1995;54:959-964.

4. Tate AR, McClure PW, Kareha S, Irwin D. Effect of the scapula reposition test on shoulder impingement symptoms and elevation strength in overhead athletes. *J Orthop Sports Phys Ther.* 2008;38:4-11.

5. Ludewig PM, Reynolds JF. The association of scapular kinematics and glenohumeral joint pathologies. *J Orthop Sports Phys Ther.* 2009;39:90-104.

6. Neer CS II. Impingement lesions. *Clin Orthop Relat Res.* 1983;173:70-77.

7. Seitz AL, McClure PW, Finucane S, et al. Mechanisms of rotator cuff tendinopathy: intrinsic, extrinsic, or both? *Clin Biomech.* 2011;26:1-12.

8. Bigliani LU, Ticker JB, Flatow EL, et al. The relationship of acromial architecture to rotator cuff disease. *Clin Sports Med.* 1991;10:823-838.

9. Epstein RE, Schweitzer ME, Frieman BG, et al. Hooked acromion: prevalence on MR images of painful shoulder. *Radiology.* 1993;187:479-481.

10. Gill TJ, McIrvin E, Kocher MS, et al. The relative importance of acromial morphology and age with respect to rotator cuff pathology. *J Shoulder Elbow Surg.* 2002;11:327-330.

11. Ogawa K, Yoshida A, Inokuchi W, Naniwa T. Acromial spur: relationship to aging and morphologic changes in the rotator cuff. *J Shoulder Elbow Surg.* 2005;14:591-598.

12. Aoki M, Ishii S, Usui M. The slope of the acromion and rotator cuff impingement. *Orthop Trans.* 1986;10:228.

13. Edelson JG. The 'hooked' acromion revisited. *J Bone Joint Surg Br.* 1995;77:284-287.

14. Toivonen D, Tuite MJ, Orwin JF. Acromial structure and tears of the rotator cuff. *J Shoulder Elbow Surg.* 1995;4:376-383.

15. Vaz S, Soyer J, Pries P, Clarac JP. Subacromial impingement: influence of coracoacromial arch geometry on shoulder function. *Joint Bone Spine.* 2000;67:305-309.

16. Farley TE, Neumann CH, Steinbach LS, Petersen SA. The coracoacromial arch: MR evaluation and correlation with rotator cuff pathology. *Skeletal Radiol.* 1994;23:641-645.

17. Nicholson GP, Goodman DA, Flatow EL, Bigliani LU. The acromion: morphologic condition and age-related changes. A study of 420 scapulas. *J Shoulder Elbow Surg.* 1996;5:1-11.

18. Tahran O, Yesilyaprak SS. Effects of modified posterior shoulder stretching exercises on shoulder mobility, pain and dysfunction in patient with subacromial impingement syndrome. *Sports Health.* Mar/Apr 2020;12:139-148.

19. Harryman DT 2nd, Sidles JA, Clark JM, et al. Translation of the humeral head in the glenoid with passive glenohumeral motion. *J Bone Joint Surg Am.* 1990;72:1334-1343.

20. Turgut E, Duzgun I, Baltaci G. Stretching exercises for subacromial impingement syndrome: effects of 6-week program on shoulder tightness, pain, and disability status. *J Sports Rehabil.* 2018;27:132-137.

21. Borstad JD, Ludewig PM. The effect of long versus short pectoralis minor resting length on scapular kinematics in healthy individuals. *J Orthop Sports Phys Ther.* 2005;35:227-238.

22. Iannotti JP, Zlatkin MB, Esterhai JL, et al. Magnetic resonance imaging of the shoulder. Sensitivity, specificity, and predictive value. *J Bone Joint Surg Am.* 1991;73:17-29.

23. Milgrom C, Schaffler M, Gilbert S, van Holsbeeck M. Rotator-cuff changes in asymptomatic adults. The effect of age, hand dominance and gender. *J Bone Joint Surg Br.* 1995;77:296-298.

24. Sher JS, Uribe JW, Posada A, et al. Abnormal findings on magnetic resonance images of asymptomatic shoulders. *J Bone Joint Surg Am.* 1995;77:10-15.

25. Tempelhof S, Rupp S, Seil R. Age-related prevalence of rotator cuff tears in asymptomatic shoulders. *J Shoulder Elbow Surg.* 1999;8:296-299.

26. Biberthaler P, Wiedemann E, Nerlich A, et al. Microcirculation associated with degenerative rotator cuff lesions. In vivo assessment with orthogonal polarization spectral imaging during arthroscopy of the shoulder. *J Bone Joint Surg Am.* 2003;85-A:475-480.

27. Brooks CH, Revell WJ, Heatley FW. A quantitative histological study of the vascularity of the rotator cuff tendon. *J Bone Joint Surg Br.* 1992;74:151-153.

28. Fukuda H, Hamada K, Yamanaka K. Pathology and pathogenesis of bursal-side rotator cuff tears viewed from en bloc histologic sections. *Clin Orthop Relat Res.* 1990;254:75-80.

29. Goodmurphy CW, Osborn J, Akesson EJ, et al. An immunocytochemical analysis of torn rotator cuff tendon taken at the time of repair. *J Shoulder Elbow Surg.* 2003;12:368-374.

30. Rudzki JR, Adler RS, Warren RF, et al. Contrast-enhanced ultrasound characterization of the vascularity of the rotator cuff tendon: age-and activity-related changes in the intact asymptomatic rotator cuff. *J Shoulder Elbow Surg.* 2008;17:96S-100S.

31. Kumagai J, Sarkar K, Uhthoff HK. The collagen types in the attachment zone of rotator cuff tendons in the elderly: an immunohistochemical study. *J Rheumatol.* 1994;21:2096-2100.

32. Riley GP, Harrall RL, Constant CR, et al. Glycosaminoglycans of human rotator cuff tendons: changes with age and in chronic rotator cuff tendinitis. *Ann Rheum Dis.* 1994;53:367-376.

33. Riley GP, Harrall RL, Constant CR, et al. Tendon degeneration and chronic shoulder pain: changes in the collagen composition of the human rotator cuff tendons in rotator cuff tendinitis. *Ann Rheum Dis.* 1994;53:359-366.

34. Bey MJ, Song HK, Wehrli FW, Soslowsky LJ. Intratendinous strain fields of the intact supraspinatus tendon: the effect of glenohumeral joint position and tendon region. *J Orthop Res.* 2002;20:869-874.

35. Herbert LJ, Moffet H, McFadyen BJ, Dionne CE. Scapular behavior in shoulder impingement syndrome. *Arch Phys Med Rehabil.* 2002;83:60-69.

36. Hung CJ, Jan MH, Lin YF, et al. Scapular kinematics and impairment features for classifying patients with subacromial impingement syndrome. *Man Ther.* 2010;15:547-551.

37. Reilly P, Amis AA, Wallace AL, Emery RJ. Mechanical failures in the initiation and propagation of tears of the rotator cuff. Quantification of strains of the supraspinatus tendon in vivo. *J Bone Joint Surg Br.* 2003;84:594-599.

38. Tuoheti Y, Itoi E, Pradhan RL, et al. Apoptosis in the supraspinatus tendon with stage II subacromial impingement. *J Shoulder Elbow Surg.* 2005;14:535-541.

39. Yuan J, Murrell GA, Wei AQ, Wang MX. Apoptosis in rotator cuff tendinopathy. *J Orthop Res.* 2002;20:1372-1379.

40. Lake SP, Miller KS, Elliott DM, Soslowsky JL. Effect of fiber distribution and realignment on the nonlinear and inhomogeneous mechanical properties of human supraspinatus tendon under longitudinal tensile loading. *J Orthop Res.* 2009;27:1596-1602.

41. Cholewinski JJ, Kusz DJ, Wojciechowski P, et al. Ultrasound measurement of rotator cuff thickness and acromio-humeral distance in the diagnosis of subacromial impingement syndrome of the shoulder. *Knee Surg Sports Traumatol Arthrosc.* 2007;16:408-414.

42. Kelly SM, Wrightson PA, Meads CA. Clinical outcomes of exercise in the management of subacromial impingement syndrome: a systemic review. *Clin Rehabil.* 2010;24:99-109.

43. Wainner RS, Fritz JM, Irrgang JJ, et al. Reliability and diagnostic accuracy of the clinical examination and patient self-report measures for cervical radiculopathy. *Spine.* 2003;28:52-62.

44. Ludewig PM, Cook TM. Alterations in shoulder kinematics and associated muscle activity in people with symptoms of shoulder impingement. *Phys Ther.* 2000;80:276-291.

45. Kendall FP, Provance PG, McCreary EK. *Muscles, Testing and Function: With Posture and Pain.* 4th ed. Baltimore: Lippincott, Williams and Wilkins; 1993.

46. Kebaetse M, McClure P, Pratt NA. Thoracic position effect on shoulder range of motion, strength, and three-dimensional scapular kinematics. *Arch Phys Med Rehabil.* 1999;80:945-950.

47. McClure P, Tate AR, Kareha S, et al. A clinical method for identifying scapular dyskinesis, part 1: reliability. *J Athl Train.* 2009;44:160-164.

48. Borstad JD. Resting position variables at the shoulder: evidence to support a posture-impairment association. *Phys Ther.* 2006;86:549-557.

49. Huang CY, Wang VM, Pawluk RJ, et al. Inhomogeneous mechanical behavior of the human supraspinatus tendon under uniaxial loading. *J Orthop Res.* 2005;23:924-930.

50. Borich MR, Bright JM, Lorello DJ, et al. Scapular angular positioning at end range internal rotation in cases of glenohumeral internal rotation deficit. *J Orthop Sports Phys Ther.* 2006;36:926-934.

51. Wang CH, McClure P, Pratt NE, Nobilini R. Stretching and strengthening exercises: their effect on three-dimensional scapular kinematics. *Arch Phys Med Rehabil.* 1999;80:923-929.

52. Tate AR, McClure P, Kareha S, et al. A clinical method for identifying scapular dyskinesis, part 2: validity. *J Athl Train.* 2009;44:165-173.

53. Lewis JS, Wright C, Green A. Subacromial impingement syndrome: the effect of changing posture on shoulder range of movement. *J Orthop Sports Phys Ther.* 2005;35:72-87.

54. McQuade KJ, Dawson J, Smidt GL. Scapulothoracic muscle fatigue associated with alterations in scapulohumeral rhythm kinematics during maximum resistive shoulder elevation. *J Ortho Sports Phys Ther.* 1998;28:74-80.

55. Tate AR, McClure PW, Kareha S, Irwin D. Effect of the Scapula Reposition Test on shoulder impingement symptoms and elevation strength in overhead athletes. *J Orthop Sports Phys Ther.* 2008;38:4-11.

56. Magee DJ. *Orthopedic Physical Assessment.* 3rd ed. Philadelphia, PA: WB Saunders Co; 1997.

57. Kelly SM, Brittle N, Allen GM. The value of physical tests for subacromial impingement syndrome: a study of diagnostic accuracy. *Clin Rehabil.* 2010;24:149-158.

58. Calis M, Akgun K, Birtane M, et al. Diagnostic values of clinical diagnostic tests in subacromial impingement syndrome. *Ann Rheum Dis.* 2000;59:44-47.

59. Bernhardsson S, Klintberg IH, Wendt GK. Evaluation of an exercise concept focusing on eccentric strength training of the rotator cuff for patients with subacromial impingement syndrome. *Clin Rehabil.* 2011;25:69-78.

60. Pieters L, Lewis J, Kuppens K, et al. An update of systematic reviews examining the effectiveness of conservative physical therapy interventions for subacromimal shoulder pain. *J Orthop Sports Phys Ther.* 2020;50:131-140.

Shoulder Labral Tear

Lane Bailey
Ellen Shanley

CASE 2

A 16-year-old elite-level volleyball player was participating in a regional tournament when she sustained an injury to her dominant left upper extremity while attempting to spike a ball. The patient continued to play despite complaints of left shoulder pain, a feeling of the left shoulder "slipping in and out," and a decrease in striking power. Immediately after the tournament, she sought care from her family physician who performed X-rays, which were negative for shoulder dislocation and bony pathology. The athlete's medical history was positive for vague left shoulder pain over the past season and an eating disorder, for which she is currently under the care of a sports psychiatrist. She now presents to physical therapy 3 days after the injury with a referring diagnosis of a "SLAP tear." The patient's goal is to safely return to volleyball activities.

- ▶ What are the examination priorities?
- ▶ What are the key examination tests that should be performed to identify the specific pathology and impairments?
- ▶ What are the most appropriate physical therapy interventions?
- ▶ What precautions should be taken *during* physical therapy?
- ▶ What are possible complications interfering with the patient's progress in physical therapy?

KEY DEFINITIONS

BICEPS-LABRAL COMPLEX: Integration of the long head of the biceps tendon into the superior glenoid labrum

CONCAVITY-COMPRESSION: Stabilizing mechanism in which compression provided by the rotator cuff muscles is applied through the convex humeral head into the concave glenoid fossa, thereby resisting translational forces

SHOULDER INSTABILITY: Clinical condition in which excessive translation of the humeral head occurs on the glenoid fossa, potentially resulting in subluxation or dislocation

Objectives

1. Understand the functional anatomy of the glenohumeral joint and biceps-labral complex.
2. Ask relevant patient history questions to elucidate the prognosis and plan of care.
3. Identify reliable and valid physical examination tools to aid in patient diagnosis and prognosis.
4. Provide appropriate interventions that will allow the patient to safely return to sport.
5. Determine when the athlete is prepared to return to volleyball competition with functional return-to-sport tests.

Physical Therapy considerations during management of the athlete with a labral tear:

▶ **General physical therapy plan of care/goals:** Protect patient from incurring subsequent injury; identify anatomical source(s) of pathology; improve muscular balance and flexibility to restore shoulder stability

▶ **Physical therapy interventions:** Patient education regarding local anatomy, pathomechanics, and activity modifications; modalities to manage pain; manual therapy and selective stretching to improve identified areas of hypomobility; increase joint stability through rotator cuff and periscapular muscle strengthening

▶ **Precautions during physical therapy:** Avoid aggressive overhead activity that places excessive stress on the labrum in early phases of therapy; careful progression from a neutral position to full overhead-elevation as strength and symptoms allow

▶ **Complications interfering with physical therapy:** Components of patient's current and past medical history (*e.g.*, eating disorder, poor nutrition/diet) that may impact the treatment plan and prognosis; difficulty in establishing collaborative lines of communication with the patient and other healthcare professionals involved in her care

Understanding the Health Condition

The glenohumeral joint is highly mobile allowing for wide ranges of motion to occur about the shoulder. As a result, the natural stability of the joint is decreased due to a lack of bony congruency. Glenohumeral stability is dependent on a crucial balance of both passive and active restraints. Passive restraints include the osseous congruency between the glenoid fossa and humeral head and contributions from the capsuloligamentous structures. The rotator cuff muscles improve joint stability through muscular contraction by tightening the capsule, which forces the humeral head to compress into the glenoid. This action provides increased dynamic stability at the joint. Scapular position is an extrinsic factor that influences shoulder stability by positioning the glenoid fossa for maximal osseous congruency during dynamic movements. Scapular position impairments have been associated with individuals who have postural deficits and shoulder pathology.

The glenoid fossa covers approximately 20% to 30% of the humeral head[1] and serves as the socket to the glenohumeral joint. The fibrocartilaginous glenoid labrum enhances joint congruency by increasing the depth of the socket by up to 50%.[2,3] The labrum attaches along the peripheral edges of the pear-shaped glenoid fossa and acts to improve joint stability by providing a lateral "bumper" to keep the humeral head centered on the glenoid fossa. The labrum also improves shoulder stability by increasing concavity-compression by up to 10%[4] and by maintaining negative intra-articular pressure. The thin film of synovial fluid contained between the articular surfaces produces a negative pressure within the enclosed joint capsule. This negative pressure acts as a vacuum to resist distraction forces of the humerus, thereby maintaining normal arthrokinematics. Labral defects can allow fluid exchange between the joint and adjacent tissues, resulting in a loss of negative intra-articular pressure and joint stability.

The labrum also serves as an attachment site for the glenohumeral joint capsule and the ligaments that stabilize the glenohumeral joint, particularly in extreme ranges of motion. The glenohumeral ligaments are fibrous bands intrinsic to the joint capsule that resist translational forces that oppose their anatomical positions. Rotator cuff tendons blend with the glenohumeral joint capsule prior to their attachment to the humerus. This blending of muscular tissues with the inert capsule helps increase stability by tensioning the joint capsule during contraction, causing the humeral head to approximate within the glenoid fossa. The muscles of the rotator cuff maintain a delicate balance of both the anterior-posterior and superior-inferior force couples that are responsible for proper joint alignment. Deficits in any of these relationships can jeopardize the integrity of glenohumeral joint stability.

Injuries to the superior labrum that extend anterior to posterior at the proximal biceps insertion were first described by Andrews et al.[5] in 1985 and later by Snyder et al.,[6] who coined the term superior labrum anterior to posterior (SLAP) to describe these lesions. Research suggests that the incidence[7] and prevalence[8] of SLAP lesions are higher among active individuals, particularly those who engage in overhead activities.[9,10] The mechanical impact of SLAP lesions has been studied using cadaver models that showed significant increases in humeral head translation when compared to those with intact labrums.[3,11] Several mechanisms that may contribute to superior labral injury have been proposed. These mechanisms include: traction overload of the biceps during the deceleration phase of throwing[5]; shear forces on the biceps-labral complex during the maximal cocking phase of throwing[12]; posterior shoulder tightness[13]; and compression shearing caused by a fall on outstretched hand.[14] SLAP lesions can result in pain and loss of function with potential for significant disability and decreased performance.

There are 4 basic types of SLAP lesions based on anatomical variance,[6] though additional classifications have been proposed.[15,16] Type I through Type IV SLAP lesions established by Snyder et al.[6] are the most commonly used within the literature.

A Type I SLAP lesion refers to fraying of the inner rim of the superior glenoid labrum. This lesion type is considered to be degenerative in nature due to decreased blood supply associated with increased age.[17] Type II tears are the most common and clinically significant, accounting for the majority of SLAP lesions found in overhead athletes.[18-21] Type II tears occur when the superior labrum is detached from the biceps insertion at the superior glenoid tubercle. These tears may be further divided into anterior, posterior, or a combination of anterior and posterior relative to the long head of biceps tendon.[22] As a result of the traction force being applied by the biceps (e.g., deceleration during throwing activities), these injuries commonly result in elevation of the labrum away from the glenoid fossa. Concomitant injuries of shoulder instability and rotator cuff pathology may also be present with SLAP lesions, warranting thorough physical screening. Type III SLAP lesions are bucket-handle tears of the superior labrum that extend from anterior to posterior on the face of the glenoid fossa.[17] These lesions alone do not cause superior elevation of the labrum away from the glenoid fossa; however, entrapment and joint "locking" may ensue if the lesion is severe. Type IV SLAP lesions are also classified as bucket-handle tears. These defects extend into the biceps tendon, resulting in a split proximal attachment. Type III and IV SLAP lesions are often the result of episodes of traumatic instability.[23,24] Additional categories have been expanded to include lesions associated with the presence of shoulder instability,[15] loose bodies, and articular damage.[25] For details regarding other varieties of SLAP lesions, the reader is encouraged to seek other resources.[15,16]

It has been estimated that a high-level volleyball athlete performs up to 40,000 spikes in a single season.[26] Considering this large volume of repetitive stress, it is not surprising that 62% of these athletes report shoulder pain within the hitting zone (the arc of motion the athlete uses for impacting the ball).[27] In addition, volleyball-related overuse shoulder injuries result in an average of 6.5 weeks of lost training and/or competition time.[28] These factors suggest the need for addressing functional deficits and restoring proper mechanics for safe return to sport. Functionally, the ideal initiation of the overhand spike originates from the torso, which is responsible for the majority of the forces imparted to the ball. These forces are then potentiated up the kinetic chain to the hand. Thus, the upper extremity relies on sufficient core muscle strength to generate the forces necessary to produce the desired performance outcome. The scapula serves as a "funnel" for the efficient transfer of this kinetic energy from the trunk to the upper extremity, and is responsible for providing a stable base of support so that the hand can be properly positioned in space at the moment of impact.[29]

There are biomechanical similarities between various overhead sports such as volleyball and baseball. However, the contact point in the volleyball spiking motion is much higher than the release point of a baseball pitcher, resulting in greater maximal glenohumeral abduction for the volleyball spiker.[30] During the acceleration phase of the spike, the trunk uncoils, elevating and externally rotating the shoulder joint, which generates high tension in the inferior joint capsule.[30] The inferior glenohumeral ligament (IGHL) is maximally stressed in this elevated position, which increases the potential of capsular avulsion injuries as a result of repetitive microtrauma.[30]

Functionally, volleyball athletes have decreased external rotation strength of the dominant hitting arm compared to the opposite arm.[27] Thirty percent of these athletes also exhibit infraspinatus muscle atrophy on physical examination.[27]

Suprascapular nerve pathology (*e.g.*, paralabral cysts, neuropraxia) has been offered as a rationale for these asymmetries due to repetitive neural tension and/or compression at the spinoglenoid notch.[31] Sufficient external rotation strength is vital to the deceleration phase of overhead throwing and spiking. Decreased strength of the external rotators is thought to contribute to the high prevalence of shoulder injury within this population. Therapeutic interventions should focus on addressing identified deficits prior to returning to play.

Physical Therapy Patient/Client Management

The conservative management of shoulder pain must be tailored to the individual's symptoms, clinical presentation, and functional goals. Therapeutic interventions that have proven beneficial for nonoperative treatment of SLAP lesions include scapular stabilization exercises, rotator cuff strengthening, and posterior-inferior capsule stretching.[8] Depending on the extent of soft tissue and joint inflammation, the patient may also benefit from physician-prescribed nonsteroidal anti-inflammatory drugs (NSAIDs) and/or intra-articular glucocorticoid injection. Predicting which patients will respond positively to conservative care is often difficult and poorly understood. Surgical intervention is indicated if physical therapy interventions fail to improve patient symptoms, strength, joint stability, and shoulder function. The choice for operative care is usually a collective decision made by the entire orthopedic team; however, the final decision is often made by the patient and treating physician.

Examination, Evaluation, and Diagnosis

A thorough patient history is the foundation of the clinical examination and provides valuable information regarding the mechanism of injury, likely impairments, and rehabilitation prognosis. Individuals with SLAP lesions commonly complain of diffuse shoulder pain, instability, and "clicking" or "popping" that is exacerbated with overhead activity.[23] When evaluating a patient with a suspected SLAP lesion, it is helpful to be aware that active individuals[24] and overhead athletes[32] exhibit a high prevalence of this type of injury. Based on the mechanism of injury, the physical therapist may also be able to gain insight into the specific tissue involvement. For example, falls on outstretched hands (FOOSH injuries) are likely to be traction injuries of the biceps-labral complex resulting from an inferior humeral subluxation or dislocation episode.[33] In contrast, the eccentric load placed on the biceps during pitching is often a shear or traction type of injury that causes the superior labrum to "peel–back" from the glenoid (Type II lesion).[13] Reports of a traumatic unstable event, severe weakness, and/or intense pain may indicate the presence of concomitant pathologies. Additional injuries associated with SLAP lesions have been well documented.[23,24,32] These injuries include partial- and full-thickness rotator cuff tears, as well as Bankart and Hill-Sachs lesions. If additional injury is suspected, the physical therapist should examine the integrity of these specific tissues. Patients' subjective reports are useful in guiding the clinical examination by revealing potential injury and diminishing the necessity to investigate unlikely pathologies.

For competitive and recreational athletes, the only functional sign of a SLAP lesion may be a sudden decrease in physical performance such as a loss in striking power, throwing velocity, target accuracy, or level of consistency. Other relevant questions to ask are those specifically related to diet and the presence of systemic disease. These factors can significantly influence tissue healing rates and prognosis, thereby demanding modification of the rehabilitation timeline. Based on the severity of comorbidities, the patient may require referral to other healthcare disciplines (e.g., physician, psychiatrist, registered dietitian) for services outside the scope of physical therapy practice. In this case, the patient's eating disorder may delay tissue healing and significantly impact the overall prognosis by lengthening the time required to safely return to sport. Interviews should be adapted to glean this type of relevant information, which helps direct the physical examination and tailor the plan of care.

The physical examination begins with careful observation of the patient's posture, scapular position, and assessment of muscle volume. Procedures include superficial palpation to provide feedback and reinforcement to support (or contradict) the therapist's clinical observations. Although a rare complication of labral pathology, spinoglenoid cysts can cause significant infraspinatus muscle atrophy due to neural compression exerted at the spinoglenoid notch. Magnetic resonance imaging may be ordered to confirm the presence of a cyst. Careful neurovascular and cervical exam helps clarify any involvement of the cervical and upper thoracic spine.

The physical exam includes assessment of active and passive range of motion, flexibility, passive physiologic joint mobility, strength, tissue irritability, and apprehension. The therapist should carefully observe active range of motion (AROM) of the shoulders for symmetrical quantity and quality. Motion is also observed for normal kinematics and contributions from the thoracic spine, scapulothoracic articulation, and glenohumeral joint. Cardinal plane AROM is typically preserved in isolated SLAP lesions.[33] However, pain is often noted in positions of rotator cuff impingement and end-range humeral rotation. Previous investigators have found that thoracic posture influences scapular position, resulting in altered movement patterns of the upper extremity during shoulder elevation.[34] Altered scapular position such as medial border winging and inferior angle prominence are physical exam findings of scapular dyskinesis, which has been associated with labral pathology.[35] It remains unclear whether scapular dyskinesis is the predisposing impairment or the consequence of labral pathology. The presence of these impairments is suggestive of scapular instability and/or excessive muscle tightness.[36] Although it is standard practice to suggest that the patient's scapular dyskinesis might benefit from therapeutic interventions to improve scapular position and decrease risk for injury, there is no empirical evidence to confirm this assumption. Qualitative observational evaluations of scapular dyskinesis have been reported to reliably associate with kinematic analyses.[37-39]

Deficits in passive range of motion of the shoulder may also cause altered movement patterns and create compensatory strategies. Restrictions common in overhead athletes include glenohumeral internal rotation deficit (GIRD), decreased cross-body adduction, and scapular dyskinesis.[13] Overhead athletes, including volleyball players,[40] have shown a higher frequency of GIRD in the dominant arm. Presence of GIRD and decreased cross-body adduction are clinical measures of posterior shoulder tightness that have been associated with a higher incidence[41] and prevalence of injury.[42] These impairments can influence range of motion and function by placing excessive stress on the labrum. Factors thought to influence these motions include posture, posterior-inferior capsular tightness, and humeral torsion.[13,33,43,44] If these limitations are not identified and addressed, the patient may be unable to reach optimal level of performance, and possibly be at increased risk for subsequent injury.[41]

Next, the physical therapist should use manual joint glides to clinically assess the resting glenohumeral relationship as well as the degree of capsular extensibility. Individuals with posterior shoulder tightness have demonstrated excessive anterior humeral resting positions on the glenoid fossa.[45,46] Contributions to altered positions are thought to result from increased stiffness of the IGHL and posterior capsule.

Due to the loss of negative intra-articular pressure and excessive translation of the humeral head that can occur with a SLAP tear, the passive stability of the glenohumeral joint may be impaired. Table 2-1 lists common physical examination tests to aid in the diagnosis of a SLAP lesion or glenohumeral joint instability.[47] Principles of diagnostic test sensitivity and specificity should be employed to accurately identify specific impairments and pathology. For example, tests that are more sensitive should be performed first to help focus the physical exam by avoiding performance of unnecessary procedures.

Based on criteria established by Richards *et al.*[48], the load and shift test and the sulcus sign are graded on a 0-III scale. For anterior/posterior translations: Grade I equals 0 to 1 cm translation up the glenoid face; Grade II equals 1 to 2 cm translation, or to the glenoid rim; and, Grade III equals greater than 2 cm translation over the rim.[49] For an inferior sulcus sign, Grade 0 equals no translation; Grade I equals 0 to 1 cm translation; Grade II equals 1 to 2 cm translation; and, Grade III equals greater than 2 cm translation.[49]

Careful muscular strength and endurance testing is critical because individuals with labral pathology, shoulder pain, and joint instability often display weakness, particularly in the scapular stabilizers (*e.g.*, rhomboids, serratus anterior) and rotator cuff muscles.[33] Neuromuscular control and endurance testing are additional components of muscle integrity that should be incorporated. Deficits that are not apparent during maximal isometric contraction may become evident following fatiguing tasks. Handheld dynamometry is an objective measurement tool that can effectively convey strength deficits to the patient. Anecdotally, the presence of night pain in addition to weakness is *not* consistent with an isolated SLAP tear and may be indicative of a concomitant rotator cuff pathology.[23] Further diagnostic testing is required if this clinical presentation is present.

During the physical examination, tissue irritability and patient apprehension may negatively influence the outcomes of other tests. As a general rule, selective tissue testing should begin with procedures that are less aggravating, reserving those that are more provocative to the end of the examination. For example, patients with SLAP lesions and concomitant shoulder instability may become highly fearful and reactive when placed in an "apprehension test" position (Table 2-1). Eliciting these symptoms earlier in the exam may result in excessive guarding and the inability to fully investigate the patient's entire pathological involvement. These guidelines also aid in gaining patient trust and participation compliance.

Table 2-1	PHYSICAL EXAMINATION TESTS FOR SHOULDER INSTABILITY AND SLAP LESIONS			
Test (Purpose)	Patient Position	Performance of Test	Sensitivity	Specificity
Sulcus sign (Joint stability)	Seated or standing	Therapist grasps the elbow and produces an inferior traction force	17%	93%
Biceps Load I (SLAP tear)	Supine with 90° of shoulder abduction and 90° of elbow flexion	Therapist resists elbow flexion at maximal shoulder external rotation	91%	97%
Biceps Load II (SLAP tear)	Supine with shoulder in 120° of abduction and 90° of elbow flexion	Therapist resists elbow flexion at maximal shoulder external rotation	90%	97%
Speed's test (Labral tear)	Standing with elbow fully extended and forearm fully supinated	Therapist resists shoulder flexion from 0° to 60°	9%-18%	74%-87%
Load and shift (Joint stability)	Supine with examiner stabilizing the clavicle and superior border of the scapula	Therapist provides humeral compression into the glenoid fossa and applies posteriorly and anteriorly directed forces at glenohumeral joint	Not available	Not available
Apprehension test (Joint stability)	Supine with humerus hanging off of the table and maximally externally rotated in 90° of abduction	Therapist provides anteriorly directed force through the posterior shoulder	30%-40%	63%-87%
Surprise test (Joint stability)	Supine with shoulder at edge of treatment table	With one hand, therapist provides posteriorly directed force through humeral head. With the other hand, therapist grasps patient's forearm, moving the shoulder to 90° abduction and externally rotating to end range. Then, therapist releases posterior force on humeral head.	64%-92%	89%-99%
Crank test (Labral tear)	Supine or seated with shoulder in 160° of elevation in the scapular plane	Therapist applies compression and then rotates between internal and external rotation	58%-91%	72%-93%
Clunk test (Labral tear)	Supine with shoulder maximally abducted	Therapist applies a posterior to anterior force to the shoulder while maintaining humeral external rotation	44%	68%

Plan of Care and Interventions

The rehabilitation program of a patient presenting with a SLAP lesion should be focused on restoring and enhancing the dynamic stability of the glenohumeral joint. Emphasis should be placed on improving scapular mechanics and addressing any deficits within the kinetic chain (*e.g.*, core stability, balance, and lower extremity strength). A clear understanding of the pathology and mechanism of injury should be considered prior to developing the plan of care. For example, the treatment of compressive injuries (*e.g.*, FOOSH) should be modified to avoid excessive joint loading, while the treatment of traction injuries should discourage biceps activation due to potential migration of the superior labrum.

Several investigators have reported successful postoperative outcomes after SLAP repair.[19,50-53] However, **little evidence exists regarding the effectiveness of conservative physical therapy management for these lesions.** Edwards *et al.*[8] documented that 49% of individuals with SLAP lesions treated nonoperatively with physical therapy had successful outcomes as determined by subjective measures and functional return-to-sport participation. Approximately 67% of the overhead athletes who were effectively treated with nonoperative care were able to return to the same or higher level of competition. These findings are difficult to reconcile with the results reported in surgical intervention studies. The therapeutic interventions in this study included **selective tissue stretching of the posterior-inferior capsule.** Sleeper and cross-body adduction stretches have been recommended for overhead athletes to improve the clinical impairments of posterior shoulder tightness commonly seen within this population.[54] Research investigating the effects of these stretches suggests a resolution of shoulder pain in overhead athletes following a course of therapy (~7 weeks).[55] Table 2-2 describes several flexibility exercises commonly prescribed for individuals with SLAP lesions.

Table 2-2 SOFT TISSUE FLEXIBILITY INTERVENTIONS FOR POSTERIOR SHOULDER TIGHTNESS		
Intervention	**Patient Position**	**Exercise Performance**
Cross-body stretch	Sidelying on affected side with shoulder flexed to 90°. The table (with a wedge, if necessary) should be used to block the scapula. (Fig. 2-1A)	Patient applies passive overpressure into horizontal adduction until a gentle stretch is felt. This position is held for 30 s and 3 sets are performed.
Sleeper stretch	Sidelying on affected side with the shoulder flexed to 90°. The table (with a wedge, if necessary) should be used to block the scapula. (Fig. 2-1B)	Patient applies passive overpressure into humeral internal rotation until a gentle stretch is felt. This position is held for 30 s and 3 sets are performed.
Prayer latissimus dorsi stretch	Quadruped with hands positioned above head. (Fig. 2-1C)	Patient sits back onto heels until a gentle stretch is felt. This position is held for 30 s and 3 sets are performed.
Latissimus dorsi and subscapularis mobilizations with foam roller	Sidelying on affected side with foam roller positioned under axillary fold. The top leg is crossed in front to provide mobility. (Figs. 2-1D and E)	Patient uses the top leg to move up and down the foam roll to provide passive mobilization. Humeral internal and external rotation should be performed when over the subscapularis.

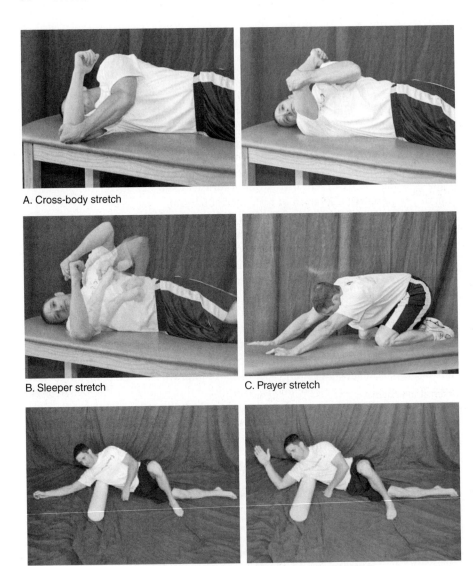

A. Cross-body stretch

B. Sleeper stretch

C. Prayer stretch

D. Foam roll—latissimus

E. Foam roll—subscapularis

Figure 2-1. Soft tissue flexibility interventions for posterior shoulder tightness.

In addition to stretching, soft tissue and joint mobilization techniques may be helpful in restoring passive mobility to the posterior shoulder. Glides directed toward the posterior and inferior joint capsule provide valuable feedback regarding the mobility of the posterior capsule and IGHL. Individuals with excessive or asymmetrical stiffness may benefit from manual joint mobilizations and selective tissue stretching of the posterior shoulder. Tightness of the dynamic posterior restraints of glenohumeral stability (teres minor, latissimus dorsi, and infraspinatus) is thought to contribute to motion restrictions.[13,56] Foam roller mobilizations are useful to selectively mobilize and potentially lengthen these active restraints.

Overhead motions place large distraction forces on the humerus. Because so much stress is repetitively exerted on the upper extremity, the athlete must have adequate flexibility, strength, and stability to safely return to sport after injury. **Scapular stabilization exercises, rotator cuff strengthening, and kinetic chain activities have been effectively used to conservatively manage overhead athletes with SLAP lesions.**[8] Table 2-3 presents strengthening exercises for individuals with SLAP lesions. Initially, muscular function goals should focus on improving scapular control and rotator cuff muscle strength with the elbow at the individual's side prior to progressing to more elevated humeral positions. As strength increases, the volume of resisted exercise must be increased to prepare the patient for the muscular endurance required for the repetitive demands of overhead sports. Once acceptable rotator cuff strength and scapular stability has been established, the treatment plan should advance to plyometric and closed kinetic chain activities that promote joint and core stability. The closed kinetic chain upper extremity stability test (CKCUEST) was initially developed as a field test to determine readiness for return to sport in those with upper extremity injuries.[57] However, this activity can also be used as a clinical treatment tool to enhance both core and scapular stability. Last, progressive sports-specific programs should be applied to

Table 2-3 STRENGTHENING INTERVENTIONS FOR INDIVIDUALS WITH SLAP LESIONS		
Intervention	**Patient Position**	**Exercise Performance**
Internal and external humeral rotation	Standing holding the band with towel roll under a 90° flexed elbow • Internal rotation starts with humerus in neutral rotation. (Fig. 2A) • External rotation begins with affected arm tucked in at the abdomen. (Fig. 2B)	The shoulder is actively internally rotated to the abdomen for internal rotation and externally rotated just past neutral for external rotation. Progression of these activities should be performed at 90° of shoulder flexion.
Scapular stabilizations: I's, T's, and Y's	Prone on floor, table, or stability ball with upper extremities in the coronal plane. • I's—Arms are held out to the side at ~30° humeral abduction. (Fig. 7-13) • T's—Arms are held out to the side at 90° of horizontal abduction. (Fig. 7-14) • Y's—Arms are held out to ~150-160° flexion. (Fig. 7-15)	• I's—Shoulders are extended (~10°-20°) while simultaneously performing full scapular retraction and depression. • T's—Shoulders are horizontally abducted (~10°-20°) while simultaneously performing full scapular retraction and depression. • Y's- Shoulders are flexed and abducted (~10°-20°) while simultaneously performing full scapular retraction and depression.
Closed kinetic chain upper extremity stability exercise	Plank (push-up) position with the hands placed 15 inches apart for smaller individuals, and 36 inches apart for larger individuals. (Fig. 2F)	While maintaining scapular protraction, the patient alternates tapping one hand with the opposite hand. This exercise is progressed in 15-s increments for up to a minute.

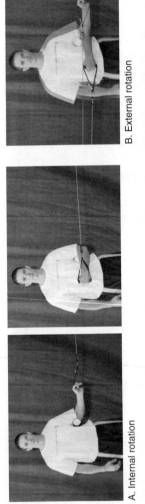

A. Internal rotation

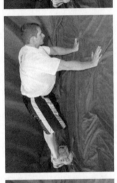

B. External rotation

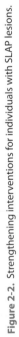

C. Closed kinetic chain upper extremity stability exercise

Figure 2-2. Strengthening interventions for individuals with SLAP lesions.

safely prepare the athlete for the physical demands required by her activity. When the patient is completely asymptomatic and has demonstrated sufficient strength, endurance, and dynamic joint stability, she is ready to return to sport.

Evidence-Based Clinical Recommendations

SORT: Strength of Recommendation Taxonomy

A: Consistent, good-quality patient-oriented evidence
B: Inconsistent or limited-quality patient-oriented evidence
C: Consensus, disease-oriented evidence, usual practice, expert opinion, or case series

1. Nonoperative treatment is moderately effective for returning athletes with SLAP tears to sport. **Grade B**
2. Posterior shoulder stretching decreases pain in those overhead athletes who experience shoulder pain. **Grade B**
3. Rotator cuff and scapular stability strengthening improves function and decreases pain in overhead athletes with SLAP lesions. **Grade B**

COMPREHENSION QUESTIONS

2.1 A high-school volleyball player presents with left shoulder pain during a "maximal cocking" mechanism of injury. What would MOST likely be the patient's classification of SLAP lesion?

  A. Type I
  B. Type II
  C. Type III
  D. Type IV

2.2 Which of the following concomitant pathologies is MOST likely to be present in younger overhead athletes with a Type II SLAP lesion?

  A. Rotator cuff tear
  B. Avascular necrosis of the humeral head
  C. Anterior shoulder instability
  D. Spinoglenoid cysts

ANSWERS

2.1 **B.** Type II lesions are the most common form of SLAP tear within athletic populations. The eccentric load applied to the biceps during maximal cocking is thought to result in a peel-back lesion of the superior labrum and a type II defect. Type I lesions are associated with degeneration to the inner rim of the labrum and not common in younger populations (option A). Type III and IV SLAP lesions are bucket handle tears thought to be the result of fall on outstretched hand (FOOSH) mechanism of injury rather than traction to the biceps-labral complex (options C and D).

2.2 **C.** Excessive anterior joint instability or laxity and contracture of the posterior capsule is thought to result from repetitive overhead throwing activities. During maximal cocking, the humeral head translates anteriorly, stressing the anterior joint capsule. Due to the arthromechanics and repetitive nature of this activity, some authors maintain that anterior instability may result over time. The prevalence of rotator tears is low in younger overhead athletes (option A). Avascular necrosis is the result of severe vascular insufficiency associated with traumatic shoulder dislocations that can rupture the circumflex humeral arteries (option B). Spinoglenoid cysts are insidious in nature and result from suprascapular nerve palsy (option D).

REFERENCES

1. Costouras J, Warner J. Classification, clinical assessment, and imaging of glenohumeral instability. In: Galatz LM, ed. *Orthopedic Knowledge Update: Shoulder and Elbow, No. 3.* Rosemont, IL: American Academy of Orthopedic Surgeons; 2008:67-81.

2. Howell SM, Galinat BJ. The glenoid-labral socket. A constrained articular surface. *Clin Orthop Relat Res.* 1989;243:122-125.

3. Park M. Anatomy and function of the shoulder structures. In: Galatz LM, ed. *Orthopedic Knowledge Update: Shoulder and Elbow No. 3.* Rosemont, IL: American Academy of Orthopedic Surgeons; 2008.

4. Halder AM, Kuhl LG, Zorbitz ME, An KN. Effects of the glenoid labrum and glenohumeral abduction on stability of the shoulder joint through concavity-compression: an in vitro study. *J Bone Joint Surg Am.* 2001;83-A:1062-1069.

5. Andrews JR, Carson WG Jr, McLeod WD. Glenoid labrum tears related to the long head of the biceps. *Am J Sports Med.* 1985;13:337-341.

6. Snyder SJ, Karzel RP, Del Pizzo W, et al. SLAP lesions of the shoulder. *Arthroscopy.* 1990;6:274-279.

7. Kampa RJ, Clasper J. Incidence of SLAP lesions in a military population. *J R Army Med Corps.* 2005;151:171-175.

8. Edwards SL, Lee JA, Bell JE, et al. Nonoperative treatment of superior labrum anterior posterior tears: improvements in pain, function, and quality of life. *Am J Sports Med.* 2010;38:1456-1461.

9. Handelberg F, Willems S, Shahabpour M, et al. SLAP lesions: a retrospective multicenter study. *Arthroscopy.* 1998;14:856-862.

10. Kim TK, Queale WS, Cosgarea AJ, McFarland EG. Clinical features of the different types of SLAP lesions: an analysis of one hundred and thirty-nine cases. *J Bone Joint Surg Am.* 2003;85-A:66-71.

11. Pagnani MJ, Deng XH, Warren RF, et al. Effect of lesions of the superior portion of the glenoid labrum on glenohumeral translation. *J Bone Joint Surg Am.* 1995;77:1003-1010.

12. Jobe CM. Posterior superior glenoid impingement: expanded spectrum. *Arthroscopy.* 1995;11: 530-536.

13. Burkhart SS, Morgan CD, Kibler WB. The disabled throwing shoulder: spectrum of pathology Part I: pathoanatomy and biomechanics. *Arthroscopy.* 2003;19:404-420.

14. Clavert P, Bonnomet F, Kempf JF, et al. Contribution to the study of the pathogenesis of type II superior labrum anterior-posterior lesions: a cadaveric model of a fall on the outstretched hand. *J Shoulder Elbow Surg.* 2004;13:45-50.

15. Maffet MW, Gartsman GM, Moseley B. Superior labrum-biceps tendon complex lesions of the shoulder. *Am J Sports Med.* 1995;23:93-98.

16. Powell SE, Nord KD, Ryu RKN. The diagnosis, classification, and treatment of SLAP lesions. *Oper Tech Sports Med.* 2004;12:99-110.

17. Barber F. Superior labrum anterior and posterior injury. In: Galatz L, ed. *Orthopedic Knowledge Update: Shoulder and Elbow, No. 3.* Rosemont IL: American Academy of Orthopedic Surgeons; 2008:327-335.

18. Bey MJ, Elders GJ, Huston LJ, et al. The mechanism of creation of superior labrum, anterior, and posterior lesions in a dynamic biomechanical model of the shoulder: the role of inferior subluxation. *J Shoulder Elbow Surg.* 1998;7:397-401.

19. Nam EK, Snyder SJ. The diagnosis and treatment of superior labrum, anterior and posterior (SLAP) lesions. *Am J Sports Med.* 2003;31:798-810.

20. Snyder SJ, Banas MP, Karzel RP. An analysis of 140 injuries to the superior glenoid labrum. *J Shoulder Elbow Surg.* 1995;4:243-248.

21. Boileau P, Parratte S, Chuinard C, et al. Arthroscopic treatment of isolated type II SLAP lesions: biceps tenodesis as an alternative to reinsertion. *Am J Sports Med.* 2009;37:929-936.

22. Burkhart SS, Morgan CD. The peel-back mechanism: its role in producing and extending posterior type II SLAP lesions and its effect on SLAP repair rehabilitation. *Arthroscopy.* 1998;14:637-640.

23. Dodson CC, Altchek DW. SLAP lesions: an update on recognition and treatment. *J Orthop Sports Phys Ther.* 2009;39:71-80.

24. Mileski RA, Snyder SJ. Superior labral lesions in the shoulder: pathoanatomy and surgical management. *J Am Acad Orthop Surg.* 1998;6:121-131.

25. Choi NH, Kim SJ. Avulsion of the superior labrum. *Arthroscopy.* 2004;20:872-874.

26. Kugler A, Kruger-Franke M, Reininger S, et al. Muscular imbalance and shoulder pain in volleyball athletes. *Br J Sports Med.* 1996;30:256-259.

27. Lajtai G, Pfirrmann CW, Aitzetmuller G, et al. The shoulders of professional beach volleyball players: high prevalence of infraspinatus muscle atrophy. *Am J Sports Med.* 2009;37:1375-1383.

28. Verhagen EA, Van der Beek AJ, Bouter LM, et al. A one season prospective cohort study of volleyball injuries. *Br J Sports Med.* 2004;38:477-481.

29. Reeser JC, Verhagen E, Briner WW, et al. Strategies for the prevention of volleyball-related injuries. *Br J Sports Med.* 2006;40:594-600.

30. Taljanovic MS, Nisbet JK, Hunter TB, et al. Humeral avulsion of the inferior glenohumeral ligament in college female volleyball players caused by repetitive microtrauma. *Am J Sports Med.* 2011;39:1067-1076.

31. Safran MR. Nerve injury about the shoulder in athletes, part 1: suprascapular nerve and axillary nerve. *Am J Sports Med.* 2004;32:803-819.

32. Andrews J, Carson W. The arthroscopic treatment of glenoid labrum tears in the throwing athlete. *Orthop Trans.* 1984;8:44.

33. Keener JD, Brophy RH. Superior labral tears of the shoulder: pathogenesis, evaluation, and treatment. *J Am Acad Orthop Surg.* 2009;17:627-637.

34. Thigpen CA, Padua DA, Michener LA, et al. Head and shoulder posture affect scapular mechanics and muscle activity in overhead tasks. *J Electromyogr Kinesiol.* 2010;20:701-9.

35. Kibler WB. The role of the scapula in athletic shoulder function. *Am J Sports Med.* 1998;26:325-337.

36. Laudner KG, Moline MT, Meister K. The relationship between forward scapular posture and posterior shoulder tightness among baseball players. *Am J Sports Med.* 2010;38:2106-2112.

37. Kibler WB, Uhl TL, Maddux JW, et al. Qualitative clinical evaluation of scapular dysfunction: a reliabililty study. *J Shouder Elbow Surg.* 2002;11:550-566.

38. Tate AR, McClure P, Kareha S, et al. A clinical method for identifying scapular dyskinesis, part 2: validity. *J Athl Train.* 2009;44:165-173.

39. McClure P, Tate AR, Kareha S, et al. A clinical method for identifying scapular dyskinesis, part 1: reliability. *J Athl Train.* 2009;44:160-164.

40. Schwab LM, Blanch P. Humeral torsion and passive shoulder range in elite volleyball players. *Phys Ther Sport.* 2009;10:51-56.

41. Shanley E, Rauh MJ, Michener LA, et al. Shoulder range of motion measures as risk factors for shoulder and elbow injuries in high school softball and baseball players. *Am J Sports Med.* 2011;39:1997-2006.

42. Wilk KE, Macrina LC, Fleisig GS, et al. Correlation of glenohumeral internal rotation deficit and total rotational motion to shoulder injuries in professional baseball pitchers. *Am J Sports Med;* 39:329-335.

43. Harryman DT 2nd, Sidles JA, Clark JM, et al. Translation of the humeral head on the glenoid with passive glenohumeral motion. *J Bone Joint Surg Am.* 1990;72:1334-1343.

44. Myers JB, Laudner KG, Pasquale MR, et al. Glenohumeral range of motion deficits and posterior shoulder tightness in throwers with pathologic internal impingement. *Am J Sports Med.* 2006;34:385-391.

45. Yang JL, Lu TW, Chou FC, et al. Secondary motions of the shoulder during arm elevation in patients with shoulder tightness. *J Electromyogr Kinesiol.* 2009;19:1035-1042.

46. Lin JJ, Lim HK, Yang JL. Effect of shoulder tightness on glenohumeral translation, scapular kinematics, and scapulohumeral rhythm in subjects with stiff shoulders. *J Orthop Res.* 2006;24:1044-1051.

47. Cook C, Hegedus E. *Orthopedic Physical Examination Tests: An Evidence-Based Approach.* Upper Saddle River, NJ: Prentice Hall; 2008.

48. Richards RR, An K, Bigliani LU, et al. A standardized method for the assessment of shoulder function. *J Shoulder Elbow Surg.* 1994;3:347-352.

49. Hawkins RJ, Schutte JP, Janda DH, Huckell GH. Translation of the glenohumeral joint with the patient under anesthesia. *J Shoulder Elbow Surg.* 1996;5:286-292.

50. Pagnani MJ, Speer KP, Altchek DW, et al. Arthroscopic fixation of superior labral lesions using a biodegradable implant: a preliminary report. *Arthroscopy.* 1995;11:194-198.

51. O'Brien SJ, Allen AA, Coleman SH, Drakos MC. The trans-rotator cuff approach to SLAP lesions: technical aspects for repair and a clinical follow-up of 31 patients at a minimum of 2 years. *Arthroscopy.* 2002;18:372-377.

52. Cohen DB, Coleman S, Drakos MC, et al. Outcomes of isolated type II SLAP lesions treated with arthroscopic fixation using a bioabsorbable tack. *Arthroscopy.* 2006;22:136-142.

53. Yoneda M, Hirooka A, Saito S, et al. Arthroscopic stapling for detached superior glenoid labrum. *J Bone Joint Surg Br.* 1991;73:746-750.

54. Laudner KG, Sipes RC, Wilson JT. The acute effects of sleeper stretches on shoulder range of motion. *J Athl Train.* 2008;43:359-363.

55. Tyler TF, Nicholas SJ, Lee SJ, et al. Correction of posterior shoulder tightness is associated with symptom resolution in patients with internal impingement. *Am J Sports Med.* 2009;38:114-119.

56. Pappas AM, Zawacki RM, McCarthy CF. Rehabilitation of the pitching shoulder. *Am J Sports Med.* 1985;13:223-235.

57. Goldbeck TG, Davies GJ. Test-Retest reliability of the closed kinetic chain upper extremity stability test: a clinical field test. *J Sport Rehabil.* 2000;9:35-45.

Acute Shoulder Instability

Nathan R. Neff
Thomas J. Olson
Paul E. Westgard

CASE 3

A 22-year-old female snowboard instructor is referred to an outpatient physical therapy clinic from a medical center with a diagnosis of right shoulder pain. She fell while snowboarding 3 days ago and reports that her shoulder "popped out and went back in again." She attempted to teach today but was unable to continue due to pain and a sense that her shoulder would "come out again" if she tried to help one of her fallen clients stand up. Plain film images taken at the clinic showed no obvious bony abnormality; no additional imaging was performed. The patient's medical history is otherwise unremarkable. Signs and symptoms are consistent with anterior shoulder dislocation. The patient's goal is to continue snowboarding and teaching for the rest of the season.

- ▶ What examination signs may be associated with this diagnosis?
- ▶ What are the most appropriate examination tests?
- ▶ What precautions should be taken during physical therapy examination and interventions?
- ▶ What are the most appropriate physical therapy interventions?
- ▶ What referral may be appropriate based on her condition?
- ▶ What is her rehabilitation prognosis?

KEY DEFINITIONS

ALPSA LESION: Acronym for anterior labroligamentous periosteal sleeve avulsion; an anteroinferior labral detachment associated with a stripped, but continuous glenoid periosteum

BANKART LESION: Avulsion of the labrum and inferior glenohumeral ligament from the anteroinferior glenoid rim[1]

HAGL LESION: Acronym for humeral avulsion of the anterior glenohumeral ligament

HEMARTHROSIS: Bleeding into a joint

HILL-SACHS LESION: Impression fracture of the posterosuperior articular surface of the humeral head caused by translation of the humeral head over the glenoid rim[2]

SHOULDER DISLOCATION: Complete disruption of the humeral head from the glenoid fossa due to a force that overcomes the joint's static, capsulolabral, and dynamic restraints[3]

SHOULDER SUBLUXATION: Increased excursion of the humeral head on the glenoid fossa without complete displacement; also known as an incomplete or partial dislocation[3]

SLAP LESION: Tear of the superior labrum, anterior to posterior

Objectives

1. Describe the mechanism of injury and the resulting pathoanatomy associated with an anterior shoulder dislocation.
2. Identify the risk factors for primary and secondary dislocations.
3. Describe the benefits and risks related to conservative treatment and surgical intervention following a first-time anterior shoulder dislocation.
4. Prescribe an appropriate therapeutic exercise program for a patient who elects conservative treatment following a first-time anterior shoulder dislocation.

Physical Therapy Considerations

Physical therapy considerations during management of the individual with a diagnosis of acute anterior shoulder instability:

▶ **General physical therapy plan of care/goals:** Decrease pain; minimize loss of neuromuscular control and strength; restore functional joint stability

▶ **Physical therapy interventions:** Patient education regarding functional anatomy and injury pathomechanics; patient education regarding treatment options; sling for comfort; modalities and manual therapy to decrease pain; periscapular and rotator cuff neuromuscular retraining; resistance exercises to increase muscular endurance and strength; functional bracing for return to activity

▶ **Precautions during physical therapy:** Initial avoidance of shoulder abduction and external rotation (ER) to prevent continued anterior instability

▶ **Complications interfering with physical therapy:** Impaired neurovascular status; reoccurrence of dislocation

Understanding the Health Condition

The shoulder is designed to maximize mobility, and as a result, it possesses the greatest range of motion of any joint in the human body.[2] However, this freedom comes at a price. The glenohumeral joint is also the body's most commonly dislocated joint.[4,5] Approximately 70,000 shoulder dislocations present to hospital emergency departments annually, and many more are seen by primary care physicians and orthopedic specialists.[6] Overall, shoulder dislocations occur in 1.7% of the general population[7] though the occurrence among athletes and military personnel is significantly higher.[8,9] Shoulder dislocations can be traumatic or atraumatic and can occur in either the anterior or posterior direction, but traumatic, anterior dislocations are the most common, occurring in 96% and 98% of all cases, respectively.[10]

Sports and recreation-related injuries account for nearly half of all shoulder dislocations in the United States.[6,7,11-14] Between one-quarter and one-third of all reported upper extremity injuries occurring in football, soccer, basketball, and wrestling are shoulder dislocations.[6,15] Nontraditional sports like surfing, skiing, and snowboarding also result in a significant number of shoulder dislocations.[16,17] Contact between competitors and contact with the playing surface are responsible for 75% of these dislocations, with the classic mechanism of injury described as a forceful twisting of the arm into abduction and ER at or above shoulder level.[15] However, falls on an outstretched arm, forced end-range shoulder flexion, or a direct blow to the shoulder are also causes of anterior dislocation in athletes.[3,9,11,13,18] Males are two to three times more likely to incur a shoulder dislocation than females,[6,7,10] and younger athletes appear to be at the highest risk with 20% to 27% of dislocations occurring before 20 years of age.[10,13] College athletes are also at substantial risk: 47% of all shoulder dislocations occur among individuals 15 to 29 years of age.[6]

The glenohumeral joint's inherent instability is due to a lack of bony congruency and the disparity in size between the articulating surfaces of the large humeral head and the small, shallow glenoid fossa. Consequently, the joint is reliant on the support of both static and dynamic elements that function together to provide the shoulder stability necessary for function.[19]

The static stabilizers of the shoulder include the glenoid fossa, labrum, joint capsule, and ligaments. The glenoid labrum is a fibrocartilage ring that deepens the glenoid fossa and provides a vacuum seal to help center the head of the humerus on the glenoid fossa.[2,3] In addition, the labrum serves as the attachment site for the joint capsule and glenohumeral ligaments. The glenohumeral ligaments are thickenings of the joint capsule and are divided into individual superior, middle, and inferior entities, each with a slightly different stabilizing role.[20] The superior glenohumeral ligament originates from the superior glenoid tubercle, the upper part of the labrum, and the base of the coracoid process and inserts between the lesser tuberosity and anatomical neck of the humerus. It assists in preventing inferior displacement of the humeral head when the upper extremity is in a neutral position. The middle glenohumeral ligament is a wide ligament that lies under the tendon of the subscapularis muscle. It originates from the anterior glenoid rim and passes laterally to attach to the anatomic neck and lesser tuberosity of the humerus. The middle glenohumeral ligament works along with the subscapularis tendon to reinforce the anterior glenohumeral joint and limit ER of the humerus in mid-ranges of abduction. Finally, the inferior glenohumeral ligament, formed by anterior and posterior bands separated by a redundancy known as the axillary pouch, reinforces the anterior and inferior aspects of the joint capsule, particularly in the upper ranges of abduction.[2,3] The coracohumeral ligament adds stability to the joint. It originates from the coracoid process and passes inferolaterally to the humerus, blending with the supraspinatus muscle and joint capsule. It separates into two bands that attach to the greater and lesser tuberosities of the humerus, providing a tunnel through which the long head of the biceps tendon passes. It reinforces the superior joint capsule and stabilizes the tendon of the long head of the biceps brachii.[2,3]

The dynamic stability of the glenohumeral joint is provided by the compressive forces generated during co-contraction of the rotator cuff muscles. The force-couple created by co-contraction of supraspinatus, subscapularis, infraspinatus, and teres minor compresses the humeral head into the glenoid fossa, stabilizing the joint during activation of the shoulder's prime movers including the deltoid, pectoralis major, and latissimus dorsi muscles. Activation of a second force couple consisting of the upper, mid, and lower portions of the trapezius, along with the serratus anterior produces upward rotation of the scapulothoracic joint during upper extremity elevation. This activation also helps maintain the humeral head more centrally within the glenoid fossa, further increasing glenohumeral stability during functional movements above shoulder height.[21]

Acute anterior shoulder dislocations are caused by forceful disruptions of the joint's static and dynamic stabilizers that are observed either via diagnostic imaging or through arthroscopic evaluation. The aggressive anteroinferior translation of the humeral head associated with anterior dislocation may result in damage to the labrum, joint capsule, and ligaments, as well as to the bony surfaces of the humerus and glenoid fossa. When these injuries occur, a hemarthrosis develops more than 90% of the time and may interfere with healing.[11,22-25]

There are several common concomitant bony and soft tissue lesions associated with anterior shoulder dislocations. The most frequently observed lesion occurring in an acute anterior dislocation (68%-100% of cases) is called a Bankart lesion.[9,11,14,18,22-24,26] A Bankart lesion is also the predominant pathology in those who experience recurrent dislocation.[27] The ALPSA lesion involves the anteroinferior labrum and capsuloligamentous complex. In this injury, the anterior band of the inferior glenohumeral ligament, labrum, and the anterior scapular periosteum are stripped and displaced in a sleeve-type fashion, medially on the neck of the glenoid fossa. In a study by Antonio et al.,[28] the ALPSA lesion was found in roughly 40% of all anteroinferior labral avulsions. Lateral detachment of the anterior band of the inferior glenohumeral ligament from the humeral neck is called a HAGL lesion.

In the late 1990s, Taylor *et al.*[23] reported that HAGL lesions are associated with only 1.6% of acute anterior shoulder dislocations. However, Liavaag and colleagues[1] have suggested HAGL lesions are more common, occurring in almost a quarter of individuals following anterior dislocation. In addition to soft tissue injuries, bony lesions can also occur during anterior glenohumeral disruption. The "bony Bankart lesion" is an avulsion of the anterior inferior glenoid that occurs in 11.4% of traumatic anterior dislocations.[5] This injury can lead to a reduced resistance to anterior translation of the humeral head on the glenoid, much like a golf ball attempting to rest on a broken tee.[29] The most common bony lesion is the Hill-Sachs lesion. This is an impression fracture on the posterior humeral head resulting from a collision with the anterior glenoid rim as the humeral head comes to rest in the subcoracoid position following displacement. Hill-Sachs lesions occur in 38% to 100% of all traumatic anterior shoulder dislocations.[9-11,14,18,22-24,26] Despite being a near pathognomonic indicator of an anteroinferior glenohumeral dislocation, a Hill-Sachs lesion typically does not contribute significantly to the joint instability normally experienced following injury because this lesion occurs in the superior posterior aspect of the humeral head. However, when the glenohumeral joint is in the end range of combined abduction and ER, the superior posterior aspect of the humeral head comes into contact with the anterior glenoid; if there is also bone loss of the anterior glenoid that is ≥25% of the inferior glenoid diameter, the Hill-Sachs lesion can become an "engaging" or "off-track" lesion that contributes to anterior instability.[30]

Other pathologies associated with acute anterior shoulder dislocation include SLAP lesions, glenoid rim fractures, greater tuberosity fractures, rotator cuff tears, long head of the biceps tears, capsular tears, and nerve injuries. These injuries are less common, presenting in less than a quarter of all cases but can substantially increase glenohumeral instability in the presence of an anteroinferior labral lesion.[10,11,14,18,22-24]

Physical Therapy Patient/Client Management

Recurrent instability is common after anterior shoulder dislocation. The recurrence rate in patients without stabilization surgery is between 66% and 95% for those less than 20 years of age and between 40% and 74% for those between 20 and 40 years old.[7,8,10,13,14,18,22-24,26,27,31-35] Further, in those individuals less than 20 years of age whose initial dislocation occurred while participating in a sport, the recurrence rate can jump to greater than 80%.[36] These same individuals also demonstrate a shorter time period between the first and second dislocation compared to nonathletes.[5] **Age and activity level are two of the most important factors that predict recurrence**: athletes less than 30 years old at the time of their first dislocation are at greatest risk.[5,13,31,32] Clearly, the primary goal following anterior shoulder dislocation is to decrease the likelihood of recurrence while allowing a return to normal activity with as few restrictions as possible.

Traditionally, conservative care following acute shoulder instability has involved dislocation reduction, sling immobilization, and physical therapy to restore range of motion and strength.[37,38] Given the high rates of recurrence, this approach has not been particularly successful. As a result, **surgical intervention is considered an**

appropriate alternative for first-time dislocators. Almost 30 years ago, Jobe and Jobe suggested that throwing athletes with a history of even one dislocation should undergo surgical repair to restore normal anatomy.[39] In a 2004 Cochrane Review, Handoll *et al.*[40] examined five studies comparing surgical and conservative treatment for acute anterior shoulder dislocation and reported a relative risk reduction of 68% to 80% for recurrent instability in those treated surgically. In addition, they noted that half of those initially treated nonoperatively eventually sought surgical intervention. They concluded that surgical stabilization was warranted for young, active individuals following first-time traumatic shoulder dislocation.[40] This conclusion is supported by a review published in 2009. Brophy and Marx[41] described that at 2-year follow-up, surgically treated patients showed a significantly lower rate of recurrent instability (7%) compared to those that received nonoperative care (46%). This trend was consistent at a 10-year follow-up, with recurrence of 10% to 58%, respectively.[41] Based on these findings, a treatment algorithm has been proposed in which surgery is advocated for patients 15 to 25 years of age and a trial of physical therapy is recommended for patients 25 to 40 years of age with surgical intervention reserved to address recurrent dislocation. Finally, nonoperative care is endorsed for patients over 40 years of age secondary to low recurrence rates in this age group.[37]

Despite this evidence-based algorithm, controversy regarding immediate surgical care for the first-time dislocator persists. Hovelius *et al.*[42] have shown that out of 229 anterior shoulder dislocations followed over 25 years, 49% of shoulders did not experience a second dislocation, and 20% of those who were 12 to 22 years old at the time of primary dislocation had one or fewer subluxations or dislocations. Thus, if the proposed treatment algorithm was followed, 30% to 50% of patients would have endured unnecessary surgery. A frequently cited work by Aronen and Regan[43] reported a 75% rate of stabilization at 3-year follow-up after patients completed a regimented conservative treatment protocol combining activity modification with focused strengthening of the shoulder internal rotators and adductors.

Though the outcomes of the Aronen and Regan[43] protocol have not been duplicated and recurrence rates seem to respond favorably to early surgical intervention, the debate regarding surgical or nonsurgical stabilization for first-time traumatic shoulder dislocation continues. As a result, providing education to the patient about the cost/benefit ratio for surgery versus conservative intervention is a large component of the physical therapist's role in managing a patient following an episode of acute anterior shoulder instability. Understanding the patient's lifestyle, including work responsibilities, recreational pursuits, and functional goals in the context of risk factors and prognosis following shoulder dislocation, allows the physical therapist to accurately counsel a patient and create an appropriate, individualized plan of care.

Examination, Evaluation, and Diagnosis

The examination of a patient who has experienced an anterior glenohumeral dislocation depends on how recently the injury occurred. If a physical therapist is providing medical coverage for a sporting event and the athlete presents with significant pain and is holding the arm in slight abduction and neutral rotation, diagnosis is relatively apparent and the examination may be brief. The mechanism of injury was likely witnessed, and an obvious deformity may be visible and palpable over the athlete's anterolateral chest just inferior to the coracoid process. Deformation or a "flattening/squaring off" of the deltoid musculature can also be appreciated as the acromion process becomes the most lateral structure of the shoulder. After an anterior dislocation, traction and compression of chest and shoulder soft tissue can compromise the neurovascular status of the upper extremity. A rapid, but thorough evaluation of sensation and motor function is imperative. Radial and brachial pulse identification,[44,45] dermatomal assessment of sensation to light touch or sharp/dull differentiation, with special attention given to the C5 region supplied by the often affected axillary nerve,[3,44,46] and a distal myotome strength evaluation of wrist and intrinsic finger strength should be performed and compared bilaterally. Joint reduction should then be attempted by a physician.[18] Restoration of normal anatomic alignment should be done within an hour of dislocation to decrease the chance for neuropraxia or vascular trauma.[16] Following reduction, the neurovascular examination should be repeated,[44,45] the arm stabilized using a sling, and the patient referred to a physician for definitive care, including plain film imaging to assess for bony and capsulolabral injury. If reduction cannot be successfully performed at the event, the shoulder should be stabilized in the position found, and the patient should be rapidly transported to an emergency department for additional medical evaluation and treatment.

Occasionally, a dislocated shoulder spontaneously reduces, and a patient may be unsure of exactly what happened. If a patient presents to the clinic with a spontaneously relocated shoulder several days after a traumatic event, a thorough subjective history and physical examination helps differentially diagnose an anterior shoulder dislocation or subluxation[1] versus a shoulder separation or acromioclavicular joint disruption. When patients describe the mechanism of injury involving the provocative position of abduction and ER, indirect forces applied to the distal upper extremity increasing torque at the shoulder joint,[3,16] and/or report a "dead-arm," generalized shoulder pain, and limitations in motion due to fear, the physical therapist should strongly suspect anterior instability.[3,47] On physical examination, tenderness to palpation through the deltopectoral interval and over the bicipital groove, decreased active motion above 90° in flexion and abduction, plus pain and/or weakness with manual muscle testing of the shoulder rotators further suggests an anterior dislocation.

Several special tests can be selected to help confirm the presence of anterior instability following dislocation or subluxation. First, the physical therapist assesses the presence of a sulcus sign bilaterally with the upper extremity in a neutral position to assess general laxity and competency of the superior glenohumeral and coracohumeral ligaments (Fig. 3-1). To assess the integrity of the middle glenohumeral ligament, the rotator interval, and the glenoid rim, the therapist performs an anterior/posterior load and shift test.[48] Here, the therapist applies a force to centralize the humeral head in the glenoid fossa. Then, the therapist applies anteromedial and posterolateral directional stresses to the humeral head with the scapula stabilized. The amount of translation is noted and again compared bilaterally. Patients with

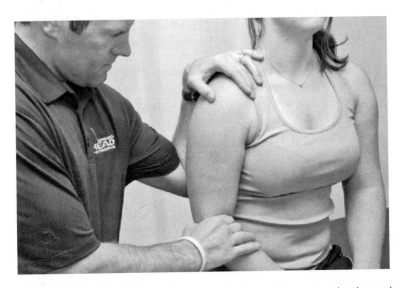

Figure 3-1. Sulcus sign to assess general laxity and competency of the superior glenohumeral and coracohumeral ligaments. Therapist grasps proximal to elbow and produces an inferior traction force. This assessment may also be performed in the supine position.

anterior shoulder instability may demonstrate increased anterior translation on the affected side.[49] Finally, apprehension, relocation, and anterior release tests may be performed on the involved upper extremity. Table 3-1 describes the three most common tests and their corresponding diagnostic accuracy statistics to help distinguish shoulder dislocation/subluxation versus impingement.

The psychometric properties listed in Table 3-1 represent the test results when a "positive" test is operationally defined as apprehension. Apprehension can be defined by verbal acknowledgement of the shoulder "shifting, moving, dislocating"[54] as well as by facial grimacing or a reluctance to assume the test position.[55] It is critical to note that the presence or absence of pain alone does not accurately predict anterior shoulder instability.[50,51,54] Individually, the apprehension and anterior release tests appear to be most effective for ruling in the diagnosis of anterior shoulder dislocation or subluxation. The physical therapist must be careful because the anterior release test can dislocate the glenohumeral joint by replicating the original mechanism of injury. If the therapist chooses to perform the anterior release test, it should be performed *after* the apprehension and relocation tests so the therapist has an impression of the patient's shoulder instability and possibility for dislocation.[50] However, when the **apprehension and relocation tests** are performed consecutively and their results are clustered, the sensitivity is reported at 68% and specificity increases to 100% with a positive predictive value of 100%.[54] Thus, the results of this test cluster make the additional inclusion of the anterior release test difficult to justify.

If the physical therapist suspects a diagnosis of post-traumatic anterior shoulder dislocation/subluxation, referral to a physician is warranted for imaging. Plain film

Table 3-1   DESCRIPTION OF SPECIAL TEST PERFORMANCE AND PSYCHOMETRIC PROPERTIES[a]

Test	Positioning	Findings	Psychometrics[50,51]
Apprehension (Fig. 3-2)	Patient is supine (or sitting) with scapula on treatment table for stabilization. Upper extremity is passively moved into 90° abduction and maximum external rotation. Therapist applies anteriorly directed force to posterior humeral head.[39,47,52]	*Apprehension*: positive for dislocation/ subluxation[39] *Pain*: positive for impingement[39]	Sen: 53%-72% Spec: 96%-99% PPV: 98% NPV: 73% +LLR: 20.2
Relocation (Fig. 3-3)	Patient is supine with scapula on treatment table for stabilization. Upper extremity is passively moved into 90° abduction and maximum external rotation. Therapist applies posteriorly directed force to anterior humeral head.[52]	If the *apprehension* caused by increased external rotation is relieved by the posteriorly directed force: positive for dislocation/ subluxation[52] If the *pain* caused by increased external rotation is relieved by the posteriorly directed force: positive for impingement[52]	Sen: 32%-81% Spec: 54%-100% PPV: 44% NPV: 56% +LLR: 10.4
Anterior release or "Surprise" (Fig. 3-4)	Patient is supine with scapula on treatment table for stabilization. Upper extremity is passively moved into 90° abduction and maximum external rotation. Therapist applies posteriorly directed force applied to anterior humeral head. External rotation is passively taken to end range and pressure is released from humeral head.[53]	Return of *apprehension*: positive for dislocation/ subluxation[50]	Sen: 64% Spec: 99% PPV: 98% NPV: 78%

[a]LLR, likelihood ratio; NPV, negative predictive value; PPV, positive predictive value; Sen, sensitivity; Spec, specificity.

images including three anteroposterior views: one in neutral (Grashey view), and one each in internal and ER. In addition, a transscapular (scapular "Y" view) and an axillary view are commonly obtained. These images help confirm dislocation and identify the presence of bony abnormalities of the humeral head or glenoid rim.[2,56] A Striker Notch view can also be beneficial to specifically diagnose the Hill-Sachs lesion and the bony Bankart lesion that commonly accompany anterior dislocations.[56] Magnetic resonance imaging (MRI) is often performed to determine the presence

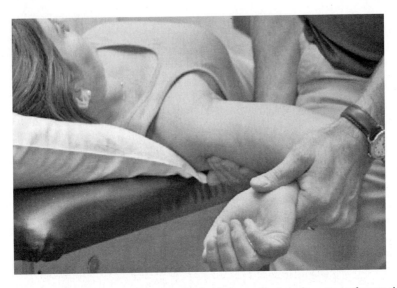

Figure 3-2. Apprehension test originally described with the application of an anterior force to the posterior humeral head. Care must be taken to protect a patient's shoulder from re-dislocation during performance of this test; therefore, the therapist may forego the anterior force if apprehension is appreciated with the positioning alone.

and extent of the anterior inferior labral lesions associated with 73% of glenohumeral dislocations.[1,28] MRI images also allow the inspection of the integrity of the rotator cuff musculature that is frequently compromised in individuals over 40 years of age who experience an anterior dislocation.[3,28] Reviewing these images and radiologist reports can help the physical therapist counsel the patient and establish an appropriate plan of care.

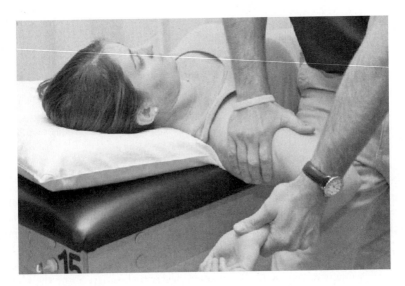

Figure 3-3. Relocation test.

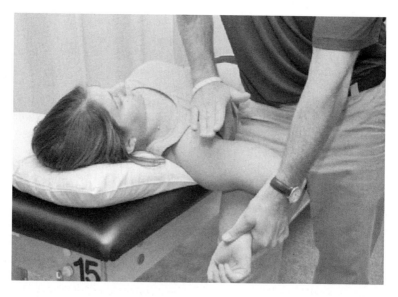

Figure 3-4. Anterior release test. This test should only be performed after the apprehension and relocation tests (if at all) secondary to potential for re-dislocation.

Plan of Care and Interventions

If a patient elects to pursue conservative treatment following an episode of acute anterior shoulder instability, the physical therapist's first goal is to protect the healing tissue. This is usually accomplished through sling immobilization, customarily with the shoulder positioned in internal rotation (IR). There is no consensus regarding the proper duration or positioning for upper extremity immobilization following dislocation. A timeframe of 6 weeks is often proposed based on physiologic healing times of soft tissue, but evidence suggests this may be too long. Hovelius *et al.*[35] compared a group of first-time dislocators immobilized in IR for 3 to 4 weeks with a group instructed to wear a sling as needed for up to 1 week. At 2- and 5-year follow-ups, recurrent dislocation was the same in both groups. A meta-analysis of level I and II evidence compared dislocation recurrence rates for individuals younger than 30 years immobilized for ≤1 week with those immobilized for ≥3 weeks and concluded there was no benefit to conventional sling immobilization for longer than 1 week.[38]

As far as position of immobilization, shoulder IR is typically selected for patient comfort and compliance. Nevertheless, a cadaveric study, several MRI studies, and a preliminary clinical trial suggest that **shoulder immobilization** with the shoulder in abduction and 10° of *external* rotation provides tension on anterior soft tissue structures, decreases hemarthrosis, and increases approximation of the labrum and capsule to the glenoid rim.[25,57-61] A meta-analysis and a randomized controlled trial comparing internal and external immobilization indicate that immobilization in ER is superior to IR at reducing recurrence of dislocation.[38,62] In 2009, McNeil *et al.*[63] recommended that immobilization in

ER be included in the standard of care for first-time traumatic anterior shoulder dislocations. However, a clinical investigation by Finestone and colleagues[46] in the same year contradicted this suggestion, reporting that those immobilized in ER experienced recurrence rates similar to those immobilized in IR. A 2019 Cochrane Review concluded that current evidence is insufficient to inform the choice of immobilization in ER versus IR to prevent recurrent anterior shoulder dislocation.[64] Regardless of time and position selected for immobilization, the physical therapist must address range of motion and strength impairments of the patient with anterior shoulder instability following immobilization. **Reactivation of the dynamic stabilizers of the glenohumeral joint**, including both the rotator cuff and periscapular musculature is essential.[3,43,52,65,66] Initially, isolated submaximal isometric exercises and closed chain activities that promote rotator cuff and periscapular muscle co-contraction performed below 90° of shoulder elevation are appropriate.[65,67] The therapist needs to closely monitor the patient's performance of these exercises. Until the patient has developed appropriate neuromuscular control, the therapist needs to provide verbal and tactile feedback to minimize the recruitment of the prime movers (pectoralis major, latissimus dorsi, upper trapezius) that may contribute to further joint destabilization (Figs. 3-5 and 3-6). An early emphasis on posture and scapular positioning is also important to promote normal muscular firing patterns during upper extremity movement.

As range of motion normalizes, patients can be advanced to progressive isotonic resistance training. Some therapists may be tempted to focus on strengthening the subscapularis muscle at this time as a way to reinforce the anteroinferior glenohumeral capsulolabral complex and prevent recurrent dislocation. However, a cadaveric study by Werner et al.[68] demonstrated that although the subscapularis

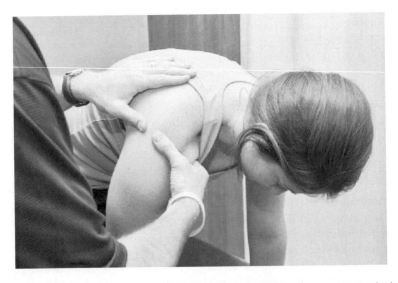

Figure 3-5. Isometric closed chain shoulder protraction for activating the serratus anterior in quadruped. Patient is cued to protract scapula while therapist provides tactile cueing to prevent compensatory pectoralis major contraction.

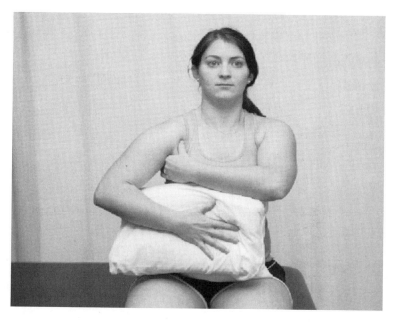

Figure 3-6. Isometric subscapularis activation. Patient performs isometric shoulder internal rotation while applying tactile cueing to prevent pectoralis major compensation.

primarily produces a stabilizing force by compressing the humeral head into the glenoid fossa, tension produced by the inferior segments of the muscle dislocated the joint in some specimens when the upper extremity was abducted and externally rotated. Consequently, a comprehensive strengthening program focusing on dynamic stabilizers and periscapular muscles should be implemented. Table 3-2

Table 3-2 EXERCISES FOR OPTIMUM ROTATOR CUFF AND PERISCAPULAR MUSCLE ACTIVATION	
Targeted Muscles	**Exercise**
Mid/lower trapezius	Prone position: horizontal abduction with external rotation[69,70] (Fig. 3-7)
Serratus anterior	Standing: band-resisted punch plus with shoulder ≥90° flexion[69,71]
	Push-up plus position: progression from vertical (*i.e.,* standing wall push-up position) to horizontal (*i.e.,* traditional prone push-up position)[71]
Supraspinatus	Prone position: horizontal abduction with external rotation[72] (Fig. 3-7)
	Prone position: external rotation at 90° abduction; this exercise must be performed only during the later phases of rehabilitation due to the provocative position required.[72,73]
Infraspinatus/teres minor	Sidelying: shoulder external rotation[72]
Subscapularis	Sidelying shoulder IR. Progress to standing position with shoulder elevated to 90° in scapular plane performing IR against resistance with elastic band.
	Push-up plus position: progression from standing against vertical surface to horizontal surface[71]

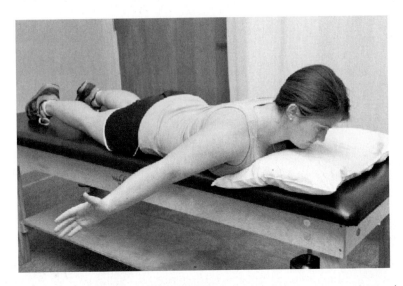

Figure 3-7. Prone horizontal abduction with shoulder external rotation to activate and strengthen middle and lower trapezius and supraspinatus muscles.

describes exercises that result in significant electromyographic activity for the key dynamic stabilizers of the shoulder. Exercise prescription for this patient should emphasize high repetitions to build endurance of the stabilizing muscles and avoid compensation by prime movers in response to excessive loads.[65]

Proprioceptive training for muscular co-contraction should also be continued, not only to promote joint compression and stability but also to address kinesthetic deficits associated with anterior shoulder instability. Smith and Brunolli[74] demonstrated that joint position sense and joint movement perception are impaired following dislocation. The cause of these impairments may be related to receptor damage in the muscles and capsule surrounding the joint, or to a decrease in afferent input from stretch receptors secondary to increased laxity. Regardless of the cause, the presence of these deficits may contribute to abnormal neuromuscular control and increased risk of recurrent instability.[74] Closed chain exercises performed with upper extremity weightbearing through an unstable surface promote reflexive neuromuscular control and improve joint position sense.[65] Exercises in which the involved upper extremity control an oscillating device (*e.g.,* Bodyblade, Thera-Band FlexBar) may be valuable in stimulating mechanoreceptors in both the dynamic and static stabilizers of the shoulder.[75] Exercises that require shoulder hyperextension like full push-ups, dips, latissimus pull downs, and bench press should be avoided to limit stress on the anterior capsule and labrum.[52]

Sport-specific training can be initiated when symmetric motion and strength have been restored, with an expected to return to sport 3 to 4 months following injury.[43] Athletes injured during the competitive season may not be willing or able to delay their return to competition for this duration, but combining physical therapy with the use of a functional brace that prevents upper extremity movement into the provocative position of abduction and ER can often allow them to complete their seasons. Buss *et al.*[76] used this approach and were able to return 87% of high school and college athletes to their sports in 0 to 30 days over a 2-year period. Despite this success, the risk of recurrent dislocation remained high and 37% of the athletes experienced at least one additional episode of instability during the remainder of their season. Almost half then underwent surgical stabilization during the off season.[76]

The methods for surgical repair of anterior glenohumeral instability fall into two categories: anatomic and nonanatomic reconstruction. Anatomic reconstruction focuses on restoring normal anatomy to the shoulder, whereas nonanatomic reconstruction involves creating new structures to contain the humeral head.[77] The non-anatomic reconstruction procedures are typically reserved for patients who require a second stabilization procedure. The anatomic reconstruction procedure most often selected for first-time stabilization is the Bankart repair, which is designed to address the Bankart lesion common in patients with anterior instability. This repair restores tension to the anteroinferior capsule and inferior glenohumeral ligament complex by reattaching the anteroinferior labrum and capsuloligamentous tissue to the glenoid with suture anchors[78] (Fig. 3-8). Similar outcomes have been reported with open repairs and arthroscopic approaches.[41] In patients who demonstrate excessive capsular laxity, a capsular shift or rotator interval closure may also be performed in conjunction with the standard Bankart repair.

Postoperative care after a Bankart repair varies depending on the surgical technique used, the surgeon's preferences, and the patient's goals. Bottoni *et al.*[24] described a three-phase, 12-week postoperative protocol. Phase I consists of immobilization for 4 weeks with therapist-supervised pendulum and isometric exercises.

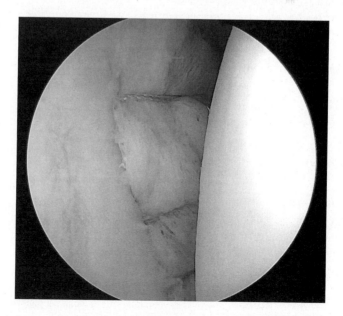

Figure 3-8. Arthroscopic Bankart repair using a 3 suture anchor technique. (Reproduced with permission from Dr. Peter Millett MD, MSc; The Steadman Clinic, Vail, Colorado.)

Phase II emphasizes progressive passive motion followed by active assisted motion. Phase III focuses on full active motion and progressive resistance exercises. Contact sports, overhead, and heavy lifting are restricted until 4 months postoperatively. Wang et al.[79] have described a slightly more conservative program with immobilization for 6 weeks. Active range of motion is emphasized during weeks 6 to 12. Resistance training is introduced about 12 weeks after surgery—after patients had achieved full, painless range of motion. Sport-specific exercises begin between weeks 16 to 20 and patients can expect to be cleared for return to contact sports between 20 and 24 weeks postoperatively.[79] These two programs are similar to postoperative guidelines published by the American Society of Shoulder and Elbow Therapists (ASSET) that include a 4-week period of absolute immobilization, a staged recovery of full range of motion over a 3-month period, a strengthening progression beginning at week 6, and a functional progression for return to athletic activities between 4 and 6 months.[80]

Historically, postoperative protocols and timelines of progression after a Bankart repair progress through phases of rehabilitation that have been predetermined and time-based. Two recently published postoperative approaches combine initial immobilization and (passive and active) range of motion restrictions per surgeon protocol with criteria-based benchmarks to assist the physical therapist with the decision-making process after shoulder instability surgical procedures.[81,82] Each phase of rehabilitation has criteria and associated passing scores for appropriate progression to the next phase (Table 3-3).

Table 3-3 CRITERIA TO PROGRESS TO ACTIVE RANGE OF MOTION AND MUSCULAR ENDURANCE EXERCISES

Criteria Item	Passing Score
Pain	<3/10 at rest
Quick DASH[a] Score	<60%
PROM	Flexion 120°, abduction 90°, external rotation 30°
Scapular Control	Able to perform scapular clock
CRITERIA TO PROGRESS TO INITIAL RESISTANCE STRENGTHENING	
Pain	<3/10 with active motion
Quick DASH Score	<40%
AROM	Flexion 120°, abduction 120°, external rotation 45°
Scapular Dyskinesis	Demonstrates normal scapular movement
Repeated AROM Fatigue	Able to perform 20 repetitions of: scapular plane elevation to 90°, abduction to 90°, sidelying external rotation to 0°
CRITERIA TO PROGRESS TO ADVANCED STRENGTHENING	
Quick DASH	<20
AROM	Flexion, abduction, external rotation >90% of contralateral side
Strength	MMT or handheld dynamometer: 4/5 or greater or >80% in all planes

(Continued)

Table 3-3 **CRITERIA TO PROGRESS TO ACTIVE RANGE OF MOTION AND MUSCULAR ENDURANCE EXERCISES (CONTINUED)**	
CRITERIA TO PROGRESS TO POWER EXERCISES	
Strength	MMT or hand-held dynamometer: 5/5 or >90% in all planes ER/IR strength ratio >70% at 90°
CRITERIA TO RETURN TO SPORT—FUNCTIONAL TESTING	
Various tests	Completion of 60-second 2-lb medicine ball bounce at 165 beats per minute during Wall Med Ball Plyometric Bounce[b]
	Complete 6-lb Single Arm Shot Put Throw[c] >90% distance of contra-lateral side
	Complete >21 touches in 15 seconds of Closed Kinetic Chain Upper Extremity Test[d]
	Score >90% distance of contralateral side during Upper Extremity Y Balance Test[e]

[a]Quick DASH is subjective outcome measure that rates patient's severity of shoulder symptoms and ability to perform functional tasks.
[b]Wall Med Ball Plyometric Bounce assesses overhead shoulder stability and endurance.
[c]Single Arm Shot Put Throw assesses patient's ability to produce overhead power.
[d]Closed Kinetic Chain Upper Extremity Test assesses closed chain endurance.
[e]Upper Extremity Y Balance Test assesses closed chain control through maximal distance while reaching.

Evidence-Based Clinical Recommendations

SORT: Strength of Recommendation Taxonomy

A: Consistent, good-quality patient-oriented evidence
B: Inconsistent or limited-quality patient-oriented evidence
C: Consensus, disease-oriented evidence, usual practice, expert opinion, or case series

1. Athletic males less than 30 years of age are at greatest risk of experiencing acute and recurrent anterior shoulder instability. **Grade A**

2. Surgical intervention for young active individuals following traumatic first-time anterior shoulder dislocation significantly reduces the rate of recurrent dislocation. **Grade A**

3. The apprehension and relocation tests have the best diagnostic accuracy to confirm a suspicion of acute anterior shoulder instability in patients with suggestive history and mechanism of injury. **Grade A**

4. Shoulder immobilization in ER after acute glenohumeral dislocation increases the approximation of the capsulolabral complex with the glenoid fossa and reduces the rate of recurrent dislocation. **Grade B**

5. Nonsurgical intervention focused on reestablishing neuromuscular control and strength of the shoulder's dynamic stabilizers provides patients with acute anterior shoulder instability the best chance to limit recurrent dislocation. **Grade C**

COMPREHENSION QUESTIONS

3.1 A physical therapist completed an examination of a young, active snowboard instructor that suffered an acute anterior shoulder dislocation 3 days ago. The therapist reviewed the X-ray and MRI reports to determine what underlying pathologies may be present. Which of the following pathologies is MOST likely to be seen in this patient?

A. Rotator cuff lesion

B. Bankart lesion

C. Hill-Sachs lesion

D. Bony Bankart lesion

3.2 A snowboard instructor decides she cannot undergo surgical intervention for an acute anterior shoulder dislocation due to financial constraints. She elects to pursue conservative treatment in an attempt to return to work as soon as possible. What is the MOST appropriate plan of care to assist her in achieving this goal?

A. Immobilization for 1 week, global rotator cuff and periscapular muscle strengthening below shoulder level, proprioceptive training in open and closed kinetic chain positions, functional bracing to prevent abduction and external rotation during work, education regarding prognosis in the event of recurrent dislocation

B. Immobilization for 1 week, joint mobilization to maximize range of motion, strength training to include dips, bench press, and behind-the-neck latissimus pull-downs, return to unrestricted activity

C. Immobilization for 3 weeks, isolated subscapularis muscle strengthening below shoulder level, proprioceptive training in open kinetic chain positions only, functional bracing to prevent abduction and external rotation during work, education regarding prognosis in the event of recurrent dislocation

D. Immobilization for 3 weeks, muscle strengthening in abduction and external rotation to increase stability and prevent recurrent dislocation, reassurance that dislocations are typically a single occurrence and should not be an issue in the future

3.3 A snowboard instructor has decided on surgical intervention for an acute anterior shoulder dislocation. At 10 weeks post-anterior labral repair, her involved shoulder active range of motion is 95% of her contralateral side and the physical therapist does not observe scapular dyskinesia. Manual muscle testing for shoulder abduction, scaption, IR (at 0° abduction), and ER (at 0° abduction) were rated as a 4+/5. Which type of therapeutic exercise is MOST appropriate for the next phase of rehabilitation?

A. Aggressive end-range stretching

B. Advanced overhead strengthening

C. Return to on-the-snow training

D. Submaximal isometric strengthening

ANSWERS

3.1 **B.** The Bankart lesion is considered the essential lesion of the acute anterior shoulder dislocation and can lead to recurrent anterior instability. This injury is characterized by the separation of the anterior glenohumeral ligaments and glenoid labrum from the articular surface of the anterior inferior glenoid neck and can lead to increased anterior translation of the humeral head, particularly when the arm is in the abducted and externally rotated position.

3.2 **A.** Initial protection of the joint to minimize inflammation and pain is essential, but controversy persists regarding position and duration. If an internally rotated position is selected, Paterson et al.[38] suggest that there is no benefit to immobilization for longer than 1 week. However, if an externally rotated position is selected, 3 weeks appears to be more appropriate. Strength training focused only on the subscapularis muscle may actually destabilize the glenohumeral joint further in positions of abduction and external rotation (option C). Therefore, a balanced strength program addressing all the rotator cuff and periscapular musculature is recommended. Though open kinetic chain proprioceptive training is beneficial to restore kinesthetic awareness, closed chain exercises are also beneficial to promote joint stability through co-contraction of the glenohumeral dynamic stabilizers.

3.3 **B.** Current timeframes and objective testing suggest that the patient is ready to progress to the advanced overhead strengthening phase of her rehabilitation. At this time, aggressive end-range stretching, returning to work, and sport-specific training on-the-snow are too advanced (options A and C), whereas submaximal isometric strengthening is too conservative (option D).

REFERENCES

1. Liavaag S, Stiris MG, Svenningsen S, et al. Capsular lesions with glenohumeral ligament injuries in patients with primary shoulder dislocation: magnetic resonance imaging and magnetic resonance arthrography evaluation. *Scand J Med Sci Sports*. 2011;21:1-7.

2. Omoumi P, Teixeira P, Lecouvet F, Chung CB. Glenohumeral joint instability. *J Magn Reson Imaging*. 2011;33:2-16.

3. Glousman RE, Jobe FW. How to detect and manage the unstable shoulder. *J Musculoskel Med*. 1989;7:93-110.

4. Kazár B, Relovszky E. Prognosis of primary dislocation of the shoulder. *Acta Orthop Scand*. 1969;40:216-224.

5. Rhee YG, Cho NS, Cho SH. Traumatic anterior dislocation of the shoulder: factors affecting the progress of the traumatic anterior dislocation. *Clin Orthop Surg*. 2009;1:188-193.

6. Zacchilli MA, Owens BD. Epidemiology of shoulder dislocations presenting to emergency departments in the United States. *J Bone Joint Surg Am*. 2010;92:542-549.

7. Hovelius L. Incidence of shoulder dislocation in Sweden. *Clin Orthop Relat Res*. 1982;166:127-131.

8. Hovelius L. Shoulder dislocation in Swedish ice hockey players. *Am J Sports Med*. 1978;6:373-377.

9. Owens BD, Duffey ML, Nelson BJ, et al. The incidence and characteristics of shoulder instability at the United States Military Academy. *Am J Sports Med*. 2007;35:1168-1173.

10. Rowe CR. Prognosis in dislocations of the shoulder. *J Bone Joint Surg*. 1956;38-A:957-977.

11. Baker CL, Uribe JW, Whitman C. Arthroscopic evaluation of acute intitial anterior shoulder dislocations. *Am J Sports Med*. 1990;18:25-28.

12. Hovelius L. Anterior dislocations of the shoulder in teenagers and young adults. *J Bone Joint Surg*. 1987;69:393-399.

13. Simonet WT, Cofield RH. Prognosis in anterior shoulder dislocation. *Am J Sports Med*. 1984;12:19-24.

14. Kirkley A, Griffin S, Richards C, et al. Prospective randomized clinical trial comparing the effectiveness of immediate arthroscopic stabilization versus immobilization and rehabilitation in first traumatic anterior dislocations of the shoulder. *Arthroscopy*. 1999;15:507-514.

15. Bonza JE, Fields SK, Yard EE, et al. Shoulder injuries among United States high school athletes during the 2005-2006 and 2006-2007 school years. *J Athl Train*. 2009;44:76-83.

16. McCall D, Safran MR. Injuries about the shoulder in skiing and snowboarding. *Br J Sports Med*. 2009;43:987-992.

17. Yamauchi K, Wakahara K, Fukuta M, et al. Characteristics of upper extremity injuries sustained by falling during snowboarding: a study of 1918 cases. *Am J Sports Med*. 2010;38:1468-1474.

18. Arciero RA, Wheeler JH, Ryan JB, McBride JT. Arthroscopic Bankart repair versus nonoperative treatment for acute, initial anterior shoulder dislocations. *Am J Sports Med*. 1994;22:589-594.

19. Abboud JA, Soslowsky LJ. Interplay of the static and dynamic restraints in glenohumeral instability. *Clin Orthop Rel Res*. 2002;400:48-57.

20. Burkart AC, Debski RE. Anatomy and function of the glenohumeral ligaments in anterior shoulder instability. *Clin Orthop Rel Res*. 2002;400:32-39.

21. Paine RM, Voight M. The role of the scapula. *J Orthop Sports Phys Ther*. 1993;18:386-391.

22. Wheeler JH, Ryan JB, Arciero RA, Molinari RN. Arthroscopic versus nonoperative treatment of acute shoulder dislocations in young athletes. *Arthroscopy*. 1989;5:231-237.

23. Taylor DC, Arciero RA. Pathologic changes associated with shoulder dislocation: arthroscopic and physical examination findings in first-time, traumatic anterior dislocations. *Am J Sports Med*. 1997;25:306-311.

24. Bottoni CR, Wilckens JH, DeBerardino TM, et al. A prospective, randomized evaluation of arthroscopic stabilization versus nonoperative treatment in patients with acute, traumatic, first-time shoulder dislocations. *Am J Sports Med.* 2002;30:576-580.

25. Miller BS, Sonnabend DH, Hatrick C, et al. Should acute anterior dislocations of the shoulder be immobilized in external rotation? A cadaveric study. *J Shoulder Elbow Surg.* 2004;13:589-592.

26. Henry JH, Genung JA. Natural history of glenohumeral dislocation—revisited. *Am J Sports Med.* 1982;10:135-137.

27. Larrain MV, Botto GJ, Montenegro HJ, Mauas DM. Arthroscopic repair of acute traumatic anterior shoulder dislocation in young athletes. *Arthroscopy.* 2001;17:373-377.

28. Antonio GE, Griffith JF, Yu AB, et al. First-time shoulder dislocation: high prevalence of labral injury and age-related differences revealed by MR arthrography. *J Magn Reson Imaging.* 2007;26:983-991.

29. Bushnell BD, Creighton RA, Herring MM. Bony instability of the shoulder. *Arthroscopy.* 2008;24:1061-1073.

30. Di Giacomo G, Itoi E, Burkhart SS. Evolving Concept of Bipolar Bone Loss and the Hill-Sachs Lesion: From "Engaging/Non-Engaging" Lesion to "On-Track/Off-Track" Lesion. *Arthroscopy.* 2014;30:90-98.

31. Sachs RA, Lin D, Stone ML, et al. Can the need for future surgery for acute traumatic anterior shoulder dislocation be predicted? *J Bone Joint Surg.* 2007;89:1665-1674.

32. Rowe CR, Sakellarides HT. Factors related to recurrences of anterior dislocations of the shoulder. *Clin Orthop.* 1961;20:40-48.

33. McLaughlin HL, MacLellan DI. Recurrent anterior dislocation of the shoulder. II. A comparative study. *J Trauma.* 1967;7:191-201.

34. McLaughlin HL, Cavallaro WU. Primary anterior dislocation of the shoulder. *Am J Surg.* 1950;80:615-621.

35. Hovelius L, Eriksson K, Fredin H, et al. Recurrences after initial dislocation of the shoulder. Results of a prospective study of treatment. *J Bone Joint Surg Am.* 1983;65:343-349.

36. Deitch J, Mehlman CT, Foad SL, et al. Traumatic anterior shoulder dislocation in adolescents. *Am J Sports Med.* 2003;31:758-763.

37. Boone JL, Arciero RA. First-time anterior shoulder dislocations: has the standard changed? *Br J Sports Med.* 2010;44:355-360.

38. Paterson WH, Throckmorton TW, Koester M, et al. Position and duration of immobilization after primary anterior shoulder dislocation: a systematic review and meta-analysis of the literature. *J Bone Joint Surg Am.* 2010;92:2924-2933.

39. Jobe FW, Jobe CM. Painful athletic injuries of the shoulder. *Clin Orthop Relat Res.* 1983;173:117-124.

40. Handoll HH, Almaiyah MA, Rangan A. Surgical versus non-surgical treatment for acute anterior shoulder dislocation. *Cochrane Database Syst Rev.* 2004;(1):CD004325.

41. Brophy RH, Marx RG. The treatment of traumatic anterior instability of the shoulder: nonoperative and surgical treatment. *Arthroscopy.* 2009;25:298-304.

42. Hovelius L, Olofsson A, Sandström B, et al. Nonoperative treatment of primary anterior shoulder dislocation in patients forty years of age and younger: a prospective twenty-five-year follow-up. *J Bone Joint Surg Am.* 2008;90:945-952.

43. Aronen JG, Regan K. Decreasing the incidence of recurrence of first time anterior shoulder dislocations with rehabilitation. *Am J Sports Med.* 1984;12:283-291.

44. Caudevilla Polo S, Estébanez de Miguel E, Lucha López O, et al. Humerus axial traction with acromial fixation reduction maneuver for anterior shoulder dislocation. *J Emerg Med.* 2011;41:282-284.

45. Sahin N, Oztürk A, Özkan Y, et al. A comparison of the scapular manipulation and Kocher's technique for acute anterior dislocation of the shoulder. *Eklem Hastalik Cerrahisi.* 2011;22:28-32.

46. Finestone A, Milgrom C, Radeva-Petrova DR, et al. Bracing in external rotation for traumatic anterior dislocation of the shoulder. *J Bone Joint Surg Br.* 2009;91:918-921.

47. Rowe CR, Zarins B. Recurrent transient subluxation of the shoulder. *J Bone Joint Surg Am.* 1981;63:863-872.

48. Hawkins RJ, Schutte JP, Janda DH, Huckell GH. Translation of the glenohumeral joint with the patient under anesthesia. *J Shoulder Elbow Surg.* 1996;5:286-292.

49. Faber KJ, Homa K, Hawkins RJ. Translation of the glenohumeral joint in patients with anterior instability: awake examination versus examination with the patient under anesthesia. *J Shoulder Elbow Surg.* 1999;8:320-323.

50. Lo IK, Nonweiler B, Woolfrey M, et al. An evaluation of the apprehension, relocation, and surprise tests for anterior shoulder instability. *Am J Sports Med.* 2004;32:301-307.

51. Farber AJ, Castillo R, Clough M, et al. Clinical assessment of three common tests for traumatic anterior shoulder instability. *J Bone Joint Surg Am.* 2006;88:1467-1474.

52. Jobe FW, Kvitne RS, Giangarra CE. Shoulder pain in the overhand or throwing athlete. The relationship of anterior instability and rotator cuff impingement. *Orthop Rev.* 1989;18:963-975.

53. Gross ML, Distefano MC. Anterior release test. A new test for occult shoulder instability. *Clin Orthop Relat Res.* 1997;339:105-108.

54. Speer KP, Hannafin JA, Altchek DW, Warren RF. An evaluation of the shoulder relocation test. *Am J Sports Med.* 1994;22:177-183.

55. Rowe CR. Dislocations of the shoulder. In: Rowe CR, ed. *The Shoulder.* New York, NY: Churchill Livingstone; 1988:165-292.

56. Sanders TG, Zlatkin M, Montgomery J. Imaging of glenohumeral instability. *Semin Roentgenol.* 2010;45:160-179.

57. Itoi E, Hatakeyama Y, Urayama M, et al. Position of immobilization after dislocation of the shoulder. A cadaveric study. *J Bone Joint Surg Am.* 1999;81:385-390.

58. Itoi E, Sashi R, Minagawa H, et al. Position of immobilization after dislocation of the glenohumeral joint. A study with use of magnetic resonance imaging. *J Bone Joint Surg Am.* 2001;83-A:661-667.

59. Itoi E, Hatakeyama Y, Kido T, et al. A new method of immobilization after traumatic anterior dislocation of the shoulder: a preliminary study. *J Shoulder Elbow Surg.* 2003;12:413-415.

60. Siegler J, Proust J, Marcheix PS, et al. Is external rotation the correct immobilisation for acute shoulder dislocation? An MRI study. *Orthop Traumatol Surg Res.* 2010;96:329-333.

61. Scheibel M, Kuke A, Nikulka C, et al. How long should acute anterior dislocations of the shoulder be immobilized in external rotation? *Am J Sports Med.* 2009;37:1309-1316.

62. Taskoparan H, Kılınçoğlu V, Tunay S, et al. Immobilization of the shoulder in external rotation for prevention of recurrence in acute anterior dislocation. *Acta Orthop Traumatol Turc.* 2010;44:278-284.

63. McNeil NJ. Postreduction management of first-time traumatic anterior shoulder dislocations. *Ann Emerg Med.* 2009;53:811-813.

64. Braun C, McRobert CJ. Conservative management following closed reduction of traumatic anterior dislocation of the shoulder. *Cochrane Database Syst Rev.* 2019;5(5):CD004962.

65. Jaggi A, Lambert S. Rehabilitation for shoulder instability. *Br J Sports Med.* 2010;44:333-340.

66. Burkhead WZ Jr, Rockwood CA Jr. Treatment of instability of the shoulder with an exercise program. *J Bone Joint Surg Am.* 1992;74:890-896.

67. Kibler WB. The role of the scapula in athletic shoulder function. *Am J Sports Med.* 1998;26:325-337.

68. Werner CM, Favre P, Gerber C. The role of the subscapularis in preventing anterior glenohumeral subluxation in the abducted, externally rotated position of the arm. *Clin Biomech.* 2007;22:495-501.

69. Ekstrom RA, Donatelli RA, Soderberg GL. Surface electromyographic analysis of exercises for the trapezius and serratus anterior muscles. *J Orthop Sports Phys Ther.* 2003;33:247-258.

70. Cools AM, Dewitte V, Lanszweert F, et al. Rehabilitation of scapular muscle balance: which exercises to prescribe? *Am J Sports Med.* 2007;35:1744-1751.

71. Decker MJ, Hintermeister RA, Faber KJ, Hawkins RJ. Serratus anterior muscle activity during selected rehabilitation exercises. *Am J Sports Med.* 1999;27:784-791.

72. Reinold MM, Wilk KE, Fleisig GS, et al. Electromyographic analysis of the rotator cuff and deltoid musculature during common shoulder external rotation exercises. *J Orthop Sports Phys Ther.* 2004;34:385-394.

73. Boettcher CE, Ginn KA, Cathers I. Which is the optimal exercise to strengthen supraspinatus? *Med Sci Sports Exerc.* 2009;41:1979-1983.

74. Smith RL, Brunolli J. Shoulder kinesthesia after anterior glenohumeral joint dislocation. *J Orthop Sports Phys Ther.* 1990;11:507-513.

75. Buteau JL, Eriksrud O, Hasson SM. Rehabilitation of a glenohumeral instability utilizing the body blade. *Physiother Theory Pract.* 2007;23:333-349.

76. Buss DD, Lynch GP, Meyer CP, et al. Nonoperative management for in-season athletes with anterior shoulder instability. *Am J Sports Med.* 2004;32:1430-1433.

77. Wilk KE, Reinold MM, Andrews JR. *The Athlete's Shoulder.* 2nd ed. Philadelphia, PA: Churchill Livingston Elsevier; 2009.

78. Romeo AA, Cohen BS, Carreira DS. Traumatic anterior shoulder instability. *Orthop Clin North Am.* 2001;32:399-409.

79. Wang RY, Arciero RA, Mazzocca AD. The recognition and treatment of first-time shoulder dislocation in active individuals. *J Orthop Sports Phys Ther.* 2009;39:118-123.

80. Gaunt BW, Shaffer MA, Sauers EL, et al. American Society of Shoulder and Elbow Therapists. The American Society of Shoulder and Elbow Therapists' Consensus Rehabilitation Guideline for Arthroscopic Anterior Capsulolabral Repair of the Shoulder. *J Orthop Sport Phys Ther.* 2010;40:155-168.

81. Bradley H, Lacheta L, Goldenberg BT, et al. Latarjet Procedure for the Treatment of Anterior Glenohumeral Instability in the Athlete: Key Considerations for Rehabilitation. *Int J Sports Phys Ther.* 2021;16:259–269.

82. Goldenberg BT, Goldsten P, Lacheta L, et al. Rehabilitation following posterior shoulder stabilization. *Int J Sports Phys Ther.* 2021;16:930–940.

Surgical Stabilization for Shoulder Instability: Return-to-Sport Rehabilitation

Laura S. Pietrosimone
Ellen Shanley

CASE 4

Four months ago, a 16-year-old high school multisport athlete (football quarterback/defensive back and baseball shortstop/relief pitcher) was injured in a football game. He sustained a glenohumeral dislocation when a defensive lineman contacted his arm at maximal cocking (90° of abduction and external rotation [ER]). He was unable to continue the game and needed reduction of his dislocation in the emergency department. This was his second instability episode. He was diagnosed with a Bankart and Hill-Sachs lesion of his right (dominant) shoulder. Ten days after the dislocation, he had arthroscopic fixation of the Bankart lesion, anterior capsule plication, and remplissage. The patient was referred to physical therapy on postoperative day one (POD 1) by his orthopedic surgeon. The patient hopes to be ready for varsity baseball season. He is starting shortstop and relief pitcher (throws right-handed and is a switch hitter). However, his primary goal is to earn the starting role as quarterback for the upcoming football season. The patient is now 4 months postsurgery and able to begin return-to-sport rehabilitation.

▶ Based on the patient's diagnosis and surgical intervention, what criteria are critical for progression to the return-to-sport program for baseball?
▶ What examination techniques could be used to clarify the athlete's readiness for the tasks of the sport?
▶ What are the most appropriate interventions at this stage of the rehabilitation program?
▶ What are possible complications that may delay the athlete's return to full participation?

KEY DEFINITIONS

BANKART LESION: Described as the "essential lesion" of the shoulder by Bankart in 1923[1]; includes an avulsion of the anteroinferior labrum from its glenoid attachment, generally resulting from an anterior shoulder dislocation

CRITICAL INSTANTS OF FORCE PRODUCTION: The moment during a throwing motion at which peak force is required from the dynamic muscular stabilizers to resist glenohumeral distraction

HILL-SACHS LESION: Impact fractures of the posterolateral aspect of the humeral head usually caused by anterior dislocation of the glenohumeral joint; this fracture may contribute to recurrent shoulder instability[2]

PLICATION: Surgical tightening of soft tissue structures of the shoulder joint; purpose is to reduce the joint volume and looseness to make the joint tighter

REMPLISSAGE: Surgical technique involving transfer of the posterior capsule and infraspinatus tendon into the Hill-Sachs lesion to prevent engagement of the lesion with the glenoid fossa when the arm is abducted and externally rotated to 90°[3]

Objectives

1. Identify risk factors for shoulder dislocation related to sport participation and recurrent instability episodes.

2. Prescribe appropriate interventions to restore the athlete's upper extremity motion, strength, endurance, and joint proprioception by the end of traditional rehabilitation, but prior to returning to sport.

3. Determine appropriate criteria for advancement into a return-to-sport progression based on the imposed demands of each sport in which the athlete participates.

Physical Therapy Considerations

Physical therapy considerations during management of the athlete following surgical shoulder stabilization:

▶ **General physical therapy plan of care/goals:** Restore pain-free range of motion (ROM); increase dynamic shoulder girdle muscular strength and endurance; sport-related functional biomechanical assessment; return athlete to sport

▶ **Physical therapy interventions:** Patient education related to involved anatomy and surgical procedure; manual therapy to restore ROM and joint mobility; flexibility exercises; resistance training to increase rotator cuff and scapular strength to provide dynamic stability; core and lower extremity strength and endurance training to provide stability and power

▶ **Precautions during physical therapy:** Consideration of postsurgical timeline regarding tissue healing properties and appropriate selection and dosage of therapeutic exercise

▶ **Complications interfering with physical therapy:** Patient noncompliance, premature phase progression, poor tissue healing, and psychosocial challenges

Understanding the Health Condition

The anatomical structure of the shoulder girdle (clavicle, scapula, and humerus) permits multiplanar ROM. As a result, it requires a balance between stability and mobility to allow functional activities, which is achieved through coordinated activity of both passive and active structures (Table 4-1). Glenohumeral instability is traditionally classified into two categories: traumatic and multidirectional. Instability is a term used to describe a pathological condition involving unwanted and uncontrolled translation within the joint, often following trauma to the shoulder. Laxity is a nonpathological, objective finding of capsuloligamentous integrity, concerning the degree of passive translation without associated symptoms.[4,5]

Traumatic shoulder injury can result in damage to multiple structures about the shoulder girdle, including soft tissue (muscle-tendon unit) rupture, capsular tearing, and glenoid and/or humeral head fracture (Fig. 4-1). **An individual's age plays a**

Table 4-1	ANATOMICAL COMPONENTS OF SHOULDER STABILITY
Static/Passive	**Dynamic/Active**
Bony structures	Rotator cuff
Glenoid labrum	Long head of biceps
Capsular structures	Scapular positioning
Negative intra-articular pressure	Concavity compression
Coefficient of friction	Neuromuscular control

ANATOMIC LESIONS

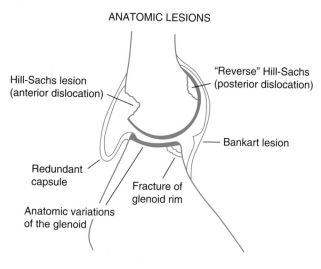

Hill-Sachs lesion (anterior dislocation)

"Reverse" Hill-Sachs (posterior dislocation)

Bankart lesion

Redundant capsule

Fracture of glenoid rim

Anatomic variations of the glenoid

Figure 4-1. Anatomic lesions producing shoulder instability. (Reproduced with permission from Skinner HB. Current Diagnosis & Treatment in Orthopedics, 4th ed. NY: McGraw-Hill; 2006.)

profound role in risk of recurrent instability, with recurrence rates upward of 85% to 95% in individuals younger than 25 years.[6-9] **Higher activity level has also been proposed as a risk factor.** Simonet et al.[10] showed that 82% of young athletes had recurrent dislocation compared to only 30% of nonathletes of similar age. Interestingly, greater than 90% of young athletes undergoing shoulder stabilization expect to return to sport, and the majority of patients with these high expectations report participating in high-risk sports (i.e., collision sports).[11] Therefore, systematic and detailed treatment and return-to-sport planning are critical to optimize patient outcomes.

Acute traumatic anterior shoulder dislocations are more common than traumatic posterior dislocations.[4,12] When associated bony injury to the humeral head (Hill-Sachs lesion) is present in conjunction with anteroinferior capsulolabral disruption, immediate surgical intervention is indicated to restore anatomical alignment and glenohumeral joint arthrokinematics.

Physical Therapy Patient/Client Management

After arthroscopic anterior stabilization of the shoulder, rehabilitation with return-to-sport goals must include intentional planning and thorough communication of appropriate timelines and criteria for advancement. The physical therapist should consider healing time of involved tissues and specific imposed demands of the desired sport(s) in forming the plan of care and counseling for return to sport. Table 4-2 outlines the sports-specific considerations for each position that this athlete plays.

Evidence-based recommendations for the necessary shoulder ROM and strength have been established for the athletic population. For the postsurgical athlete, obtaining and maintaining the proper shoulder girdle kinematics should be a focus throughout the rehabilitation process. In football players, arthroscopic treatment of anterior shoulder instability has allowed athletes to return to play within 1 year of their surgery.[13] In this study, none of the athletes returning to football lost more than 15° of ER on side-to-side comparison and the average ER loss was only 5°.[13]

Critical instants of force production during pitching tend to occur just before maximal ER during the late cocking phase and immediately after ball release.[14] In adult pitchers, ER at maximum cocking has been reported to reach 165° to 180° of motion.[15] This total arc of approximately 180° is necessary to move from maximum ER to maximal internal rotation (IR).[16] Loss of glenohumeral IR in pitchers has been related to posterior-inferior capsular thickening and potential pathomechanical

Table 4-2 SPORT-SPECIFIC CONSIDERATIONS DURING REHABILITATION	
Sport (Position)	**Specific Considerations**
Football (quarterback)	Throwing Contact Protection: bracing
Baseball (starting shortstop, relief pitcher)	Throwing Pitching Hitting

compromise of rotator cuff, biceps tendon, and labral integrity.[17] One of the primary roles of the physical therapist is to help the athlete successfully return to sport, which may depend on restoration of functional shoulder rotational ROM.

Examination, Evaluation, and Diagnosis

Considering the extent of surgical stabilization required for the athlete in this case, a conservative return-to-activity program is recommended. For the first 4 months after surgery, the athlete is guided through the first two phases of rehabilitation. The first phase emphasizes pain control, protection of surgical repair to promote tissue healing, and normalization of ROM and neuromuscular control. The second phase progresses the athlete to activities focused on re-establishing coordinated upper extremity movement and muscular endurance.

At 4 months postsurgical stabilization, the physical therapist would expect this athlete to present with full, pain-free active ROM without compensation patterns, good scapular control during motion and strengthening activities, and the ability to perform all prescribed strengthening exercises with little to no pain ($\leq 2/10$ on the visual analog scale).[18] The next phase of rehabilitation should emphasize enhancing glenohumeral and scapular muscular endurance, as well as overall neuromuscular control of the shoulder girdle during sport-specific movement patterns and positions. It is essential that the physical therapist carefully considers, modifies, and monitors the stresses placed on each reconstructed tissue to ensure protection of the surgical repair while promoting progression in functional ability. Following anterior stabilization, the anteroinferior capsule is most notably stressed when the shoulder is placed in ER above 90° of abduction.[18] Therefore, ER motion must be obtained systematically following an intentional progression, particularly for an overhead athlete who requires this mobility for his sport. In the earlier rehabilitation phase, the athlete demonstrated the necessary physical performance, including functional motion, muscular strength and endurance, and appropriate body control. Now, as the athlete is preparing for return to his sports, it is appropriate to begin stressing these tissues in *overhead* ranges of motion.

When designing a return-to-play program for this athlete, utilization of objective, validated tests and measures is necessary to assess psychological and physical readiness to handle the demands of each of his sports and minimize risk of future injury. In 2022, Otley et al.[19] described a criterion-based testing continuum, which provides an evidence-based guide for rehabilitation and return-to-sports testing following shoulder stabilization procedures. The selective use of psychological readiness and performance tests during the return-to-sport phase of rehabilitation is warranted to compare to presurgical findings and assess resolution of instability. Table 4-3 describes three common tests to determine shoulder instability.[19,20]

Passive shoulder ROM, including ER, IR, and horizontal adduction, should also be evaluated when making return-to-play decisions. Myers et al.[22] demonstrated superior reliability and validity when measuring shoulder ROM in supine versus sidelying. The supine position is also more sensitive in identifying changes in overhead athletes who tend to demonstrate greater posterior shoulder tightness than non-overhead athletes.

Table 4-3 SPECIAL TESTS ASSOCIATED WITH SHOULDER INSTABILITY[2]

Test	Direction of Instability	Technique	Findings
Apprehension	Anterior	Patient lies supine on edge of table; therapist stands at the involved side. Therapist positions shoulder at 90° abduction, grasps forearm and wrist, and externally rotates the humerus.	Positive test is defined as patient report of apprehension and/or pain.
Relocation	Anterior	Performed following a *positive* apprehension test. If patient indicates apprehension or pain with humeral ER, the therapist applies a posterior force at proximal humerus.	Positive test is defined as a decrease in apprehension and/or pain when posterior force is applied.
Sulcus	Anterior, posterior, or inferior	Patient is seated and therapist stands beside patient. Therapist applies an inferior long traction force at the patient's elbow, measuring the distance (cm) between the inferior acromion and superior humeral head. Rowe modification: Patient stands and bends forward slightly with arm relaxed by side. Therapist reassesses translation.	Distance of humeral head translation[21] Grade 1: <1.5 cm Grade 2: 1.5-2 cm Grade 3: >2 cm

The therapist should utilize objective performance-based tests for determining readiness for returning to sport. For a pitcher and quarterback, **performance testing is geared toward assessing shoulder function, including rotator cuff endurance and scapular stability in dynamic overhead positions** (Table 4-4).

Table 4-4 SAMPLE PERFORMANCE TESTS FOR ROTATOR CUFF AND SCAPULAR ENDURANCE TO HELP DETERMINE READINESS FOR SPORT PARTICIPATION

Test	Goal	Technique	Return-to-Play Performance Criteria
ER >90°	Assess posterior rotator cuff endurance before and after sport-specific training.	Patient stands facing wall. Anchor resistance band to wall at patient's head height. Patient holds band with involved arm in 90° abduction. Patient rotates band to end-range ER while maintaining abducted position (Fig. 4-2).	Pre-throwing session: 1 minute of repetitions with medium-resistance elastic band Post-throwing session: 30 seconds of repetitions with medium-resistance elastic band. There should be no loss in timing or control during repetitions.

(Continued)

Table 4-4   SAMPLE PERFORMANCE TESTS FOR ROTATOR CUFF AND SCAPULAR ENDURANCE TO HELP DETERMINE READINESS FOR SPORT PARTICIPATION (CONTINUED)

Test	Goal	Technique	Return-to-Play Performance Criteria
Closed kinetic chain upper extremity stability test (CKCUE; hand tap test)[23]	Assess glenohumeral, scapular, and core stability through endurance-based closed-chain dynamic movement.	Place two lines on floor at distance of 3 ft apart. Patient assumes push-up position and moves hands alternately back and forth between lines as fast as possible. Record number of taps at 15 and 30 seconds (Fig. 4-3).	<u>15 seconds:</u> 18 taps (male) 20 taps (female) <u>60 seconds:</u> 90 taps
Posterior shoulder endurance test (PSET)[24,25]	Assess endurance of posterior shoulder girdle musculature.	Patient lies prone with arm off edge of treatment table holding a weight equal to 2% body weight. Patient moves arm to 90° of horizontal abduction and repeats this motion until either position or technique cannot be maintained. Modified version: Patient maintains isometric hold in the abducted position until failure.	Limb symmetry index (LSI) within 10% Modified version norms: Females: 46 seconds Males: 47 seconds
Scapular dyskinesis Test[26,27]	Assess scapular position during overhead motion.	Patient holds 5-lb dumbbell in each hand and performs 10 repetitions of overhead elevation in scapular plane.	Normal or only subtle dyskinesis following throwing session

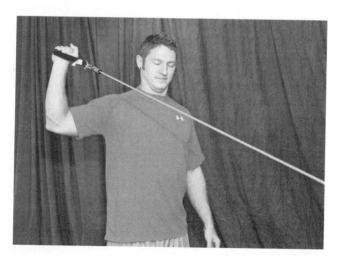

Figure 4-2. Exercise to assess right posterior rotator cuff endurance. Patient holds band with involved shoulder in 90° abduction and rotates band to end-range external rotation while maintaining the abducted position.

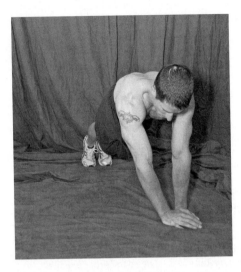

Figure 4-3. Closed Kinetic Chain Upper Extremity (CKCUE) stability test to assess glenohumeral, scapular, and core stability in an endurance task. Place two lines on floor at distance of 3 ft apart. Patient assumes push-up position and moves hands alternately back and forth between lines that are approximately 3 ft apart. The therapist records the number of taps at 15 and 30 seconds.

Plan of Care and Interventions

A strengthening program should work on acquiring dynamic stability of the rotator cuff muscles. There are three main biomechanical functions of the rotator cuff: compression of the humeral head in the glenoid fossa, rotation of the humeral head, and provision of muscular balance to limit stress placed on static joint stabilizers. The primary shoulder internal and external rotators act in concert as a muscular force couple to provide compression and centering of the humeral head within the glenoid fossa. Placing a towel roll between the patient's trunk and humerus when performing strengthening activities close to the plane of the body maximizes rotator cuff activation and subacromial space to avoid impingement and minimize hypovascularity at the muscle-tendon junction.[28] Reinold et al.[29] demonstrated a 10% increase in maximum voluntary contraction of the infraspinatus/teres minor force couple during shoulder ER at 0° abduction when healthy subjects placed a towel roll between trunk and humerus. As the athlete advances, the rotator cuff should be trained in greater planes of elevation and abduction to simulate sport-specific positions in which the athlete must demonstrate excellent dynamic stability.

When progressing upper extremity resistance band exercises, the therapist can alter the demand of the activity by altering numerous variables, including resistance level, repetitions, speed, and type of muscle contraction (isometric, concentric, eccentric). Strengthening exercises for the overhead athlete should primarily address rotator cuff and scapular stability, as well as lumbopelvic or "core" strength. Ellenbecker et al.[30] recommended increasing the isokinetic shoulder ER to IR strength ratio from 66% to 76% to increase the ER strength for patients with shoulder instability. This ER bias would help create a "posterior dominant" shoulder to increase dynamic stability and aid in preventing reinjury in throwing and racquet-sport athletes.[30]

The benefits of internal rotation and posterior shoulder stretching programs for individuals with posterior shoulder tightness and postural deficits have been well-documented. These include improved posture and scapular kinematics, decreased pain, and fewer days missed from sports participation.[31-33] In 2003, Kibler et al.[34] demonstrated increased ROM in areas at most risk of injury following an IR stretching program in young tennis players. Shanley et al.[35] showed that baseball players with a decrease of ≥25° of IR in the dominant shoulder (compared to the nondominant shoulder) were at four times *greater* risk for upper extremity injury than those who lost <25° over the course of one season.[35,36] Resolution of impingement symptoms has been demonstrated in those enrolled in a posterior shoulder stretching program.[37]

Finally, the overhead athlete needs to progress through an interval-throwing program (ITP). A separate program for baseball and football should be designed and implemented at the appropriate time. The goal of an ITP is to return the athlete to preinjury status through a stepwise progression, taking care to prevent overtraining. Although little evidence is available for the specific design of such programs, several themes must be present and consistent.[38-42] First, athletes must be educated on the importance of following the prescribed program, with the risks of poor compliance outlined in understandable terms. Athletes should understand the implication of pain during or following throwing. Soreness rules should be implemented: each athlete's subjective report of soreness defines the modification of the ITP progression.[41] For example, if the athlete experiences specific or generalized arm soreness during warm-up or throws, or if soreness lasts longer than 1 hour following a workout, the athlete should rest 1 to 2 days and not move to the next step of his ITP. An ITP should include a specific and consistent warm-up routine and should emphasize technique over quantity. The parameters (number of pitches, sets, and outings/week) should be defined based on the individual's specific pitching role (e.g., starter versus reliever) and age.[41] Each outing should be defined based on effort level, distance, and duration of throws.[43] In Table 4-5,

Table 4-5	RETURN-TO-PLAY CRITERIA
Dimension	**Expected Outcome**
Pain	No pain at rest
Range of motion	Full, pain-free rotational range of motion
Muscle strength	Manual muscle testing 5/5 in all planes
	Hand-held dynamometry: ≥90% of uninvolved UE following throwing session
Muscle performance	ER/IR ratio 2:3 (measured in pounds of force)
	(Strength of shoulder external rotators should be at least two-thirds of the strength of shoulder internal rotators of same upper extremity.)
	ER/IR at 90-90 position, repetitions for 1 minute with medium band
Scapular stability	Open chain: normal or subtle scapular dyskinesis during shoulder elevation with 3-lb dumbbells for 10 repetitions
	Closed chain: 90 repetitions in 1 minute on CKCUE stability test
Subjective outcome measures	Disability of the arm, shoulder, and hand (DASH) questionnaire: <5% disability
	DASH-sport: <10% disability

suggested return-to-play criteria are outlined based on documented clinical norms and rehabilitation progressions cited in peer-reviewed literature.[18,27,35,38,39]

The physical therapist should be prepared to counsel the athlete if he encounters obstacles as he returns to sport. Many athletes experience muscle soreness after being removed from a live athletic environment for extended recovery and rehabilitation. Progression through each stage of rehabilitation and continued participation following return to sport should be guided by subjective report of pain. The athlete must be informed that concordant shoulder pain is a flag for reassessment and that progression should be paused. However, the athlete should expect some muscle soreness each time the physical demand of sport increases. The therapist should educate the athlete on the use of appropriate modalities to address soreness. Yanagisawa et al.[44,45] showed that using ice after pitching reduced shoulder muscle soreness both immediately and 24 hours after pitching. The athlete may also experience psychological challenges as he reintegrates into sport. Use of a validated patient-reported outcome measure such as the Shoulder Instability Return to Sport Index (SIRI) provides valuable information on psychological readiness.[19] A referral to a sports psychologist may be warranted and valuable to provide psychological training regarding the athlete's perception of performance, expectation, and outcomes.

Consideration of the athlete's complete physical and psychological readiness to meet the demands of athletics following a traumatic injury and surgical repair is essential to successful participation and decreasing risk of future injury.

Evidence-Based Clinical Recommendations

SORT: Strength of Recommendation Taxonomy

A: Consistent, good-quality patient-oriented evidence
B: Inconsistent or limited-quality patient-oriented evidence
C: Consensus, disease-oriented evidence, usual practice, expert opinion, or case series

1. Younger age (<25 years) and increased activity level are positively correlated with increased risk of recurrent shoulder instability. **Grade B**

2. Both open and closed kinetic chain performance tests provide the most comprehensive assessment of an overhead athlete's functional performance after injury. **Grade C**

3. IR and posterior shoulder stretching for overhead athletes improves posture and scapular kinematics, decreases pain and risk of injury, and results in fewer days missed from sport participation. **Grade A**

COMPREHENSION QUESTIONS

4.1 A sports physical therapist is treating an overhead athlete 4 months following surgical anterior shoulder stabilization. Which of the following positions should only be incorporated during the *final* phase of the rehabilitation program?

   A. Internal rotation at 0° abduction

   B. Shoulder elevation in scapular plane

   C. External rotation at 90° abduction

   D. Horizontal adduction at 90° abduction

4.2 Which of the following combinations of tests provides the therapist with the MOST complete assessment of the athlete's readiness to resume full return to overhead sports?

   A. Number of repetitions of shoulder external and internal rotation performed in 0° abduction with medium resistance in 60 seconds

   B. Completion of interval throwing program without pain and with safe technique; CKCUE stability test

   C. Number of push-ups and pull-ups performed after a throwing session

   D. Manual muscle testing score of 5/5 for all shoulder girdle musculature following throwing session

4.3 Why might a physical therapist want to utilize a patient-reported outcome (PRO) measure to assess psychological readiness for return to sport, and which PRO is most appropriate for this athlete following anterior shoulder stabilization?

   A. Easier than performance metrics and a single measure can be used independently; pain scale

   B. Provides a valid and reliable tool to evaluate psychological readiness for returning to sport in this particular patient population; SIRI

   C. Monitors change in physical and psychological variables; Disabilities of the Arm, Shoulder, and Hand Questionnaire (DASH)

   D. Patient-reported outcome measures do not provide useful information and should not be utilized

ANSWERS

4.1 **C.** Coupling shoulder external rotation and abduction places the greatest stress across the inferior glenohumeral ligament complex. This capsuloligamentous structure was repaired surgically, and therefore, must be protected by avoiding positions that would increase tension across the tissue for at least 12 weeks. Therefore, this therapeutic intervention should be reserved for later stages of rehabilitation.

4.2 **B.** An interval throwing program and the CKCUE stability test provide the best evidence-based information for the therapist to make an objective decision on returning to sport. These two tests are also most relevant to the athlete's sports of baseball and football because they directly assess throwing biomechanics as well as global upper quarter strength, stability, and endurance.

4.3 **B.** The Shoulder Instability Return to Sport Index (SIRI) quantifies psychological readiness to return to sport and asks specific questions relevant to athletes who have undergone shoulder stabilization procedures. It includes queries on relevant positions, demands, and activities that will be required for sport and evaluates the athlete's perceptions and feelings of readiness to take on those tasks. Using PROs in conjunction with physical performance measures provides a strong and comprehensive picture of an athlete's overall health status and readiness to progress toward full unrestricted physical activity.

REFERENCES

1. Bankart ASB. The pathology and treatment of recurrent shoulder dislocation of the shoulder. *Br J Surg.* 1938;26:23-29.
2. Cho SH, Cho NS, Rhee YG. Preoperative analysis of the Hill-Sachs lesion in anterior shoulder instability: how to predict engagement of the lesion. *Am J Sports Med.* 2011;39:2389-2395.
3. Purchase RJ, Wolf EM, Hobgood ER, et al. Hill-Sachs "remplissage": an arthroscopic solution for the engaging Hill-Sachs lesion. *Arthroscopy.* 2008;24:723-726.
4. Park M. Anatomy and function of the shoulder structures. In: Galatz LM, ed. Orthopedic Knowledge Update: Shoulder and Elbow, No. 3. Rosemont, IL: American Academy of Orthopaedic Surgeons;2009.
5. Jia X, Ji JH, Petersen SA, et al. An analysis of shoulder laxity in patients undergoing shoulder surgery. *J Bone Joint Surg Am.* 2009;91:2144-2150.
6. Rowe CR, Sakellarides HT. Factors related to recurrences of anterior dislocations of the shoulder. *Clin Orthop.* 1961;20:40-48.
7. Arciero RA, Wheeler JH, Ryan JB, McBride JT. Arthroscopic Bankart repair versus nonoperative treatment for acute, initial anterior shoulder dislocations. *Am J Sports Med.* 1994;22:589-594.
8. McLaughlin HL, MacLellan DI. Recurrent anterior dislocation of the shoulder. II. A comparative study. *J Trauma.* 1967;7:191-201.
9. Murphy AI, Hurley ET, Hurley DJ, et al. Long-term outcomes of the arthroscopic Bankart repair: A systematic review of studies at 10-year follow-up. *J Shoulder Elbow Surg.* 2019;28:2084-2089.
10. Simonet WT, Cofield RH. Prognosis in anterior shoulder dislocation. *Am J Sports Med.* 1984;12:19-24.
11. Plath JE, Saier T, Feucht MJ, et al. Patients' expectations of shoulder instability repair. *Knee Surg Sports Traumatol Arthrosc.* 2018;26:15-23.
12. Rowe CR. Prognosis in dislocations of the shoulder. *J Bone Joint Surg Am.* 1956;38-A: 957-977.
13. Pagnani MJ, Dome DC. Surgical treatment of traumatic anterior shoulder instability in American football players. *J Bone Joint Surg Am.* 2002;84-A:711-715.
14. Fleisig GS, Andrews JR, Dillman CJ, Escamilla RF. Kinetics of baseball pitching with implications about injury mechanism. *Am J Sports Med.* 1995;23:233-239.
15. Fleisig GS, Dillman CJ, Andrews JA. Proper mechanics for baseball pitching. *Clin Sports Med.* 1989;1:151-170.

16. Wilk KE, Meister K, Andrews JR. Current concepts in the rehabilitation of the overhead throwing athlete. *Am J Sports Med.* 2002;30:136-151.

17. Burkhart SS, Morgan CD, Kibler WB. The disabled throwing shoulder: spectrum of pathology, part II: evaluation and treatment of SLAP lesions in throwers. *Arthroscopy.* 2003;19:531-539.

18. Gaunt BW, Shaffer MA, Sauers EL, et al. American Society of Shoulder and Elbow Therapists. The American Society of Shoulder and Elbow Therapists' consensus rehabilitation guideline for arthroscopic anterior capsulolabral repair of the shoulder. *J Orthop Sports Phys Ther.* 2010;40:155-168.

19. Otley T, Myers H, Lau BC, Taylor DC. Return to sport after shoulder stabilization procedures: a criteria-based testing continuum to guide rehabilitation and inform return-to-play decision making. *Arthrosc Sports Med Rehabil.* 2022;4:e237-e246.

20. Cook C, Hegedus EJ. *Orthopedic Physical Examination Tests: An Evidence-Based Approach.* Upper Saddle River, NJ: Pearson Prentice Hall; 2008.

21. Silliman JF, Hawkins RJ. Classification and physical diagnosis of instability of the shoulder. *Clin Orthop Relat Res.* 1993;(291):7-19.

22. Myers JB, Oyama S, Wassinger CA, et al. Reliability, precision, accuracy, and validity of posterior shoulder tightness assessment in overhead athletes. *Am J Sports Med.* 2007;35:1922-1930.

23. Goldbeck TG, Davies GJ. Test-retest reliability of the closed kinetic chain upper extremity stability test: a clinical field test. *J Sport Rehabil.* 2000;9:35-45.

24. Powell A, Williamson S, McCaig S, et al. An investigation of a Kerlan-Jobe Orthopaedic Clinic shoulder and elbow score in elite canoe slalom: establishing measurement properties to make practice recommendations. *Phys Ther Sport.* 2021;50:15-21.

25. Moore SD, Uhl TL, Kibler WB. Improvements in shoulder endurance following a baseball-specific strengthening program in high school baseball players. *Sports Health.* 2013;5:233-238.

26. Tate AR, McClure P, Kareha S, et al. A clinical method for identifying scapular dyskinesis, part 2: validity. *J Athl Train.* 2009;44:165-173.

27. McClure P, Tate AR, Kareha S, et al. A clinical method for identifying scapular dyskinesis, part 1: reliability. *J Athl Train.* 2009;44:160-164.

28. Reinold MM, Wilk KE, Hooks TR, et al. Thermal-assisted capsular shrinkage of the glenohumeral joint in overhead athletes: a 15- to 47-month follow-up. *J Orthop Sports Phys Ther.* 2003;33:455-467.

29. Reinold MM, Wilk KE, Fleisig GS, et al. Electromyographic analysis of the rotator cuff and deltoid musculature during common shoulder external rotation exercises. *J Orthop Sports Phys Ther.* 2004;34:385-394.

30. Ellenbecker TS, Davies GJ. The application of isokinetics in testing and rehabilitation of the shoulder complex. *J Athl Train.* 2000;35:338-350.

31. Thigpen CA, Padua DA, Michener LA, et al. Head and shoulder posture affect scapular mechanics and muscle activity in overhead tasks. *J Electromyogr Kinesiol.* 2010;20:701-709.

32. Lynch SS, Thigpen CA, Mihalik JP, et al. The effects of an exercise intervention on forward head and rounded shoulder postures in elite swimmers. *Br J Sports Med.* 2010;44:376-381.

33. Wang CH, McClure P, Pratt NE, Nobilini R. Stretching and strengthening exercises: their effect on three-dimensional scapular kinematics. *Arch Phys Med Rehabil.* 1999;80:923-929.

34. Kibler WB, Chandler TJ. Range of motion in junior tennis players participating in an injury risk modification program. *J Sci Med Sport.* 2003;6:51-62.

35. Shanley E, Rauh MJ, Michener LA, et al. Shoulder range of motion measures as risk factors for shoulder and elbow injuries in high school softball and baseball players. *Am J Sports Med.* 2011;39:1997-2006.

36. Keeley DW, Hackett T, Keirns M, et al. A biomechanical analysis of youth pitching mechanics. *J Pediatr Orthop.* 2008;28:452-459.

37. Tyler TF, Nicholas SJ, Lee SJ, et al. Correction of posterior shoulder tightness is associated with symptom resolution in patients with internal impingement. *Am J Sports Med.* 2010;38:114-119.

38. Axe MJ, Snyder-Mackler L, Konin JG, Strube MJ. Development of a distance-based interval throwing program for Little League-aged athletes. *Am J Sports Med.* 1996;24:594-602.

39. Axe MJ, Windley TC, Snyder-Mackler L. Data-based interval throwing programs for collegiate softball players. *J Ath Train.* 2002;37:194-203.

40. Coleman AE, Axe MJ, Andrews JR. Performance profile-directed simulated game: an objective functional evaluation for baseball pitchers. *J Orthop Sports Phys Ther.* 1987;9:101-105.

41. Axe MJ, Wickham R, Snyder-Mackler L. Data-based interval throwing programs for Little League, high school, college, and professional baseball pitchers. *Sports Med Arthrosc Rev.* 2001;9: 24-34.

42. Love S, Aytar A, Bush H, Uhl TL. Descriptive analysis of pitch volume in southeastern conference baseball pitchers. *N Am J Sports Phys Ther.* 2010;5:194-200.

43. Olsen SJ II, Fleisig GS, Dun S, et al. Risk factors for shoulder and elbow injuries in adolescent baseball pitchers. *Am J Sports Med.* 2006;34:905-912.

44. Yanagisawa O, Miyanaga Y, Shiraki H, et al. The effects of various therapeutic measures on shoulder strength and muscle soreness after baseball pitching. *J Sports Med Phys Fitness.* 2003;43:189-201.

45. Yanagisawa O, Miyanaga Y, Shiraki H, et al. The effects of various therapeutic measures on shoulder range of motion and cross-sectional areas of rotator cuff muscles after baseball pitching. *J Sports Med Phys Fitness.* 2003;43:356-366.

Rotator Cuff Repair: Rehabilitation Weeks 1 to 4

Todd S. Ellenbecker
Brianne Lewis
David S. Bailie

CASE 5

A 55-year-old female is referred to physical therapy after an arthroscopic rotator cuff repair performed 2 weeks ago. Three months ago, the patient experienced gradually progressive shoulder pain while hitting a series of repetitive serves during a tennis match. The pain did not subside after the match and escalated such that it was present at rest, during sleep, and with all activities of daily living. The patient consulted an orthopedic surgeon who found significant weakness in the right (dominant) shoulder in external rotation and elevation and pain along the anterior and lateral margins of the acromion. An MRI scan with contrast enhancement showed a 2-cm full-thickness tear in the supraspinatus tendon extending posteriorly into the infraspinatus without a concomitant labral tear. The patient underwent an arthroscopic rotator cuff repair using suture anchors and a modest acromioplasty to address a type II acromion. She was given immediate postoperative instructions that included Codman pendulum exercises, shoulder shrugs and scapular retractions, grip-strengthening exercises, and instructions to wear a sling to protect the shoulder. Two weeks after surgery, the surgeon inspected the incisions, removed the external sutures, and referred the patient for physical therapy. The patient arrives with the right shoulder immobilized in a sling with a pillow that places the shoulder in approximately 20° of abduction in the scapular plane. She has no complaints of radiating symptoms into the distal right upper extremity and she rates her pain on the numeric pain rating scale as 2/10 at rest and 5/10 with attempted movement of the right shoulder. The patient's medical history is otherwise unremarkable for cardiovascular disease, diabetes, or neurological disorders.

▶ Based on the patient's diagnosis and surgery, what do you anticipate may be the contributors to her activity limitations?
▶ What are the most appropriate physical therapy interventions?
▶ What is her rehabilitation prognosis?

KEY DEFINITIONS

ACROMIOPLASTY: Surgical procedure whereby the surgeon removes the anterior-inferior portion of a type II or type III acromion to more closely resemble a flat type I acromion

ROTATOR CUFF TEAR: Tearing and failure of the rotator cuff tendons, most commonly those of the supraspinatus and infraspinatus muscles; tears can be full thickness (involving entire thickness of the rotator cuff) or partial thickness. Partial-thickness tears can involve the superior (bursal) surface or inferior (articular) side of the tendon. Superior partial rotator cuff tears result from abrasion and impingement of the rotator cuff tendon against the coracoacromial arch, whereas articular side partial-thickness rotator cuff tears most often result from tensile overload of the muscle tendon unit.

TYPE II ACROMION: Acromion with a curved shape from an anterior to posterior (sagittal plane) orientation that results in a narrow subacromial space

Objectives

1. Describe key and specific range of motion and glenohumeral joint mobilization interventions that can be safely applied to the patient following arthroscopic rotator cuff repair.

2. Describe safe initial scapular stabilization interventions that should be prescribed for the patient following rotator cuff repair.

3. Identify evidence-based physical therapy interventions for early-stage rehabilitation after rotator cuff repair.

4. List precautions for early rehabilitation following rotator cuff repair.

Physical Therapy Considerations

Physical therapy considerations during early postoperative management (1-4 weeks) of the individual with a surgically repaired rotator cuff tear:

▶ **General physical therapy plan of care/goals:** Decrease pain; increase active and passive range of motion; increase upper extremity rotator cuff and scapular strength

▶ **Physical therapy interventions:** Patient education regarding functional anatomy and injury pathomechanics and general precautions regarding protection of healing tendons; modalities and manual therapy to decrease pain; mobilization and passive stretching to improve joint mobility and prevent/minimize capsular restriction; submaximal resistance exercises to increase muscular strength and endurance of the rotator cuff and scapular stabilizers, home exercise instruction

▶ **Precautions during physical therapy:** Monitor neural signs and symptoms

▶ **Complications interfering with physical therapy:** Tear size; tissue quality; medical or lifestyle issues that interfere with optimal tissue healing (*e.g.*, smoking); health complications that limit the patient's ability to be positioned for range of motion or attend physical therapy sessions

Understanding the Health Condition

The etiology of rotator cuff pathologies can be described along a continuum, ranging from overuse microtraumatic tendinosis to either degenerative or macrotraumatic full-thickness rotator cuff tears. A second continuum consists of glenohumeral joint instability and primary impingement or compressive disease that leads to rotator cuff dysfunction.[1] The clinical challenge of managing the patient with a rotator cuff injury begins with a specific evaluation to gain a clear understanding of the underlying stability and integrity of not only the components of the glenohumeral joint, but also of the entire upper extremity kinetic chain.

Full-thickness rotator cuff tears can be caused by degeneration of the rotator cuff over time, as well as by repetitive loading of the tendon (*e.g.*, as occurs in an overhead athlete). Forces encountered during a traumatic event are greater than the normal tendon can tolerate. Full-thickness tears of the rotator cuff, with bony avulsions of the greater tuberosity, can occur from single traumatic episodes. According to Cofield,[2] 30% or more of the tendon must be damaged to produce a substantial reduction in strength, so minor tendon injuries may not be functionally apparent. A single traumatic event resulting in tendon failure is often reported by the patient in the subjective examination. However, repeated microtraumatic insults and degeneration over time may have substantially weakened the tendon prior to its *ultimate* failure under the heavy load described by the patient. Full-thickness rotator cuff tears can require surgical treatment and aggressive rehabilitation to achieve a positive functional outcome.[3,4]

Several etiologic factors are important to consider with respect to rotator cuff tears. The vascularity of the rotator cuff, specifically the supraspinatus, has been extensively studied. In his classic 1934 monograph on ruptures of the supraspinatus tendon, Codman described a critical zone of hypovascularity located half an inch proximal to its insertion on the greater tuberosity.[5] The biceps long head tendon was found to have a similar region of hypovascularity in its deep surface 2 cm from its insertion.[6] Rathbun and MacNab[7] reported the effects of position on the microvascularity of the rotator cuff tendons. With the glenohumeral joint in a position of adduction, they found a constant area of hypovascularity near the insertion of the supraspinatus tendon. In contrast, this consistent area of hypovascularity was not observed with the arm in a position of abduction. These investigators termed this observation the "wringing out phenomenon" and this pattern was also noticed in the long head tendon of the biceps. This positional influence on blood flow to the rotator cuff tendons has clinical ramifications for both immobilization and exercise positioning. Using quantitative histologic analysis more than 20 years later, Brooks *et al.*[8] reported hypovascularity—or a critical zone—in the tendinous insertions of both the supraspinatus and infraspinatus.

Swiontowski et al.[9] measured vascularity by laser Doppler flowmetry in individuals with rotator cuff tendinitis from subacromial impingement. In this population, blood flow was greatest in the previously identified area of hypovascularity compared with other parts of the tendon.

Several primary types of rotator cuff tears are commonly described in the literature. Full-thickness tears consist of tears that comprise the entire thickness (from top to bottom) of the rotator cuff tendon or tendons. Full-thickness tears are often initiated in the critical zone of the supraspinatus tendon and can extend to include the infraspinatus, teres minor, and subscapularis tendons.[10] A tear in the subscapularis tendon is often associated with a subluxation of the biceps long head tendon from the intertubercular groove, or either a partial or complete tear of the biceps tendon. Histologically, full-thickness rotator cuff tears show various findings ranging from almost entirely acellular and avascular margins to neovascularization with cellular infiltrate.[10]

In cadaveric studies, Loehr et al.[11] evaluated the effects of a full-thickness rotator cuff tear on stability of the glenohumeral joint by selective division of the supraspinatus or infraspinatus tendons. While a one-tendon lesion of either the supraspinatus or infraspinatus did not influence movement patterns of the glenohumeral joint, a two-tendon lesion induced notable changes compatible with glenohumeral joint instability.[11] Therefore, individuals with full-thickness rotator cuff tears may have additional stress placed on the dynamic stabilizing function of the remaining rotator cuff tendons because of increased humeral head translation and resulting instability.

Miller and Savoie[12] examined consecutive patients with full-thickness tears of the rotator cuff to determine the incidence of associated intra-articular injuries. Seventy-four of 100 patients had one or more coexisting intra-articular abnormalities: anterior labral tears were noted in 62 patients and biceps tendon tears were noted in 16 patients. These results clearly indicate the importance of a thorough clinical examination of the patient with a rotator cuff injury.

Physical Therapy Patient/Client Management

Patients presenting for physical therapy following arthroscopic rotator cuff repair can benefit from modalities for pain control. The use of manual therapy in addition to submaximal therapeutic exercise is of tremendous benefit in restoring the range of motion, increasing strength, and improving shoulder function. Knowledge of the tissue stresses following rotator cuff repair helps the physical therapist to optimize shoulder range of motion early in the postoperative phase of rehabilitation without jeopardizing tissue healing.

Examination, Evaluation, and Diagnosis

Key highlights for examination of the postoperative shoulder consist of neurologic screening and passive range of motion (PROM) measurement of the involved extremity and active ROM measurement of the uninvolved extremity. These serve as important baseline parameters for goal setting for the injured shoulder. The physical therapist should view the patient from the posterior aspect to inspect for atrophy of the scapular and rotator cuff muscles, which is appreciated more easily when the patient places hands on hips.[13] Ellenbecker *et al.*[14] have noted the common prevalence of atrophy in the infraspinous fossa of the dominant arm in elite tennis players, which may be indicative of external rotation weakness and the degree of infraspinatus muscle weakness. When inspecting the resting position of the scapula, the therapist should assess for prominence of the inferior or medial borders of the scapula, which indicates the need for scapular stabilization interventions.[15,16] During the initial examination, assessment of active glenohumeral rhythm is *not* indicated due to the acute postoperative status. However, static scapular posture can reveal asymmetries between the injured and uninjured extremity and serve as an early warning sign of scapular dysfunction that may be revealed when a more robust active evaluation can be assessed in later stages of the rehabilitation process.[15,16]

Examination of glenohumeral joint stability is imperative. Tests like the load and shift[17] and multidirectional instability (MDI) sulcus sign[18] (see Case 2, Table 2-1) should be performed bilaterally and compared. At this initial stage, identification of excessive hypermobility or excessive capsular tightness has critical ramifications for the plan of care. The patient in this case has significant atrophy of the infraspinatus muscle evident by atrophy in the infraspinous fossa as well as inferior angle prominence of the right scapula at rest and in the hands-on-hips position. There is no evidence of instability with grade I anterior-posterior translation noted during the load and shift test. The MDI sulcus test is negative bilaterally.

Plan of Care and Interventions

Initial postsurgical rehabilitation focuses on increasing shoulder ROM to prevent capsular adhesions while protecting the surgically repaired tissues. Some postsurgical rehabilitation protocols specify ROM limitations during the first 6 weeks of rehabilitation. Several basic science studies have provided rationale for the safe application of passive glenohumeral joint ROM and the movements that allow joint excursion and capsular lengthening, yet provide safe and protective inherent tensions in the repaired tendon.

In human cadavers, Hatakeyama *et al.*[19] repaired 1 × 2 cm supraspinatus tears and studied the effects of humeral rotation on the tension in the supraspinatus in 30° of arm elevation in the coronal, scapular, and sagittal planes. Compared to tension in a position of neutral rotation, 30° and 60° of external rotation *decreased* the tension within the supraspinatus muscle tendon unit. In contrast, 30° and 60° of internal rotation *increased* tension within the supraspinatus tendon. This study provides important insight into the safety of performing early PROM into external rotation following rotator cuff repair. During the period of postsurgical immobilization, most patients are placed in positions of internal rotation. This study suggests that this postsurgical immobilization positioning provides increased tension onto the repaired supraspinatus tendon. Controlled tension in the repair is advocated to improve tendon strength and healing without jeopardizing healing or tendon-bone congruity. Based on the study by Hatakeyama et al.,[19] physical therapists should understand that moving the shoulder up to 60° of external rotation in 30° of elevation in the scapular or coronal plane provides *less* tissue tension than the position of typical immobilization (30°-60° of internal rotation).

Another aspect of clinical relevance that can be derived from the study by Hatakeyama et al.[19] was the comparison of the intrinsic tensile load in the repaired supraspinatus tendon between the coronal, scapular, and sagittal planes during humeral rotation. Significantly higher loading was present in the supraspinatus tendon during humeral rotation in the sagittal plane compared to both the coronal and scapular planes. Therefore, based on this study, early PROM should be performed into the directions of both external and internal humeral rotation using the *scapular plane* position to minimize tensile loading in the repaired tendon.[19] Figure 5-1 shows a technique used to perform humeral rotation ROM with the glenohumeral joint placed in the scapular plane. The use of a platform or the therapist's leg provides a supported position in the scapular plane allowing the therapist's hands to be free to provide both scapular stabilization support and to mobilize the humeral head.

Another cadaveric study provides guidance for ROM application in the early postoperative phase. Muraki et al.[20] studied the effects of passive upper extremity motion on tensile loading of the supraspinatus tendon. They found no significant increases in strain in either the supraspinatus or infraspinatus tendons at 60° of shoulder flexion during the movement of horizontal adduction. However, internal rotation performed at 30° and 60° of flexion increased tension in the inferiormost portion of the infraspinatus tendon compared to the resting or neutral position. This study provides additional guidance that the performance of internal rotation

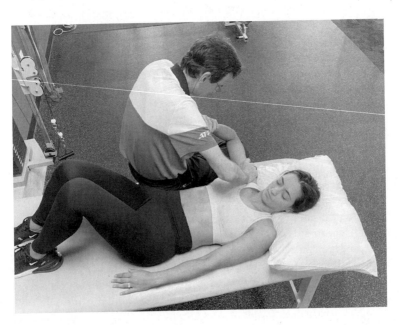

Figure 5-1. Right glenohumeral rotation ROM in the scapular plane.

and cross arm adduction ranges of motion can be performed with minimal strain placed on the repaired supraspinatus tendon. This study also illustrated the importance of knowing the degree of tendon involvement and repair because posteriorly based rotator cuff repairs (those involving the infraspinatus and teres minor) may be subjected to increased tensile loads if early internal rotation is applied during postoperative rehabilitation. Therefore, communication between the surgeon and treating physical therapist is of vital importance to ensure that optimal range of motion is performed following repair.

Muraki *et al.*[21] investigated the strain in the repaired supraspinatus tendon with glenohumeral joint anterior, posterior, and inferior glide mobilizations in 30° of glenohumeral joint abduction. The cadaveric specimens showed no loading of the supraspinatus tendon with these glenohumeral joint mobilizations when performed in this position. Therefore, clinicians can provide early joint mobilizations after rotator cuff repair, within approximately 30° of glenohumeral joint abduction (Fig. 5-2).

An area of concern early after rotator cuff repair is when to progress from PROM to active-assisted range of motion (AAROM) and eventually active range of motion (AROM). From intramuscular electromyographic (EMG) recordings in adults with no history of shoulder pathology, McCann *et al.*[22] compared the degree of supraspinatus activation during supine-assisted flexion range of motion and seated elevation with the use of a pulley. While both activities produce low levels of supraspinatus activation, the seated upright pulley activity produced significantly more EMG activity than the comparable activity in the supine position. This study clearly demonstrated the effect of patient positioning on supraspinatus

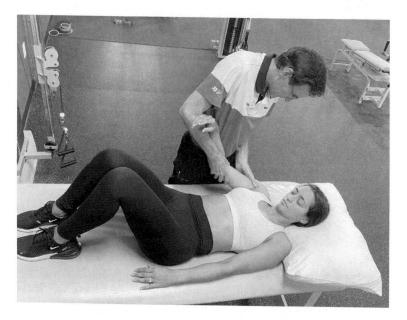

Figure 5-2. Glenohumeral joint mobilizations (anterior/posterior) performed with the shoulder in the scapular plane and 20° of abduction to decrease tension on the repaired rotator cuff tendon.

activation and provides the therapeutic rationale for using supine, active-assisted shoulder flexion exercise in the early phase following rotator cuff repair to protect the healing tendon.

Ellsworth et al.[23] measured shoulder EMG activity in adults with and without shoulder pathology and found minimal EMG activity in the rotator cuff musculature during the commonly prescribed Codman pendulum exercise. Muscular activity was unchanged with and without weight application during the performance of pendulum exercises. However, **the rotator cuff musculature is still activated during the Codman pendulum exercise,** *especially* in individuals with shoulder pathology. Many therapists (including the authors of this case) do not recommend the use of weight application in the hand during pendulum exercises due to the potential for unwanted anterior glenohumeral translation. Because pendulum exercises (with or without weight) activate rotator cuff musculature, it calls into question their prescription in the early post-surgery phase in cases when only passive movements may be indicated.

Early versus delayed ROM is likely one of the areas of greatest controversy and variation in rehabilitation following rotator cuff repair. Given the increase in the number of arthroscopic rotator cuff repairs being performed, rehabilitation professionals and surgeons have been investigating this particular issue for some time. In 2009, a systematic review found insufficient evidence to provide an evidence-based conclusion or recommendation regarding immobilization versus early passive ROM for rotator cuff repair rehabilitation.[24] In 2011, Koo et al.[25] identified patients from a large population that were particularly vulnerable to ROM loss after rotator cuff repair: those who simultaneously underwent superior labrum anterior-posterior (SLAP) repair, had preoperative adhesive capsulitis, calcific tendonitis, and/or had only single tendon rotator cuff repairs. In the subset of patients with any of these identified risk factors, the authors prescribed an active-assisted exercise called a table slide (Fig. 5-3). This exercise—performed daily early in the first week of the postoperative rehabilitation protocol—ultimately prevented ROM loss in all patients in this vulnerable subgroup. Based on this study, prescription of this exercise that uses a controlled motion into overhead elevation through torso-initiated movement is indicated in the early rehabilitation phase to prevent loss of shoulder ROM in a patient particularly vulnerable to loss of shoulder ROM.

Five randomized controlled trials (RCTs) have compared early passive ROM to sling immobilization following arthroscopic rotator cuff repair[25-29] and a subsequent meta-analysis synthesized the findings.[30] While advocates of early passive ROM following surgery cite postoperative stiffness (the most common complication following arthroscopic rotator cuff repair) as the primary rationale for early mobilization and movement,[31,32] opponents cite the high incidence of re-tear.[33,34] The meta-analysis concluded that early postoperative passive ROM (in the first 4 to 6 weeks) results in significant increases in shoulder *flexion* at 3, 6, and 12 months after surgery compared with immobilization.[30] Although *external rotation* ROM increased across the early passive ROM groups, this increase was only significant at 3 months after surgery. Perhaps most important, early passive ROM did *not* result in increased rotator cuff re-tear rates at a minimum follow-up of 1 year. The studies included in this meta-analysis excluded massive rotator cuff tears.

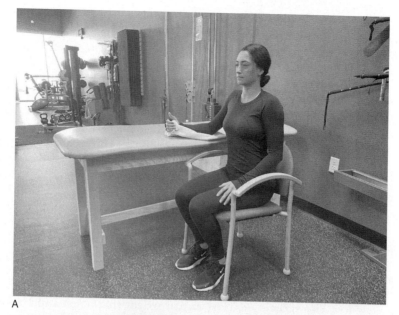

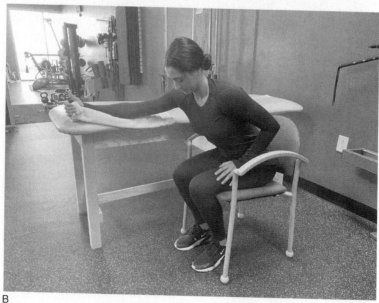

Figure 5-3. Table slide exercise for early active-assisted closed-chain shoulder flexion range of motion. From starting position **A**, patient flexes forward at the hips to ending position **B**.

These results indicate that early passive ROM is not a significant risk factor for increased re-tear rates following arthroscopic rotator cuff repairs. The early motion performed in these studies included pendulum exercises and manual passive ROM performed by a physical therapist. A 2013 study showed that therapist-performed passive ROM does not produce EMG activity in the supraspinatus and infraspinatus above baseline levels (postural standing at rest).[35] This finding, coupled with increased ROM in elevation and external rotation demonstrated in the meta-analysis,[30] supports the use of early passive ROM following rotator cuff repair.

These studies give objective guidance for the application of passive and active-assisted ROM activities that can be applied safely in early postsurgical rehabilitation following rotator cuff repair. As further research becomes available, physical therapists will be able to make evidence-based decisions regarding the appropriateness of specific rehabilitation exercises based on their inherent muscular activation. Rehabilitation in the first 2 to 4 weeks following rotator cuff repair typically consists of the use of truly passive, as well as several minimally active or active-assisted exercises for the rotator cuff such as active-assisted flexion using overhead pulleys and pendulum exercises. To recruit rotator cuff and scapular muscles, the patient can use the "balance point" position (90° of shoulder flexion) in supine; the patient is cued to perform small active motions of flexion/extension from the 90° starting position. These exercises should be coupled with early scapular stabilization via manual resistance techniques using direct hand contacts on the scapula to bypass force application to the rotator cuff and optimize trapezius, rhomboid, and serratus anterior muscular activation (Fig. 5-4). Kibler *et al.*[36] measured EMG activity during low-level closed chain exercises such as weight shifting on a rocker board (patient in a standing position with upper extremity resting on a rocker board sitting on a tabletop). They showed that this activity produced low levels of activation (<10%) of the rotator cuff and scapular musculature. An open-chain exercise credited to Kibler *et al.*[37] called the "robbery" exercise is an active upper extremity exercise. This exercise involves minimal glenohumeral joint motion, but emphasizes

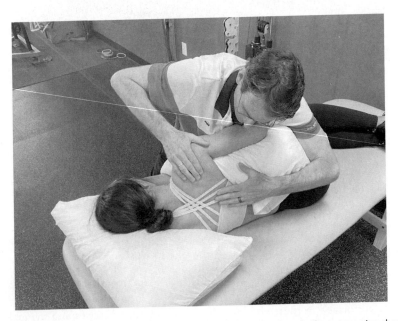

Figure 5-4. Therapist applying manual resistance on patient's scapula to facilitate trapezius, rhomboid, and serratus anterior muscular activation.

scapular retraction and recruits the scapular stabilizers for early scapular stabilization (Fig. 5-5).

One study has compared the effects of simulated shoulder AROM on the integrity of a cadaveric supraspinatus repair performed using either transosseous tunnels or suture anchors.[38] Their findings showed no difference between these two types of surgical repair following repetitive loading, indicating that an arthroscopically based suture anchor fixation method can withstand active loading similarly to a transosseous repair used during mini-open and open rotator cuff repair. Future research may identify the effects of simulated submaximal loads on different rotator cuff repair constructs to allow for optimal application of resistive exercise sequences.

In a 2021 systematic review and meta-analysis of 8 studies with 756 participants who had undergone rotator cuff repair, Silveira *et al.*[39] concluded that there was **high-certainty evidence favoring early versus delayed AROM for the movements of flexion (elevation), abduction, and external rotation.** Concomitant with increased ROM was the consistent finding that **early AROM did not compromise the integrity**

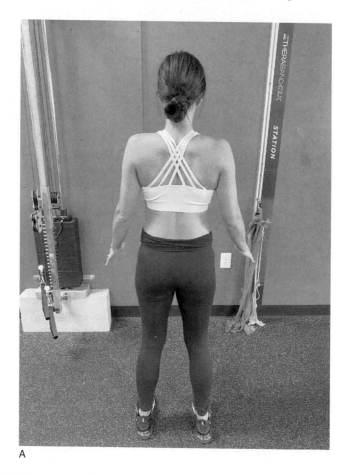

A

Figure 5-5. Robbery exercise for scapular stabilization. **A,** Patient starts with both hands down and **B,** raises them up to end position while performing scapular retraction.

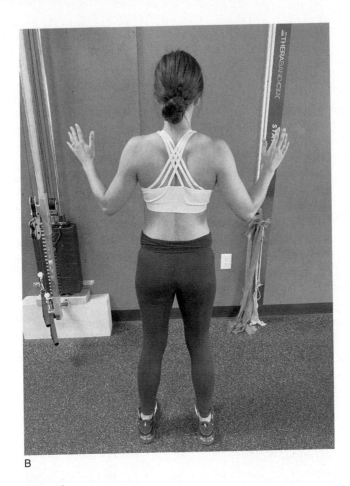

B

Figure 5-5. (Continued)

of the surgical repair. Two RCTs from a single institution[40,41] suggest that early active ROM also does not compromise postoperative strength, quality of life, or repair integrity. When early active motion is indicated through the available motion, assisted elevation techniques can bridge the transition from PROM to AROM. Figure 5-6 shows that the use of the Upper Extremity Ranger device (Rehab Innovations Inc., Omaha, Nebraska) provides assistance via leverage to reinforce the passive motion gained by the therapist in the first stages of rehabilitation following rotator cuff repair.

In the initial phase of rehabilitation (1-4 weeks postsurgery), care must be taken regarding strengthening because the priority is to optimize shoulder ROM, protect the repair, and initiate scapular stabilization. The use of AROM exercises such as sidelying external rotation against gravity with little or no weight application can be prescribed to begin activating the posterior rotator cuff musculature (Fig. 5-7). EMG studies have confirmed that this exercise activates the infraspinatus and teres minor muscles.[42,43] Additional movements such as active shoulder flexion can also be done in sidelying to decrease shoulder loads[44] (Fig. 5-8).

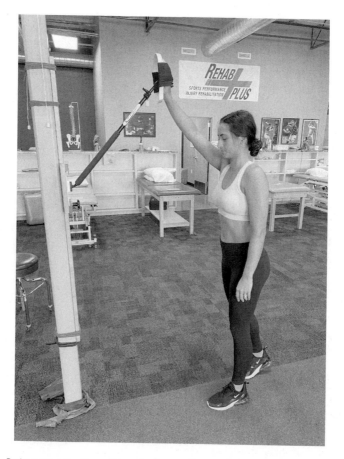

Figure 5-6. Patient using the Upper Extremity Ranger device (Rehab Innovations Inc., Omaha, Nebraska) to provide assistance with shoulder flexion.

As the patient progresses, emphasis shifts to strengthening the entire rotator cuff complex. In this early phase, exercises are also applied with elastic resistance to provide an isometric contraction of the internal and external humeral rotators (rotator cuff) through the use of an exercise commonly called "dynamic isometrics" or step-outs (Fig. 5-9). A small towel roll is placed under the axilla during the exercise to place the shoulder in the scapular plane.[7] The use of elastic resistance bands or tubing allows the physical therapist to ensure that the patient is not exercising with loads exceeding her present tolerance due to the standardized elongation parameters of the colored tubing progression (e.g., TheraBand, Performance Health, Akron OH). Elastic resistance is preferred over other methods of isometric exercise using a wall or pillow because the physical therapist has less ability to control or monitor the patient's exercise intensity.

Key components of rehabilitation in the first month following rotator cuff repair include the use of early shoulder ROM, glenohumeral joint mobilization, submaximal rotator cuff and scapular active movement, and gentle resistance. Basic science

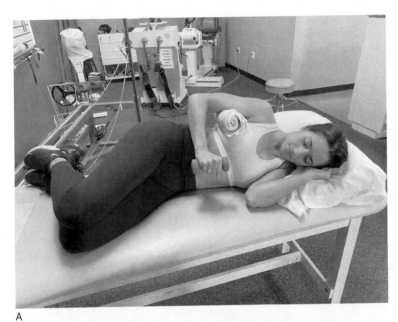

A

B

Figure 5-7. Sidelying external rotation against gravity with small dumbbell weight to begin activating posterior rotator cuff musculature. **A.** starting position. **B.** ending position.

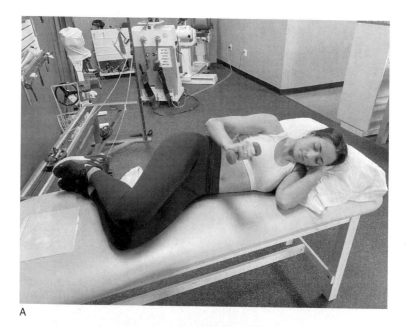

A

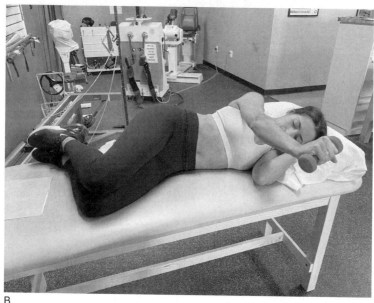

B

Figure 5-8. Sidelying shoulder flexion exercise. **A.** starting position. **B.** ending position.

research can be applied during this initial stage to ensure that appropriate loading is provided to the postsurgical tissue to produce successful ROM and strength outcomes following rehabilitation. Future research will further elucidate optimal loading and immobilization periods following surgical repair of the rotator cuff.

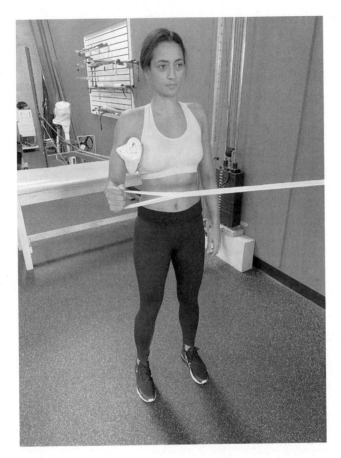

Figure 5-9. Resistance exercise for right humeral rotator cuff complex. With a roll under the axilla to keep the shoulder in the scapular plane, the patient takes a step away (or, a "step out") from the band's attachment site while maintaining the same upper extremity position.

Evidence-Based Clinical Recommendations

SORT: Strength of Recommendation Taxonomy

A: Consistent, good-quality patient-oriented evidence
B: Inconsistent or limited-quality patient-oriented evidence
C: Consensus, disease-oriented evidence, usual practice, expert opinion, or case series

1. Codman pendulum exercises (with or without weight) that are typically prescribed in the early postsurgery phase when active movements are contraindicated may not be appropriate because this exercise still activates rotator cuff musculature. **Grade B**

2. In the first 4 weeks after surgical rotator cuff repair, a rehabilitation program emphasizing early shoulder ROM, glenohumeral joint mobilization, submaximal rotator cuff activation, and active scapular movement with subtle resistance produces good patient outcomes for range of motion, muscular strength, and shoulder function and without jeopardizing repair integrity. **Grade A**

COMPREHENSION QUESTIONS

5.1 In the first 4 weeks following rotator cuff repair, humeral rotation range of motion should be done in which of the following planes to minimize loading and tension on the repair?

A. Sagittal plane

B. Scapular plane

C. Coronal plane

D. Transverse plane

5.2 Which of the following is NOT a component of early rehabilitation following rotator cuff repair?

A. Scapular stabilization exercise

B. Glenohumeral joint mobilization

C. Aggressive strengthening of the supraspinatus

D. Submaximal activation of the posterior rotator cuff

ANSWERS

5.1 **B.** In human cadaver studies, Hatakeyama et al.[19] have shown that humeral rotation exercise performed in the scapular plane produces less tensile loading than similar ranges of motion performed in the sagittal plane.

5.2 **C.** Care must be taken when implementing loading strategies to the repaired rotator cuff following surgical repair in the early postoperative period.[38] Aggressive loading of the rotator cuff has been shown to produce failures in traditional transosseous repairs and single- and double-row suture anchor fixation methods.

REFERENCES

1. Jobe FW, Kvitne RS, Giangarra CE. Shoulder pain in the overhand or throwing athlete. The relationship of anterior instability and rotator cuff impingement. *Orthop Rev.* 1989;28:963-975.

2. Cofield RH. Current concepts review of rotator cuff disease of the shoulder. *J Bone Joint Surg Am.* 1985;67:974-979.

3. Andrews JR, Alexander EJ. Rotator cuff injury in throwing and racquet sports. *Sports Med Arthroscop Rev.* 1995;3:30-38.

4. Neer CS II. Impingement lesions. *Clin Orthop Relat Res.* 1983;173:70-77.

5. Codman EA. *The Shoulder*. 2nd ed. Brooklyn, NY: Miller & Medical;1934.

6. Chansky HA, Iannotti JP. The vascularity of the rotator cuff. *Clin Sports Med*. 1991;10:807-822.

7. Rathbun JB, Macnab I. The microvascular pattern of the rotator cuff. *J Bone Joint Surg Br*. 1970;52:540-553.

8. Brooks CH, Revell WJ, Heatley FW. A quantitative histological study of the vascularity of the rotator cuff tendon. *J Bone Joint Surg Br*. 1992;74:151-153.

9. Swiontowski MF, Iannotti JP, Boulas HJ, Esterhai JL. Intraoperative assessment of rotator cuff vascularity using laser Doppler flowmetry. In: Post M, Morrey BF, Hawkins RJ, eds. *Surgery of the Shoulder*. St. Louis, MO: Mosby Year Book;1990:208-212.

10. Iannotti JP. Lesions of the rotator cuff: pathology and pathogenesis. In: Matsen FA, Fu FH, Hawkins RJ, eds. *The Shoulder: A Balance of Mobility and Stability*. Rosemont, IL: American Academy of Orthopaedic Surgeons;1993.

11. Loehr JF, Helmig P, Sojbjerg JO, Jung A. Shoulder instability caused by rotator cuff lesions. An in vitro study. *Clin Orthop Relat Res*. 1994;304:84-90.

12. Miller C, Savoie FH. Glenohumeral abnormalities associated with full-thickness tears of the rotator cuff. *Orthop Rev*. 1994;23:159-162.

13. Ellenbecker TS. *Clinical Examination of the Shoulder*. St. Louis, MO: W.B. Saunders; 2004.

14. Ellenbecker TS, Dines DM, Renstrom PA, Windler GS. Visual observation of apparent infraspinatus muscle atrophy in male professional tennis players. *Orthop J Sports Med*. 2020;27;8:2325967120958834.

15. Kibler WB. Role of the scapula in the overhead throwing motion. *Contemp Orthop*. 1991;22:525-532.

16. Kibler WB, Uhl TL, Maddux JW, et al. Qualitative clinical evaluation of scapular dysfunction: a reliability study. *J Shoulder Elbow Surg*. 2002;11:550-556.

17. Gerber C, Ganz R. Clinical assessment of instability of the shoulder. With special reference to anterior and posterior drawer tests. *J Bone Joint Surgery*. 1984;66:551-556.

18. McFarland EG, Torpey BM, Curl LA. Evaluation of shoulder laxity. *Sports Med*. 1996;22:264-272.

19. Hatakeyama Y, Itoi E, Urayama M, et al. Effect of superior capsule and coracohumeral ligament release on strain in the repaired rotator cuff tendon. A cadaveric study. *Am J Sports Med*. 2001;29: 633-640.

20. Muraki T, Aoki M, Uchiyama E, et al. The effect of arm position on stretching of the supraspinatus, infraspinatus, and posterior portion of deltoid muscles: a cadaveric study. *Clin Biomech*. 2006;21: 474-480.

21. Muraki T, Aoki M, Uchiyama E, et al. Strain on the repaired supraspinatus tendon during manual traction and translational glide mobilization on the glenohumeral joint: a cadaveric biomechanics study. *Man Ther*. 2007;12:231-239.

22. McCann PD, Wooten ME, Kadaba MP, Bigliani LU. A kinematic and electromyographic study of shoulder rehabilitation exercises. *Clin Orthop Rel Res*. 1993;288:178-188.

23. Ellsworth AA, Mullaney M, Tyler TF, et al. Electromyography of selected shoulder musculature during un-weighted and weighted pendulum exercises. *N Am J Sports Phys Ther*. 2006;1:73-79.

24. Baumgarten KM, Vidal AF, Wright RW. Rotator cuff rehabilitation: a level I and II systematic review. *Sports Health*. 2009;1:125-130.

25. Koo SS, Parsley BK, Burkhart SS, Schoolfield JD. Reduction of postoperative stiffness after arthroscopic rotator cuff repair: results of a customized physical therapy regimen based on risk factors for stiffness. *Arthroscopy*. 2011;27:155-160.

26. Cuff DJ, Pupello DR. Prospective randomized study of arthroscopic rotator cuff repair using an early versus delayed postoperative physical therapy protocol. *J Shoulder Elbow Surg*. 2012;21:1450-1455.

27. Kim YS, Chung SW, Kim JY, et al. Is early passive motion exercise necessary after arthroscopic rotator cuff repair? *Am J Sports Med*. 2012;40:815-821.

28. Lee BG, Cho NS, Rhee YG. Effect of two rehabilitation protocols on range of motion and healing rates after arthroscopic rotator cuff repair: aggressive versus limited early passive exercises. *Arthroscopy*. 2012;28:34-42.

29. Keener JD, Galatz LM, Stobbs-Cucchi G, et al. Rehabilitation following arthroscopic rotator cuff repair. A prospective randomized trial of immobilization compared with early motion. *J Bone Joint Surg Am*. 2014;96:11-19.

30. Riboh JC, Garrigues GE. Early passive motion versus immobilization after arthroscopic rotator cuff repair. *Arthroscopy*. 2014;30:997-1005.

31. Brislin KJ, Field LD, Savoie FH III. Complications after arthroscopic rotator cuff repair. *Arthroscopy*. 2007;23:124-128.

32. Namdari S, Green A. Range of motion limitation after rotator cuff repair. *J Shoulder Elbow Surg*. 2010;19:290-296.

33. Galatz LM, Ball CM, Teefey SA, et al. The outcome and repair integrity of completely arthroscopically repaired large and massive rotator cuff tears. *J Bone Joint Surg Am*. 2004;86:219-224.

34. Tashjian RZ, Hollins AM, Kim HM, et al. Factors affecting healing rates after arthroscopic double-row rotator cuff repair. *Am J Sports Med*. 2010;38:2435-2442.

35. Murphy CA, McDermott WJ, Petersen RK, et al. Electromyographic analysis of the rotator cuff in postoperative shoulder patients during passive rehabilitation exercises. *J Shoulder Elbow Surg*. 2013;22:102-107.

36. Kibler WB, Livingston B, Bruce R. Current concepts in shoulder rehabilitation. In: Stauffer RN, Erlich MG. *Advances in Operative Orthopaedics*. Vol 3. St Louis, MO: Mosby; 1995:249-297.

37. Kibler WB, Sciascia AD, Uhl TL, et al. Electromyographic analysis of specific exercises for scapular control in early phases of shoulder rehabilitation. *Am J Sports Med*. 2008;36:1789-1799.

38. Tashjian RZ, Levanthal E, Spenciner DB, et al. Initial fixation strength of massive rotator cuff tears: in vitro comparison of single-row suture anchor and transosseous tunnel constructs. *Arthroscopy*. 2007;23:710-716.

39. Silveira A, Luk J, Kang SH, et al. Move it or lose it? The effects of early active movement on clinical outcomes following rotator cuff repair: a systematic review with meta-analysis. *J Orthop Sports Phys Ther*. 2021;51:331-344.

40. Sheps DM, Boulian M, Styles-Tripp F, et al. Early mobilisation following mini-open cuff repair: a randomized control trial. *Bone Joint J*. 2015; 97-B(9):1257-1263.

41. Sheps DM, Silveira A, Beaupre L, et al. Shoulder and Upper Extremity Research Group of Edmonton (SURGE). Early active motion versus sling Immobilization after arthroscopic rotator cuff repair: a randomized control trial. *Arthroscopy*; 2019;35:749-760.

42. Townsend H, Jobe FW, Pink M, Perry W. Electromyographic analysis of the glenohumeral muscles during a baseball rehabilitation program. *Am J Sports Med*. 1991;19:264-272.

43. Reinold MM, Macrina LC, Wilk KE, et al. Electromyographic analysis of the supraspinatus and deltoid muscles during 3 common rehabilitation exercises. *J Athl Train*. 2007;42:464-469.

44. Struyf F, Cagnie B, Cools A, et al. Scapulothoracic muscle activity and recruitment timing in patients with shoulder impingement symptoms and glenohumeral instability. *J Electromyogr Kinesiol*. 2014;24:277-284.

Adhesive Capsulitis

Jason Brumitt

A 44-year-old female with a 5-month history of right (dominant) shoulder pain was referred to an outpatient physical therapy clinic by her orthopedic surgeon. She reports first experiencing pain while fastening her bra. The patient denies any trauma. Pain intensity has increased since onset and regularly affects her ability to sleep on her right side. In addition to pain, she is unable to clean her house, reach overhead, or reach behind her back because her shoulder "just won't move." The patient's history, symptoms, and examination findings are consistent with a diagnosis of primary (idiopathic) adhesive capsulitis. Her right shoulder passive range of motion (PROM) is limited to 100° of flexion, 40° of extension, 85° of abduction, 10° of external rotation (ER), and 50° of internal rotation (IR). The PROM of her left (uninvolved) shoulder is normal: flexion 170°, extension 40°, abduction 170°, ER 90°, and IR 70°. Palpation of the right shoulder reveals tenderness at the greater tubercle (rotator cuff insertion site), intertubercular groove, and the coracoid (positive coracoid pain test).

▶ Based on the patient's suspected diagnosis, what do you anticipate may be the contributing factors to her condition?
▶ What are the most appropriate examination tests?
▶ Describe a physical therapy plan of care based on each stage of the health condition.
▶ Based on the patient's diagnosis, what are appropriate physical therapy interventions?

KEY DEFINITIONS

AXILLARY FOLD: Region of the armpit in which the anterior border includes a portion of the pectoralis major muscle and the posterior border includes portions of the latissimus dorsi and teres major muscles

KALTENBORN MOBILIZATION GRADING SCALE: Mobilization scale consisting of 3 grades: grade I is a traction mobilization performed to decrease pain; grade II is a glide or traction mobilization performed to decrease pain and increase joint play; grade III is performed to increase joint play at the end range of motion.[1]

MAITLAND MOBILIZATION GRADING SCALE: Mobilization scale consisting of 5 grades: oscillatory mobilizations are performed in grades I to IV, whereas grade V consists of a high-velocity low-amplitude thrust. The purpose of grades I and II mobilizations is to decrease pain, whereas the purpose of grades III to V mobilizations is to increase joint mobility.[2]

MOBILIZATION: Skilled, passive movement of a synovial joint performed by a clinician for the purpose of decreasing pain and/or improving joint range of motion

MULLIGAN MOBILIZATIONS WITH MOVEMENT: Joint mobilization technique in which the patient performs an active movement while the clinician provides a mobilization force

PRIMARY (IDIOPATHIC) ADHESIVE CAPSULITIS: Musculoskeletal condition of the shoulder of unknown etiology marked by significant restriction in shoulder active and passive range of motion[3,4]

ROTATOR INTERVAL: Triangular region of the anterior shoulder that contains the coracoid process, supraspinatus and subscapularis tendons, long head of the biceps tendon, and the superior glenohumeral and coracohumeral ligaments

Objectives

1. Describe the differences between primary (idiopathic) and secondary adhesive capsulitis.

2. Describe the pathophysiology and clinical presentation associated with primary adhesive capsulitis.

3. Describe appropriate clinical examination tests that help rule in primary adhesive capsulitis.

4. Describe appropriate physical therapy interventions to treat primary adhesive capsulitis.

5. Assess the reported outcomes between treatment approaches for primary adhesive capsulitis.

6. Describe treatments for primary adhesive capsulitis that may be prescribed or performed by orthopedic physicians.

Physical Therapy Considerations

Physical therapy considerations during examination of the individual with suspected primary adhesive capsulitis:

▶ **General physical therapy plan of care/goals:** Decrease pain; increase flexibility; increase or prevent loss of shoulder range of motion; increase upper quadrant strength; prevent or minimize loss of aerobic fitness

▶ **Physical therapy tests and measures:** Observation of the upper quadrant; active and passive range of motion testing; passive accessory joint motion testing; coracoid pain test, palpation; patient education regarding functional anatomy and injury pathomechanics; modalities and manual therapy to decrease pain; flexibility and self-mobilization exercises to increase range of motion; resistance exercises to increase endurance of the scapular stabilizers and to increase strength of the upper extremity muscles; aerobic exercise program

▶ **Differential diagnoses:** Rotator cuff strain, rotator cuff tendinosis, subacromial impingement, osteoarthritis, tumor, fracture

▶ **Precautions during physical therapy:** Monitor vital signs; adhere to postsurgical restrictions if patient has had a surgical release or manipulation under anesthesia; monitor patient response to therapist-performed stretching and/or manual therapy

Understanding the Health Condition

Adhesive capsulitis (also known as frozen shoulder) affects up to 5% of the general population and upward of 30% of those with diabetes mellitus.[4,5] Adhesive capsulitis (AC) primarily affects women between 40 and 65 years of age.[6,7] The onset of AC is associated with several endocrine, neurologic, and cardiovascular conditions including diabetes, cerebrovascular accident, Dupuytren's contracture, ischemic heart disease, post-cardiac surgery, hyperlipidemia, Parkinson's disease, and thyroid disease.[4] AC is considered a self-limiting condition with some individuals experiencing a gradual resolution of symptoms without treatment. There are two types of AC: primary (idiopathic) and secondary. Primary AC is characterized by pain and stiffness without history of trauma or surgery, whereas secondary AC is preceded by trauma or surgery in the shoulder region. It is currently believed that the two types are unique entities sharing only the similarities in pain and loss of shoulder range of motion.[4]

Physicians have developed a three-stage model and a four-stage model that describe the clinical presentation and pathoanatomical features associated with primary AC.[4,8-13] Both models describe stages that vary in length and can overlap other stages.[8-13] A three-stage model emphasizes clinical features highlighting pain severity, motion loss, and restoration of function (Table 6-1).[9,10,14] The first stage in this model—*the freezing or painful stage*—is associated with an insidious, gradual onset of pain and stiffness in the shoulder. The patient may describe increased pain at night, especially when attempting to sleep on the involved shoulder. The second stage—*the frozen or adhesive stage*—is associated with less shoulder pain, except for increased

Table 6-1	THREE STAGES OF PRIMARY ADHESIVE CAPSULITIS	
Stage	**Duration**	**Clinical Features**
1. Freezing (painful)	2.5-9 mo[9,10]	Constant pain; worse at night Gradual loss of motion
2. Frozen (adhesive)	4-12 mo[9,10]	Joint stiffness (loss of motion) Pain may decrease, but intensifies at end ranges of motion
3. Thawing (resolution)	5-26 mo[9] 12-42 mo[10]	Restoration of motion and function

pain intensity at the end ranges of available motion. During the final stage—*the thawing or resolution phase*—a patient may experience a gradual and spontaneous restoration of pain-free motion. The more frequently used four-stage model was developed by Neviaser and Hannafin.[11-13] This model combines clinical features with patho-anatomical findings observed during arthroscopy and histopathological findings from tissue biopsies (Table 6-2).[11,12] These models of AC help the physical therapist appreciate the stages of disease progression that occur with changes in clinical

Table 6-2	FOUR-STAGE MODEL OF PRIMARY ADHESIVE CAPSULITIS			
	Symptoms	**Signs**	**Arthroscopic Appearance**	**Biopsy**
Stage 1	Pain referred to deltoid insertion Pain at night	Capsular pain on deep palpation Empty end feel at extremes of motion Full motion under anesthesia	Fibrinous synovial inflammatory reaction No adhesions or capsular contracture	Rare inflammatory cell infiltrate Hypervascular hypertrophic synovitis Normal capsular tissue
Stage 2	Severe night pain Stiffness	Motion restricted in forward flexion, abduction, internal and external rotation Some motion loss under anesthesia	Christmas tree synovitis Some loss of axillary fold	Hypertrophic, hypervascular synovitis Perivascular, subsynovial capsular scar
Stage 3	Profound stiffness Pain only at the end range of motion	Significant loss of motion Tethering at ends of motion No improvement under anesthesia	Complete loss of axillary fold Minimal synovitis	Hypercellular, collagenous tissue with a thin synovial layer Similar features to other fibrosing conditions
Stage 4	Profound stiffness Pain minimal	Significant motion loss Gradual improvement in motion	Fully mature adhesions Identification of intra-articular structures difficult	Not reported

presentation. However, a caveat is that appreciation of the patient's stage of AC may not help guide treatment because there is currently a lack of evidence to accurately prescribe effective interventions based on stage of disease progression.

Our understanding of the pathophysiology associated with primary AC has evolved from Codman's (1934) and Neviaser's (1945) initial descriptions.[15,16] Based on early surgical findings, the loss of shoulder motion was thought to be the result of the axillary fold adhering to itself and to the anatomical neck of the humerus.[4,16] However, AC is now believed to be the result of synovial inflammation and fibrosis of the capsule.[4,13,17] Cytokines, which are proteins involved in regulating inflammation, appear to play a role in the development of AC.[18-20] Excessive cytokine activity has been shown to increase the activity of fibroblasts, which may cause thickening and contracture of the anterior shoulder capsule.[21] Researchers are investigating the role of growth factors, immune cells, and matrix metalloproteinases in the onset of AC.[20] There may also be a genetic predisposition for the condition, though more research is needed to confirm initial findings.[22,23] Identifying pathoanatomical factors associated with AC may improve therapeutic options in the future. The loss of shoulder motion results from contracture of the coracohumeral ligament, rotator interval, and the anterior and inferior capsules.[4] In individuals with diabetes, the pathogenesis of AC may include unique biochemical components.[4]

Examination, Evaluation, and Diagnosis

Diagnosis is based on patient history and motion testing of the shoulder.[7,14,24] Observation may reveal disuse atrophy of the deltoid muscle. The patient may hold her arm in a position of comfort against the side of the body.[10] A clinical practice guideline (CPG) published by the American Academy of Orthopaedic Physical Therapy (AAOPT) recommends administering functional outcome measures at the start of treatment and at discharge. The three specific tools recommended include the Disabilities of the Arm, Shoulder, and Hand (DASH), the American Shoulder and Elbow Surgeons Standardized Shoulder Assessment Form, and the Shoulder Pain and Disability Index (SPADI).[7]

Patients with AC present with significant loss of active and passive shoulder range of motion. Classically, the **glenohumeral loss of motion pattern** is ER presenting the greatest loss of motion (as a percentage of the contralateral uninvolved shoulder), followed by loss of abduction, and finally loss of IR.[25,26] However, recent reports suggest that there is *not* a consistent pattern of motion loss; the loss of ER motion is the primary restriction observed in all patients with AC.[24,26-28] Assessment of glenohumeral (GH) passive range of motion is performed with the patient lying supine. The physical therapist supports the involved upper extremity to assess passive ER of the GH joint (Fig. 6-1). The end feel associated with AC is a firm (capsular) end point that is reproducible. Passive motion testing and goniometry should be performed for all cardinal motions.

Carbone *et al.*[29] have proposed a clinical test to diagnose AC. The **coracoid pain test** (CPT) is performed by applying digital pressure to the coracoid process (Fig. 6-2). A positive test is associated with pain at the coracoid process that

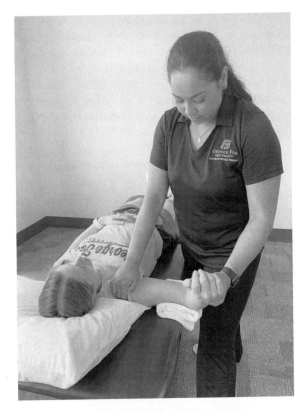

Figure 6-1. Physical therapist assessing glenohumeral external rotation passive range of motion.

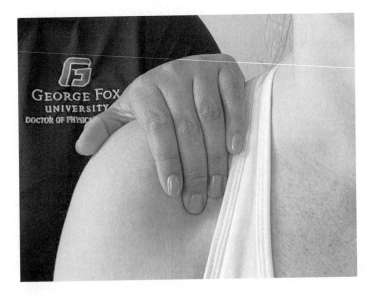

Figure 6-2. Coracoid pain test.

is greater than pain experienced when applying digital pressure to the ipsilateral acromioclavicular joint and to the anterolateral subacromial region (by ≥3 points on a 0-10 visual analog scale). When compared to asymptomatic adults, the CPT had a sensitivity of 99% (95% CI = 0.99-1.00) and a specificity of 98% (95% CI = 0.97-0.99). When compared to adults with other common shoulder conditions (*e.g.*, calcific tendonitis, rotator cuff tear, acromioclavicular arthritis, GH arthritis), the CPT had a sensitivity of 96% and a specificity of 87% to 89%.[29] The diagnostic accuracy of the CPT has not been reevaluated since initially reported in 2010.

Plan of Care and Interventions

Individuals with AC are traditionally referred to physical therapy by their primary care provider or an orthopedic surgeon. Nonoperative treatments include physical therapy (exercise, manual therapy, modalities), nonsteroidal anti-inflammatory drugs, oral or injected glucocorticoids, and sodium hyaluronate injections.[4,7,10,13,24,30-41] Often, patients are receiving more than one nonoperative treatment concurrently. If a patient fails to improve with conservative measures, an orthopedic physician may consider manipulation under anesthesia or a surgical release.[4,10,13,42]

Therapeutic modalities (*e.g.*, ultrasound, moist heat, cryotherapy, electrical stimulation) **are frequently used as an adjunct to therapeutic exercise and manual therapy techniques.**[43] For example, thermal agents may be used at the beginning of a treatment session to increase collagen extensibility prior to manual therapy or performance of therapeutic exercise.[44,45] Cryotherapy and electrical modalities may be used at the end of a treatment session to help decrease pain.[36]

Joint mobilization techniques have traditionally been included in the plan of care for the patient with AC. It is thought that mobilization techniques help the excursion of the adhered capsule. Table 6-3 describes the **manual therapy techniques that have been shown to improve shoulder range of motion (ROM) in patients with AC** (Table 6-3).

Table 6-3 MANUAL THERAPY-BASED STUDIES FOR THE TREATMENT OF PRIMARY ADHESIVE CAPSULITIS

Author(s) (Year)	Study Design	Participants (symptom duration)	Manual Techniques (and additional treatments)	Outcomes
Vermeulen *et al.* (2000)	Case series	7 patients (3 women; mean age 50.2 ± 6.0 y) with AC diagnosed by orthopaedic surgeon Symptom duration: mean 8.4 mo; range 3-12 mo	End-range GH mobilization (grades III and IV)	Improvements in GH AROM and PROM

(Continued)

Table 6-3 MANUAL THERAPY-BASED STUDIES FOR THE TREATMENT OF PRIMARY ADHESIVE CAPSULITIS (CONTINUED)

Author(s) (Year)	Study Design	Participants (symptom duration)	Manual Techniques (and additional treatments)	Outcomes
Wies (2005)	Case series	8 patients (6 women) with AC diagnosed by a rheumatologist Symptom duration ≥3 mo	Soft tissue mobilization: effleurage, prolonged soft-tissue approximation, cross-friction, sustained pressure; HEP: stretching and strengthening exercises	Significant improvement in AROM (flexion, abduction, ER, and composite total)
Vermeulen et al. (2006)	RCT	100 patients: HGMT (n = 49; mean age 51.6 ± 7.6 y) and LGMT (n = 51; 51.7 ± 8.6 y) Symptom duration: HGMT 8 mo (range 5-14.5 mo); LGMT 8 mo (range 6-14 mo)	HGMT (grades III and IV) and LGMT (grades I and II) to GH joint	HGMT: significant improvement in passive abduction range and active and passive ER
Johnson et al. (2007)	RCT	18 patients (14 women) with AC diagnosed by orthopaedic physicians Symptom duration (median and range): Group 1: 8.4 mo (2-12 mo); Group 2: 10.9 mo (4-60 mo)	Group 1: anterior GH mobilization; Group 2: posterior GH mobilization (Both groups received ultrasound prior to mobilization and 3 minutes UBE after mobilization)	Group 2 (posterior mobilization) experienced significant increase in shoulder ER
Yang et al. (2007)	RCT, multiple-treatment trial	28 patients with primary AC; Group 1: mean age 53.3 ± 6.5 y; Group 2: mean age 58 ± 10.1 y. Symptom duration: Group 1: 18 ± 8 mo; Group 2: 22 ± 10 mo)	End-range mobilization (ERM), mid-range mobilization (MRM), and mobilization with movement (MWM)	ROM gains statistically greater ERM and MWM techniques
Agarwal et al. (2016)	RCT	30 patients with primary AC; Group 1 (n = 15): mean age 48.7 ± 6.4 y; Group 2 (n = 2): mean age 52.5 ± 9.6 y. Symptom duration (range): group 1: 4.6 mo (2.9, 6.2 mo); 5 mo (3-7 mo)	Group 1: reverse distraction technique; Group 2: Kaltenborn's caudal and posterior glides (grades III and IV. Both groups received hot pack to shoulder for 15-20 minutes and home exercise program of pendulum and stretching exercises into flexion, ER, IR, and horizontal adduction).	Both groups had significant improvements in ER and abduction AROM and PROM, pain, and functional outcome score. Group 1 had significant improvements in pain, abduction ROM, and functional scores over Group 2.

Abbreviations: ER, external rotation; GH, glenohumeral; HEP, home exercise program; HGMT, high-grade mobilization techniques; LGMT, low-grade mobilization techniques; RCT, randomized controlled trial; UBE, upper body ergometry

The manual therapy techniques that have been studied on patients with AC include low-grade and high-grade GH mobilizations (Maitland grades I-IV), sustained end-range mobilizations (Kaltenborn grade III), mobilizations with movement (Mulligan), and effleurage and other soft tissue mobilization techniques.[44,46-50] Johnson et al.[44] randomized adults with primary AC into two groups: a group receiving anterior glide mobilizations to the GH joint ($n = 10$) and a group receiving posterior glide mobilizations to the GH joint ($n = 8$). The protocol consisted of thermal ultrasound to the shoulder capsule, followed by shoulder mobilizations, and 3 minutes of upper body ergometry. Stretch mobilizations (Kaltenborn grade III) were performed in either an anterior (Fig. 6-3) or posterior (Fig. 6-4) direction (with the shoulder positioned into end-range abduction and ER). Each sustained mobilization was held for 1 minute. A total of 15 mobilization repetitions were performed during each of the 6 treatment sessions. Although anterior glide mobilizations might have been expected to provide superior ROM gains (because anteriorly directed force should have a greater effect on the fibrotic anterior capsule), the subjects in the *posterior* glide mobilization group experienced statistically significant mean improvement in shoulder ER (31°), whereas those in the anterior glide mobilization group experienced an insignificant improvement of only 3° in shoulder ER.

Oscillatory mobilization techniques have also been reported to improve ROM in patients with AC. Vermeulen et al.[46] performed grades III and IV (Maitland)

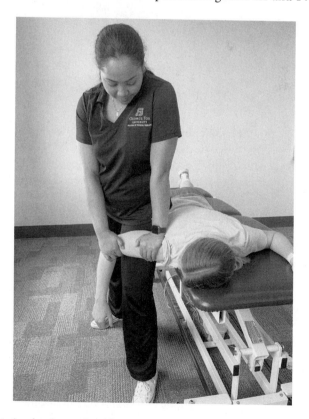

Figure 6-3. Anterior glenohumeral mobilization.

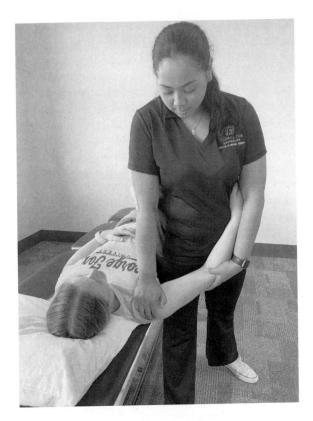

Figure 6-4. Posterior glenohumeral mobilization.

mobilizations to the GH joint for 30 minutes, twice per week for 3 months. Improvements in active range of motion (AROM), PROM, and GH joint capacity (measured by arthrography) occurred at the end of the 3-month treatment period. A subsequent study compared outcomes between groups based on mobilization intensity.[47] One group was treated with high-grade mobilization techniques (HGMT: Maitland grades III and IV) and the other group was treated with low-grade mobilization techniques (LGMT: Maitland grades I and II). Patients were treated for 30 minutes, twice per week, for up to 12 weeks. Subjects in the HGMT group had significant improvements in shoulder active and passive ER and passive abduction. Although the HGMT group had greater ROM improvements compared to the LGMT group in these motions, the authors suggested that for patients who wish to avoid the pain that may be associated with HGMT, a LGMT approach may still improve ROM.[47] Agarwal et al.[50] randomized adults with AC to a reverse distraction mobilization technique group or to a Kaltenborn mobilization (caudal and posterior glides) group. Subjects participated in 18 treatment sessions over a 6-week period receiving "conventional physical therapy" (hot pack applied to the shoulder for 15 to 20 minutes and therapeutic exercises) and either reverse distraction mobilizations or Kaltenborn mobilizations. Subjects also performed the therapeutic exercise program, consisting of the pendulum exercise and shoulder stretching (four positions: flexion, ER, IR, and horizontal adduction) to be performed 2 to 3 sessions per day with each stretch held up to 5 seconds. Both groups experienced significant improvements in pain, active and passive ER and abduction ROM, and functional outcome scores. However, the reverse distraction group experienced significantly greater gains in pain scores, abduction ROM, and functional outcome scores.[50] The AAOPT's CPG recommends utilizing joint mobilization techniques (though not any specific technique) to increase range of motion and to reduce pain in patients with AC.[7]

Based on the evidence, manual therapy techniques should be included in the plan of care for patients with primary AC. However, there are two major limitations to these studies.[51] First, subjects were not homogeneous based on their symptom *duration*. There are three (or four) stages of primary AC: freezing, frozen, and thawing. Each stage varies in length and can overlap other stages. These studies do not allow conclusions to be drawn regarding the effect of manual therapy on a patient in a particular stage of AC. It is possible that some subjects in the freezing or frozen stages failed to experience changes in AROM or PROM with treatment, whereas subjects in the thawing phase may have experienced increases in ROM due to the natural history of the condition and not due to the manual techniques performed. The second limitation to these studies is the lack of either a nonmanual therapy comparison group or a placebo group. The lack of a nonmanual therapy comparison group limits the ability to determine the effectiveness of these treatments within a comprehensive therapy program. The lack of a placebo group limits the ability to interpret the effectiveness of these treatments with the natural history of this condition.

Therapeutic exercises—specifically stretching and self-mobilization—are frequently prescribed to patients with AC.[4,13,24,34,40,45,52,53] Miller *et al.*[45] reported that a two-phase conservative treatment program successfully restored ROM in most patients with AC. Phase I consisted of rest and the use of a sling, moist heat, and prescription anti-inflammatory and/or opiate medications. The purpose of Phase I was to decrease pain prior to initiating the exercises in Phase II. Phase II exercises included PROM and active assisted ROM exercises (*i.e.*, wall climb, posterior capsule stretch, pendulum, overhead pulley, and cane exercises for flexion, extension, IR, and ER). Griggs *et al.*[52] assessed the benefits of a stretching program in patients who were diagnosed with stage II AC (frozen stage). Seventy-five adults (58 females) with a mean duration of 9.2 months (range, 1.3-47 months) of pain were prescribed the following four shoulder stretches: flexion, ER, and horizontal adduction in a supine position and behind-the-back IR in standing. The majority of patients (90%) reported satisfactory outcomes (significant improvements in AROM and PROM), with only 5 individuals requiring arthroscopic capsular release or manipulation under anesthesia to regain ROM.

These two studies demonstrated the potential value of prescribing stretching exercises to patients with AC. However, they share similar internal validity threats to those in the manual therapy studies. To date, only one investigation has compared a stretching program against a more "aggressive" physical therapy routine. Diercks *et al.*[53] compared the effects of a "supervised neglect" program and a "standardized treatment protocol." Subjects in the supervised neglect group were educated about the natural course of AC, prescribed passive pendulum and active exercises within a pain-free range, and advised to continue participation in all other activities as tolerated. For subjects in the standardized treatment group, a physical therapist passively stretched and manipulated the affected GH joint. All subjects were prescribed an exercise program consisting of active exercises to be performed *above* their pain threshold. The authors concluded that a program of supervised neglect was superior to the standard treatment program. After 1 year, 64% of the supervised neglect group had achieved a good outcome (score of 80 on the Constant Score test), whereas none of the subjects in the standardized treatment group reached this goal. At 2 years, 89% in the supervised neglect group and only 63% in the standardized treatment group achieved this goal. The Diercks et al.[53] study appears to be the first to compare a pain-free self-stretching program to an intensive, pain-provoking physical therapy program. Despite the study's strengths (*e.g.*, longitudinal, comparison between groups), threats to internal validity may have introduced bias. First, this was a quasi-experimental study of successive cohorts instead of a randomized controlled trial. Second, the authors did not provide details regarding the mobilization techniques or grades employed or adequate descriptions of the prescribed exercises. Third, the number of treatment sessions was not reported for either group. Finally, the authors prescribed anti-inflammatory medication and/or analgesics to patients in each group as needed; however, details regarding how many subjects were prescribed medications or dosages actually taken were not provided.

Additional investigations are warranted to identify the best treatment or combination of treatments for patients with primary AC. A major question to be answered is whether there are specific treatment strategies based on the stage of the condition. Kelley et al.[24] have proposed a treatment strategy based on the irritability (high, moderate, or low) of the joint. They recommended that a highly irritable joint should be treated with modalities, pain-free PROM, and active-assisted ROM exercises (Figs. 6-5 to 6-8; Table 6-4) and low-grade (grades I and II) mobilizations.

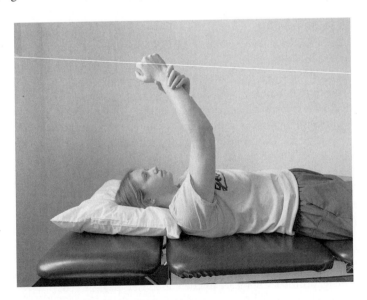

Figure 6-5. Supine overhead stretch using opposite arm.

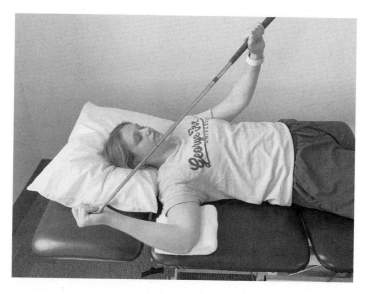

Figure 6-6. Supine external rotation stretch with wand.

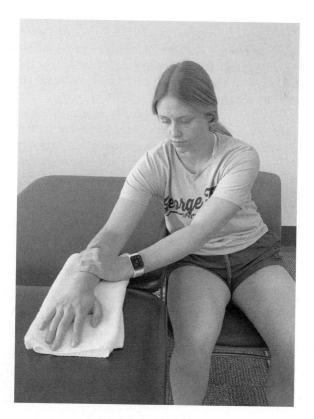

Figure 6-7. Sitting with arm supported on table to perform shoulder flexion PROM.

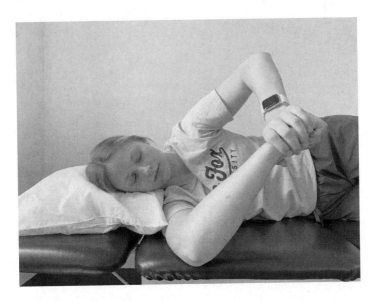

Figure 6-8. Sleeper stretch.

As the tissue becomes less irritable (moderate stage), the intensity of ROM/ stretching exercises may be progressed along with progression from low-grade to high-grade (Maitland grades III and IV) mobilizations. Finally, at the low irritability stage, high-grade mobilizations (Maitland) and sustained holds (Kaltenborn) can be added.[24] This proposed strategy incorporates the successful treatment programs that have used either pain-free ROM exercises or manual therapy techniques. To determine the efficacy of a stage-specific therapeutic program, researchers will need to progress patients based on specific diagnostic criteria. In this way, therapists can implement treatments based on evidence-based criteria, rather than their impression of the patient's stage.

Table 6-4 STRETCHING/ROM EXERCISES FREQUENTLY PRESCRIBED TO PATIENTS WITH PRIMARY AC	
Exercise	**Alternate Positions/Strategies**
Pendulum exercises	Pendulum exercise with hand of involved shoulder weight bearing on Physioball
Supine overhead stretch using opposite arm (Fig. 6-5)	1. Sitting: arm supported on table (Fig. 6-7) 2. Standing: shoulder flexion with arms placed on Physioball
Supine external rotation stretch with wand (Fig. 6-6)	Sitting: arm supported on table and using wand to assist shoulder external rotation
Overhead pulleys	Wall walks
Sleeper stretch (Fig. 6-8)	1. Cross arm adduction stretch 2. Arm behind back stretch

Evidence-Based Clinical Recommendations

SORT: Strength of Recommendation Taxonomy

A: Consistent, good-quality patient-oriented evidence
B: Inconsistent or limited-quality patient-oriented evidence
C: Consensus, disease-oriented evidence, usual practice, expert opinion, or case series

1. There is a consistent pattern of glenohumeral joint range of motion loss associated with adhesive capsulitis. **Grade C**

2. The coracoid pain test accurately identifies patients with adhesive capsulitis. **Grade B**

3. Modalities increase shoulder ROM and/or decrease pain in patients with adhesive capsulitis. **Grade C**

4. Sustained stretch or oscillatory mobilization techniques increase shoulder ROM in patients with AC. **Grade B**

5. Stretching exercises (self-mobilization) are superior to manual therapy techniques in increasing shoulder ROM and improving function in patients with AC. **Grade B**

COMPREHENSION QUESTIONS

6.1 Which of the cardinal motions of the shoulder experiences the greatest loss of passive motion (as a percentage of the contralateral shoulder) in adhesive capsulitis?

   A. Abduction
   B. External rotation
   C. Internal rotation
   D. Flexion

6.2 Which of the following statements correctly identifies the differences between primary and secondary adhesive capsulitis (AC)?

   A. Primary AC is due to trauma whereas secondary AC is due to surgery.
   B. In general, the pain experienced by those with a diagnosis of secondary AC is greater than the pain intensity experienced by those with primary AC.
   C. Primary AC is idiopathic and secondary AC is due to either surgery or trauma.
   D. External rotation is significantly decreased in those with secondary AC, but not in those with primary AC.

6.3 Joint mobilization techniques are used to increase shoulder PROM and AROM in patients with AC. Which technique used by Johnson et al.[44] significantly increased shoulder ER?

A. Anterior glide end-range mobilizations (Kaltenborn grade III)

B. Posterior glide low-grade mobilizations (Maitland grades I and II)

C. Anterior glide low-grade mobilizations (Maitland grades I and II)

D. Posterior glide end-range mobilizations (Kaltenborn grade III)

6.4 Patients with primary AC present with significant loss of ROM, especially shoulder ER. During the first treatment session, the physical therapist wants to prescribe a stretch to increase shoulder ER. The patient is unable to assume a supine position secondary to a pre-existing low back injury. Of the following four exercises, which one would be MOST appropriate to address shoulder ER deficits?

A. Sitting with involved extremity supported on table (elbow at 90°) using a wand to passively mobilize the shoulder into ER

B. Overhead pulleys

C. Sleeper stretch

D. Wall walks

ANSWERS

6.1 **B.** In AC, the greatest overall loss of motion is in shoulder external rotation due to contracture of the anterior and inferior shoulder structures (coracohumeral ligament, rotator interval, and anterior and inferior capsules). Arthroscopic surgical release of the rotator interval may help to rapidly restore external rotation range of motion.

6.2 **C.** Primary AC is idiopathic in nature; there is no known trauma related to the onset of the condition.

6.3 **D.**

6.4 **A.** The other positions are performed to increase shoulder elevation/flexion (options B and D) or IR (option C).

REFERENCES

1. Kaltenborn FM, Evjenth O, Kaltenborn TB, Vollowitz E. *The Spine. Basic Evaluation and Mobilization Techniques.* 2nd ed. Oslo, Norway: Olaf Norlis Bokhandel; 1993.

2. Hengeveld E, Banks K, Maitland GD. *Maitland's Peripheral Manipulation.* 4th ed. Edinburgh, United Kingdom: Butterworths Heinemann;2005.

3. Zuckerman J, Rokito S. Frozen shoulder: a consensus approach. *J Shoulder Elbow Surg.* 2011;20:322-325.

4. Hsu JE, Anakwenze OA, Warrender WJ, Abboud JA. Current review of adhesive capsulitis. *J Shoulder Elbow Surg.* 2011;20:502-514.

5. Balci N, Balci MK, Tuzuner S. Shoulder adhesive capsulitis and shoulder range of motion in type II diabetes mellitus: association with diabetic complications. *J Diabetes Complications.* 1999;13:135-140.

6. Hand C, Clipsham K, Rees JL, Carr AJ. Long-term outcome of frozen shoulder. *J Shoulder Elbow Surgery.* 2008;17:231-236.

7. Kelley MJ, Shaffer MA, Kuhn JE, et al. Shoulder pain and mobility deficits: adhesive capsulitis. *J Orthop Sports Phys Ther.* 2013;43:A1-A31.

8. Reeves B. The natural history of the frozen shoulder syndrome. *Scand J Rheumatol.* 1975;4:193-196.

9. Rizk TE, Pinals RS. Frozen shoulder. *Semin Arthritis Rheum.* 1982;11:440-452.

10. Dias R, Cutts S, Massoud S. Frozen shoulder. *BMJ.* 2005;331:1453-1456.

11. Neviaser RJ, Neviaser TJ. The frozen shoulder: diagnosis and management. *Clin Orthop Relat Res.* 1987;223:59-64.

12. Hannafin JA, DiCarlo EF, Wickiewicz TL, Warren RF. Adhesive capsulitis: capsular fibroplasia of the glenohumeral joint. *J Shoulder Elbow Surg.* 1994;3(Suppl 5):435.

13. Neviaser AS, Hannafin JA. Adhesive capsulitis: a review of current treatment. *Am J Sports Med.* 2010;38:2346-2356.

14. Manske RC, Prohaska D. Diagnosis and management of adhesive capsulitis. *Curr Rev Musculoskelet Med.* 2008;1:180-189.

15. Codman EA. *The Shoulder; Rupture of the Supraspinatus Tendon and Other Lesions in or About the Subacromial Bursa.* Thomas Todd Co., Boston:1934.

16. Neviaser JS. Adhesive capsulitis of the shoulder: a study of pathological findings in periarthritis of the shoulder. *J Bone Joint Surg Am.* 1945;27:211-222.

17. Le HV, Lee SJ, Nazarian A, Rodriguez EK. Adhesive capsulitis of the shoulder: review of pathophysiology and current clinical treatments. *Shoulder Elbow.* 2017;9:75-84.

18. Rodeo SA, Hannafin JA, Tom J, et al. Immunolocalization of cytokines and their receptors in adhesive capsulitis of the shoulder. *J Orthop Res.* 1997;15:427-436.

19. Bunker TD, Reilly J, Baird KS, Hamblen DL. Expression of growth factors, cytokines and matrix metalloproteinases in frozen shoulder. *J Bone Joint Surg Br.* 2000;82:768-773.

20. Cho CH, Song KS, Kim BS, et al. Biological aspect of pathophysiology for frozen shoulder. *Biomed Res Int.* 2018;7274517.

21. Gharaee-Kermani M, Phan SH. Role of cytokines and cytokine therapy in wound healing and fibrotic diseases. *Curr Pharm Des.* 2001;7:1083-1103.

22. Prodromidis AD, Charalambous CP. Is there a genetic predisposition to frozen shoulder?: A systematic review and meta-analysis. *JBJS Rev.* 2016;4:e4.

23. Green HD, Jones A, Evans JP, et al. A genome-wide association study identifies 5 loci associated with frozen shoulder and implicates diabetes as a causal risk factor. *PLoS Genet.* 2021;7:e1009577.

24. Kelley MJ, McClure PW, Leggin BG. Frozen shoulder: evidence and a proposed model guiding rehabilitation. *J Orthop Sports Phys Ther.* 2009;39:135-148.

25. Neviaser RJ, Neviaser TJ. The frozen shoulder. Diagnosis and management. *Clin Orthop Relat Res.* 987;223:59-64.

26. Mitsch J, Casey J, McKinnis R, et al. Investigation of a consistent pattern of motion restriction in patients with adhesive capsulitis. *J Man Manip Ther.* 2004;12:153-159.

27. Rundquist PJ, Anderson DD, Guanche CA, Ludewig PM. Shoulder kinematics in subjects with frozen shoulder. *Arch Phys Med Rehabil.* 2003;84:1473-1479.

28. Rundquist PJ, Ludewig PM. Patterns of motion loss in subjects with idiopathic loss of shoulder range of motion. *Clin Biomech.* 2004;19:810-818.

29. Carbone S, Gumina S, Vestri AR, Postacchini R. Coracoid pain test: a new clinical sign of shoulder adhesive capsulitis. *Int Orthop.* 2010;34:385-388.

30. Buchbinder R, Hoving JL, Green S, et al. Short course prednisolone for adhesive capsulitis (frozen shoulder or stiff painful shoulder): a randomised, double blind, placebo controlled trial. *Ann Rheum Dis.* 2004;63:1460-1469.

31. Lorbach O, Anagnostakos K, Scherf C, et al. Nonoperative management of adhesive capsulitis of the shoulder: oral cortisone application versus intra-articular cortisone injections. *J Shoulder Elbow Surg.* 2010;19:172-179.

32. Bal A, Eksioglu E, Gulec B, et al. Effectiveness of corticosteroid injection in adhesive capsulitis. *Clin Rehabil.* 2008;22:503-512.

33. Bell AD, Conaway D. Corticosteroid injections for painful shoulders. *Int J Clin Pract.* 2005;59:1178-1186.

34. Blanchard V, Barr S, Cerisola FL. The effectiveness of corticosteroid injections compared with physio-therapeutic interventions for adhesive capsulitis: a systematic review. *Physiotherapy.* 2010;96:95-107.

35. Calis M, Demir H, Ulker S, et al. Is intraarticular sodium hyaluronate injection an alternative treatment in patients with adhesive capsulitis? *Rheumatol Int.* 2006;26:536-540.

36. Cheing GL, So EM, Chao CY. Effectiveness of electroacupuncture and interferential electrotherapy in the management of frozen shoulder. *J Rehabil Med.* 2008;40:166-170.

37. Gulick DT, Borger A, McNamee L. Effect of analgesic nerve block electrical stimulation in a patient with adhesive capsulitis. *Physiother Theory Pract.* 2007;23:57-63.

38. Levine WN, Kashyap CP, Bak SF, et al. Nonoperative management of idiopathic adhesive capsulitis. *J Shoulder Elbow Surg.* 2007;16:569-573.

39. Lorbach O, Anagnostakos K, Scherf C, et al. Nonoperative management of adhesive capsulitis of the shoulder: oral cortisone application versus intra-articular cortisone injections. *J Shoulder Elbow Surg.* 2010;19:172-179.

40. Harrast MA, Rao AG. The stiff shoulder. *Phys Med Rehabil Clin N Am.* 2004;15:557-573.

41. Yilmazlar A, Turker G, Atici T, et al. Functional results of conservative therapy accompanied by interscalene brachial plexus block and patient-controlled analgesia in cases with frozen shoulder. *Acta Orthop Traumatol Turc.* 2010;44:105-110.

42. Tasto JP, Elias DW. Adhesive capsulitis. *Sports Med Arthrosc.* 2007;15:216-221.

43. Jewell DV, Riddle DL, Thacker LR. Increased or decreased likelihood of pain reduction and improved function in patients with adhesive capsulitis: a retrospective cohort study. *Phys Ther.* 2009;89:419-429.

44. Johnson AJ, Godges JJ, Zimmerman GJ, Ounanian LL. The effect of anterior versus posterior glide joint mobilization on external rotation range of motion in patients with shoulder adhesive capsulitis. *J Orthop Sports Phys Ther.* 2007;37:88-99.

45. Miller MD, Wirth MA, Rockwood CA Jr. Thawing the frozen shoulder: the "patient" patient. *Orthopedics.* 1996;19:849-853.

46. Vermeulen HM, Obermann WR, Burger BJ, et al. End-range mobilization techniques in adhesive capsulitis of the shoulder joint: a multiple-subject case report. *Phys Ther.* 2000;80:1204-1213.

47. Vermeulen HM, Rozing PM, Obermann WR, et al. Comparison of high-grade and low-grade mobilization techniques in the management of adhesive capsulitis of the shoulder: randomized controlled trial. *Phys Ther.* 2006;86:355-368.

48. Wies J. Treatment of eight patients with frozen shoulder: a case study series. *J Bodyw Mov Ther.* 2005;9:58-64.

49. Yang JL, Chang CW, Chen SY, et al. Mobilization techniques in subjects with frozen shoulder syndrome: randomized multiple-treatment trial. *Phys Ther.* 2007;87:1307-1315.

50. Agarwal S, Raza S, Moiz JA, et al. Effects of two different mobilization techniques on pain, range of motion and functional disability in patients with adhesive capsulitis: a comparative study. *J Phys Ther Sci.* 2016; 28:3342-3349.

51. Brumitt J. [Commentary on] The effect of anterior versus posterior glide joint mobilization on external rotation range of motion in patients with shoulder adhesive capsulitis. *NZ J Physiother.* 2008;36:29-30.

52. Griggs SM, Ahn A, Green A. Idiopathic adhesive capsulitis. A prospective functional outcome study of nonoperative treatment. *J Bone J Surg.* 2000;82-A:1398-1407.

53. Diercks RL, Stevens M. Gentle thawing of the frozen shoulder: a prospective study of supervised neglect versus intensive physical therapy in seventy-seven patients with frozen shoulder syndrome followed up for two years. *J Shoulder Elbow Surg.* 2004;13:499-502.

Chronic Cervical Spine Pain

Jake Bleacher

CASE 7

A 43-year-old female was referred to outpatient physical therapy for chronic neck pain by her family physician. The patient has worked as an administrative assistant for the past 20 years. Her initial onset of neck pain was 2 years ago with a significant increase in pain in the past 6 months. On the numerical pain rating scale, she reports a pain score of 2/10 at the beginning of the day, which worsens to 10/10 by the end of the day. She describes her symptoms as "tightness" and "aching" extending from the superior scapula and shoulder up toward her neck and occipital area. Recently, she has had headaches and an "aching" pain radiating into her dominant right arm by the end of the day. Her day consists of sitting at a computer 75% of the time and using the computer mouse 50% of that time. Her workload has increased 2 to 3 hours per day (overtime) due to staffing shortages over the past 6 months. She denies any significant medical history or trauma to the cervical spine and her cervical x-rays are unremarkable. She reports a small improvement in her symptoms over the last week since she started taking a non-steroidal anti-inflammatory medication and a muscle relaxant prescribed by her family physician. She states that she has been exercising less frequently during the past 2 years due to her busy schedule.

▶ Based on the patient's diagnosis, what do you anticipate may be the contributing factors to her condition?
▶ What are the most appropriate physical therapy outcome measures for neck pain?
▶ What are the concerns regarding the pain radiating into her arm and shoulder?
▶ What are the most appropriate physical therapy interventions?
▶ Would this patient benefit from PNE (pain neuroscience education)?

KEY DEFINITIONS

CENTRAL SENSITIZATION: An increased response by the central nervous system to a normal or subthreshold pain stimulus

ELONGATED MUSCLE: Lengthening of a muscle secondary to being in a sustained elongated position for prolonged period of time

ERGONOMIC INTERVENTION: Workstation assessment to determine risk or extent of injury, followed by implementation of workstation modifications to decrease musculoskeletal symptoms

FORWARD HEAD POSTURE: Position of the head that is markedly anterior to an imaginary line bisecting the glenohumeral joint resulting in mid- and lower-cervical spine flexion and upper cervical spine extension

NEUROMUSCULAR CONTROL: Integration of peripheral sensations relative to joint position to produce an effective efferent motor response

PAIN NEUROSCIENCE EDUCATION (PNE): Educational approach designed to inform patient regarding underlying mechanisms of pain, decrease the perceived threat of their pain, and provide better coping strategies

POSTURAL NECK PAIN: Pain associated with sustained static loading of the cervical spine and shoulder girdle during occupational or leisure activities

POSTURE: Segmental alignment of the body at rest or in equilibrium with the forces acting on the body

TRIGGER POINT: Knots or nodes that form within a taut band of muscle or at myotendinous junctions

TRIGGER POINT DRY NEEDLING: Insertion and manipulation of a thin monofilament needle into taut muscular bands within skeletal muscle with the intent to treat musculoskeletal pain and movement impairments

VALSALVA TEST: Test used to diagnose cervical radiculopathy, whereby a forced expiration against a closed glottis slightly increases intraspinal pressure. The test is positive if it exacerbates symptoms associated with nerve impingement.

Objectives

1. Describe postural neck pain and its contributing factors.
2. Describe components of the musculoskeletal examination that would assist in ruling in postural neck pain and ruling out cervical and/or shoulder conditions.
3. Prescribe appropriate treatment interventions for the patient with postural neck pain.
4. Identify factors complicating the treatment of patients with postural neck pain.
5. Describe key elements in designing a work-style intervention for a patient with postural neck pain.
6. List risk factors for the development of postural neck pain.

Physical Therapy Considerations

Physical therapy considerations during management of the individual with postural cervical pain:

▶ **General physical therapy plan of care/goals:** Decrease pain; increase muscular flexibility and strength; improve postural awareness and correction strategies

▶ **Physical therapy interventions:** Manual therapy, including the use of dry needling, to decrease pain, decrease circulatory stasis and improve muscle and joint flexibility; patient education regarding symptoms and cause and effect of chronic sustained postures; postural and movement correction strategies to minimize postural stress; exercises to improve muscular strength and endurance in cervical and shoulder girdle stabilizing muscles; stress management; work and computer station modifications to minimize postural strain

▶ **Precautions during physical therapy:** Rule out the possibility of significant cervical pathology including cervical disc herniation, spondylosis, thoracic outlet syndrome, cervical stenosis, and nonmusculoskeletal causes of pain; monitor vital signs; address precautions or contraindications for exercise; bruising, bleeding, infection, and a vagal response are risks associated with dry needling

▶ **Complications interfering with physical therapy:** Patient's inability to minimize continuous hours at the computer or to take substantial rest periods; potential development of chronic pain

Understanding the Health Condition

Postural neck pain (PNP) is associated with low levels of static stress to musculoskeletal tissues with very little to no relaxation.[1] PNP is common in individuals who work primarily on computers or at video display terminals. Based on studies in Australia and Sweden, prevalence ranges from 20% to 63% with a higher rate in female office workers.[2] Epidemiologic studies examining risks associated with musculoskeletal disorders of the neck and shoulder have found strong correlations between longer duration of computer usage and higher prevalence rates of neck and arm symptoms.[3-5] In a study of more than a thousand high school computer users, frequent computer exposure was the one consistent predictor of developing neck pain.[5] Additional risk factors for the development of PNP are psychosocial stress, wearing bifocal lenses, using a computer mouse for extended periods of time, and prolonged bouts of computer use without a rest period.[4] Recent systematic reviews have found that **females or a history of neck pain are the strongest and most consistent risk factors for new onset of neck pain** in office workers and in the general population.[6,7] McClean et al.[6] identified additional risk factors for nonspecific neck pain including high job demands, smoking history, and low social support.

The physical demands of computer work include low-level static exertions in which there is little to no relaxation phase for the muscles involved. Muscles that are commonly painful in individuals with PNP include splenius capitis and cervicis, upper trapezius, levator scapulae, sternocleidomastoid, and the scalenes. The head and neck postures typically adopted with prolonged computer use affect these muscles because they span the shoulder girdle and cervical and thoracic spinal regions. The effects of sustained low-load forces can cause creep—the time-dependent deformation to soft tissues.[5,8] This low-level mechanical tissue deformation may cause inflammation, stimulation of nociceptors in affected tissues, and the development of myofascial trigger points.[1] When these low-level stresses are applied over a long period of time, it can cause excessive wear to articular surfaces, stretching of ligaments, and development of osteophytes and bone spurs.[9] Over a period of time, central sensitization can also occur. In central sensitization, there is a hypervigilant response to a (painful) stimulus that is partially due to malfunction of descending inhibitory pain pathways.[10] Central sensitization is observed in chronic pain conditions such as osteoarthritis, fibromyalgia, and in computer users with significant neck and shoulder pain.[11]

Symptom chronicity also contributes to altered neuromuscular recruitment and activation patterns in muscles that are frequently affected in patients with PNP. Szeto et al.[12] found that individuals with neck pain related to computer use had aberrant muscle activation patterns in the upper trapezius as well as frequent scapular protraction compared to an asymptomatic control group. In fact, postural muscles of symptomatic individuals work *harder* and *longer* when using a computer mouse. Using electromyography (EMG), Szeto et al.[12,13] found that individuals with PNP had significantly higher levels of muscle contraction and fewer periods of rest in the upper trapezius and erector spinae compared to asymptomatic individuals with similar exposure working at a computer. Falla et al.[14] found that when subjects with chronic PNP performed a functional reach test, there was an increased latency in the feed-forward contraction of the deep cervical flexors (longus colli and longus capitis) necessary for joint support and control. In addition, the superficial muscles (scalenes and sternocleidomastoid) of those with PNP exhibited increased activity and fatigability along with a lack of coordinated activation with the deep cervical flexors.[14]

Individuals with chronic PNP also exhibit poor postural and kinesthetic awareness. Edmondston et al.[15] found that individuals with chronic PNP had a different perception of "good posture" than those without symptoms. Symptomatic individuals demonstrated a protracted head position and more upper cervical extension than the asymptomatic group. Falla et al.[16] demonstrated similar findings: individuals with PNP had a reduced ability to maintain an erect neutral spine posture when performing a typing task.

Key **intrinsic factors** contributing to the perpetuation of chronic postural cervical pain include differences in neuromuscular control and decreased postural awareness.[17] **Extrinsic factors** contributing to PNP include the workstation setup (*e.g.*, seating, keyboard, monitor, mouse), frequency and duration of time spent at the computer, and psychosocial factors such as stress involved with high work demands and decreased rest periods.[18-20]

Physical Therapy Patient/Client Management

Physical therapy management of patients with chronic PNP may include the use of modalities, soft tissue and joint mobilization, therapeutic exercises, postural correction strategies, and ergonomic interventions.[2,4,6] In 2017, the Orthopaedic

Section of the American Physical Therapy Association revised the clinical practice guidelines (CPGs) for chronic neck pain.[21] The CPGs reiterated a multimodal approach including cervical and thoracic joint mobilizations and manipulations, neuromuscular exercises for the cervical spine and scapular regions, dry needling, postural education, and cognitive affective training.[21]

At the beginning of treatment sessions, passive treatments (*e.g.*, electrical stimulation, ultrasound, soft tissue and joint mobilization, and dry needling) are often used to decrease pain and muscle guarding. Therapeutic exercises should initially focus on re-educating the deep cervical flexors and postural muscles with general strengthening exercises introduced later.[16] This treatment approach is similar to that used when treating a patient with low back pain in which the initial focus is on activating the local stabilizing muscles (transversus abdominis and multifidi) followed by the prescription of general and functional strengthening exercises.[17] To prevent *recurrence* of PNP, appropriate management strategies need to be implemented. These include teaching proper ergonomic workstation setup and implementing rest periods and preventative exercises.[17,22] Behavioral modifications to reduce stress and to monitor total time working on the computer are essential.[14,19,23]

Examination, Evaluation, and Diagnosis

Individuals presenting with PNP tend to have symptoms of low to moderate intensity that do not preclude them from performing functional and work-related tasks. Symptoms of PNP are generally chronic in nature, lacking a history of acute onset or significant trauma. Due to the insidious onset of symptoms, the physical therapist must rule out systemic pathology through a thorough medical history, including any recent health status changes (*e.g.*, unexplained weight loss), nonmechanical pain, and/or history of cancer.[24] A mechanical source of symptoms has predictable pain patterns and symptoms should be intermittent and mitigated when the underlying stressors are decreased or eliminated. Symptoms of PNP should be worse during sustained activities or postures at computer workstations, and diminished when not performing these activities.[24] Use of a **self-report outcome questionnaire such as the NDI (Neck Disability Index) is recommended** at initial examination and at intervals during the plan of care to determine prognosis and change over time. Schellingerhout *et al.*[25] found the NDI to have adequate measurement properties and is one of the most frequently used outcome measures for neck pain.

When PNP symptoms radiate into the arm, it is important to rule out more serious pathology including, but not limited to cervical disc herniation, degenerative joint disease, or foraminal stenosis. A neurologic examination including testing of deep tendon reflexes, manual muscle testing of the cervical myotomes, and sensory testing for dermatomal changes must be performed. One of the differential diagnoses that the physical therapist must rule out is cervical radiculopathy (Table 7-1). A clinical prediction rule (CPR) for assisting in the diagnosis of cervical radiculopathy has been established and found to be reliable.[26] The CPR for diagnosis of cervical radiculopathy consists of positive findings on several tests: ipsilateral cervical rotation <60°, positive cervical spine compression and distraction (Figs. 7-1 and 7-2), positive Spurling's test (Fig. 7-3), and positive Upper Limb

Table 7-1	SPECIAL TESTS TO RULE IN CERVICAL RADICULOPATHY	
Tests	**Patient Position**	**Findings**
Cervical compression	Patient is seated. Therapist stands behind patient with hands folded and resting on crown of head. Therapist gently applies axial load downward. (Fig. 7-1)	Reproduction of pain in the arm or shoulder constitutes a positive test.
Cervical distraction	Patient is seated. Therapist stands behind patient. With the heels of hands under mandible, therapist applies upward vertical distraction force on head on neck. (Fig. 7-2)	Relief of shoulder or upper extremity pain constitutes a positive test.
Spurling's test	Patient is seated. Therapist stands behind patient. Patient actively side bends head *toward* affected side. Therapist then applies an axial load on the head in the side bent position. (Fig. 7-3)	Reproduction of arm or neck pain on same side of compression constitutes a positive test.
Upper Limb Tension Test I	Patient is supine. Therapist stands facing patient at shoulder level. Therapist depresses shoulder girdle, abducts glenohumeral joint to ~110°. With patient's elbow flexed at 90°, forearm in neutral rotation and wrist slightly extended, the therapist gently extends elbow wrist and fingers at same time while supinating the forearm. (Fig. 7-4)	Reproduction of upper extremity symptoms constitutes a positive test.

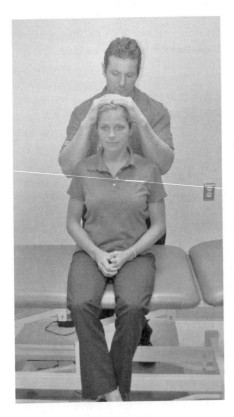

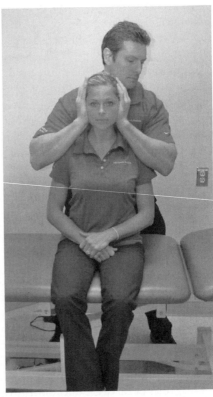

Figure 7-1. Cervical compression.

Figure 7-2. Cervical distraction.

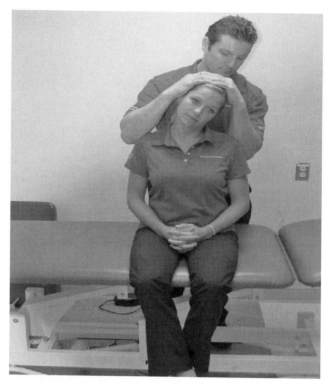

Figure 7-3. Spurling's test.

Tension Test (ULTT I; Fig. 7-4).[26] The recent 2017 CPGs also recommend use of the Valsalva test for cervical radiculopathy because of its high specificity (0.94).[21] In individuals presenting with chronic PNP, these tests are typically *negative* for reproducing peripheral symptoms because the source of chronic PNP is myofascial and not neurovascular.[26,27]

It is critical to observe the patient in her natural posture to be able to gather information on typical postural awareness and habits. Valuable information can be gathered by observing the patient in the waiting area as well as during the subjective history, when she is less aware that her posture is being assessed.

A detailed standing postural assessment should be performed from anterior, posterior, and lateral views observing for postural deviations and muscular asymmetries.[9] In the *ideal* posture, the ear bisects the acromion and the bodies of the cervical vertebrae. A common posture observed in the person with PNP is a forward head posture in which the head is anterior to the acromion, shoulders are rounded anteriorly, scapulae are protracted, and the mid- and lower-cervical spine are flexed with compensatory upper cervical extension (Fig. 7-5).

Active range of motion (ROM) of the cervical spine is measured in all directions, noting any limitations and painful responses. The cervical range of motion device (CROM; Performance Attainment Associates, St. Paul, MN) is a device worn by the patient as a head and spectacle frame with a shoulder-mounted piece. It consists

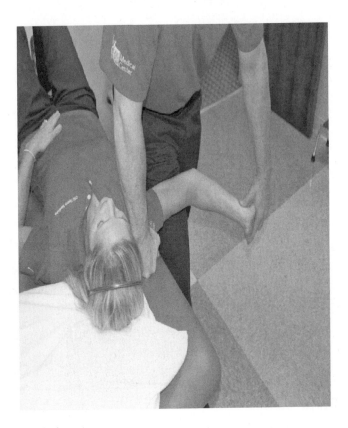

Figure 7-4. Upper limb tension test.

of three gravity-driven dial meters to measure cervical ROM in three axes of movement.[26] The CROM device has good reliability and validity in measuring cervical ROM in asymptomatic and symptomatic individuals.[21,26]

Muscle length or flexibility tests, as well as palpation tests, should be performed to confirm adaptively shortened or lengthened muscles and to identify trigger points. The muscles that typically present with decreased flexibility (adaptive shortening) due to a chronic forward head posture are levator scapulae, sternocleidomastoids, scalenes, suboccipitals, upper trapezius, and pectoralis major and minor. Chronic forward head posture typically lengthens lower cervical and thoracic erector spinae, middle and lower trapezius, rhomboids, and deep cervical flexors. Lengthened muscles are typically weaker due to the altered relationship of the contractile elements (actin and myosin) when the muscles are in sustained stretched positions.[28] This pattern of opposing muscle tightness and weakness has been referred to as "upper crossed syndrome." The habitual "poking" chin of the forward head posture causes tightness in upper cervical region and weakness in deep neck flexors, tightness in the anterior chest and shoulders, and weakness in the scapular stabilizers (Fig. 7-5).[8,9,26] Manual muscle testing must be performed to confirm the weakness in the muscles commonly lengthened (middle and lower trapezius, rhomboids, and deep neck flexors) in patients presenting with chronic forward head posture.

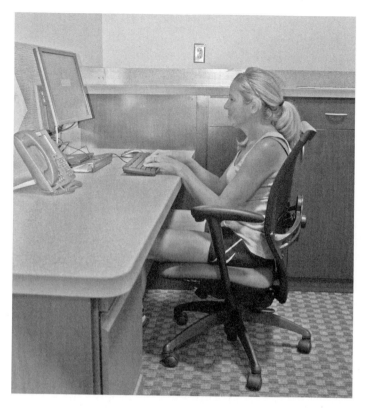

Figure 7-5. Forward head sitting posture.

Due to the importance of the deep cervical flexors in maintaining ideal cervical posture, an assessment of the strength and endurance of the deep cervical flexors should be performed. The supine capital flexion test is performed by having the patient lie supine and raise her head approximately two inches off the table while keeping the chin tucked. The physical therapist records the time she is able to maintain the chin in a tucked position.[22,29] Jull et al.[30] have modified the test by placing a pressure sensor (stabilizer or blood pressure cuff) in the suboccipital region while the patient performs a head nod, and holds this position for 5 to 10 seconds in five incremental stages starting at a baseline of 20 mm Hg and working to a final level of 30 mm Hg (craniocervical flexion test, Fig. 7-6). If the patient is unable to perform neck flexion with incremental increases in pressure and maintain the position for the allotted time without compensation of the superficial neck flexors (resorting to retraction), this indicates decreased neuromuscular control and endurance of the deep neck flexors.

Joint mobility assessment must be performed to determine areas of cervical and thoracic spine hypomobility. In patients with chronic forward head posture, mobility restrictions are common in the upper cervical and upper- and mid-thoracic regions.[31,32] Fernandez-de-las-Penas et al.[31] found that subjects with forward head posture had significantly decreased mean craniovertebral angles and limitations in

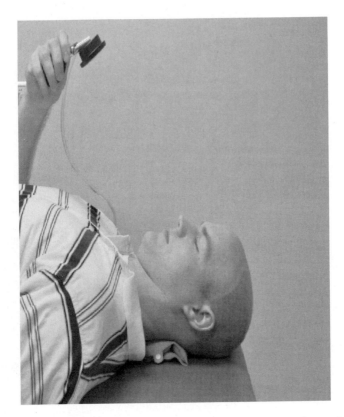

Figure 7-6. Test position for the craniocervical flexion test. The exercise for the deep neck flexors is also performed in this position.

cervical ROM in almost all directions compared to a control group. Typically, palpation and spring tests to the involved joint segments are hypomobile and elicit a painful response with accessory motion testing. Jull *et al.*[33] found excellent interexaminer reliability between experienced manual therapists in identifying dysfunctional symptomatic joints in the cervical spine.

Palpation of the levator scapulae and the upper trapezius is recommended to determine which muscles are contributing to the patient's neck pain. The updated CPGs for chronic cervical spine pain found that pressure algometry has excellent intra-rater reliability ($ICC_{2,1} = 0.96$) and its use is recommended to classify pain.[21] In the event that clinicians do not have access to a pressure algometer, graded palpatory pressure to the muscle(s) should be performed to determine the extent of muscular involvement.

Last, the physical therapist needs to assess how the patient performs her occupation. A work style assessment includes looking at the interaction of ergonomic and psychosocial risk factors affecting the development and maintenance of shoulder and neck pain in office workers. There is a complex interaction between biomechanical stressors resulting from poor ergonomics and psychosocial stressors involved with high-volume workload.

Plan of Care and Interventions

A standardized program of 12 physical therapy sessions over 4 to 6 weeks is recommended to address musculoskeletal impairments, correct faulty posture, and implement appropriate ergonomic interventions.[33-38]

Restoring pain-free ROM through the use of modalities, active range of motion (AROM) exercises, dry needling, and joint mobilizations to the cervical and thoracic spine may alleviate pain, muscle guarding, and circulatory stasis.[37] Loss of cervical AROM, especially retraction and rotation, is common in patients with PNP. Loss of these motions is due to chronic forward head posture and muscular tightness in the superficial cervical and axial skeletal muscles. The performance of frequent gentle cervical retraction and cervical rotation (up to 5 times per day) in a neutral spine position helps restore cervical AROM.[23] If excessive pain or muscle guarding prevents the patient from being able to perform the exercises in a weight-bearing position, exercises may be initiated in supine and progress to sitting. To regain normal postural control and alignment, muscles that have become adaptively shortened in the axial skeleton and upper cervical spine need to have adequate muscle flexibility. Table 7-2 outlines static stretching exercises for the

Table 7-2   POSTURAL EXERCISES FOR THE PATIENT WITH POSTURAL NECK PAIN

Exercise	Starting Position	Exercise Technique
Cervical retraction	Sitting with fingertips placed on chin. (Fig. 7-7)	Push head straight backward until stretch is felt in neck and upper thoracic region. Hold 5-10 seconds.
Cervical rotation	Sitting with head in a neutral position (not in forward head posture)	Rotate head as far as possible in one direction without pain and apply slight overpressure with your hand in a pain-free range. Hold 5 seconds. Repeat to other side.
Suboccipital stretch	Supine with 2-3 inch towel roll placed at base of occiput (Fig. 7-8)	Slide occiput superiorly, maintaining contact of head on table. Hold position 10 seconds.
Pectoralis stretch	Standing in a corner with elbows at shoulder height. (Fig. 7-9)	Lean toward corner slowly until stretch is felt in anterior chest. Hold 30 seconds.
Upper trapezius stretch	Sitting with one arm behind back, slightly depressing shoulder, rest opposite hand on side of head. (Fig. 7-10)	Using hand on top of head, gently pull head laterally while depressing opposite shoulder until stretch is felt trapezius. Hold for 30 seconds.
Levator scapulae stretch	Sitting with one arm behind back and other arm on occipital area. (Fig. 7-11)	Gently pull head down toward axilla until stretch is felt in levator scapulae. Hold for 30 seconds.
Upper extremity wall slides	Standing with back and against wall (arms close to a 90°/90° position). (Fig. 7-12)	Slide arms upward as far as possible, while always maintaining contact of arms against wall.

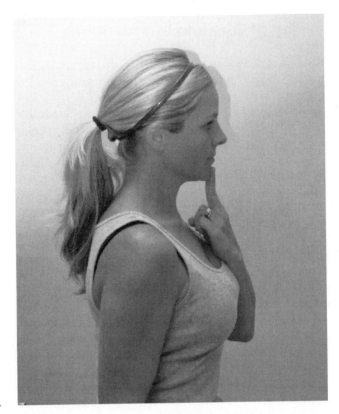

Figure 7-7. Cervical retraction (chin tuck).

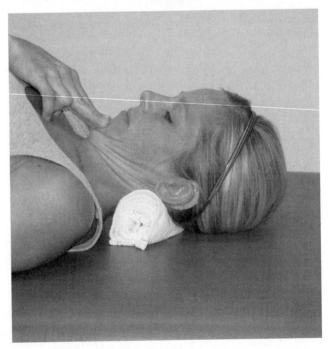

Figure 7-8. Suboccipital stretch.

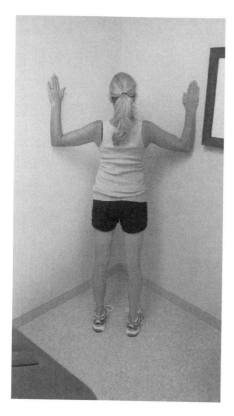

Figure 7-9. Corner pectoralis stretch.

patient with PNP. Typically, each stretch should be performed for 30 seconds for 2 repetitions, performed 3 times per day. Dry needling is an emerging physical therapy modality that may alleviate neck pain resulting from muscular tightness. Cerezo-Tello et al.[39] randomized 130 patients with chronic nonspecific neck pain to one of two treatments groups. Over a 2-week period, the experimental group performed stretching exercises and received 4 sessions of dry needling, whereas the control group only performed the stretching exercises. At 15, 30, 90, and 180 days after completion of the study, the experimental group had significantly greater improvements in ROM, mechanical hyperalgesia, neck muscle strength, and disability scores compared to the control group.

Patients with PNP demonstrate impaired activation patterns and decreased endurance in the deep cervical flexors, similar to the dysfunctional activation patterns of the transverse abdominis displayed by patients with low back pain. Jull et al.[30] demonstrated the importance of **improving neuromuscular control and endurance in the deep cervical flexors in maintaining cervical posture and stabilizing the cervical spine** when performing reaching and upper extremity tasks. The training program consisted of low-load activation of the deep flexors using a pressure gauge (Stabilometer, Chattanooga Group Inc, Hixson, TN). Each repetition was held for up to 10 seconds to increase endurance of the deep flexors and avoid activating the superficial cervical muscles. The gauge was set at 20 mm Hg pressure

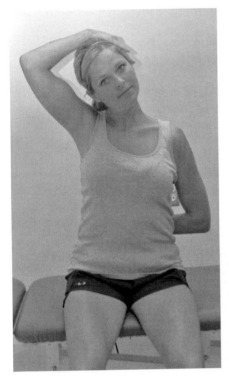

Figure 7-10. Upper trapezius stretch.

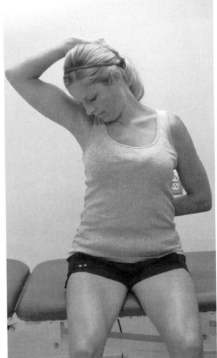

Figure 7-11. Levator scapulae stretch.

with 10-second holds and increased by incremental steps of 2 mm Hg using color-coded stripes for visual feedback[30] (Fig. 7-6).

Strengthening exercises to improve scapular orientation and muscle recruitment patterns should be prescribed to individuals with PNP. Chronic forward head posture decreases activation in the scapular stabilizers due to aberrant positioning of the scapula from midline. Frequently, the middle and lower trapezius, rhomboids, and serratus anterior have decreased activation patterns in patients experiencing cervical and shoulder pain.[12,38] The stabilizing muscles of the scapulae can be adequately trained with low-load exercises and the use of visual or verbal cues for scapular positioning (Table 7-3). Using EMG recordings, Wegner *et al.*[38] showed that patients with chronic PNP who demonstrated altered scapular activation patterns during a typing task significantly improved activation of the middle trapezius by following simple instructions and feedback to position their scapulae in midline. For example, patients presenting with a downwardly rotated scapula were instructed to "gently lift the tip of your shoulder" to improve scapular orientation and muscle activation.

Joint mobilizations to the cervical spine and manipulation to the thoracic spine also improves cervical ROM and decreases pain in patients with PNP.[22,31,36,40] A systematic Cochrane review comparing manipulation versus mobilization for

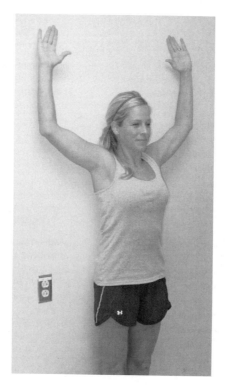

Figure 7-12. Upper extremity wall slides.

patients with neck pain concluded there was moderate quality evidence that both treatments produced similar improvements in pain, function, and patient satisfaction at a 6-month follow-up.[41]

Identifying and addressing risk factors contributing to chronic PNP is an important component for achieving long-term success. Once discharged from physical therapy, most patients return to the same pursuits, likely spending a significant amount of work and leisure time at video display terminals in sustained postures.[4,19] An ergonomic assessment and intervention should be performed to address improper workstation setup. An adjustable chair that is appropriately fitted can significantly reduce shoulder and neck pain.[2] Proper seat height allows for comfortable resting positions of the spine and lower extremities by helping maintain a lumbar lordosis. The hips should be slightly elevated above the level of the knees with the feet resting on the floor.[2] The keyboard should be placed at or below the height of the elbows. Forearms should rest on the desk or chair armrests to allow for neutral shoulder, elbow, and wrist postures. This neutral upper extremity posture has consistently demonstrated reduced muscle activity in the upper extremities, thereby decreasing the risk of developing musculoskeletal disorders.[4,19] The computer mouse should be positioned to avoid excessive shoulder abduction and scapular protraction. The monitor should be directly in front of the individual's

Table 7-3 SCAPULAR STABILIZATION STRENGTHENING EXERCISES

Scapular Exercise	Starting Position	Exercise Technique
Prone retraction	Lying prone with small towel roll under forehead, arms at side with palms facing down	Initiate movement by squeezing shoulder blades together, then externally rotate and slightly extend shoulders. Hold for 5-10 seconds. (Fig. 7-13)
Prone middle trapezius	Lying prone with small towel roll under forehead, arms at a 90° angle ("T" position), thumbs pointed up	Initiate movement by squeezing shoulder blades together, then raise both arms parallel to body position. Hold for 5-10 seconds. (Fig. 7-14)
Prone lower trapezius	Lying prone with small towel roll under forehead, arms at a 135° angle ("Y" position), thumbs pointing up	Initiate movement by squeezing shoulder blades together, then raise arms to parallel to body position. Hold for 5-10 seconds. (Fig. 7-15)
Seated row	Seated position and holding resistance band with arms close to body	Allow arms to extend out in front to chest level. Initiate movement by squeezing shoulder blades together, then pull arms to sides.
Serratus wall slide	Standing with forearms in neutral rotation, resting on foam roll at chest level against the wall.	Shift weight forward. Using scapular muscles, slide roll to overhead position. (Fig. 7-16)

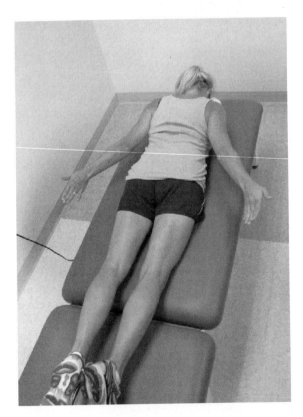

Figure 7-13. Prone scapular retraction.

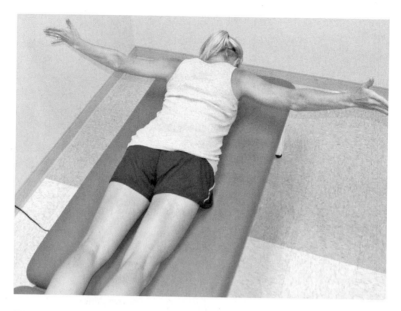

Figure 7-14. Prone middle trapezius.

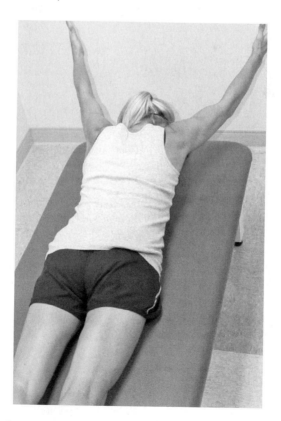

Figure 7-15. Prone lower trapezius.

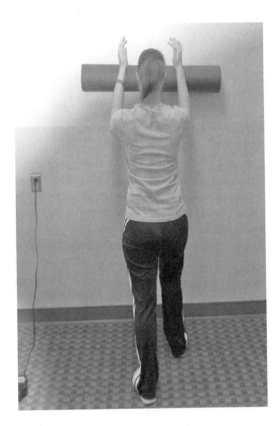

Figure 7-16. Serratus wall slide.

face (at a distance of ~66 cm) and the top of the monitor should be adjusted to eye level to allow for a neutral head position.[38] Less than a 3° upward or downward tilt of the head from a neutral position can have a significant effect on reducing head and neck symptoms.[1]

Postural education and retraining is a necessary component for achieving successful outcomes in patients with PNP. Symptomatic subjects typically demonstrate an increased forward head and shoulder posture[1] and have an increased load in the cervical muscles while performing typing and mousing tasks on the computer.[12] Achieving a neutral spine posture helps equalize load-sharing. This can decrease stress on pain-sensitized structures and improve activation of the deep neck flexors required to maintain cervical lordosis and postural form.[30] To offset the adverse effect of prolonged computer use, the patient should be advised to take 20- to 30-second "microbreaks" every 30 minutes, and not exceed 2 hours while working on the computer. During the microbreaks, the patient should perform basic exercises such as cervical and scapular retraction, thoracic extension, and upper extremity stretching to provide relief to the muscles and joints in the sustained postures.[23]

Falla et al.[16] reported improved activation of spinal stabilizing muscles when subjects sat erect with a neutral posture versus a slumped posture. Instructing an individual to "sit straight up" without cueing was less effective than specific verbal and manual cues to achieve an erect but neutral spine posture. Cueing for achieving a neutral spine posture resulted in significantly greater activation of lumbar multifidi and deep neck flexors than instructions to "sit straight up."[16,39] To achieve the erect neutral posture, subjects were first instructed to achieve the ideal lumbopelvic sitting posture by gently rolling their pelvis forward to rest on the ischial tuberosities, followed by a slight sternal lift, avoiding excessive thoracolumbar extension. Finally, subjects were instructed to lift the occiput minimally to position the head in neutral and to reduce upper cervical extension. The control group was instructed to sit up straight the best they knew how, which resulted in significantly less recruitment of the cervical and lumbar stabilizing muscles. Maintaining a neutral spine posture for prolonged postural activities not only decreases the amount of deleterious stress to the musculoskeletal structures, but also optimally aligns the spine for activation of the deep cervical flexors and lumbar multifidi responsible for maintaining ideal postural form.

In recent years, treatment has focused not only on the biomechanical aspects underlying the development of chronic neck pain, but also on the psychosocial stressors for long-term management of symptoms. **Work style** takes into consideration both the biomechanical and the psychosocial risk factors contributing to the perpetuation of chronic neck pain arising from the imbalance between workload and capacity. A long-term study analyzing the effects of work style interventions showed that a **combined intervention of ergonomic and behavioral changes to manage workload resulted in significant long-term reductions in neck and shoulder pain and recovery rate.** The behavioral changes included training and education regarding taking adequate rest breaks, strategies to cope with high work demands, and increased body awareness with posture.[18,19] In a study aimed to address ergonomic issues and psychosocial issues, Bernaards et al.[18,19] found that when ergonomic interventions were coupled with counseling for behavioral modifications to cope with high work demands, office workers had long-term improvements in neck and shoulder pain. More recently, evidence has shown the benefit of providing **pain neuroscience education (PNE) to patients exhibiting signs of central sensitization such as pain catastrophizing or high self-reported symptoms.** In a multicenter randomized controlled trial with adults with chronic spinal pain, Malfliet et al.[34] compared PNE (experimental group) versus neck/back school (control group) over 3 sessions. Although there was no difference between groups for pain disability (primary outcome measure), only the PNE group experienced significant improvement in kinesiophobia (secondary outcome measure). In the PNE group, pain catastrophizing was significantly decreased in those with high self-reported central sensitization symptoms.

The development of chronic PNP is multifaceted and involves both intrinsic and extrinsic factors contributing to the perpetuation of symptoms. For long-term success, treatment should involve addressing musculoskeletal impairments with traditional physical therapy interventions and ergonomic and psychosocial issues that often contribute to perpetuating the condition.

Evidence-Based Clinical Recommendations

SORT: Strength of Recommendation Taxonomy
A: Consistent, good-quality patient-oriented evidence
B: Inconsistent or limited-quality patient-oriented evidence
C: Consensus, disease-oriented evidence, usual practice, expert opinion, or case series

1. Intrinsic factors such as altered muscular control in the cervical and scapular muscles and decreased postural and kinesthetic awareness contribute to the development of postural neck pain. **Grade B**

2. Extrinsic factors such as poor workstation setup and increased duration of time spent on a video display unit contribute to the development of postural neck pain. **Grade B**

3. Use of an outcome measure with adequate measurement properties, such as the Neck Disability Index (NDI), helps determine prognosis and change over time in patients with neck pain. **Grade A**

4. Exercises aimed at improving deep neck flexor strength improve the ability to maintain cervical posture and stabilize the cervical spine when performing reaching and upper extremity tasks. **Grade B**

5. Interventions aimed at improving an individual's "work style" improve the long-term success of treating postural neck pain. **Grade C**

6. Including PNE in a comprehensive treatment program for individuals with neck pain decreases kinesiophobia. **Grade C**

COMPREHENSION QUESTIONS

7.1 Individuals with chronic postural neck pain typically present with *which* of the following postural positions of the shoulder and neck?

    A. Rounded forward shoulders, scapular retraction, mid- and lower-cervical extension, and upper-cervical flexion

    B. Rounded forward shoulders, scapular protraction, mid- and lower-cervical flexion, and upper-cervical flexion

    C. Depressed shoulders, scapular retraction, mid- and lower-cervical extension, and upper-cervical extension

    D. Rounded forward shoulders, scapular protraction, mid- and lower-cervical flexion, and upper-cervical extension

7.2 When *initiating* an exercise program for individuals with chronic postural neck pain, early focus should be on *which* of the following?

A. General cardiovascular exercises

B. Isometric cervical and shoulder girdle exercises

C. Strengthening and retraining of the deep cervical flexors

D. Low-load high repetition neck extension exercises

7.3 Which list represents individual risk factors for chronic postural neck pain?

A. Female, wearing bifocals, use of a computer mouse for extended periods, psychosocial stressors

B. Male, psychosocial stressors, use of computer mouse, lower chair

C. Female, contact lenses, right-hand dominant, infrequent rest breaks

D. Male, psychosocial stressors, bifocals, infrequent rest breaks

7.4 Which of the following patients would MOST likely benefit from pain neuro-science education (PNE)?

A. 38-year-old female office worker with 3-week insidious onset of neck and shoulder pain with a numeric pain rating of 9/10 by the end of the work day

B. 45-year-old female office worker with 3-year history of neck pain, history of anxiety, and consistent pain rating of 8/10 in neck and shoulder area with some radiation into arm while working at computer terminal

C. 22-year-old female administrative assistant with 3-month history of neck and shoulder pain with a numeric pain rating of 4/10

D. 60-year-old male information technology worker with 5-month history of daily headaches and neck pain (numeric pain rating 4/10) after working long hours on a project and he has not missed any work.

ANSWERS

7.1 **D.** Postural adaptations typically found in the frequent computer user are the forward rounded shoulders and protracted scapulae, mid- and lower-cervical flexion, and compensatory upper-cervical extension. Frequently, these postural adaptations are due to inadequate workstation setup and decreased attention to maintaining a neutral spine posture.

7.2 **C.** Research has shown the importance of training the deep cervical flexors to maintain postural control and alignment for feed-forward stabilization of the cervical spine with upper extremity use.[2,9]

7.3 **A.** Risk factors for developing postural neck pain in office workers include female sex, frequent computer usage with a computer mouse, eyewear, and psychosocial stressors.[14]

7.4 **B.** The chronicity of symptoms (3 years) with consistently high pain levels (9/10) with relatively low pain stimulus (sitting at desk) are characteristics of individuals with central sensitivity that have been shown to benefit from PNE.

REFERENCES

1. Hoyle JA, Marras WS, Sheedy JE, Hart DE. Effects of postural and visual stressors on myofascial trigger point development and motor unit rotation during computer work. *J Electromyogr Kinesiol.* 2011;21:41-48.

2. Fabrizio P. Ergonomic intervention in the treatment of a patient with upper extremity and neck pain. *Phys Ther.* 2009;89:351-360.

3. Andrews JR, Harrelson GL, Wilk KE. *Physical Rehabilitation of the Injured Athlete.* 3rd ed. Philadelphia, PA: Saunders; 2004.

4. Gerr F, Marcus M, Monteilh C. Epidemiology of musculoskeletal disorders among computer users: lesson learned from the role of posture and keyboard use. *J Electromyogr Kinesiol.* 2004;14:25-31.

5. Johnston V, Souvlis T, Jimmieson NL, Jull G. Associations between individual and workplace risk factors for self-reported neck pain and disability among female office workers. *Appl Ergon.* 2008;39:171-182.

6. McLean SM, May S, Klaber-Moffett J, et al. Risk factors for the onset of non-specific neck pain: a systematic review. *J Epidemiol Community Health.* 2010;64:565-572.

7. Paksaichol A, Janwantanakul P, Purepong N, et al. Office workers' risk factors for the development of non-specific neck pain: a systematic review of prospective cohort studies. *Occup Environ Med.* 2012;69:610-618.

8. Smith L, Louw Q, Crous L, Grimmer-Somers K. Prevalence of neck pain and headaches: impact of computer use and other associative factors. *Cephalgia.* 2009;29:250-257.

9. Magee DJ. *Orthopedic Physical Assessment.* 4th ed. Philadelphia, PA: Saunders; 2002.

10. Malfliet A, Kregel J, Coppeieters I, et al. Effect of pain neuroscience education combined with cognition-targeted motor control training on chronic spinal pain: a randomized clinical trial. *JAMA Neurol.* 2018;75:808-817.

11. Heredia-Riza AM, Petersen KK, Madeleine P, Arendt-Neilsen L. Clinical outcomes and central pain mechanisms are improved after upper trapezius eccentric training in female computer users with chronic neck/shoulder pain. *Clin J Pain.* 2019;35:65-76.

12. Szeto GP, Straker LM, O'Sullivan PB. A comparison of symptomatic and asymptomatic office workers performing monotonous keyboard work–1: neck and shoulder muscle recruitment patterns. *Man Ther.* 2005;10:270-280.

13. Szeto GP, Straker LM, O'Sullivan PB. During computing tasks symptomatic female office workers demonstrate a trend towards higher cervical postural muscle load than asymptomatic office workers: an experimental study. *Aust J Physiother.* 2009;55:257-262.

14. Falla D, Bilenkij G, Jull G. Patients with chronic neck pain demonstrate altered patterns of muscle activation during performance of a functional upper limb task. *Spine.* 2004;29:1436-1440.

15. Edmondston SJ, Chan HY, Ngai GC, et al. Postural neck pain: an investigation of habitual sitting posture, perception of "good" posture and cervicothoracic kinaesthesia. *Man Ther.* 2007;12:363-371.

16. Falla D, O'Leary S, Fagan A, Jull G. Recruitment of the deep cervical flexor muscles during a postural-correction exercise performed in sitting. *Man Ther.* 2007;12:139-143.

17. Caneiro JP, O'Sullivan P, Burnett A, et al. The influence of different sitting postures on head/neck posture and muscle activity. *Man Ther.* 2010;15:54-60.

18. Bernaards CM, Ariens GA, Hildebrandt VH. The cost-effectiveness of a lifestyle physical activity intervention in addition to a work style intervention on the recovery from neck and upper limb symptoms in computer workers. *BMC Musculoskelet Disord.* 2006;7:80.

19. Bernaards CM, Ariens GA, Knol DL, Hildebrandt VH. The effectiveness of a work style intervention and a lifestyle physical activity intervention on the recovery from neck and upper limb symptoms on computer workers. *Pain.* 2007;132:142-153.

20. Falla D. Unravelling the complexity of muscle impairment in chronic neck pain. *Man Ther.* 2004;9:125-133.

21. Blanpied PR, Gross AR, Elliott JM, et al. Neck pain: revision 2017. *J Orthop Sports Phys Ther.* 2017;47(7):A1-A83.

22. Grimmer K. Measuring endurance capacity of the cervical short flexor muscle group. *Aust J Physiother.* 1994;40:251-254.

23. Kisner C, Colby LA. *Therapeutic Exercise: Foundation and Techniques.* 5th ed. Philadelphia, PA: FA Davis Company; 2007.

24. Porterfield JA, DeRosa C. *Mechanical Low Back Pain: Perspectives in Functional Anatomy.* Philadelphia, PA: Saunders;1991.

25. Schellingerhout JM, Heymans MW, Verhagen AP, et al. Measurement properties of translated versions of neck-specific questionnaires: a systematic review. *BMC Med Res Methodol.* 2011;11:87.

26. Wainner RS, Fritz JM, Irrgang JJ, et al. Reliability and diagnostic accuracy of the clinical examination and patient self-report measures for cervical radiculopathy. *Spine.* 2003;28:52-62.

27. Waldrop MA. Diagnosis and treatment of cervical radiculopathy using a clinical prediction rule and a multimodal intervention approach: a case series. *J Orthop Sport Phys Ther.* 2006;36:152-159.

28. Sahrmann S. *Diagnosis and Treatment of Movement Impairment Syndromes.* St. Louis, MO: Mosby; 2002.

29. Edmonston SJ, Wallumrod ME, Macleid F, et al. Reliability of isometric muscle endurance tests in subjects with postural neck pain. *J Manipulative Physiol Ther.* 2008;31:348-354.

30. Jull G, Barrett C, Magee R, Ho P. Further clinical clarification of the muscle dysfunction in cervical headache. *Cephalalgia.* 1999;19:179-185.

31. Fernandez-de-las Penas C, Alonso-Blanco C, et al. Forward head posture and neck mobility in chronic tension-type headache: a blinded, controlled study. *Cephalalgia.* 2006;26:314-319.

32. Paris SV, Loubert PV. *Foundations of Clinical Orthopaedics.* St. Augustine, FL: Institute Press;1999.

33. Jull G, Treleaven J, Versace G. Manual examination: is pain provocation a major cue for spinal dysfunction. *Aust J Physiother.* 1994;40:159-165.

34. Malfliet A, Kregel J, Meeus M, et al. Patients with chronic spinal pain benefit from pain neuroscience education regardless the self-reported signs of central sensitization: secondary analysis of a randomized controlled multicenter trial. *PMR.* 2018;10:1330-1343.

35. D'Sylva J, Miller J, Gross A, et al. Cervical Overview Group. Manual therapy with or without physical medicine modalities for neck pain: a systematic review. *Man Ther.* 2010;15:415-433.

36. Miller J, Gross A, D'Sylva J, et al. Manual therapy and exercise for neck pain: a systematic review. *Man Ther.* 2010;15:334-354.

37. Wang WT, Olson SL, Campbell AH, et al. Effectiveness of physical therapy for patients with neck pain: an individualized approach using a clinical decision-making algorithm. *Am J Phys Med Rehabil.* 2003;82:203-218.

38. Wegner S, Jull G, O'Leary S, Johnston V. The effect of scapular postural correction strategy on trapezius activity in patients with neck pain. *Man Ther.* 2010;15:562-566.

39. Cerezo-Tellez E, Torres-Lacomba I, Fuentes-Gallardo, et al. Effectiveness of dry needling for chronic nonspecific neck pain: a randomized, single–blinded, clinical trial. *Pain.* 2016.15;1905-1917.

40. Falla D, Jull G, Russell T, et al. Effect of neck exercise on sitting posture in patients with chronic neck pain. *Phys Ther.* 2007;87:408-417.

41. Gross A, Miller J, D'Sylva J, et al. Manipulation or mobilisation for neck pain: a Cochrane Review. *Man Ther.* 2010;15:315-333.

Mechanical Neck Pain: Thoracic Spine Manipulation

Dan Kang
Jason Brumitt

CASE 8

A 34-year-old male agricultural worker presents to an outpatient physical therapy clinic with a referral from his primary care provider (PCP) to evaluate and treat pain in the cervical and thoracic spine. The patient reports experiencing a sharp pain followed by a feeling of "his midback locking up" that occurred when using a cultivator 3 days ago. He reports experiencing neck pain, stiffness, and occasional headaches. He also reports that the pain in his midback increases when he raises his arms and when he looks down or to the side. He has missed work since the aggravating episode. Lying supine on an ice pack provides some pain relief. He reports that this is his first episode of neck and back pain. The patient's PCP diagnosed his injury as a cervical and thoracic strain and did not order any imaging studies. The PCP instructed him to take two 200-mg ibuprofen tablets twice per day until his symptoms resolve or until his follow-up visit in 3 weeks.

▶ Based on the patient's diagnosis, what are the contributing factors to the condition?

▶ What examination signs may be associated with this diagnosis?

▶ What are the most appropriate physical therapy interventions?

▶ What precautions should be taken during physical therapy interventions?

KEY DEFINITIONS

CAVITATION: The audible pop associated with gas bubble implosion during a spinal manipulation technique

HIGH-VELOCITY LOW-AMPLITUDE THRUST (HVLAT): Another term for a joint manipulation

HYPOMOBILE: Decrease in the arthrokinematic motion available at a joint

JOINT MANIPULATION: Passive high-velocity and low-amplitude thrust applied to a joint complex within its anatomical limit with the intent to restore optimal motion, function, and/or to reduce pain

JOINT MOBILIZATIONS: Manual therapy techniques comprising a continuum of skilled passive movements to the joint complex that are applied at varying speeds and amplitudes

STRAIN: Muscle injury that results in tearing of the muscle-tendon unit and is associated with pain and loss of function

Objectives

1. Define a strain injury.
2. Perform a musculoskeletal evaluation for the cervical and thoracic spine.
3. Describe the use of high-velocity low-amplitude thrust techniques to the thoracic spine.
4. Identify contraindications and precautions associated with a high-velocity low-amplitude thrust manipulation in the thoracic spine.
5. Prescribe therapeutic exercise to restore range of motion deficits.

Physical Therapy Considerations

Physical therapy considerations during management of the individual with cervical and thoracic strain:

▶ **General physical therapy plan of care/goals:** Decrease pain, increase flexibility

▶ **Physical therapy interventions:** Patient education regarding functional anatomy and injury pathomechanics; manual therapy and modalities to decrease pain; therapeutic exercises to improve muscular flexibility; home exercise program

▶ **Precautions during physical therapy:** Monitor vital signs; address precautions and contraindications to spinal manipulation or therapeutic exercise

Understanding the Health Condition

Injury to the cervical and thoracic spine is common. The yearly incidence of neck pain may be as high as 50% with a lifetime prevalence over 60%,[1-4] while pain in the thoracic spine is associated with a lifetime prevalence above 30%.[5] The seven cervical vertebrae and associated musculature support and orient the head in space and protect the spinal column. The thoracic spine, situated between the cervical spine and the lumbar spine, consists of 12 vertebrae, 12 ribs bilaterally, and associated musculature. The thoracic vertebrae and ribs provide protection to the heart and lungs and serve as attachment sites for muscles of respiration, create movement at the cervical spine and upper extremities, and contribute to posture. Although examination and treatment of cervical and lumbar spine impairments have received more attention in the literature, thoracic spinal pain can be severe, resulting in medical and physical therapy visits and time lost from work or sport.[6-9]

A muscular strain is an injury resulting in a partial or complete tear of the muscle-tendon unit. Strain injuries are categorized into three grades. A grade I strain is marked by pain during movement of the involved muscle with microtearing of some muscle fibers. There may be minimal swelling with little to no loss of strength or range of motion (ROM). A grade II strain results in increasing pain with movement and a greater disruption (*i.e.*, tearing) of muscle fibers. This injury is associated with moderate swelling, loss of ROM, and some loss of strength. A grade III strain is a rupture of the muscle belly, the musculotendinous junction, and/or the osseotendinous junction. A patient with a grade III strain experiences intense pain during the injury that may decrease after the initial injury if associated nerve fibers are also destroyed. Individuals with grade III strains experience major swelling and significant loss of both ROM and strength. Muscle spasm may occur in response to a strain in the cervical and/or thoracic spine.[10] It is generally thought that a muscle spasm occurs to protect the injured area from further damage; however, the spasm itself can cause significant pain and further limit ROM.

Pain is the primary subjective complaint from individuals who have experienced a strain in the cervical and/or thoracic region. Pain may increase with raising the arms or moving the neck (*e.g.*, looking down or rotating the head side to side). Minor strains (*e.g.*, grade I) cause pain, but the individual may still be able to work and perform activities of daily living (ADLs) as usual. A person with a grade II or III strain will experience increasing pain which may limit the ability to tolerate normal work responsibilities and ADLs.

Physical Therapy Patient/Client Management

Following a thorough evaluation to rule out differential diagnoses, a conservative treatment approach for patients with a cervical and/or thoracic strain consists of manual therapy, including **high-velocity, low-amplitude thrust (HVLAT) techniques, therapeutic exercise, and modalities to reduce pain and restore function.**

Examination, Evaluation, and Diagnosis

The physical examination begins with a review of the patient's subjective history. The history informs the physical therapist as to the patient's relevant medical history including prior episodes of neck or back pain, the mechanism of current injury, and contraindications for physical therapy treatment. For this case, the patient did not present with any significant medical history.

During the subjective and objective examination, the physical therapist must rule out potential non-musculoskeletal sources of pain. The musculoskeletal examination should find positive signs associated with a cervical and/or thoracic strain. Differential diagnoses associated with cervical spine pain include: injury to the spinal cord, cervical myelopathy, vertebral artery dissection, neoplasm, fracture, systemic disease, and infection. Differential diagnoses associated with thoracic spine pain include: cardiac ischemia, dissecting thoracic aneurysm, peptic ulcer, cholecystitis, renal infection, kidney stones, fracture, neoplastic conditions, inflammatory disorders (*e.g.*, ankylosing spondylitis, sacroiliitis), and systemic disease.

The physical examination starts with an observation of the patient's posture. The exposed torso is viewed anteriorly, posteriorly, and sagittally. The patient may present with a forward head (*i.e.*, protraction of the head marked by extended upper cervical spine and flexed mid- to lower cervical spine) and thoracic kyphosis. While considered a deviation from an optimal postural position, the forward head posture is commonly observed in the general population.[11-15] People usually do not seek care for pain associated with postural dysfunction, but do so only after experiencing a strain. The postural presentation of this patient may provide clues to underlying muscular tightness (*e.g.*, upper trapezius, levator scapulae, pectoralis major and minor, suboccipitals, and sternocleidomastoids) unrelated to the presence of muscular spasms.[11,12]

Cervical and thoracic spinal ROM testing may provide an indication of the severity of the muscle strain. There are published normal ranges for cervical and thoracic active ROM (AROM). For cervical AROM, these are: flexion (45°-50°), extension (85°), rotation (90°), and lateral flexion (approximately 40°). For thoracic AROM, normal ranges are: flexion (30°-40°), extension (20°-25°), lateral flexion (25°), and rotation (30°).[16] These movements should be measured using an inclinometer with the patient in a seated position.[17,18] Cervical and/or thoracic ROM may be limited due to a strained muscle in a reflexive spasm. Cervical and/or thoracic ROM may also be limited by joint hypomobility with or without associated muscle spasms.

AROM of the glenohumeral joints and lumbar spine must be assessed to rule out pain originating from these sites. The therapist assesses the patient's ability to flex and abduct bilateral shoulders. Next, the therapist assesses lumbar spine active ROM. If the patient reports pain during these activities, the therapist must ascertain the location of pain. The therapist can rule out involvement of the glenohumeral joints and lumbar spine if pain is reproduced in the cervical or thoracic spine. A neurologic screen consisting of myotomal, dermatomal, and reflex testing of both the cervical spine and the lumbar spine is warranted in all cases of spinal injury.

Special tests are performed next to help rule out neurologic injury in the cervical or thoracic regions. To assess the cervical spine, special tests appropriate for this case include Spurling's compression test, cervical distraction test, and the upper limb tension test (see Cases 7 and 10 for test descriptions). Table 8-1 describes special tests for the thoracic spine, along with their reported diagnostic accuracy. Although the thoracic compression and thoracic distraction tests have been reported to assess compression on nerve roots, the diagnostic accuracy for these

Table 8-1   SPECIAL TESTS FOR THE THORACIC SPINE AND DIAGNOSTIC ACCURACY

Special Tests	Test Performance	Diagnostic Accuracy
Thoracic compression	Patient is seated. Standing behind the patient, the therapist places their hands on bilateral upper trapezius/shoulder region and applies an inferiorly directed pressure. *Reproduction of patient's pain* is reported to indicate decreased foraminal space for the nerve root or tissue injury.	Unknown
Thoracic distraction	Patient sits with arms crossed across chest. Therapist stands behind patient and grasps the patient's forearms, leans back and lifts the patient. *Pain reduction* during the test suggests that distraction is relieving compression on the nerve roots.	Unknown
Adson's	Patient sits with arms horizontally abducted 15°. The therapist, standing from behind, palpates a single radial pulse. The patient is asked to inhale, hold a breath, extend and rotate the neck toward the side being assessed. *A diminished or absent radial pulse and a patient report of paresthesia* is a positive test for thoracic outlet syndrome.	Sensitivity: 0.50-0.79[21,22] Specificity: 0.16-1.00[21-25]
Roos	Patient sits with the arm abducted 90° and externally rotated 90°. Patient opens and closes their fingers for 1 minute. *Reproduction of usual symptoms* is a positive test for thoracic outlet syndrome.	Sensitivity: 0.82-0.84[21,26] Specificity: 0.30-1.00[21,25,26]
Hyperabduction	Patient sits while therapist palpates the radial pulse. Patient abducts and externally rotates both shoulders to 90° and holds this position for 1 minute. *A diminished or absent pulse and the patient reporting paresthesia* is a positive test for thoracic outlet syndrome.	Sensitivity: Paresthesia: Unknown Change in pulse: 0.52[22] Specificity: Paresthesia: 0.64-0.90[22-24] Change in pulse: 0.38-0.90[22-24]

two tests has not been established. If the patient complains of pain into the shoulder or arm, impaired sensation or "pins and needles" in the upper extremity, and/or cold sensitivity, tests for thoracic outlet syndrome (*e.g.*, Adson's test, Roos test, hyperabduction test) should be performed.[19,20] The patient in this case did not report symptoms indicating a need to perform tests for thoracic outlet syndrome. There are no special tests for a muscle strain injury.

Next, the therapist performs joint mobility (*i.e.*, joint play) testing for the cervical and thoracic spine with the patient alternating between the supine and prone positions. Pain and/or hypomobility during testing is common in patients who have experienced a strain injury. With the patient supine, the physical therapist assesses physiological side glides of the cervical spine. The therapist's hand is used

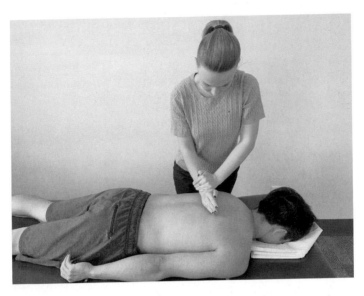

Figure 8-1. Central posterior-anterior (PA) joint mobility testing in thoracic spine, using one-handed technique.

to apply a translatory force to one segment of the cervical spine while the opposite hand provides a blocking force to the inferior segment. With the patient prone, the therapist performs central and unilateral posterior-anterior (PA) testing of the cervical spine to evaluate for pain provocation and/or hypomobility. Using thumbs only, the therapist applies a PA force on each side of the spinous process, for a central PA, or to the facet, for a unilateral PA.

With the patient still prone on the treatment table, joint mobility testing for the thoracic spine is performed. Posterior-anterior testing can be performed central to the segment or unilaterally. The central PA technique is performed by applying a force, with one or two hands, to each vertebral segment. A one-handed approach is performed by applying the hypothenar eminence, whereas a two-handed approach is performed with the pisiforms applied lateral to the spinous process (Figs. 8-1 and 8-2). Normal joint play presents as a springy motion at the vertebral segment, whereas a hypomobile region lacks this excursion. Pain, with possible muscle guarding, may also occur during joint mobility testing. As part of a comprehensive examination of the patient with pain in the thoracic spine, the therapist must also evaluate the costovertebral joints for pain and/or hypomobility with the rib spring test. The therapist orients their hand 45° to the vertical axis of the patient. The therapist assesses each rib for normal, hypomobile, or hypermobile (less likely) excursion. Palpation of the cervical and thoracic region is reserved for the final component of the physical examination because symptom provocation during palpation of injured tissues may limit the patient's tolerance to some of the aforementioned tests. Palpating the soft tissue allows the therapist to identify the muscles that are in spasm and appreciate which tissues are painful.

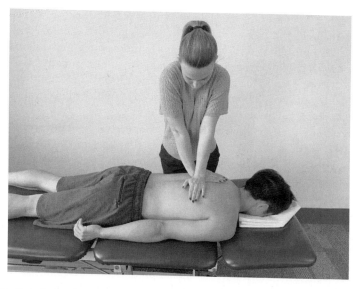

Figure 8-2. Central posterior-anterior (PA) joint mobility testing in thoracic spine, using two-handed technique. This approach is also used for the high-velocity, low-amplitude thrust (HVLAT) manipulation technique to the thoracic spine.

Plan of Care and Interventions

There are two primary treatments for patients with a thoracic strain: manual therapy including joint mobilization and manipulation (*i.e.*, HVLAT) and therapeutic exercise. **Other treatments, such as moist heat or cryotherapy, may also be used though evidence is lacking for their efficacy.**

Manual therapy techniques may be indicated to reduce pain and muscle spasm and to normalize joint mobility. Although the effectiveness of massage has been debated,[27-29] when performed at the start of a treatment session, soft tissue mobilization may reduce pain and spasming prior to spinal manipulation techniques.

Manual therapy directed to the cervical and thoracic spine is effective at reducing pain and normalizing joint play. Manipulation to the thoracic spine may also improve pain associated with cervical and lumbar spine conditions.[30-40] Gonzalez-Iglesias *et al.*[36] randomized patients with mechanical neck pain to either an experimental or control group for 5 treatment sessions. The experimental group received a thoracic spine thrust manipulation (only in 3 sessions), infrared lamp therapy (250 W) to the neck for 15 minutes, and transcutaneous electrical nerve stimulation (100 Hz, 250-ms pulses) for 20 minutes at the C7 level, whereas the control group received only the modalities. The experimental group experienced significantly greater improvements in pain (visual analog scale), cervical spine ROM, and disability (Northwick Neck Pain Questionnaire) at the fifth visit and at the 2- and 4-week follow-ups.

Researchers have attempted to develop a clinical prediction rule (CPR) to identify individuals with neck pain that would benefit from thoracic spine manipulation.[37,38] Cleland *et al.*[37] reported that patients who presented with 3 out of 6 variables had a greater chance of having a positive outcome with thoracic spine manipulation. These 6 variables were: symptoms for <30 days; no symptom aggravation with looking up; Fear-Avoidance Beliefs Questionnaire physical activity subscale score <12; <30° of cervical extension ROM; no symptoms distal to the shoulder region; and, diminished upper thoracic spine kyphosis. However, two subsequent studies have not validated this CPR.[38,39]

To determine the effects of cervical versus thoracic manipulation on adults with neck pain, Puentedura *et al.*[39] enrolled patients that presented with 4 out of 6 of the CPR variables outlined by Cleland *et al.*[37] Patients were randomized to either a *thoracic* manipulation plus exercise group or to a *cervical* manipulation plus exercise group. Both groups received manipulation techniques for 2 sessions and the same therapeutic exercise program. Patients that received manipulation to the cervical spine experienced significantly greater improvements in Neck Disability Index scores, Fear-Avoidance Beliefs Questionnaire physical activity subscale scores, and numeric pain rating scale scores.[39] This study highlights the potential benefits associated with including manipulation to the *cervical* spine as part of the manual therapy treatment program for individuals with neck pain. Dunning *et al.*[40] reported that a treatment program consisting of HVLAT (*i.e., manipulation*) techniques to the cervical and thoracic spine was superior in reducing pain and disability scores than treatment with *nonthrust* joint mobilization techniques for patients with mechanical neck pain.

There are several types of HVLAT techniques that can be administered to the thoracic spine of a patient with cervical and/or thoracic spinal pain due to a strain. Selection of HVLAT techniques is often based on the physical therapist's comfort with the manipulation approach as well as the patient's tolerance to the treatment position (*i.e.,* prone, supine, sitting). If the patient is unable to initially tolerate the application of a HVLAT technique, the therapist may choose to perform joint mobilization techniques performed at different speeds and amplitudes.

HVLAT techniques can be safe and effective; however, it is important for the physical therapist to screen the patient for contraindications associated with this treatment.[41] Absolute contraindications to spinal manipulation include: recent fracture or dislocation, segmental instability, malignancy to the bone, bone infection, disorders of the central nervous system, osteoporosis, and an active infection. Relative contraindications to spinal manipulation include: spondylolisthesis, joint hypermobility, benign bone tumors, post-surgical joints, nerve root compression, and pregnancy.

Techniques to manipulate hypomobile segments in the midthoracic spine can be performed in prone, supine, and sitting. With the patient prone on the treatment table, a posterior-anterior (PA) HVLAT manipulation can be performed (Fig. 8-2). The physical therapist's hands are placed at the level of the hypomobile segment. Prior to performing the manipulation, the therapist places their hands at the level of the hypomobile segment and performs a "skin lock." The skin lock is performed by applying a force to the soft tissue while performing a twisting motion with the therapist's upper extremity. If the therapist is positioned to the left side of the treatment table, the left hand is placed on the right side of the hypomobile segment and the right hand is placed on the left side of the segment. To perform the skin lock with the left hand, start with palm placed at the level of the hypomobile segment and the fingers pointing toward the buttocks. Visualizing a clock superimposed on the posterior anatomical structures of the body, with the head in the 12 o'clock position and the buttocks in the 6 o'clock position will help guide the movement of the therapist's hands when performing the skin locks. Next, the left hand is rotated in a counter-clockwise direction with the fingers pointing toward the 3 o'clock position. The right-hand skin lock is performed by placing the palm at the level of hypomobile segment with the fingers pointing toward 9 o'clock. Next, the right hand is rotated in the clockwise direction with the fingers pointing toward the head (*i.e.*, 12 o'clock position). Once the skin lock is finished, the therapist asks the patient to take a deep breath followed by a complete exhalation. The therapist provides the manipulation at the end of the exhalation. Failure to achieve a cavitation[42-44] may result from the patient guarding and/or the manipulation thrust being applied too early. If the first manipulation attempt was not successful due to one of the aforementioned reasons, a second attempt should be performed. A lack of cavitation does not mean that the manipulation was unsuccessful.[45] Research evaluating the effectiveness of spinal manipulation to the lumbar spine suggests that a person can experience decreased pain after a manipulation that lacked an audible pop.[45]

The PA manipulation to the *midthoracic* spine (*e.g.*, T4-T8) can also be performed with the patient supine with their arms crossed against their chest. To identify the level of the hypomobile segment, the therapist rolls the patient toward them. A pistol grip is used as a fulcrum with the desired thoracic segment (Fig. 8-3). The therapist asks the patient to take in a deep breath followed by a complete exhalation. At the point of full exhalation, the therapist uses their

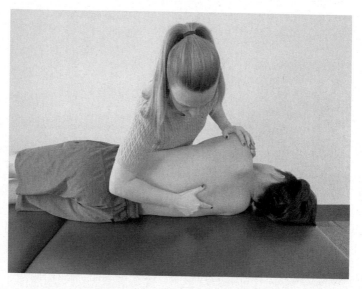

Figure 8-3. Hand placement (pistol grip) used as fulcrum at hypomobile thoracic segment for supine anterior-posterior manipulation technique to the thoracic spine.

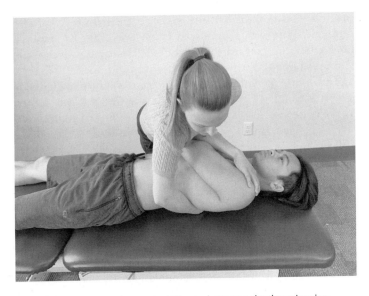

Figure 8-4. Supine anterior-posterior manipulation technique to the thoracic spine.

body to push through the patient's arms to perform a high-velocity thrust in an anterior to posterior direction to the thoracic segments (Fig. 8-4). Manipulation to the midthoracic spine can also be performed with the patient seated (Fig. 8-5). The therapist wraps her arms around the patient with the patient's midthoracic region positioned against the therapist's chest. Next, the therapist flexes the patient's thoracic spine and at the point where tension is perceived, applies a distraction thrust in an upward direction.

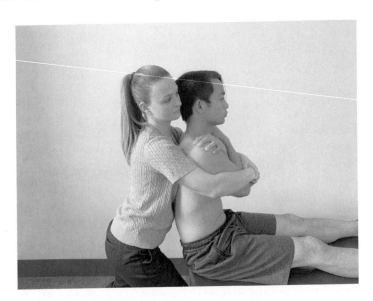

Figure 8-5. Position for thoracic spine distraction thrust manipulation.

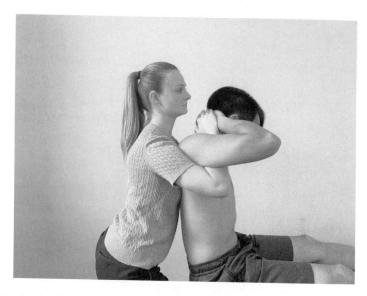

Figure 8-6. Position for cervical thoracic manipulation ("full nelson").

To manipulate hypomobile segments in the *upper thoracic* spine, the cervical-thoracic junction HVLAT can be used. This manipulation is also known as the full-nelson technique, or the cervicothoracic joint distraction technique. The patient is positioned in long sitting with buttocks near the edge of the treatment table. The patient places his hands, with fingers intertwined, behind his head. The therapist stands behind the patient with her chest positioned against the patient's back. The therapist positions her forearms in the patient's axillae and places her hands on top of the patient's hands. Once in this "full nelson" position, the therapist slightly leans the patient backward toward her and applies a distraction thrust (Fig. 8-6). Some therapists do not have long enough arms to assume the traditional full nelson position. If this is the case, the therapist can grasp each of the patient's wrists. The therapist slightly extends the patient's upper thoracic spine and applies the manipulative force in a cephalic direction (*i.e.*, toward the head).

Therapeutic exercise is prescribed to address limitations in flexibility and hypomobile vertebral segments. As previously mentioned, many patients present with a forward head posture and a kyphotic thoracic spine and this postural abnormality is *likely* unrelated to the current injury episode. However, patients with this posture likely have tightness in the suboccipital muscles, upper trapezius, levator scapulae, and pectoralis major and minor. Stretching exercises can be prescribed as part of the home exercise program (HEP). These exercises can help reduce pain and improve cervical and thoracic range of motion.[46]

Self-mobilization techniques to improve the mobility at hypomobile joints can also be prescribed as part of the HEP. Classic examples include thoracic extension sitting in a chair (Fig. 8-7) or thoracic extension in supine (Fig. 8-8). **Although evidence regarding their effectiveness is lacking, performance of self-mobilization may benefit patients who are unable to initially tolerate HVLAT techniques.**

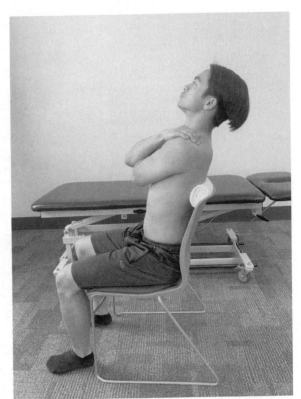

Figure 8-7. Thoracic extension self-mobilization technique in sitting. Towel roll is placed below the targeted hypomobile segment. Patient crosses arms across chest and leans backward for multiple repetitions (*e.g.,* 10-20), attempting to facilitate thoracic extension at the region superior to the towel placement. A hold time, up to 10 seconds, can be used per repetition; however, there is no evidence to guide optimal dose.

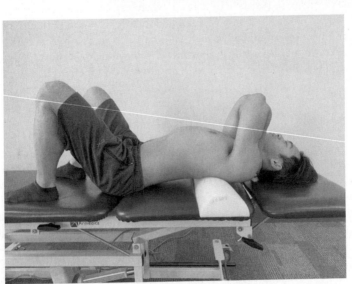

Figure 8-8. Thoracic extension self-mobilization technique in supine. A half foam roll (or a large towel roll) is placed below the targeted hypomobile segment. Patient crosses arms across chest and leans backward. Multiple repetitions (*e.g.,* 10-20) are performed to facilitate thoracic extension at the region superior to the towel placement.

Evidence-Based Clinical Recommendations

SORT: Strength of Recommendation Taxonomy

A: Consistent, good-quality patient-oriented evidence
B: Inconsistent or limited-quality patient-oriented evidence
C: Consensus, disease-oriented evidence, usual practice, expert opinion, or case series

1. High-velocity, low-amplitude thrust (HVLAT) manipulation techniques directed at the thoracic spine reduce pain in individuals with cervical and/or thoracic spine pain. **Grade B**

2. Adjunct treatments such as moist heat or cryotherapy reduce pain in individuals with thoracic strain. **Grade C**

3. Self-mobilization techniques improve joint mobility in patients with hypomobile spinal segments. **Grade C**

COMPREHENSION QUESTIONS

8.1 Which of the following is NOT a common postural deviation in the cervical-thoracic region?

A. Thoracic lordosis

B. Extended upper cervical spine

C. Forward head posture

D. Muscular tightness in the suboccipitals

8.2 During the musculoskeletal examination, the therapist determines that the patient's T4-T5 segment is hypomobile. Which of the following tests would help confirm this finding?

A. Adson's test

B. Joint mobility testing

C. Roos test

D. Thoracic compression test

ANSWERS

8.1 **A.** Lordosis describes the inward curving of the spine. An individual with a normal posture would present with lordosis in the cervical and lumbar spines and kyphosis in the thoracic spine. Patients with thoracic pain may present with excessive *kyphosis.*

8.2 **B.** Joint mobility testing is performed with the patient in a prone position on the treatment table to determine joint play. The Adson's and Roos tests are performed to assess for thoracic outlet syndrome. The thoracic compression test is performed to assess for nerve root injury.

REFERENCES

1. Cote P, Cassidy DJ, Carroll LJ, Kristman V. The annual incidence and course of neck pain in the general population: a population-based cohort study. *Pain.* 2004;112(3):267-273.

2. Cote P, Cassidy JD, Carroll L. The Saskatchewan health and back pain survey. The prevalence of neck pain and related disability in Saskatchewan adults. *Spine.* 1998;23(15):1689-1698.

3. Borghouts J, Janssen H, Koes B, et al. The management of chronic neck pain in general practice. A retrospective study. *Scand J Prim Health Care.* 1999;17(4):215-220.

4. Haldeman S, Carroll L, Cassidy JD. Findings from the bone and joint decade 2000 to 2010 task force on neck pain and its associated disorders. *J Occup Environ Med.* 2010;52(4):424-427.

5. Briggs AM, Smith AJ, Straker LM, Bragge P. Thoracic spine pain in the general population: prevalence, incidence and associated factors in children, adolescents and adults. A systematic review. *BMC Musculoskelet Disord.* 2009;10:77.

6. Delitto A, George SZ, Van Dillen L, et al; Orthopaedic Section of the American Physical Therapy Association. Low back pain. *J Orthop Sports Phys Ther.* 2012;42:A1-A57.

7. Blanpied PR, Gross AR, Elliott JM, et al. Neck pain: revision 2017. *J Orthop Sports Phys Ther.* 2017;47:A1-A83.

8. Huang P, Anissipour A, McGee W, Lemak L. Return-to-play recommendations after cervical, thoracic, and lumbar spine injuries: a comprehensive review. *Sports Health.* 2016;8:19-25.

9. Menzer H, Gill GK, Paterson A. Thoracic spine sports-related injuries. *Curr Sports Med Rep.* 2015;14:34-40.

10. Saunders HD. Classification of musculoskeletal spinal conditions*. *J Orthop Sports Phys Ther.* 1979;1:3-15.

11. Janda V. Proximal crossed syndrome. In: Hutson M, Ellis R, eds. *Textbook of Musculoskeletal Medicine.* New York, NY: Oxford University Press; 2006:48-49.

12. Moore MK. Upper crossed syndrome and its relationship to cervicogenic headache. *J Manipulative Physiol Ther.* 2004;27:414-420.

13. Szeto GP, Straker LM, O'Sullivan PB. A comparison of symptomatic and asymptomatic office workers performing monotonous keyboard work-2: neck and shoulder kinematics. *Man Ther.* 2005;10:281-291.

14. Harman K, Hubley-Kozey CL, Butler H. Effectiveness of an exercise program to improve forward head posture in normal adults: a randomized, controlled ten-week trial. *J Man Manip Ther.* 2005;13:163-176.

15. Falla D, Jull G, Russell T, et al. Effect of neck exercise on sitting posture in patients with chronic neck pain. *Phys Ther.* 2007;87:408-417.

16. Neumann D. *Kinesiology of the Musculoskeletal System: Foundations for Physical Rehabilitation.* St. Louis, MO: Mosby; 2002.

17. Takatalo J, Ylinen J, Pienimaki T, Hakkinen A. Intra- and inter-rater reliability of thoracic spine mobility and posture assessments in subjects with thoracic spine pain. *BMC Musculoskelet Disord.* 2020;21:529.

18. Williams MA, McCarthy CJ, Chorti A, et al. A systematic review of reliability and validity studies of methods for measuring active and passive cervical range of motion. *J Manipulative Physiol Ther.* 2010;33(2):138-155.

19. Dessureault-Dober I, Bronchti G, Bussieres A. Diagnostic accuracy of clinical tests for neurogenic and vascular thoracic outlet syndrome: a systematic review. *J Manipulative Physiol Ther.* 2018;41:789-799.

20. Watson LA, Pizzari T, Balster S. Thoracic outlet syndrome part 1: clinical manifestations, differentiation and treatment pathways. *Man Ther.* 2009;14:586-595.

21. Lee AD, Agarwal S, Sadhu D. Doppler Adson's test: predictor of outcome of surgery in non-specific thoracic outlet syndrome. *World J Surg.* 2006;30:291-292.

22. Gillard J, Perez-Cousin M, Hachulla E, et al. Diagnosing thoracic outlet syndrome: contribution of provocative tests, ultrasonography, electrophysiology, and helical computed tomography in 48 patients. *Joint Bone Spine*. 2001;68:416-424.

23. Rayan GM, Jensen C. Thoracic outlet syndrome: provocative examination maneuvers in a typical patient. *J Shoulder Elbow Surg*. 1995;4:113-117.

24. Plewa MC, Delinger M. The false-positive rate of thoracic outlet syndrome shoulder maneuvers in healthy patients. *Acad Emerg Med*. 1998;5:337-342.

25. Nord KM, Kapoor P, Fisher J, et al. False positive rate of thoracic outlet syndrome diagnostic maneuvers. *Electromyogr Clin Neurophysiol*. 2008;48:67-74.

26. Howard M, Lee C, Dellon AL. Documentation of brachial plexus compression (I the thoracic inlet) utilizing provocative neurosensory and muscular testing. *J Reconstr Microsurg*. 2003;19:303-312.

27. Furlan AD, Giraldo M, Baskwill A, et al. Massage for low-back pain. *Cochrane Database Syst Rev*. 2015;9:CD001929.

28. Chou R, Deyo R, Friedly J, et al. Nonpharmacologic therapies for low back pain: a systematic review for an American College of Physicians Clinical Practice Guideline. *Ann Intern Med*. 2017;166:493-505.

29. Qaseem A, Wilt TJ, McLean RM, Forcia MA; Clinical Guidelines Committee of the American College of Physicians, et al. Noninvasive treatments for acute, subacute, and chronic low back pain: A clinical practice guideline from the American College of Physicians. *Ann Intern Med*. 2017;166:514-530.

30. Cross KM, Kuenze C, Grindstaff TL, Hertel J. Thoracic spine thrust manipulation improves pain, range of motion, and self-reported function in patients with mechanical neck pain: a systematic review. *J Orthop Sports Phys Ther*. 2011;41:633-642.

31. Cho J, Lee E, Lee S. Upper cervical and upper thoracic spine mobilization versus deep cervical flexors exercise in individuals with forward head posture: a randomized clinical trial investigating their effectiveness. *J Back Musculoskelet Rehabil*. 2019;32:595-602.

32. Huisman PA, Speksnijder CM, de Wijer A. The effect of thoracic spine manipulation on pain and disability in patients with non-specific neck pain: a systematic review. *Disabil Rehabil*. 2013;35:1677-1685.

33. Sampath KK, Botnmark E, Mani R, et al. Neuroendocrine response following a thoracic spine manipulation in healthy men. *J Orthop Sports Phys Ther*. 2017;47:617-627.

34. Sparks C, Cleland JA, Elliott JM, et al. Using functional magnetic resonance imaging to determine if cerebral hemodynamic responses to pain change following thoracic spine thrust manipulation in healthy individuals. *J Orthop Sports Phys Ther*. 2013;43:340-348.

35. Walser RF, Meserve BB, Boucher TR. The effectiveness of thoracic spine manipulation for the management of musculoskeletal conditions: a systematic review and meta-analysis of randomized controlled trials. *J Man Manip Ther*. 2009;1:237-246.

36. Gonzalez-Iglesias J, Fernandez-de-las-Penas C, Cleland JA, Gutierrez-Vega Mdel R. Thoracic spine manipulation for the management of patients with neck pain: a randomized clinical trial. *J Orthop Sports Phys Ther*. 2009;39(1):20-27.

37. Cleland JA, Childs JD, Fritz JM, et al. Development of a clinical prediction rule for guiding treatment of a subgroup of patients with neck pain: use of thoracic spine manipulation, exercise, and patient education. *Phys Ther*. 2007;87(1):9-23.

38. Cleland JA, Mintken PE, Carpenter K, et al. Examination of a clinical prediction rule to identify patients with neck pain likely to benefit from thoracic spine thrust manipulation and a general cervical range of motion exercise: multi-center randomized clinical trial. *Phys Ther*. 2010;90(9):1239-1250.

39. Puentedura EJ, Landers MR, Cleland JA, et al. Thoracic spine thrust manipulation versus cervical spine thrust manipulation in patients with acute neck pain: a randomized clinical trial. *J Orthop Sports Phys Ther*. 2011;41(4):208-220.

40. Dunning JR, Cleland JA, Waldrop MA, et al. Upper cervical and upper thoracic thrust manipulation versus nonthrust mobilization in patients with mechanical neck pain: a multicenter randomized clinical trial. *J Orthop Sports Phys Ther.* 2012;42(1):5-18.

41. Cook C. *Orthopedic Manual Therapy. An Evidence-Based Approach.* 2nd ed. Pearson Education; 2012.

42. Unsworth A, Dowson D, Wright V. 'Cracking joints'. A bioengineering study of cavitation in the metacarpophalangeal joint. *Ann Rheum Dis.* 1971;30:348-358.

43. Kawchuk GN, Fryer J, Jaremko JL, et al. Real-time visualization of joint cavitation. *PloS One.* 2015;10:e0119470.

44. Cleland JA, Flynn TW, Childs JD, Eberhart S. The audible pop from thoracic spine thrust manipulation and its relation to short-term outcomes in patients with neck pain. *J Man Manip Ther.* 2007;15:143-154.

45. Flynn TW, Fritz JM, Wainner RS, Whitman JM. The audible pop is not necessary for successful spinal high-velocity thrust manipulation in individuals with low back pain. *Arch Phys Med Rehabil.* 2003;84:1057-1060.

46. Cunha ACV, Burke TN, Franca FJR, Marques AP. Effect of global posture reeducation and static stretching on pain, range of motion, and quality of life in women with chronic neck pain: a randomized clinical trial. *Clinics.* 2008;63(6):763-770.

Cervical Radiculopathy— Upper Limb Tension Testing and Treatment

Tyler Whited

A 53-year-old female presents to physical therapy with 8 weeks of paresthesia, weakness, and pain in her left forearm and hand. She reports symptom onset following pruning and trimming plants in her garden. She was referred to outpatient physical therapy with a diagnosis of cervical radiculopathy made by her primary care physician. The primary care physician ordered radiographs of her cervical spine. The radiographs demonstrate age-related degeneration from C6-C7 and C7-T1, but no acute injuries or insidious pathologies (*e.g.*, fracture, osseous lesions). Her previous medical history includes hypertension.

▶ Based on the referred diagnosis, what are the contributing factors to the condition?

▶ What are the most appropriate examination tests?

▶ What are the most appropriate physical therapy interventions?

▶ What are the possible complications that may limit effectiveness of physical therapy?

KEY DEFINITIONS

CERVICAL RADICULOPATHY: Compression of one or more cervical nerve roots that may cause pain and reduced sensation, motor function, and/or reflexes in the upper extremity

CLUSTER TEST: Combination of tests that, when each is positive, improves diagnostic accuracy

MECHANOSENSITIVITY: Local sensations of discomfort in response to limb movements that stretch tissues (*e.g.*, nerves, muscles, joints)

NEURAL MOBILIZATION: Manual therapy interventions and/or prescribed therapeutic exercises directed at mobilizing nerve tissue and surrounding soft tissue structures with the aim of reducing pain and disability

STRUCTURAL DIFFERENTIATION: Movement of a body region (*e.g.*, the head and neck) toward or away from the area being assessed (*e.g.*, the symptomatic upper extremity) to evaluate the effect of mechanical force on nerve tissue and the patient's symptoms. These maneuvers are used to distinguish between neural and non-neural structures.

UPPER LIMB TENSION TESTS (ULTT): Sequences of movements designed to provoke mechanosensitivity of nervous tissue (*i.e.*, nerve roots or peripheral nerves)

Objectives

1. Select relevant patient history questions to guide the objective examination.
2. Describe a thorough examination process for the cervical spine.
3. Describe appropriate manual therapy interventions to reduce symptoms associated with mechanosensitivity of nervous tissue.
4. Prescribe appropriate therapeutic exercises to facilitate return to activity.

Physical Therapy Considerations

Physical therapy considerations during management of the individual with a diagnosis of cervical radiculopathy with neck and arm pain:

▶ **General physical therapy plan of care/goals**: Decrease pain and paresthesia; improve upper extremity range of motion; improve upper extremity strength

▶ **Physical therapy interventions**: Patient education regarding functional anatomy and injury pathomechanics; manual therapy to reduce pain and paresthesia; therapeutic exercise to improve nerve mobility and muscular strength; home exercise program to promote independent management of symptoms

▶ **Precautions during physical therapy**: Continue to monitor the patient for any worsening of paresthesia symptoms and presence of red flags (*e.g.*, progressive weakness, ataxia, unexplained changes in speech, swallowing, or vision).

Understanding the Health Condition

Cervical radiculopathy is caused by compression of one or more nerve roots, typically from cervical disc herniation or cervical spondylosis.[1] Annual incidence of cervical radiculopathy is reported to be 107.3 per 100,000 for men and 63.5 per 100,000 for women,[2] with peak incidence occurring between the fourth and fifth decades of life.[2,3] Individuals with cervical radiculopathy may benefit from physical therapy. Recent studies have reported that 75% to 90% of patients achieved improvement or full resolution of symptoms within a year with conservative care.[4-6], Radhakrishnan et al.[2] reported that 90% of patients, after conservative treatment, were either asymptomatic or only mildly symptomatic at 4-year follow-up.

Compression of one or more cervical nerve roots by bony encroachment or herniated cervical disc material can cause the symptoms associated with cervical radiculopathy. Most cases of cervical radiculopathy are caused by cervical spondylosis and the C6-T1 roots are most commonly involved.[1] These age-related degenerative changes include a loss of disc height and bony hypertrophy of the uncinate joints and vertebral bodies, resulting in foraminal narrowing and compression on one or more nerve roots.[1] Mechanical compression from herniated disc material can cause an increase in local ischemia and nerve damage. Proinflammatory chemical cascades triggered by contact of the nucleus pulposus on the nerve tissue can lead to further sensitization and pain.

Individuals with cervical radiculopathy may present to physical therapy with a range of symptoms including neck pain, upper extremity pain, loss of sensation, paresthesia, loss of strength, and diminished reflexes.[1,7] Usually, patients present with unilateral pain that may radiate into the ipsilateral arm. However, absence of arm pain does not exclude the diagnosis of cervical radiculopathy.[1] Patients typically present with loss of sensation in a dermatomal pattern and may present with weakness in the corresponding myotome.[1]

Nonsurgical treatment options for cervical radiculopathy include immobilization of the cervical spine (with a neck brace), therapeutic exercise, mechanical traction, manual therapy (joint manipulation and mobilization), anti-inflammatory and analgesic medications, and glucocorticoid injections.[1] **Up to 90% of patients with cervical radiculopathy report good to excellent outcomes with nonoperative management.**[1,2,8] While only 10% to 15% of cases require surgical intervention,[8] signs and symptoms that indicate early referral for surgical consultation include progressive neurological deficits, suspected cervical fracture or other signs of cervical instability, and suspected osseous lesions.[1,7] Surgical consultation may also be indicated if symptoms have not improved within 6 months of starting conservative treatment.[1] Surgical options may include discectomy, decompression, fusion, or disc arthroplasty.[1]

Physical Therapy Patient/Client Management

The physical therapist's role is to reduce pain, improve function, promote independent management, and assist the patient in returning to meaningful activities. Treatment for cervical radiculopathy typically includes a variety of techniques (*e.g.*, manual therapy, nerve mobility exercises, stretching exercises for muscles of the upper quarter) aimed at reducing mechanosensitivity to provocative movements. Once sensitivity has been reduced, therapeutic exercises to improve range of motion, increase strength, restore function, and reduce any remaining disability can be prescribed.

Examination, Evaluation, and Diagnosis

A physician or other primary care provider (PCP) may have performed an abbreviated musculoskeletal examination prior to referring the patient to physical therapy. Cervical radiculopathy is a clinical diagnosis confirmed by imaging, and often physicians order imaging prior to, or in conjunction with, a referral to physical therapy.[6] The physical therapy examination begins with obtaining the subjective history that informs the therapist of relevant medical history such as prior episodes of neck pain or upper extremity paresthesias, mechanism of injury for the current episode, aggravating or easing factors, and any red or yellow flags that may alter the patient's course of care. An individual with cervical radiculopathy often describes an inciting incident (*e.g.*, repetitive neck movements, overhead activities, or reaching tasks), especially in the case of a disc herniation.[9] Some patients report no mechanism of injury, but rather a gradual onset of symptoms.[9] This latter description may be indicative of spondylosis. Functional limitations must be discussed, as these are typically the reason the patient has sought care. One or more validated outcome tools, such as the Neck Disability Index (NDI), the Disabilities of the Arm, Shoulder, and Hand (DASH), Shoulder Pain and Disability Index (SPADI), or Patient-Reported Outcomes Measurement Information System (PROMIS), should be administered during the initial examination.[9] Psychosocial outcome tools such as the STarT MSK or Tampa Scale for Kinesiophobia may be useful to determine a patient's prognosis or to identify a patient's fear of movement, respectively. Changes in performance on outcome measures as well as functional tasks (*e.g.*, placing dishes overhead without paresthesia or pain) can be used to document progress in physical therapy.

The physical examination starts with measuring vital signs (blood pressure, pulse, oxygenation via pulse oximeter, and respiration rate) to assess general health status and check for contraindications to physical therapy interventions. The therapist begins with a visual inspection of the patient's posture. Although the patient may be seeking care for neck-related arm pain, an abnormal cervical posture may be related to complaints of upper extremity paresthesias. Next, active range of motion (AROM) of the cervical spine is assessed with an inclinometer with the patient in the sitting position.[8] Table 9-1 shows normal ranges for cervical AROM in adults.[9,10] It is possible that pain, paresthesias, or both are reproduced with cervical AROM testing. For patients with reports of upper extremity paresthesias in the forearm and hand, the therapist must investigate proximal joints (*i.e.*, distal and proximal radioulnar, humeroulnar, glenohumeral, and cervical spine segments).

A neurological screen, consisting of myotomal, dermatomal, and reflex testing, is performed next. A patient with nerve root(s) involvement presents with dermatomal and myotomal patterns of loss. In contrast, a patient with peripheral nerve involvement does not present with dermatomal and myotomal patterns of loss, but

Table 9-1   NORMATIVE ACTIVE RANGE OF MOTION (AROM) VALUES FOR ADULT CERVICAL SPINE AND THE UPPER EXTREMITIES[9,10]

Active Range of Motion	Degrees
Cervical spine	
Flexion	45-50
Extension	85
Rotation	90
Lateral flexion	40
Glenohumeral joint	
Flexion	160-180
Abduction	170-180
Extension	50-60
External rotation	80-90
Internal rotation	60-100
Radiohumeral joint	
Flexion	140-150
Extension	0-10
Wrist	
Flexion	80-90
Extension	70-90
Radial deviation	30-45
Ulnar deviation	30-45
Forearm	
Pronation	85-90
Supination	85-90

rather with abnormal sensation or decreased strength specific to the areas innervated by the involved nerve. Tables 9-2 and 9-3 show sensory and motor distributions for nerve roots and peripheral nerves of the upper extremity. Upper limb tension testing (ULTT) can further assist in distinguishing whether the primary impairment is due to compromise of the nerve root or the peripheral nerve.

To confirm the diagnosis of cervical radiculopathy and rule out other potential diagnoses, relevant special tests include ULTTs, Spurling's A, and cervical distraction.[11] There are four unique ULTTs that use specific passive sequences of movements of the upper extremity to selectively and progressively apply mechanical strain to the brachial plexus and each of the three main nerve trunks of the upper limb. As such, ULTTs are the most commonly used tests for neural mechanosensitivity. ULTT 1 and ULTT 2A are used to evaluate the median nerve. ULTT 2B is used to evaluate the radial nerve and ULTT3 is used to evaluate the ulnar nerve.[5,11] The reader should be aware that although sources have used different names for some of the ULTTs (*e.g.*, ULTT 1 or ULTT A; ULTT 2B or ULTT B),

Table 9-2 SENSORY AND MOTOR DISTRIBUTIONS FOR NERVE ROOTS[1]

Nerve Root	Key Muscles	Sensory Distribution	Reflex
C5	Deltoid	Lateral arm	Biceps
C6	Biceps brachii, wrist extensors	Lateral forearm, thumb, index finger	Brachioradialis
C7	Triceps brachii, wrist flexors	Middle finger	Triceps
C8	Finger flexors	Ring and little finger	
T1	Hand intrinsics	Medial forearm	

test performance is the same.[5,11] Table 9-4 includes photos of each ULTT with descriptions of patient position, and therapist application of sensitizing positions and structural differentiation.

A positive ULTT test is defined as causing at least partial reproduction of familiar arm and/or neck pain. In addition, a positive test must produce a change in the

Table 9-3 SENSORY AND MOTOR DISTRIBUTIONS OF PERIPHERAL NERVES[9]

Nerve	Segmental Levels	Sensory Distribution	Muscles Innervated
Musculocutaneous	C5, C6, C7	Lateral forearm	Coracobrachialis, biceps, brachialis
Lateral antebrachial cutaneous	C5, C6, C7	Lateral forearm	No motor
Median	C6, C7, C8, T1	Palmar and distal dorsal aspects of lateral 3 ½ digits and lateral palm	Flexor carpi radialis, flexor digitorum superficialis, lateral half of flexor digitorum profundus, flexor pollicis longus, pronator quadratus, pronator teres, most thenar muscles, lateral lumbricals
Anterior interosseus	C6, C7, C8, T1	No sensory	Flexor digitorum profundus, flexor pollicis longus, pronator quadratus
Ulnar	C7, C8, T1	Medial hand including medial half of fourth digit	Flexor carpi ulnaris, medial half of flexor digitorum profundus, and most small muscles in hand
Radial	C5, C6, C7, C8, T1	Posterior aspect of forearm	Triceps brachii, anconeus, brachioradialis, extensor muscles of forearm
Posterior interosseous	C5, C6, C7, C8, T1	No sensory	Abductor pollicis longus, extensor pollicis brevis and longus, extensor digitorum communis, extensor indicis, extensor digiti minimi

Table 9-4	CLUSTER TEST FOR CERVICAL RADICULOPATHY[5,11,13]	
Test	**Description[5,11]**	**Image of Final Position**
ULTT 1 (median nerve)	Patient is supine. To test the left upper extremity, therapist stands to side of patient and grasps the superior shoulder girdle with the left hand and grasps patient's hand with the right hand. Therapist stabilizes the shoulder girdle by providing inferiorly directed force. Therapist abducts and externally rotates the shoulder to 90°. Once in this position, therapist slowly extends patient's elbow, supinates the forearm, and extends the wrist and fingers. This sequence of movements is performed to the point of symptom reproduction. Cervical sidebending and/or the release of wrist extension by the therapist can be used for further structural differentiation.	
ULTT 2A (median nerve)	Patient is supine. When testing the left upper extremity, physical therapist stands to the side of the patient (facing in a caudal direction) and grasps the shoulder with the right hand and grasps the patient's hand with the left hand. Therapist stabilizes the shoulder by providing inferiorly directed force with their right hand, maintaining that force with their right thigh. Therapist next externally rotates patient's shoulder, extends the elbow, supinates the forearm, and extends the wrist and fingers. Sequence of movements is performed to the point of symptom reproduction. Cervical sidebending, release of shoulder depression, and/or release of wrist extension can be used for further structural differentiation.	

(Continued)

Table 9-4 CLUSTER TEST FOR CERVICAL RADICULOPATHY[5,11,13] (CONTINUED)

Test	Description[5,11]	Image of Final Position
ULTT 2B (radial nerve)	Patient and therapist are in the same initial position as for ULTT 2A, except that the therapist extends the patient's elbow, pronates the forearm, flexes the wrist and fingers, and abducts the shoulder. Sequence of movements is performed to point of symptom reproduction. Release of shoulder girdle depression or release of wrist flexion can be used for further structural differentiation.	
ULTT 3 (ulnar nerve)	Patient is supine. To test the left upper extremity, therapist stands to side of patient and grasps the superior shoulder girdle with left hand and grasps patient's hand with their right hand. The therapist stabilizes the shoulder girdle by providing inferiorly directed force with their left hand. Therapist abducts and externally rotates the shoulder to 90°. Therapist flexes the patient's elbow, pronates the forearm, and extends the wrist and fingers. Sequence of movements is performed to the point of symptom reproduction. Cervical sidebending, release of shoulder girdle depression, and/or release of wrist extension can be used for further structural differentiation.	
Spurling's A	Patient is seated with neck laterally flexed toward the symptomatic upper extremity. Therapist applies approximately 7 kg of compressive force to the head applied in the direction of lateral flexion.[11]	

(Continued)

Table 9-4	CLUSTER TEST FOR CERVICAL RADICULOPATHY[5,11,13] (CONTINUED)	
Test	**Description[5,11]**	**Image of Final Position**
Distraction test	Test can be performed in sitting or supine. With the patient seated, therapist stands behind the patient, applies both hands to lateral sides of the head and applies an upward traction force. With the patient supine, the therapist grasps under the patient's chin and occiput and slightly flexes neck while applying a traction force of approximately 14 lb.[11] Wainner et al.[13] used the supine test version as part of the cluster of tests.	
Cervical rotation <60° to ipsilateral side	Patient is seated and motion is measured with a goniometer.	

patient's familiar pain via *sensitizing movements*. Sensitizing movements increase or decrease the strain on neural tissue by moving structures distal to the patient's familiar pain (*e.g.*, ipsilateral or contralateral cervical lateral flexion, elbow or wrist extension/flexion, shoulder girdle elevation).[5] Use of sensitizing movements, called structural differentiation, allows the clinician to determine whether a ULTT response is related to nerve mechanosensitivity.[12]

For diagnosing cervical radiculopathy, ULTT 1 demonstrates a sensitivity of 0.97 and a specificity of 0.22, while ULTT 2B has a sensitivity of 0.72 and specificity of 0.33.[11] In 2021, Grondin *et al.*[5] reported that although individual ULTTs did not lead to acceptable likelihood ratios or post-test probabilities for diagnosing cervical radiculopathy, having 3 out of 4 positive ULTTs was specific (0.97) in ruling in the diagnosis. Wainner *et al.*[13] evaluated 82 patients with electrophysiologically confirmed diagnosis of either cervical radiculopathy or carpal tunnel syndrome. By comparing the results of 34 clinical tests with the electrophysiologic examination, they found that **the performance of a cluster of 4 tests—ULTT 1, Spurling's A test, distraction test, and cervical AROM rotation (<60°) to the ipsilateral side—was most useful in aiding clinicians in the diagnosis of cervical radiculopathy.**[11,13] For example, the specificity associated with 2 positive tests out of these 4 is 0.56 and for 3 positive tests is 0.94. If all 4 of these tests are positive, the specificity for diagnosis of cervical radiculopathy is 0.99.[11,13]

Plan of Care and Interventions

Optimal treatment of cervical radiculopathy has not been established, but many studies support multimodal treatment paradigms.[14-17] The two primary interventions aimed at reducing symptom irritability and improving function for individuals with cervical radiculopathy are manual therapy and therapeutic exercise.[11,17,18] Neural mobilization can be performed as a manual therapy technique and also prescribed as a therapeutic exercise. Research supports the use of both passive (*i.e.*, manual therapy) and active (*i.e.*, exercise prescription) neural mobilization techniques to reduce pain and improve function.[15] Neural mobilization may improve neural vascularity, nerve movement, and reduce intraneural edema.[11,19-22] Neural mobilization is indicated when a patient presents with suspected cervical root and/or peripheral nerve involvement. **Studies suggest that the addition of neural mobilization improves pain and disability compared to standard treatment and no treatment.**[18,23]

Initial interventions typically include manual therapy to the cervical spine (*e.g.*, lateral glides) and nerve mobility interventions. Evidence supports the use of mobilization and manipulation techniques directed to both the cervical and thoracic spine (See Case 8).[21] A systematic review reported that lateral cervical glides (Table 9-5) and nerve mobility exercises (Table 9-5) decreased pain in patients with cervical radiculopathy.[18] In 20 individuals with clinical signs of cervical radiculopathy (including motor and/or sensory change and radiating pain in the arm/periscapular region), Thoomes *et al.*[17] implemented a weekly program that included cervicothoracic joint mobilization, neurodynamic mobilizations, and therapeutic exercises (self-neural mobilization and endurance training of cervical musculature) with the aim of improving median nerve excursion. After 3 months, subjects demonstrated large correlations between improvements in median nerve excursion at the elbow with reduced pain intensity and functional limitations.[17]

Other manual therapy interventions include treatment of the tissues (*e.g.*, joints, muscles) adjacent to neural tissue. Multiple studies have demonstrated reduced pain and disability when neural mobilization is combined with cervical manual therapy.[14,16,24] A randomized controlled trial of 66 patients with cervical radiculopathy comparing the effects of manual cervical traction, with and without the addition of neural mobilization, found statistically significant improvements in NDI scores, pain, and active cervical rotation in the traction-plus-neural mobilization compared to a wait-list control group.[14]

Self-mobilization techniques (Table 9-5) are prescribed to the patient as part of a comprehensive home exercise program (HEP). While dosage parameters vary among protocols, initial HEP prescription is typically guided by *minimal* symptom reproduction, which depends on each patient's tolerance and irritability level. As patient irritability reduces and tolerance improves, exercises are progressed with regard to duration, intensity, and range of motion. A systematic review by Basson *et al.*[18] lists a wide range of dosing strategies for interventions, ranging from relatively low frequency (*e.g.*, 1 set of 10 mobilizations performed 3 times per week) up to high frequency (*e.g.*, 10 repetitions of mobilizations performed 5 times daily, every day of the week).[18]

Table 9-5 MANUAL THERAPY AND SELF-MOBILIZATION TECHNIQUES FOR PATIENTS WITH CERVICAL RADICULOPATHY

Technique	Description[15, 25]	Figure
Lateral cervical glide mobilization technique	Patient is supine on the treatment table with cervical spine in neutral. With one hand, the therapist supports the patient's cervical spine below the segment that will be mobilized. With the other hand on the cervical spine ipsilateral to the symptomatic upper extremity, the therapist applies a lateral glide away from the symptomatic side.	
Median nerve self-mobilization	Patient is sitting or standing with cervical spine in neutral. The patient begins by moving the symptomatic upper extremity into the starting position: shoulder abduction and external rotation, forearm supination, elbow flexion, and wrist and finger flexion. From this position, patient extends the elbow, extends the wrist/fingers, and simultaneously side bends the cervical spine toward the symptomatic side. The patient then reverses the motion by flexing the wrist/fingers, flexing elbow, and sidebending the cervical spine to the asymptomatic side.	

(Continued)

Table 9-5 MANUAL THERAPY AND SELF-MOBILIZATION TECHNIQUES FOR PATIENTS WITH CERVICAL RADICULOPATHY (CONTINUED)

Technique	Description[15, 25]	Figure
Radial nerve self-mobilization	Patient is sitting or standing with cervical spine in neutral. Patient begins by moving the symptomatic upper extremity into the starting position: shoulder girdle depression and internal rotation, elbow extension, forearm pronation, and wrist/fingers/thumb flexion. From that position, the patient abducts the shoulder while also sidebending the cervical spine away from the involved side. The patient then reverses the motion by adducting the shoulder and sidebending the cervical spine back to neutral.	
Ulnar nerve self-mobilization	Patient is sitting or standing with cervical spine in neutral. Patient begins by moving the symptomatic upper extremity into the starting position: shoulder abduction and external rotation, elbow flexion to 90°, forearm pronation, wrist and finger extension. From this position, the patient then moves into wrist flexion and cervical sidebending toward the symptomatic side. The patient then reverses the motion by extending the wrist and fingers and returning the cervical spine to neutral.	
Thoracic manipulation (high-velocity low-amplitude thrust)	See Case 8	See Figs 8-2; 8-4; 8-5; 8-6

As the patient's symptoms resolve, the therapist should prescribe therapeutic exercises to address identified deficits in motion and strength and to improve posture. Patients with chronic symptoms should be encouraged to participate in recreational exercise.[8] Cardiovascular training and resistance training have been shown in multiple studies to improve overall health.[25-28] The Centers for Disease Control and Prevention recommend that adults should perform 150 minutes of moderate-intensity aerobic exercise per week (*e.g.*, brisk walking) or 75 minutes of vigorous-intensity aerobic exercise per week, or some combination of the two.[29] For individuals with chronic neck pain (with or without radiating pain), aerobic exercise also improves neck pain and reduces disability at 6-month follow-up when combined with neck-specific exercises.[30]

Evidence-Based Clinical Recommendations

SORT: Strength of Recommendation Taxonomy

A: Consistent, good-quality patient-oriented evidence
B: Inconsistent or limited-quality patient-oriented evidence
C: Consensus, disease-oriented evidence, usual practice, expert opinion, or case series

1. Most individuals with cervical radiculopathy improve with conservative care. **Grade B**

2. The performance of a cluster of 4 clinical tests—ULLT 1, Spurling's A test, distraction test, and cervical AROM rotation (<60°) to the ipsilateral side—can be used to accurately diagnose cervical radiculopathy. **Grade A**

3. Neural mobilization techniques reduce symptom severity in individuals presenting with cervical radiculopathy. **Grade B**

COMPREHENSION QUESTIONS

9.1 A positive ULTT has which of the following components?
   A. At least partial reproduction of familiar neck and/or arm pain
   B. Reduced reflex testing
   C. Diminished cutaneous sensation
   D. Reduced cervical spine range of motion

9.2 Which of the following is NOT part of the cervical radiculopathy cluster testing?
   A. Spurling's A test
   B. Distraction test
   C. First rib test
   D. ULTT A test

ANSWERS

9.1 **A.**

9.2 **C.** The cervical radiculopathy cluster tests include Upper limb tension test A, Spurling A test, distraction test, cervical rotation <60° to the ipsilateral side.[11]

REFERENCES

1. Iyer S, Kim HJ. Cervical radiculopathy. *Curr Rev Musculoskelet Med.* 2016; 9:272-80.

2. Radhakrishnan K, Litchy WJ, O'Fallon WM, Kurland LT. Epidemiology of cervical radiculopathy. A population-based study from Rochester, Minnesota, 1976 through 1990. *Brain.* 1994;117 (Pt 2):325-335.

3. Kelsey JL, Githens PB, Walter SD, et al. An epidemiological study of acute prolapsed cervical intervertebral disc. *J Bone Joint Surg Am.* 1984;66:907-914.

4. Woods BI, Hilibrand AS. Cervical radiculopathy: epidemiology, etiology, diagnosis, and treatment. *J Spinal Disord Tech.* 2015;28:E251-259.

5. Grondin F, Cook C, Hall T, et al. Diagnostic accuracy of upper limb neurodynamic tests in the diagnosis of cervical radiculopathy. *Musculoskelet Sci Pract.* 2021;55:epub ahead of print.

6. Wong JJ, Côté P, Quesnele JJ, et al. The course and prognostic factors of symptomatic cervical disc herniation with radiculopathy: a systematic review of the literature. *Spine J.* 2014;14:1781-1789.

7. Blanpied PR, Gross AR, Elliott JM, et al. Neck Pain: Revision 2017. *J Orthop Sports Phys Ther.* 2017;47:A1-A83.

8. Nikolaidis I, Fouyas IP, Sandercock PA, Statham PF. Surgery for cervical radiculopathy or myelopathy. *Cochrane Database Syst Rev.* 2010;2010:CD001466.

9. Magee DJ. *Orthopedic Physical Assessment.* 6th ed. St. Louis, MS: Saunders Elsevier; 2014.

10. Neumann DA, Kelly ER, Kiefer CL, et al. *Kinesiology of the Musculoskeletal System: Foundations for Rehabilitation.* 2nd ed. St. Louis, MO: Elsevier; 2017.

11. Cleland JA, Koppenhaver S. *Netter's Orthopaedic Clinical Examination. An Evidence-Based Approach.* 2nd ed. Philadelphia, PA: Elsevier; 2015.

12. Nee RJ, Jull GA, Vicenzino B, Coppieters MW. The validity of upper-limb neurodynamic tests for detecting peripheral neuropathic pain. *J Orthop Sports Phys Ther.* 2012;42:413-424.

13. Wainner RS, Fritz JM, Irrgang JJ, et al. Reliability and diagnostic accuracy of the clinical examination and patient self-report measures for cervical radiculopathy. *Spine.* 2003;28:52-62.

14. Savva C, Vasileios K, Efstathio M, Karagiannis C. Cervical traction combined with neural mobilization for patients with cervical radiculopathy: A randomized control trial. *J Bodyw Mov Ther.* 2021;26:279-289.

15. Ayub A, Osama M, Shaki-ur-Rehman, Ahmad S. Effects of active versus passive upper extremity neural mobilization combined with mechanical traction and joint mobilization in females with cervical radiculopathy: A randomized controlled trial. *J Back Musculoskelet Rehabil.* 2019;32:725-730.

16. Ranganath PNU, Dowle P, Chandrasekhar P. Effectiveness of MWM, neurodynamics and conventional therapy versus neurodynamics and conventional therapy in unilateral cervical radiculopathy: A randomized control trial. *Indian J Physiother Occup Ther.* 2018;12:101-106.

17. Thoomes E, Ellis R, Dilley A, et al. Excursion of the median nerve during a contra-lateral cervical lateral glide movement in people with and without cervical radiculopathy. *Musculoskelet Sci Pract.* 2021;52:102349. Epub ahead of print.

18. Basson A, Olivier B, Ellis R, et al. The effectiveness of neural mobilization for neuromusculoskeletal conditions: a systematic review and meta-analysis. *J Orthop Sports Phys Ther.* 2017;47:593-615.

19. Mersy DJ. Health benefits of aerobic exercise. *Postgrad Med.* 1991;90:103-112.

20. Boudier-Revéret M, Gilbert KK, et al. Effect of neurodynamic mobilization on fluid dispersion in median nerve at the level of the carpal tunnel: A cadaveric study. *Musculoskelet Sci Pract.* 2017;31:45-51.

21. Brown CL, Gilbert KK, Brismee JM, et al. The effects of neurodynamic mobilization on fluid dispersion within the tibial nerve at the ankle: an unembalmed cadaveric study. *J Man Manip Ther.* 2011;19:26-34.

22. Gilbert KK, Roger James C, Apte G, et al. Effects of simulated neural mobilization on fluid movement in cadaveric peripheral nerve sections: implications for the treatment of neuropathic pain and dysfunction. *J Man Manip Ther.* 2015;23:219-225.

23. Rodríguez-Sanz D, López-López D, Unda-Solano F, et al. Effects of median nerve neural mobilization in treating cervicobrachial pain: A randomized waiting list-controlled clinical trial. *Pain Practice.* 2017;18:431-442.

24. Kim DG, Chung SH, Jung HB. The effects of neural mobilization on cervical radiculopathy patients' pain, disability, ROM, and deep flexor endurance. *J Back Musculoskelet Rehabilit.* 2017;30:951-959.

25. Fernández-de-Las-Peñas C, Arias-Buría JL, Cleland JA, et al. Manual therapy versus surgery for carpal tunnel syndrome: 4-year follow-Up from a randomized controlled trial. *Phys Ther.* 2020;100: 1987-1996.

26. Ruiz JR, Sui X, Lobelo F, et al. Association between muscular strength and mortality in men: prospective cohort study. *BMJ.* 2008;337(7661):a439.

27. Kamada M, Shiroma EJ, Buring JE, et al. Strength training and all-cause, cardiovascular disease, and cancer mortality in older women: a cohort study. *J Am Heart Assoc.* 2017;6:e007677.

28. García-Hermoso A, Cavero-Redondo I, Ramírez-Vélez R, et al. Muscular strength as a predictor of all-cause mortality in an apparently healthy population: a systematic review and meta-analysis of data from approximately 2 million men and women. *Arch Phys Med Rehabil.* 2018;99:2100-2113.e5.

29. Centers for Disease Control and Prevention. How much physical activity do adults need? https://www.cdc.gov/physicalactivity/basics/adults/index.htm. Published October 7, 2020. Accessed October 27, 2021.

30. Daher A, Carel RS, Tzipi K, et al. The effectiveness of an aerobic exercise training on patients with neck pain during a short- and long-term follow-up: a prospective double-blind randomized controlled trial. *Clin Rehabil.* 2020;34:617-629.

Neck Dissection for Cancer: Postsurgical Rehabilitation

Douglas Lauchlan

CASE 10

A right-hand dominant 46-year-old self-employed carpenter presents to an outpatient physical therapist with a referral from a head and neck surgeon. The patient has been complaining of increasing pain in the right shoulder region following a right-sided neck dissection performed 3 months ago. Six months ago, the patient was diagnosed with squamous cell carcinoma of the mucosal lining of the head and neck and he has been undergoing intervention for this condition since. Surgical clearance of Levels I to IV of the posterior triangle of the neck was performed and the patient completed 5 weeks of daily radiotherapy to this region. The patient's previous medical history is otherwise unremarkable. The patient has been complaining of an inability to fully elevate his right upper limb since the surgery and increasing pain has also caused his sleep to become disturbed. He is aware that he "lacks strength" in his right upper limb in a variety of activities of daily living (ADLs). He reports that his social encounters with other individuals who have undergone head and neck surgery have made him fearful that his physical function will continue to deteriorate and he is concerned about his future quality of life.

▶ What are the examination priorities?
▶ Based on his health condition, what do you anticipate may be the contributors to activity limitations?
▶ What are possible complications that may limit the effectiveness of physical therapy?
▶ What is his rehabilitation prognosis?
▶ Describe a physical therapy plan of care based on each stage of the health condition.
▶ How might the patient's emotional condition affect rehabilitation?

KEY DEFINITIONS

HEAD AND NECK CANCER: Cancer of the mucosal lining of the head and neck, most commonly involving the lymph nodes of the neck

NECK DISSECTION: Surgical clearance of all cancerous cells and relevant lymph nodes of the region; commonly called "Levels I to IV clearance" based on the anatomical division of lymph nodes of the neck into distinct groups

QUALITY OF LIFE (QOL): Relates not only to the ability of an individual to perform activities of daily living (ADLs), but also to social interactions with others; commonly takes into consideration physical, mental, and emotional health

SHOULDER: Includes both the glenohumeral and scapulothoracic complex and associated musculature that control position and range of motion (ROM) of the upper limb

Objectives

1. Outline the anticipated physical presentation of the individual at 3 months postsurgical neck dissection and identify the adaptive processes that have likely occurred.

2. Understand the interaction of different neuromusculoskeletal structures causing dysfunction at the shoulder region.

3. Identify appropriate clinical objective measures to monitor change and evaluate the impact of physical therapy interventions.

4. Identify outcome measures for both functional and QOL status for this patient population.

5. Outline the possible emotional and behavioral issues that are likely to impact rehabilitation and recovery.

6. Describe the benefits of a holistic philosophy of care for this patient population.

Physical Therapy Considerations

Physical therapy considerations during management of the head and neck cancer survivor with the development of shoulder region pain and disability several months after neck dissection:

▶ **General physical therapy plan of care/goals:** Prevent or minimize loss of ROM of the glenohumeral joint in particular, but also the neck and scapulothoracic regions; restore (as close as possible) local muscle recruitment and static/dynamic postural controls; encourage functional strength gains in associated global muscles of the shoulder region; restore ability to perform ADLs, as able; improve QOL

▶ **Physical therapy interventions:** Patient education regarding regular maintenance of shoulder ROM; stretching; joint mobilization; exercises to promote scapular control; postural and functional re-education resistance training; promotion and reintegration of social and physical activity

▶ **Precautions during physical therapy:** Skin viability and impact of physical therapy to skin flaps/grafts at neck; potential onset of adhesive capsulitis of the glenohumeral joint; ongoing medical health status

▶ **Complications interfering with physical therapy:** Social and lifestyle factors that may impact compliance/engagement of individual to regular physical therapy sessions; postsurgical activity modifications

Understanding the Health Condition

Despite recent surgical advances, there is still a high mortality rate in individuals requiring surgical clearance of the posterior triangle for head and neck cancer.[1] Although survival rates are improving, survivors face significant issues relating to shoulder disability and its impact on QOL. Almost one in every two patients recovering from head and neck cancer surgery quit working solely due to shoulder disability; three in every four patients report difficulty returning to everyday tasks with regard to social and recreational activity.[2] Despite the evolution of surgical procedures for this condition, shoulder disability is considered an unavoidable by-product of surgery.[2,3] Although its etiology and pathogenesis are debated, postoperative shoulder disability following neck dissection is widely accepted. Patten and Hillel[4] first suggested that postoperative shoulder disability may be due to adhesive capsulitis of the glenohumeral joint (GHJ) that is associated with nonuse of the upper limb on the side of surgery during the postoperative period. More recent work in this field has shown that abnormal scapular control due to temporary or permanent damage to the spinal accessory nerve (CN XI) results in altered GHJ mechanics with resulting pain and disability.[5,6] The spinal accessory nerve arises from two sources: the cranial roots from the medulla and the spinal roots from the first five segments of the spinal cord. The nerve makes its passage through the posterior triangle of the neck to innervate both the sternocleidomastoid and the lower fibers of the trapezius. Thus, radical surgical clearance of the neck often has an impact on associated neuromusculoskeletal structures of the neck and shoulder region that can result in symptomatic and asymptomatic movement disorders.

Physical therapy management of shoulder disability following neck dissection is aimed at creating a holistic and balanced approach to functional return and promotion of normal movement of the shoulder region. Due to the adaptable nature of the neuromusculoskeletal system, developmental movement disorders may require time to become established. Shoulder disability commonly presents over weeks and months following surgery. Early literature on the development of shoulder problems following neck dissection suggested that partial injury and entrapment of the spinal accessory nerve (primary motor innervation to lower fibers of trapezius muscle) is the reason for a delayed onset in shoulder disability.[7] This hypothesis has been supported in recent literature describing that patients commonly do not report symptoms until *weeks* postsurgery.[8] Although the role of the spinal accessory nerve and resulting lower trapezius paresis is recognized, it has been proposed that the latent onset of pain is more attributable to adhesive capsulitis of the GHJ.[4] The concept that adhesive capsulitis of the GHJ can result from sustained altered mechanics of the scapulothoracic muscles (regardless of initial etiology) is well recognized in the physical therapy literature.[9-11] Furthermore, the establishment of adhesive capsulitis significantly reduces the effectiveness of physical therapy interventions.[9] The post-neck dissection patient population, therefore, appears at risk of developing shoulder pain and disability with subsequent resistance to effective physical therapy interventions. Many authors have attempted to throw more light on the nature of this postsurgical shoulder phenomenon termed "radical neck dissection/11th nerve syndrome." However, its etiology remains difficult to elucidate due to the developing nature of the disability. Early after surgery, patients are commonly in pain and demonstrate paresis of the lower trapezius muscle, but there is rarely any capsular shortening or adaptations until 6 to 12 months following surgery.[1,2,4] Recognizing that radical neck dissection/11th nerve syndrome may be due to the emergence of adhesive capsulitis is significant, but understanding what movement adaptations lead to this clinical state is still unknown.

Panjabi[12] has proposed a model for physical therapists to understand normal movement and the neuromusculoskeletal factors that may lead to dysfunction. This model suggests that injury to structures belonging to one or more subsystems results in overall system dysfunction. Figure 10-1 shows how this model can be adapted to the pathodynamics and development of postoperative shoulder disability following neck dissection.

Given that there is a 50% chance of injury to the spinal accessory nerve postsurgery, there are often complex maladaptive movement patterns that arise through these subsystem interactions which relate to eventual shoulder pain and disability.[3,6] Despite the development of shoulder pain and disability, it is important to recognize the individual and their immediate healthcare needs. Surviving cancer and the subsequent surgical clearance can have a profound impact on the physical

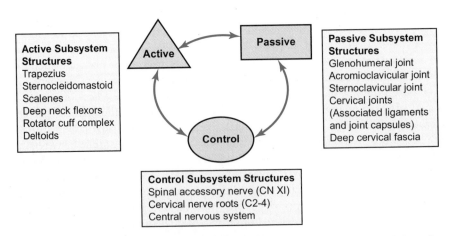

Figure 10-1. A subsystem-based approach to rehabilitation of the shoulder following neck dissection surgery (Adapted from Panjabi MM. The stabilizing system of the spine. Part I. Function, dysfunction, adaptation, and enhancement. *J Spinal Disord.* 1992;5:383-389.)

and emotional well-being of this patient population.[13] Therefore, it is of great importance to consider strategies of engagement and participation when establishing a rehabilitation program. The physical therapist should evaluate the person holistically as they improve not only their functional status, but also their social participation in typical vocational and habitual environments.

Physical Therapy Patient/Client Management

Physical therapy management of this population can be divided into three domains following the International Classification of Function, Disability and Health: impairments, activity limitations, and participation restrictions.[14] Postsurgical inpatient management is aimed at the main impairment: injury to neuromusculoskeletal tissues in the aftermath of surgical clearance. Management includes respiratory and airway monitoring, postural advice, and maintenance of active ROM of the shoulder and neck region. After surgery, treatment commonly involves a period of outpatient radiotherapy directed toward the neck/shoulder area. This approach to cancer management is typified by a period of change in the patient's social and daily routines that must incorporate a demanding schedule of treatment. It is important that the physical therapist engages the patient in his shoulder/neck rehabilitation during this period, emphasizing maintenance of GHJ ROM to avoid capsular tightening.[15] During the next phase of rehabilitation, impairments and activity limitations need to be addressed. There is a need to maximize active ROM and return strength and power of the muscles affecting the shoulder and neck region. It is critical at this stage to recognize the impact of the neural control subsystem and likely adaptive scapular mechanics due to abnormal neuromuscular control. The typical postsurgical adaptations and potential for postsurgical upper limb disuse have a significant impact on the balance and integration of the other subsystems. The third phase of management focuses on lifestyle participation and reintegration of ADLs including work, hobbies, and typical social interaction.

Examination, Evaluation, and Diagnosis

The physical therapist starts the examination by observing the head, neck, and shoulder structures. Although there are numerous notable observations 3 months following neck dissection surgery (*e.g.*, skin grafting), many of these features are unlikely to impact shoulder function at this stage and will not be discussed. On the side of the neck dissection, decreased muscle mass around the shoulder creates the classic "square-edge" to the deltoid due to the bony prominence of the acromion process being more easily visible. Another common bony point to assess is the spine of the scapula, where significant wasting of the supraspinatus and infraspinatus muscles can be apparent due to disuse atrophy. The patient will most likely adopt the "forward head posture" position with a similarly protracted and elevated scapula. This leads to two significant postural adaptations: lengthened deep neck flexors (similar adaptation seen post-whiplash[16]) and a reduced subacromial space due to a lack of dynamic stability as the humeral head migrates in a cephalad direction.[11]

Shoulder active range of motion (AROM) should be measured with a goniometer and compared between the affected and unaffected limbs. The affected shoulder often shows reduced glenohumeral elevation with abnormal scapular control due to denervation of the lower trapezius and resulting compensatory *hyperactive* fibers of the upper trapezius.[10] Depending on the stage of adaptive shortening of the GHJ capsule, loss of functional upper limb elevation is likely associated with a combined loss of physiological flexion and abduction of the GHJ. This may also be associated with a tight elastic end feel and pain on testing passive ROM (PROM) of the GHJ. The most limited movements are likely to follow the capsular pattern of restriction at the GHJ (lateral rotation is most restricted, followed by abduction, flexion, and then extension).[17]

Strength testing is unlikely to be painful, but the patient may have selective or global weakness (especially in shoulder abduction) due to lack of scapular control. The physical therapist must evaluate the postsurgical motor involvement of the spinal accessory nerve. An inability to actively shrug the affected shoulder (upper trapezius fibers) and/or an inability to control the scapulothoracic fixation during active elevation of the upper limb—commonly seen as "winging" of the inferior angle of the scapula (lower trapezius fibers) clearly highlight the presence of an impaired motor output and the likelihood of spinal accessory nerve damage.[18] Thorough neurologic testing should be conducted because the patient may present with decreased or absent sensation, numbness, and/or an associated hypoalgesia or hyperalgesia around the site of the surgery and skin graft. There may also be adaptive proprioceptive loss as the subsystems attempt to correct the adaptive imbalances postsurgery.[11]

Significant restrictions in AROM and PROM in the cervical spine are likely to be present due to superficial facial and neck scarring (from the skin graft) and deeper scarring due to the surgical clearance technique. The most affected movements are side bending away from the affected side and rotation toward the affected side. As previously described, a loss of local muscle control (deep neck flexor recruitment) often leads to muscle system imbalances of the head and neck (*e.g.*, hyperactive sternocleidomastoid and upper trapezius). This pattern further contributes to the loss of cervical spine AROM. Often, there is adaptive stiffness and discomfort on palpation and with passive accessory movements of C3 to C5 vertebrae.

Several tests and outcome measures, including goniometry, pain ratings, and passive end feels can be used to identify impairments. Although more commonly used in populations presenting with a traumatic shoulder injury, the shoulder assessment devised by Constant and Murley[19] is a robust tool that could be used to measure the impact of the postsurgical impairment on the individual. QOL can be measured using a variety of instruments. A cancer-specific tool such as the University of Washington QOL scale can be used to measure the impact of rehabilitation on recovery,[20] or a more generic QOL measure (SF-36) may be considered for participation.[21] The **Functional Assessment of Cancer Therapy—Head and Neck (FACTH&N)** has been used to specifically evaluate the impact of rehabilitation with this population.[5] The FACTH&N is a multidimensional 39-question self-report QOL outcome measure that allows the therapist to gain insight regarding the functional status of the individual and the presence and extent of risk factors which may be associated with an emerging shoulder dysfunction. Because the FACTH&N has been designed for this population, its value and response has more validity than the use of non-disease-specific evaluative tools or disease-specific tools that do not focus on functional return. Regardless of the outcome measure selected for monitoring effectiveness of clinical care, measurement of QOL is of great value in determining the meaningfulness of survival to the individual.[22, 23]

Plan of Care and Interventions

Because the GHJ capsule tightens due to pain and disuse,[9] the **most important aspect of the physical therapy plan of care with respect to the shoulder impairment is to maintain active and passive shoulder ROM.** However, emerging evidence reflects that **progressive resistance training should be included to promote return to presurgical levels of function.**[24] Heat, soft tissue massage, and cervical mobilizations can be directed to the neck and upper quadrant in an effort to reduce pain and hyperactivity of the global muscle system.[25] The physical therapist must caution the patient that return to normal scapular motion or control may not be possible due to denervation of lower trapezius fibers resulting from injury to the spinal accessory nerve (commonly seen as "winging" of the inferior angle of the scapula).[10]

Results from the objective examination should help the therapist rule in or rule out the presence of adhesive capsulitis. Passive GHJ capsular stretches should be performed to directly address any adaptive shortening of the soft tissues of the shoulder. Maintenance of the available shoulder ROM is essential through this phase to avoid the changes associated with disuse. Although active assisted ROM (AAROM) exercises are commonly used in physical therapy sessions, the ability of the patient to perform these daily at home may be limited due to the nature of the typical equipment used (*i.e.*, over-the-door shoulder pulley system). Creative attempts to promote an active-assisted role in maintaining shoulder ROM should be sought, such as holding a cane or stick with both hands and using the unaffected arm to guide the affected arm through all ranges of motion. Progressive active upper extremity exercise can be augmented with graded resistance using (color-coded) therapeutic elastic bands.[5] Progressive resistance can be applied in functional patterns of movement to improve both muscle re-education and neuromuscular recruitment and timing relating to functional patterns of normal movement.[10,11] The physical therapist must also address the impact of upper trunk and cervical resting posture on available shoulder ROM. Developmental thoracic kyphosis and increased cervical lordosis should be directly addressed, as necessary.[26] Simple postural awareness and active stretching can be implemented with the goal of reducing the tendency to adopt these restrictive postures.

Task-specific rehabilitation approaches should be considered for this population. These could be directed toward vocational-related tasks, components of day-to-day duties and general lifestyle requirements, and hobbies or recreational pursuits. Patients should be actively involved in this process of problem solving and goal setting because this enhances ownership and creates shared dialogue between therapist and patient. This shared goal-setting approach should be monitored and directed by both parties as the patient's needs change. Throughout the patient's episode of care, shoulder function and strength gains should be developed through an integrative and functionally directed return to activity. This reinforces the patient's understanding of the value and importance of a progressive rehabilitation process approach. In conjunction with developing self-directed rehabilitation habits, the patient must feel that his needs are being met by any prescriptive intervention. In other words, the patient needs to positively *value* the prescriptive and general advice he has been given. To measure the impact of this rehabilitation approach on the individual, the physical therapist may use the Consultation and Relational Empathy (CARE) measure.[27] This measure is designed to evaluate the health practitioner's empathy throughout the consultation and treatment process. Not only is **empathy strongly linked with understanding the patient's condition, but it is also hugely influential on the patient's compliance with directed care.**[23] Thus, the likelihood of successful rehabilitation that is dependent on patient compliance with prescribed therapeutic interventions is linked to the degree to which the physical therapist provides empathic care.

Managing the impairment and activity limitations of patients following neck dissection surgery is merely a component of the overall rehabilitation strategy. Patients need to link these traditional physical therapy principles of management to their social inclusion and participation with others. Relationship building and support networks are vital in regaining life focus and a sense of well-being (both from a physical and mental perspective). The physical therapist can measure the patient's self-perceived QOL with the SF-36. If possible, the therapist should observe the patient's natural environment and the many complex influences involved in his sense of well-being and ability to return to performance of ADLs. The therapist should also consider the impact of the patient's reappraisal of the internal criteria that shapes his fundamental values. Many patients may *not* wish to return to the lifestyle and environments they had prior to diagnosis/surgery.[28] This should be explored on an individual basis and the rehabilitation strategy directly based on the patient's needs. Simple short-term to long-term goals should be set and re-evaluated as the rehabilitation program progresses. The supportive roles of other healthcare professionals (in particular psychologists and occupational therapists) may be helpful in this process and should be considered as part of the multidisciplinary approach to care.

Evidence-Based Clinical Recommendations

SORT: Strength of Recommendation Taxonomy

A: Consistent, good-quality patient-oriented evidence
B: Inconsistent or limited-quality patient-oriented evidence
C: Consensus, disease-oriented evidence, usual practice, expert opinion, or case series

1. The Functional Assessment of Cancer Therapy—Head and Neck (FACTH&N) is a sensitive multidimensional self-report instrument that measures quality of life and functional status in individuals after neck dissection surgery. **Grade A**

2. Maintenance of glenohumeral joint active ROM and passive capsular stretches prevent the onset of adhesive capsulitis following neck dissection surgery. **Grade C**

3. Incorporation of progressive resistance training results in more effective returns in function and daily activities. **Grade B**

4. Increased empathy on the part of the physical therapist throughout the evaluation and treatment process increases patient compliance with prescribed therapeutic interventions and the likelihood of successful rehabilitation that depends on patient compliance. **Grade B**

COMPREHENSION QUESTIONS

10.1 Following surgery for head and neck cancer, a patient visits a physical therapist for the first time due to recent emergence of shoulder pain. She is scared to move the upper limb for fear of injury and damaging her shoulder. List the following treatment goals in order of the MOST likely priority, from highest to lowest.

    A. Maintain GHJ ROM

    B. Educate on pain values and the beliefs involving pain and damage

    C. Improve muscle strength

    D. Return to typical ADLs

    E. Reduce pain

10.2 A client is referred to a physical therapy clinic by a specialist head and neck surgeon for "rehabilitation of the shoulder" 3 months after undergoing dissection and clearance of the posterior triangle of the neck. After 2 weeks of physical therapy sessions, the patient expresses a desire to stop further treatment. She is not in much pain and is managing most of her ADLs, as long as she does not need to lift her arm above her head. She has a very supportive husband who is "doing everything" for her. What is the MOST appropriate course of action for the physical therapist to pursue?

    A. Agree with the client that she has no current deficits or predictable risks for deficits in the future and immediately discharge her from physical therapy.

    B. Educate the client about the risks for decreased ROM and functional decline and suggest a strategy to resolve any conflict and move forward together with agreed goals.

    C. Insist that the client continue therapy because she has not met all the goals that the physical therapist has set for her.

    D. Educate the client about the risks for decreased ROM and functional decline, but if she does not agree with your assessment that she needs to continue physical therapy, encourage her husband to continue to perform the overhead activities that she cannot perform.

ANSWERS

10.1 Although every individual must be assessed and managed on a prioritized impairment basis, the likely prioritization here would be **B, E, A, D, C**. A main barrier to rehabilitation is the patient's attitudes and beliefs about pain and damage (option B; *i.e.*, "hurt ≠ harm"). Pain may be modifiable through the use of modalities like transcutaneous electrical nerve stimulation (option E). Maintaining the physiological range of shoulder motion is key to attempting to prevent the onset of adhesive capsulitis of the GHJ joint and the resultant long-term morbidity (option A). Although a return to work may not be possible due to postoperative health concerns and the particular duties and tasks required at work, typical ADLs should be promoted at this stage (option D). Social inclusion and a return to normal recreation and lifestyle may allow a greater sense of physical and emotional well-being, and enhance participation and control, which is commonly reduced in patients who may feel marginalized following their treatment for cancer. An attempt by the therapist to realize the classification of functional domains during the rehabilitation process (impairment, activity limitations, and participation restrictions) allows a more holistic, patient-centered approach to the care episode. This should translate to greater patient empowerment and allow more effective management/rehabilitation outcomes. Maintenance of ROM should be considered as ongoing but less essential immediately because capsular shortening and adaptation is unlikely to become established until later in the developmental process. Similarly, traditional progressive resisted global muscle strengthening is likely not an immediate priority until pain and scapular control have been addressed (option C). Establishing an empathetic relationship with the patient is of greater importance in the immediate phase of rehabilitation, in an effort to optimize patient understanding and compliance in a self-directed program of flexibility and strengthening.

10.2 **B.** The key issue to address here is the development of adaptive soft tissue changes through disuse of the upper limb. With avoidance of full shoulder ROM, there is an increased likelihood of developing adhesive capsulitis of the GHJ with associated pain and disability following a cessation of care at this stage (option A). The client has just begun physical therapy and is unlikely to have developed much adaptive soft tissue shortening at this stage. However, there may be maladaptive scapular motion and poor scapulothoracic control limiting upper limb elevation on the affected side. This may not be holding the client back functionally because she has a supportive husband who may also still be adapting psychologically to the role of caregiver. The client is only 3 to 4 months postsurgery and is likely to have many other commitments to ongoing postoperative care from consultant surgical reviews to oncology, speech and language therapy, dietician and occupational therapy appointments. At this stage, she may not realize the potential issues associated with her shoulder because the maladaptive cycle of capsular shortening and pain has not become fully established. As much as the physical therapist may wish to persevere with a traditional approach to preventing maladaptive changes at the shoulder region (options C and D), there should be more effort at this juncture to establish the therapeutic relationship—not only with the client but with her husband as well. There is often a significant sense of change with regard to the client's values and belief systems and perhaps also within the relationship she has with her husband. There needs to be acknowledgement that "doing everything" for her in this "new" postoperative predicament may not be the most appropriate strategy for the couple in the longer term, as there is a need to promote the client's active glenohumeral range and functional involvement in ADLs. Establishing informed and shared objectives for treatment is necessary not only in creating daily routines that can help prevent the onset of adhesive capsulitis but also in enhancing positive behavior toward functional independence and social interactions. There may have to be some negotiation between client and therapist with respect to the level and frequency of contact at this point postoperatively. The physical therapist must recognize the overall impact the surgery and commitment to the postoperative care is having on both the client and her husband. However, regular monitoring of clinical signs should be agreed on and the client must engage with this on a regular basis. This could be measured through both manual testing of the passive physiological movement available at the GHJ alongside a more holistic functional measure of outcome (e.g., FACTH&N). A shared goal-setting and management planning approach should aim to evaluate the effectiveness of any home program which may be undertaken as an alternative to frequent visits to the physical therapy clinic. This gives confidence to the client that her functional status is being maintained by her *self-directed* approach through promoting a return to typical ADLs where possible.

REFERENCES

1. Hillel AD, Kroll H, Dorman J, Medieros J. Radical neck dissection: a subjective and objective evaluation of postoperative disability. *J Otolaryngol.* 1989;18:53-61.

2. Shone GR, Yardley MP. An audit into the incidence of handicap after unilateral radical neck dissection. *J Laryngol Otol.* 1991;105:760-762.

3. van Wilgen CP, Dijkstra PU, van der Laan BF, et al. Shoulder complaints after neck dissection; is the spinal accessory nerve involved? *Br J Oral Maxillofac Surg.* 2003;41:7-11.

4. Patten C, Hillel AD. The 11th nerve syndrome. Accessory nerve palsy or adhesive capsulitis. *Arch Otolaryngol Head Neck Surg.* 1993;119:215-220.

5. McNeely ML, Parliament M, Courneya KS, et al. A pilot study of a randomized controlled trial to evaluate the effects of progressive resistance exercise training on shoulder dysfunction caused by spinal accessory neurapraxia/neurectomy in head and neck cancer survivors. *Head Neck.* 2004;26:518-530.

6. Lauchlan DT, McCaul JA, McCarron T. Neck dissection and the clinical appearance of post-operative shoulder disability: the post-operative role of physiotherapy. *Eur J Cancer Care.* 2008;17:542-548.

7. Gordon SL, Graham WP 3rd, Black JT, et al. Accessory nerve function after surgical procedures in the posterior triangle. *Arch Surg.* 1977;112:264-268.

8. Hillel AD, Patten C. Neck Dissection: Morbidity and Rehabilitation. In: Jacobs C, ed. *Carcinoma of the Head and Neck: Evaluation and Management.* Boston, MA: Kluwer Academic Publishers;1990.

9. Stam HW. Frozen shoulder: a review of current concepts. *Physiotherapy.* 1994;80:588-598.

10. Mottram SL. Dynamic stability of the scapula. *Man Ther.* 1997;2:123-131.

11. Hess SA. Functional stability of the glenohumeral joint. *Man Ther.* 2000;5:63-71.

12. Panjabi MM. The stabilizing system of the spine. Part I. Function, dysfunction, adaptation, and enhancement. *J Spinal Disord.* 1992;5:383-389.

13. Lauchlan DT, McCaul JA, McCarron T, et al. An exploratory trial of preventative rehabilitation on shoulder disability and quality of life in patients following neck dissection surgery. *Eur J Cancer Care.* 2011;20:113-122.

14. Ustun TB, Chatterji S, Bickenbach J, et al. The International Classification of Functioning, Disability and Health: a new tool for understanding disability and health. *Disabil Rehabil.* 2003;25:565-571.

15. Baggi F, Santoro L, Grosso E, et al. Motor and functional recovery after neck dissection: comparison of two early physical rehabilitation programmes. *Acta Otorhinolaryngol Ital.* 2014;34:230-240.

16. Jull GA. Deep cervical flexor muscle dysfunction in whiplash. *J Musculoskeletal Pain.* 2000;8:143-154.

17. Clarkson HM. *Musculoskeletal Assessment: Joint Range of Motion and Manual Muscle Strength.* 2nd ed. Philadelphia, PA: Lippincott Williams & Wilkins;2000.

18. McGarvey AC, Osmotherly PG, Hoffman GR, Chiarelli PE. Scapular muscle exercises following neck dissection surgery for head and neck cancer: a comparative electromyographic study. *Phys Ther.* 2013;93:786–797.

19. Constant CR, Murley AH. A clinical method of functional assessment of the shoulder. *Clin Orthop Relat Res.* 1987;214:160-164.

20. Rogers SN, Scott B, Lowe D. An evaluation of the shoulder domain of the University of Washington quality of life scale. *Br J Oral Maxillofac Surg.* 2007;45:5-10.

21. Ware JE Jr, Sherbourne CD. The MOS 36-item short form health survey (SF-36). I. Conceptual framework and item selection. *Med Care.* 1992;30:473-481.

22. Nibu K, Ebihara Y, Ebihara M, et al. Quality of life after neck dissection: a multicenter longitudinal study by the Japanese Clinical Study Group on Standardization of Treatment for Lymph Node Metastasis of Head and Neck Cancer. *Int J Clin Oncol.* 2010;15:33-38.

23. Morton RP, Izzard ME. Quality-of-life outcomes in head and neck cancer patients. *World J Surg.* 2003;27:884-889.

24. Harris AS. Do patients benefit from physiotherapy for shoulder dysfunction following neck dissection? A systematic review. *J Laryngol Otol.* 2020;134:104-108.

25. Ginn KA, Herbert RD, Khouw W, Lee R. A randomized, controlled clinical trial of a treatment for shoulder pain. *Phys Ther.* 1997;77:802-811.

26. Crawford HJ, Jull GA. The influence of thoracic posture and movement on range of arm elevation. *Physiother Theory Pract.* 1993;9:143-148.

27. Mercer SW, Maxwell M, Heaney D, Watt GC. The consultation and relational empathy (CARE) measure: development and preliminary validation and reliability of an empathy-based consultation process measure. *Fam Pract.* 2004;21:699-705.

28. Schwartz CE, Sprangers MA. Methodological approaches for assessing response shift in longitudinal health-related quality-of-life research. *Soc Sci Med.* 1999;48:1531-1548.

Lateral Epicondylalgia

R. Barry Dale

A 44-year-old carpenter is referred to physical therapy with a diagnosis of right lateral elbow pain. He is right-hand dominant and reports he has "worked with his hands all his life." His pain has been "off and on" over the last 6 months, but exacerbated while working overtime 2 weeks ago. His medical history is notable for hypertension and recently quitting smoking 8 months ago (0.25 pack per day for ~20 years). Four years ago, he fell from a ladder and sustained an injury to his neck that was treated with rest, a cervical collar, and massage. Recent radiographs of right elbow and shoulder are negative for obvious pathology. However, the cervical spine shows changes consistent with mild degeneration in the right apophyseal joints of C6 and C7. Last week, the patient started taking oral nonsteroidal anti-inflammatory medications. The patient presents to an outpatient physical therapy clinic for evaluation before follow-up with his orthopedic physician in 4 weeks. His current complaints are pain in the right elbow and weakness with active gripping, wrist extension, and forearm supination. Pain and weakness limit his ability to work as a carpenter. His goal is to return to work as soon as possible.

▶ Based on the patient's diagnosis, what are the contributing factors to the condition?

▶ What are the most appropriate examination tests?

▶ What are the most appropriate physical therapy interventions?

▶ What are possible complications that may limit the effectiveness of physical therapy?

KEY DEFINITIONS

CENTRAL SENSITIZATION: Changes within the central nervous system in response to chronic pain that can result in hyperalgesia (an amplified response to noxious stimuli)

COUNTER-FORCE BRACING: Circumferential orthotic usually comprised of an inelastic material worn distal to the lateral humeral epicondyle

LATERAL EPICONDYLALGIA: Pain at the lateral humeral epicondyle, typically at the common extensor tendon; associated with overuse of the wrist extensor muscles

NEOVASCULARIZATION: Growth of new capillaries associated with tissue healing; in tendinopathy, new capillaries may displace collagen and lead to tendon weakening and ultimately failure; free nerve endings accompanying new capillaries likely contribute to pain associated with chronic tendinopathy

TENDINITIS (tendonitis): Relatively *acute* manifestation of a tendon injury associated with hallmark signs and symptoms of inflammation (heat, redness, swelling, pain, and loss of function)

TENDINOPATHY: Broad condition implicating tendon dysfunction with no attribution to injury healing timeframe

TENDINOSIS: Painful *chronic* degeneration of a tendon, largely in the absence of classic inflammation; associated with disorganized collagen and neovascularization

Objectives

1. Describe lateral epicondylalgia and identify potential risk factors associated with this diagnosis.

2. Select appropriate manual therapy interventions for a patient with lateral epicondylalgia.

3. Prescribe appropriate joint range of motion, flexibility, and resistance exercises for a patient with lateral epicondylalgia.

4. Choose appropriate adjunctive interventions for a patient with lateral epicondylalgia.

Physical Therapy Considerations

Physical therapy considerations during management of the individual with a diagnosis of lateral epicondylalgia:

▶ **General physical therapy plan of care/goals:** Decrease pain; increase flexibility; maintain or prevent loss of range of motion of wrist and elbow joints; increase upper quadrant strength; prevent or minimize loss of aerobic fitness capacity

▶ **Physical therapy interventions:** Patient education regarding functional anatomy and injury pathomechanics; modalities and manual therapy to decrease pain; flexibility exercises; resistance exercises to increase muscular endurance capacity and strength of upper extremity muscles; aerobic exercise program; counterforce bracing

▶ **Precautions during physical therapy interventions:** Monitor vital signs; address precautions or contraindications for exercise, based on patient's pre-existing conditions

Understanding the Health Condition

Lateral epicondylalgia is pain experienced at the lateral humeral epicondyle, usually as a result of overuse of the wrist extensor muscles. Other commonly used terms to describe this syndrome are "tennis elbow," lateral epicondylitis, and wrist extensor tendinopathy (tendinitis, tendinosis). Lateral epicondylalgia is the term of choice because the true pathogenesis of this condition is unclear.[1] The predominant complaint for patients with lateral epicondylalgia is pain with active or resisted movements and weakness with wrist extension, supination, and gripping activities. Prevalence in the general population is ~1% to 3%, with females being slightly more likely to experience this condition.[2-4] Individuals 45 to 54 years of age are at greatest risk for developing the condition and smokers or previous smokers carry a higher risk compared to non-smokers (odds ratio 1.49).[2,3] Individuals are more likely to experience lateral epicondylalgia in their dominant upper extremity. Persons who participate in forceful and repetitive movements are 5.6 times more likely to develop the condition than those who do not.[3]

The lateral humeral epicondyle is the origin for the common wrist extensors, and the extensor carpi radialis brevis (ECRB) muscle and tendon are most commonly implicated with lateral epicondylalgia.[5,6] During gripping activities, the wrist extensors activate to oppose finger and wrist flexion (*e.g.*, when hammering a nail). The ideal wrist position for maximal grip strength is slight wrist extension (~15°-30°) because this maximizes the length-tension relationship of the finger flexors during power gripping. This partially explains the involvement of the ECRB with gripping activities.[7] Histopathology from individuals presenting with lateral epicondylalgia shows tissue degradation and collagen disorganization within the ECRB.[5,6] Neovascularization and the accompaniment of free nerve endings that give rise to pain sensation are also present.[8] Neurochemicals such as glutamate, substance P, and calcitonin gene-related peptide are abundant and contribute to tissue sensitivity.[8,9]

While the exact pathogenesis of lateral epicondylalgia is uncertain, the most commonly proposed etiologies are tendinopathies (tendinitis, tendinosis) and radial nerve entrapment.[5] Tendinopathy is distinct from nerve compression, and it is possible that some degree of tendon pathology and nerve entrapment are present with a patient diagnosed with lateral epicondylalgia. Tendons have lower oxygen consumption and collagen turnover rate than that of other tissues.[8,10]

Tissue integrity is a byproduct of the intricate balance between tissue degradation and regeneration. When this balance is disrupted by disproportionate stresses associated with excessive physical activity, tendon degradation can occur. Occupational and recreational activities (e.g., carpentry, typing, golf, tennis) may contribute to the development of tendinopathy.[3,11] Distal entrapment of the radial nerve may also contribute to symptoms associated with lateral epicondylalgia.[5,12] Innervation of the ECRB occurs either via the main branch, posterior branch, or superficial branch of the radial nerve.[5] Nayak et al.[5] examined 72 cadaver specimens and found that 29% had a tendinous arch and 11% had a muscular arch in the ECRB musculature. The presence of a more rigid tendinous arch could compress the nerve during repeated movements, which would result in an entrapment syndrome.

An integrative model of the etiology of lateral epicondylalgia suggests that changes also occur in local and central pain processing and that motor impairments often accompany local tendon pathology.[9] The affected elbow of individuals with lateral epicondylalgia may experience up to 50% reduced tolerance to pressure-related pain compared to the unaffected elbow.[9] Hypersensitivity over the lateral epicondyle is likely mediated by increased local concentration of neurochemicals such as glutamate, substance P, and calcitonin. It is also possible that central sensitization associated with altered processing in the spinal cord or brain contributes to abnormal pain sensation.[9,13,14] Central sensitization may lead to pain within neurologically related structures such as the cervical spine. Indeed, there is a high prevalence of neck pain in individuals with lateral epicondylalgia that persists despite adjustments for age and the presence of degenerative joint conditions of the neck.[1,9] Although it is important to recognize the frequent association of neck pain and lateral epicondylalgia, it is equally important to recognize that this association should not be confused with causation.

Motor changes commonly occur with tendinopathies and often lead to performance difficulty with functional and occupational activities. Grip strength is detrimentally affected and individuals with lateral epicondylalgia often report significant difficulty carrying grocery bags.[4] It is likely that there is some interaction of the pain system and motor deficits associated with lateral epicondylalgia. **Pain-free grip strength is a clinical test that is sensitive to change for patients with lateral epicondylalgia.**[15] This test quantifies the interaction between pain and muscle activation during gripping activity with a hand grip dynamometer. As patients recover from lateral epicondylalgia, maximal pain-free grip force should increase.

Physical Therapy Patient/Client Management

Patients with lateral epicondylalgia typically experience pain on palpation at the lateral epicondyle.[12] The pain may arise insidiously or suddenly during an activity that uses the common wrist extensors. In early stages, pain often resolves when the pain-inducing activity ceases, but returns with physical activity of the affected upper extremity. Progression often limits activity participation due to pain, and symptoms (pain and stiffness) may be present at rest.

Examination, Evaluation, and Diagnosis

The physical therapist must determine if the patient's complaints are localized to the origin of the wrist extensors and whether the cervical spine and/or radial nerve entrapment contribute to the patient's clinical presentation. The clinician thoroughly screens and, if necessary, examines the cervical spine to rule out its potential involvement. A thorough examination (of any joint) must at least include active range of motion, application of overpressure at end range, passive physiological movements, passive accessory movements, and resistance to movement.[16] Impairments or limitations and whether the patient's symptoms were reproduced must be noted. Provocative physical examination techniques will likely reproduce the patient's complaint of pain. Most of the examination procedures are either passive stretching or active resistive maneuvers with or without palpation of the wrist extensor muscle group or lateral epicondyle. Table 11-1 describes physical examination techniques for lateral epicondylalgia, and most can be performed with the patient sitting on a high plinth.

According to Haker[6], the presence of radial nerve entrapment may be determined by pain localized approximately two finger-breadths inferior to the elbow's flexor crease and medial to the common extensor mass. Other symptoms associated with radial nerve entrapment are night pain, motor dysfunction, and pain radiating into the forearm.[6] The radial nerve tension test determines the presence of neural tension commonly associated with entrapment.[17,18]

Plan of Care and Interventions

Although there are many interventions to treat lateral epicondylalgia, the examination should steer the physical therapist toward potentially beneficial treatments such as manual therapy, exercises, and adjunctive procedures such as modalities.

Manual therapy interventions for lateral epicondylalgia are listed in Table 11-2. **Manual therapy of the cervical and/or thoracic spine may benefit the patient with concomitant neck pathology, and there is some evidence to show a potential benefit in some individuals with lateral epicondylalgia.**[24,25] The decision to address the cervical and/or thoracic spine with mobilizations must derive from the results of the initial examination. Cleland, Flynn, and Palmer[25] performed cervical and thoracic intervertebral joint arthrokinematic assessments (described by Maitland[16]) in individuals with lateral epicondylalgia. Hypomobility limitations were treated at the involved segments with Grades III and IV passive physiological and accessory mobilizations in addition to other treatments for lateral epicondylalgia.[16,25] Patients receiving manual therapy at the cervical and/or thoracic spine improved to a greater extent than individuals that only received treatment at the elbow. However, it is noteworthy that both groups experienced "clinically meaningful" improvement over the course of rehabilitation.[25] Zunke et al.[26] also showed that thoracic costovertebral mobilization at T5 improved pain-free grip strength in individuals with lateral epicondylalgia.

Table 11-1	PHYSICAL EXAMINATION TECHNIQUES FOR LATERAL EPICONDYLALGIA		
Test	**Patient Position**	**Therapist Action**	**Findings**
Cozen's test or sign[19,20] (active resisted)	Have patient make a fist, and place elbow in 90° flexion, forearm pronation, and full wrist extension and radial deviation.	Apply maximal resistance to wrist extensors while palpating lateral epicondyle.	Test is positive if symptoms are reproduced.
Tomsen test[6] (active resisted)	Elbow in full extension with full wrist extension	Apply maximal resistance to wrist extensors while palpating lateral epicondyle.	Test is positive if symptoms are reproduced.
Handgrip strength test[7] (active resisted)	With patient seated on high plinth: shoulder in adduction and neutral rotation, elbow flexed at 90°, forearm in neutral pronation/supination, and wrist in ~15° extension. Standardize grip size for consistency (e.g., second position on Jamar™ dynamometer[6]).	Have patient squeeze dynamometer maximally, which implies that pain is *allowed* during the test (Fig. 11-1).	Record maximum force produced and compare to unaffected side.
Pain-free handgrip strength test[6,18,21,22] (active resisted)	Same as handgrip strength test	Have patient squeeze dynamometer with as much force as possible up to the point where pain is encountered. Instruct patient to report when pain first occurs (Fig. 11-1).	Record maximum "pain-free" force produced and compare to unaffected side.
Resisted middle finger Maudsley's test[23] (active resisted)	Shoulder in ~90° flexion, elbow in full extension, forearm in pronation, wrist in neutral with fingers held apart in extension	Apply resistance to tip of middle finger into flexion, and observe patient's response.	Test is positive if symptoms are reproduced.
Mill's test[19,20] (passive stretch)	Shoulder at patient's side, elbow in 90° flexion, forearm in pronation, wrist in full flexion with fingers held in full flexion	While holding the wrist in flexion, move elbow into extension and assess patient's response.	Test is positive if symptoms are reproduced.
Radial nerve tension test[17] (passive stretch)	Shoulder at patient's side, elbow in full extension, forearm in pronation, wrist in full flexion with fingers held in full flexion	Assess for symptom replication.	Test is positive if symptoms are reproduced.
Pain-pressure threshold (passive, digital pressure algometry)[24]		Using a digital pressure algometer, apply force over the origin of the common extensor tendon. Assess for symptom replication.	Record maximum force when pain is produced and compare to unaffected side.

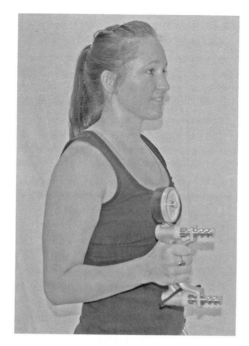

Figure 11-1. Handgrip dynamometer used to measure maximal and painfree hand grip strength (Jaymar, Clifton, NJ).

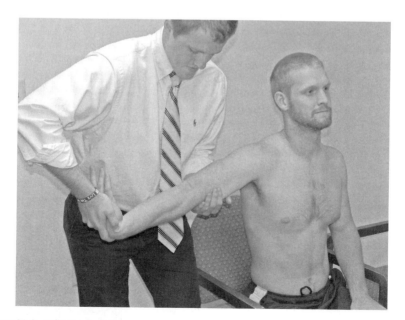

Figure 11-2. Mill's manipulation.

Table 11-2 MANUAL THERAPY INTERVENTIONS FOR LATERAL EPICONDYLALGIA		
Anatomic Region	**Technique**	**Brief Description**
Cervical spine	Lateral glides[17,24]	Place patient in supine with affected upper extremity in a position to stretch the radial nerve. Using the webspace of his/her hand, the clinician applies lateral glides at C5/C6 spinal level toward the unaffected side (*e.g.*, for affected right elbow, clinician contacts the lateral aspect of right paraspinal region at level of the C5/6 segment with his/her right hand, and then produces a straight lateral glide).
Elbow	Mill's manipulation[15]	Patient sits with arm in 90° shoulder abduction and internal rotation (enough to allow olecranon to face upward). Clinician applies small amplitude, high-velocity thrust (Grade V) at end range of elbow extension with elbow in pronation and wrist in full flexion (Fig. 11-2).
	Mulligan's Mobilizations with Movement[29]	Patient identifies an activity that recreates lateral elbow pain and clinician applies a laterally, or posterolaterally directed force (non-thrust) to the radiohumeral joint. Typically, clinician stabilizes the distal humerus with one hand while the other hand contacts the medial forearm and provides a laterally directed mobilization force (Fig. 11-3).
	Transverse friction massage[15,30]	Patient sits comfortably with affected arm placed on a table at 90° elbow flexion and forearm supination. Clinician mobilizes soft tissue either across the lateral epicondyle or 1-2 cm distal to lateral epicondyle with short strokes perpendicular to the common extensor tendon.

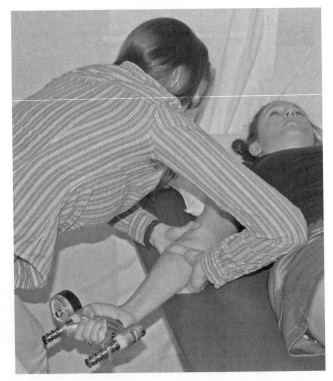

Figure 11-3. Mulligan's Mobilizations with Movement (lateral glide) while the patient performs a painful movement (gripping activity).

Several mobilization techniques at the elbow have been described for lateral epicondylalgia: Mill's manipulation (Fig. 11-2), Mulligan's Mobilization with Movement (Fig. 11-3), and transverse friction massage. Typically, a candidate for Mill's manipulation has pain at the common extensor tendon at end-range elbow extension with full wrist flexion, pain with palpation over the lateral epicondyle, and pain with gripping and resisted wrist extension.[15] Ideally, radiographs have demonstrated that the olecranon does not have osteophyte formation. In the absence of imaging, a hard end-feel noted earlier than at end range of elbow extension (especially when compared to the asymptomatic side) should warn the physical therapist to avoid aggressive maneuvers (author opinion). Vicenzino et al.[27] tested the efficacy of Mulligan's Mobilization with Movement in patients that experienced painful palpation over the lateral epicondyle, painful gripping, and pain with resistance during extension of the second or third finger. In their clinical prediction rule, Vicenzino et al.[27] identified three factors associated with improvement from a treatment program consisting of Mulligan's Mobilization with Movement and exercise: individuals with pain-free grip strength >112 N on the affected side, <336 N on the unaffected side, and younger than 49 years of age. The authors noted that more research is needed to substantiate their findings.[27] Similarly, a recent meta-analysis has shown that elbow (and regional) mobilizations can improve pain and function in individuals with lateral epicondylalgia.[28]

The benefits of joint mobilization and manipulation techniques are most likely mediated by a neurophysiological mechanism, whereas transverse friction massage facilitates tissue remodeling by physical stress.[1]

Exercise interventions for lateral epicondylalgia typically include stretching and strengthening activities (Figs. 11-4 and 11-5 and Table 11-3).[31-33] The stretching

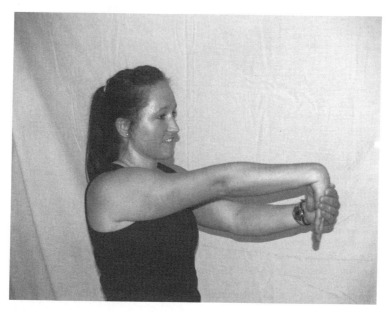

Figure 11-4. Stretching the wrist extensors with the elbow in full extension.

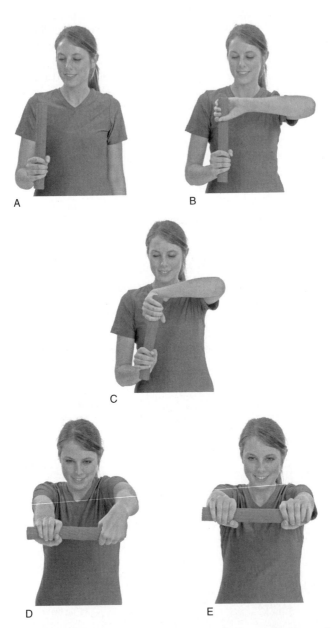

Figure 11-5. The FlexBar "Tyler Twist" regimen. Image reproduced from www.Thera-BandAcademy.com and used with kind permission from The Hygenic Corporation. © 2011 The Hygenic Corporation.

a. The FlexBar is held at the bottom end by the affected hand with the wrist placed in full extension.
b. The other end (top end) of the FlexBar is held by the unaffected hand, while the affected side is maintained in extension.
c. The unaffected hand twists the FlexBar by actively flexing the wrist.
d. The patient then moves the FlexBar to a parallel position to the floor, which places the affected elbow into extension while maintaining the wrist in extension.
e. The affected wrist slowly allows the FlexBar to "untwist" (eccentric wrist extension) while the unaffected wrist maintains a flexed position.

Table 11-3	EXERCISE INTERVENTIONS FOR LATERAL EPICONDYLALGIA	
Technique	**Muscle group**	**Brief Description**
Stretching	Wrist extensors[39]	Begin with elbow in 90° flexion, full forearm pronation, and then flex the wrist. Progress by holding the wrist in full flexion while extending the elbow (Fig. 11-4).
	Wrist flexors	Begin with elbow in 90° flexion, full forearm supination, and then extend the wrist. Progress by holding the wrist in full extension while extending the elbow.
	Forearm supinators	Begin with elbow in 90° flexion, and then pronate the forearm.
	Forearm pronators	Begin with elbow in 90° flexion, and then supinate the forearm.
	Radial nerve tension (stretch)	Have patient depress the scapula, internally rotate the shoulder, fully extend the elbow (the forearm pronates automatically when the elbow extends with the glenohumeral joint is internally rotated), and flex wrist and fingers.
Strengthening	Grip strength	Begin with gentle gripping activities (below pain threshold) with the elbow in flexion and neutral pronation/supination. Progress by increasing grip intensity, and by placing the elbow in extension and forearm in pronation.
	Wrist extension (isotonic)	Begin with elbow in 90° flexion, the forearm in full pronation, and then extend wrist with the weight of the hand only. Initially progress by increasing resistance and later by extending elbow.
	Wrist extension (eccentric-emphasis)[32,33]	Option 1: Begin with elbow in 90° flexion, the forearm in full pronation, and then extend wrist passively (use the other hand). Once wrist is extended, lower into flexion under eccentric control of wrist extensors. Initially progress by increasing resistance and later by extending elbow. Option 2: FlexBar™ regimen (Fig. 11-5).
	Wrist flexion	Begin with elbow in 90° flexion, the forearm fully supinated, and then flex wrist with the weight of the hand only. Initially progress by increasing resistance and later by extending elbow.
	Forearm supination	Begin with elbow in 90° flexion and full forearm pronation. Supinate forearm with the weight of the hand only. Progress by increasing resistance.
	Forearm supination (eccentric-emphasis)	Begin with elbow in 90° flexion and full forearm pronation. Supinate forearm passively (use the other hand, or gravity). Once forearm is supinated, lower into pronation under eccentric control of supinators. Progress by increasing resistance.
	Forearm pronation	Begin with elbow in 90° flexion and full forearm supination. Pronate forearm with the weight of the hand only. Progress by increasing resistance.
	Scapular musculature[36–38]	Lower trapezius: Prone, glenohumeral end-range flexion. Middle trapezius: Prone, scapular retraction with glenohumeral horizontal abduction and external rotation. Serratus anterior: Supine, scapular protraction; prone with push-ups and exaggerated protraction

Table 11-4 SELECTED ADJUNCTIVE INTERVENTIONS FOR LATERAL EPICONDYLALGIA

Intervention Category	Specific Intervention	Brief Description
Counter-force bracing	Proprietary orthotic	Orthotic strap placed around the affected forearm just distal to the lateral epicondyle (Fig. 11-6)
Modalities	Ultrasound[49] (low intensity)	Low-intensity ultrasound: 1.5 MHz, 20% duty cycle, spatial average intensity of 30 mW/cm^2. (Note that this is a special ultrasound application; Exogen, Smith and Nephew Inc., Memphis, TN).
	Phototherapy[22]	Polarized (waves move on parallel planes) polychromy (wide range of wavelengths, 480-3400 nm), incoherent (non-synchronized), and low-energy (40 mW/cm^2) light applied at operating distance of 5-10 cm. 3 times per week for 4 weeks may reduce patient symptoms.
	Low-level laser[43]	Wavelength of 904 nm with low output (5-50 mW) directed at tendon insertion on lateral epicondyle over area of 5 cm^2 with a dose of 0.25-1.2 J/treatment area
	Electrical therapy[50]	Patient sits comfortably and holds ground electrode in affected hand while resting the arm on a table. Therapist applies the probe electrode to local tender points around the lateral epicondyle. Noxious interrupted, low-frequency (4 Hz) DC current is applied for 30 seconds, and each tender point is stimulated 3 times for 6 treatment sessions.

prescription is usually for 30-second holds repeated for 3 to 5 repetitions at least twice per day.[31,32] Strengthening typically includes 3 sets of 5 to 15 repetitions, and the frequency is typically once per day.[31,33] Exercise provides intrinsic stress to the musculotendinous unit, which stimulates the body to adapt. Some of the beneficial adaptations include increased tissue resiliency and reduced neovascularization.[34,35] A comprehensive program should include both stretching and strengthening activities for the major muscle groups of the upper extremity including the proximal scapular musculature.[36-38]

Many adjunctive and physical modalities have been proposed to benefit lateral epicondylalgia (Table 11-4). Historically, modalities have been used to decrease local inflammation. More recent modalities such as phototherapy, low intensity ultrasound, and low-level laser attempt to stimulate changes in tissue histology and do not target inflammation, especially if the condition is chronic.[8,22,40,42–44] However, evidence regarding the effectiveness of these modalities has been mixed.[22,40,41] Multimodal treatment paradigms that include exercise, mobilizations, and physical modalities have been shown to effectively reduce dysfunction associated with lateral epicondylalgia.[36,45]

Orthotic management typically includes various forms of **counter-force bracing**.[46,47] These braces are thought to redistribute force along the common extensor tendon and away from their origin at the lateral epicondyle (Fig. 11-6).

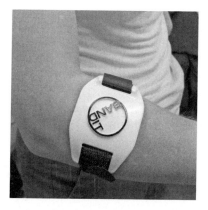

Figure 11-6. Counterforce brace (Pro Band Sports Industries, Inc., Santa Barbara, CA).

There is limited evidence demonstrating improvement with functional grip strength and pain with counter-force bracing.[38] An older comprehensive review was unable to draw definitive conclusions on the effectiveness of counter-force bracing,[46] but a 2020 systematic review concluded that orthoses can improve *pain-free* grip strength, but not necessarily *maximal* grip strength.[48] Thus, it is important to differentiate between these two types of grip strength when communicating with patients and referral sources.[48]

Evidence-Based Clinical Recommendations

SORT: Strength of Recommendation Taxonomy

A: Consistent, good-quality patient-oriented evidence
B: Inconsistent or limited-quality patient-oriented evidence
C: Consensus, disease-oriented evidence, usual practice, expert opinion, or case series

1. Pain-free grip strength is a sensitive examination sign for documenting impairment associated with lateral epicondylalgia. **Grade A**

2. Manual therapy of the cervical and/or thoracic spine is effective for management of lateral epicondylalgia for those individuals with cervical spinal pathology that contribute to their symptoms. **Grade B**

3. Mobilization techniques at the elbow and stretching and strengthening exercises are effective interventions for lateral epicondylalgia. **Grade A**

4. Adjunctive interventions such as low-intensity ultrasound, phototherapy, and low-level laser are effective treatments for lateral epicondylalgia. **Grade C**

5. Counter-force bracing is an effective component in the treatment plan for lateral epicondylalgia. **Grade B**

COMPREHENSION QUESTIONS

11.1 Patients with lateral epicondylalgia are MOST likely to have impairments with which of the following activities of daily living?

A. Reaching overhead

B. Holding a briefcase

C. Typing on a keyboard

D. Opening a drawer

11.2 Which of the following manual therapy interventions directly targets the contractile tissue of the lateral elbow?

A. Lateral glides of the cervical spine

B. Transverse friction massage of the origin of the wrist extensors

C. Wrist flexor stretch (by movement into wrist extension)

D. Mobilization with movement (lateral glide) to radiohumeral joint

11.3 Which of the following muscles is MOST commonly implicated in the tendinopathy associated with lateral epicondylalgia?

A. Extensor carpi radialis brevis

B. Flexor carpi ulnaris

C. Supinator

D. Pronator teres

ANSWERS

11.1 **B.** Holding or carrying objects requires static grip strength. In patients with lateral epicondylalgia, grip strength impairment is well documented and pain-free grip strength is considered a very useful clinical assessment measure.

11.2 **B.** While all of these interventions have some evidence to support their use in the treatment of lateral epicondylalgia, only transverse friction massage directly targets the contractile tissue of the common extensor tendon.

11.3 **A.** Extensor carpi radialis brevis is the most commonly affected muscle of the lateral elbow musculature with respect to tendinopathy.

REFERENCES

1. Vicenzino B, Cleland JA, Bisset L. Joint manipulation in the management of lateral epicondylalgia: A clinical commentary. *J Man Manip Ther*. 2007;15:50-56.

2. Sayampanathan AA, Basha M, Mitra AK. Risk factors of lateral epicondylitis: A meta-analysis. *Surg J R Coll Surg Edinb Irel*. 2020;18:122-128.

3. Shiri R, Viikari-Juntura E, Varonen H, Heliövaara M. Prevalence and determinants of lateral and medial epicondylitis: a population study. *Am J Epidemiol*. 2006;164:1065-1074.

4. Walker-Bone K, Palmer KT, Reading I, et al. Prevalence and impact of musculoskeletal disorders of the upper limb in the general population. *Arthritis Rheum.* 2004;51:642-651.

5. Nayak S, Ramanatha L, Krishnamurthy A. Extensor carpi radialis brevis origin, nerve supply and its role in lateral epicondylitis. *Surg Radiol Anat.* 2010;32:207-211.

6. Haker E. Lateral epicondylalgia: Diagnosis, treatment, and evaluation. *Crit Rev Phys Rehabil Med.* 1993;5:129-154.

7. Bhargava AS, Eapen C, Kumar SP. Grip strength measurements at two different wrist extension positions in chronic lateral epicondylitis-comparison of involved vs. uninvolved side in athletes and non athletes: a case-control study. *Sports Med Arthrosc Rehabil Ther Technol.* 2010;2:22.

8. Abate M, Silbernagel KG, Siljeholm C, et al. Pathogenesis of tendinopathies: inflammation or degeneration? *Arthritis Res Ther.* 2009;11:235.

9. Coombes BK, Bisset L, Vicenzino B. A new integrative model of lateral epicondylalgia. *Br J Sports Med.* 2009;43:252-258.

10. Vailas AC, Tipton CM, Laughlin HL, et al. Physical activity and hypophysectomy on the aerobic capacity of ligaments and tendons. *J Appl Physiol Apr.* 1978;44:542-546.

11. Smidt N, Lewis M, DA VDW, et al. Lateral epicondylitis in general practice: course and prognostic indicators of outcome. *J Rheumatol.* 2006;33:2053-2059.

12. Moradi A, Ebrahimzadeh MH, Jupiter JB. Radial Tunnel Syndrome, Diagnostic and Treatment Dilemma. *Arch Bone Jt Surg.* 2015;3:156-162.

13. Sran M, Souvlis T, Vicenzino B, Wright A. Characterisation of chronic lateral epicondylalgia using the McGill pain questionnaire, visual analog scales, and quantitative sensory tests. *Pain Clin.* 2001;13:251-259.

14. Wright A, Thurnwald P, Smith J. An evaluation of mechanical and thermal hyperalgesia in patients with lateral epicondylalgia. *Pain Clin.* 1992;5:221-227.

15. Nagrale AV, Herd CR, Ganvir S, Ramteke G. Cyriax physiotherapy versus phonophoresis with supervised exercise in subjects with lateral epicondylalgia: a randomized clinical trial. *J Man Manip Ther.* 2009;17:171-178.

16. Maitland G, Hengeveld E, Banks K, English K. *Maitland's Vertebral Manipulation.* 7th ed. Elsevier Butterworth-Heinemann; 2005.

17. Elvey R. Treatment of arm pain associated with abnormal brachial plexus tension. *Aust J Physiother.* 1986;32:225-230.

18. Vicenzino B, Neal R, Collins D, Wright A. The displacement, velocity and frequency profile of the frontal plane motion produced by the cervical lateral glide treatment technique. 1999;14:515-521.

19. Evans R. *Illustrated Orthopedic Physical Assessment, 3rd ed.* Mosby Elsevier 2009.

20. Cook C, Hegedus E. *Orthopedic Physical Examination Tests: An Evidence-Based Approach.* Pearson-Prentice Hall;2008.

21. Stratford P, Levy D. Assessing valid change over time in patients with lateral epicondylitis at the elbow. *Clin J Sport Med.* 1994;4:88-91.

22. Stasinopoulos D. The use of polarized polychromatic non-coherent light as therapy for acute tennis elbow/lateral epicondylalgia: a pilot study. *Photomed Laser Surg.* 2005;23:66-69.

23. Roles NC, Maudsley RH. Radial tunnel syndrome: resistant tennis elbow as a nerve entrapment. *J Bone Joint Surg Br.* 1972;54:499-508.

24. Vicenzino B, Collins D, Wright A. The initial effects of a cervical spine manipulative physiotherapy treatment on the pain and dysfunction of lateral epicondylalgia. *Pain.* 1996;68:69-74.

25. Cleland J, Flynn T, Palmer J. Incorporation of manual therapy directed at the cervicothoracic spine in patients with lateral epicondylalgia: A pilot clinical trial. *J Man Manip Ther.* 2005;13:143-151.

26. Zunke P, Auffarth A, Hitzl W, Moursy M. The effect of manual therapy to the thoracic spine on pain-free grip and sympathetic activity in patients with lateral epicondylalgia humeri. A randomized, sample sized planned, placebo-controlled, patient-blinded monocentric trial. *BMC Musculoskelet Disord*. 2020;21:186.

27. Vicenzino B, Smith D, Cleland J, Bisset L. Development of a clinical prediction rule to identify initial responders to mobilisation with movement and exercise for lateral epicondylalgia. *Man Ther*. 2009;14:550-554.

28. Lucado AM, Dale RB, Vincent J, Day JM. Do joint mobilizations assist in the recovery of lateral elbow tendinopathy? A systematic review and meta-analysis. *J Hand Ther*. 2019;32:262-276.e1.

29. Mulligan B R. *Manual Therapy: Nags, Snags, MWMS, etc.* 6th ed; 2010.

30. Brosseau L, Casimiro L, Milne S. Deep transverse friction massage for treating tendinitis. *Cochrane Database Syst Rev*. 2002;4:CD003528.

31. Martinez-Silvestrini J, Newcomer K, Gay R, et al. Chronic lateral epicondylitis: Comparative effectiveness of a home exercise program including stretching alone versus stretching supplemented with eccentric or concentric strengthening. *J Hand Ther*. 2005;18:411-420.

32. Svernlov B, Adolfsson L. Non-operative treatment regime including eccentric training for lateral humeral epicondylalgia. *Scand J Med Sci Sports*. 2001;11:328-334.

33. Tyler TF, Thomas GC, Nicholas SJ, McHugh MP. Addition of isolated wrist extensor eccentric exercise to standard treatment for chronic lateral epicondylosis: a prospective randomized trial. *J Shoulder Elb Surg*. 2010;19:917-922.

34. Ohberg L, Alfredson H. Effects on neovascularisation behind the good results with eccentric training in chronic mid-portion Achilles tendinosis? *Knee Surg Sports Traumatol Arthrosc*. 2004;12:465-470.

35. Ohberg L, Lorentzon R, Alfredson H. Eccentric training in patients with chronic Achilles tendinosis: normalised tendon structure and decreased thickness at follow up. *Br J Sports Med*. 2004;38:8-11.

36. Day JM, Lucado AM, Dale RB, et al. The effect of scapular muscle strengthening on functional recovery in patients with lateral elbow tendinopathy: a pilot randomized controlled trial. *J Sport Rehabil*. 2021;30:744-753.

37. Day JM, Bush H, Nitz AJ, Uhl TL. Scapular muscle performance in individuals with lateral epicondylalgia. *J Orthop Sports Phys Ther*. 2015;45:414-424.

38. Sethi K, Noohu MM. Scapular muscles strengthening on pain, functional outcome and muscle activity in chronic lateral epicondylalgia. *J Orthop Sci*. 2018;23:777-782.

39. Lucado AM, Dale RB, Kolber MJ, Day JM. Analysis of range of motion in female recreational tennis players with and without lateral elbow tendinopathy. *Int J Sports Phys Ther*. 2020;15:526-536.

40. Manias P, Stasinopoulos D. A controlled clinical pilot trial to study the effectiveness of ice as a supplement to the exercise programme for the management of lateral elbow tendinopathy. *Br J Sports Med*. 2006;40:81-85.

41. Oken O, Kahraman Y, Ayhan F, et al. The short-term efficacy of laser, brace, and ultrasound treatment in lateral epicondylitis: a prospective, randomized, controlled trial. *J Hand Ther*. 2008;21:63-67; quiz 68.

42. Kohia M, Brackle J, Byrd K, et al. Effectiveness of physical therapy treatments on lateral epicondylitis. *J Sport Rehabil*. 2008;17:119-136.

43. Bjordal JM, Lopes-Martins RA, Joensen J. A systematic review with procedural assessments and meta-analysis of low level laser therapy in lateral elbow tendinopathy (tennis elbow). *BMC Musculoskelet Disord*. 2008;975.

44. Buchbinder R, Green SE, Youd JM, et al. Shock wave therapy for lateral elbow pain. *Cochrane Database Syst Rev Online*. 2005;4:CD003524.

45. Kim YJ, Wood SM, Yoon AP, et al. Efficacy of nonoperative treatments for lateral epicondylitis: a systematic review and meta-analysis. *Plast Reconstr Surg*. 2021;147:112-125.

46. Struijs PA, Smidt N, Arola H, et al. Orthotic devices for the treatment of tennis elbow. *Cochrane Database Syst Rev.* 2002;1:CD001821.

47. Jafarian FS, Demneh ES, Tyson SF. The immediate effect of orthotic management on grip strength of patients with lateral epicondylosis. *J Orthop Sports Phys Ther.* 2009;39:484-489.

48. Heales LJ, McClintock SR, Maynard S, et al. Evaluating the immediate effect of forearm and wrist orthoses on pain and function in individuals with lateral elbow tendinopathy: A systematic review. *Musculoskelet Sci Pract.* 2020;47:102147.

49. Fu SC, Hung LK, Shum WT. In vivo low-intensity pulsed ultrasound (LIPUS) following tendon injury promotes repair during granulation, but suppresses decorin and biglycan expression during remodeling. *J Orthop Sports Phys Ther.* 2010;40:422-429.

50. Reza Nourbakhsh M, Fearon F. An alternative approach to treating lateral epicondylitis. A randomized, placebo-controlled, double-blinded study. *Clin Rehabil.* 2008;22:601-609.

Spondylolisthesis

Danny J. McMillian

An 18-year-old high school football player is referred to an outpatient physical therapy clinic for evaluation of persistent central low back pain. The orthopedist established a diagnosis of type IIB, grade II spondylolisthesis at L5/S1. The athlete reports no history of specific trauma. His pain is aggravated by prolonged standing or walking, lifting weights (especially overhead), and bending backward or twisting. Sitting or lying down with his hips and knees bent relieves the pain. His medical history is otherwise unremarkable. The patient's goal is to return to football as soon as possible.

▶ What are the examination priorities?

▶ What examination signs may be associated with this diagnosis?

▶ Based on the patient's diagnosis, what do you anticipate may be contributing factors to his condition?

▶ What are the most appropriate physical therapy interventions?

▶ What are possible complications that may limit the effectiveness of physical therapy?

▶ Identify the psychological or psychosocial factors apparent in this case.

KEY DEFINITIONS

CORE STABILITY: Ability of muscles within the "core" region (abdomen, lumbar spine, pelvis, and hips) to stabilize the lumbar spine from potentially injurious forces and to create and/or transfer forces between anatomic segments during functional movements

DYSPLASTIC SPONDYLOLISTHESIS: Translational displacement of one vertebral segment on another caused by congenital deficiency of the posterior elements of the spine

SPONDYLOLISTHESIS: Translational displacement or nonanatomic alignment of one vertebral segment on another

SPONDYLOLYSIS: Defect or abnormality of the pars interarticularis of the vertebral arch

Objectives

1. Describe spondylolisthesis and identify potential risk factors associated with this diagnosis.
2. Prescribe joint range of motion and/or muscular flexibility exercises for a patient with spondylolisthesis.
3. Prescribe motor control exercises for a young athlete with spondylolisthesis.

Physical Therapy Considerations

Physical therapy considerations during management of the individual with a diagnosis of spondylolisthesis:

▶ **General physical therapy plan of care/goals:** Decrease pain; increase pain-free range of motion and muscular flexibility; increase spine and lower quadrant strength, endurance and motor control; maintain or improve aerobic fitness capacity

▶ **Physical therapy interventions:** Patient education regarding functional anatomy and injury pathomechanics; modalities and manual therapy to decrease pain and improve joint motion; muscular flexibility exercises; resistance exercises to increase muscular strength and endurance of the core and lower extremities; aerobic exercise program

▶ **Precautions during physical therapy:** Address precautions or contraindications for exercise, based on the patient's pre-existing condition(s); identify and avoid postures and loading conditions that are likely to exacerbate the condition

▶ **Complications interfering with physical therapy:** Potential for further anterior translation of the L5 vertebra with subsequent neurologic impairment of the lower extremities

Understanding the Health Condition

Spondylolisthesis is defined as translational displacement or nonanatomic alignment of one vertebral segment on another.[1] It is most common in the lumbar spine at the L5 to S1 segment and it is usually associated with bilateral spondylolytic defects at the pars interarticularis (Fig. 12-1). In most cases, the pathology is caused by repeated mechanical stress and the condition occurs incrementally, with the spectrum ranging from a stress reaction that is undetectable with plain radiographs to a frank fracture.[2]

Mechanical stress to the pars interarticularis is greatest with spinal extension and rotational forces.[3] For this reason, spondylolysis is most commonly seen among young athletes involved in football blocking, overhead lifting, tennis serving, baseball pitching, gymnastics, and the butterfly swim stroke.[4] In fact, **spondylolysis and spondylolisthesis are the most common spinal injuries in young athletes.** The incidence of spondylolysis for young athletes seeking care for low back pain has been reported at 47% compared to 5% for the general population.[5] In contrast, the same researchers also reported an 11% incidence of disc-related back pain in adolescent athletes compared to a 48% incidence of discogenic back pain in the nonathletic adult population. The prevalence of spondylolisthesis stabilizes in adulthood, and the etiology of new occurrences after this time is usually considered to be degenerative in nature.[1] Degenerative spondylolisthesis is nearly 6 times more likely to occur

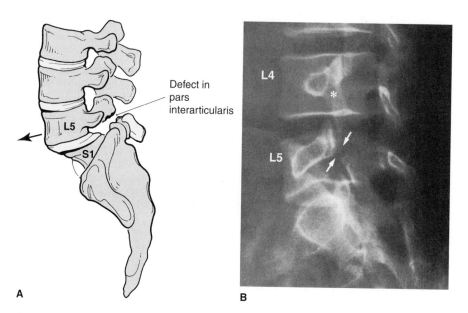

Defect in
pars
interarticularis

Figure 12-1. A. Diagram of spondylolisthesis of L5 over S1 caused by spondylolysis of L5. **B.** Oblique plain film of lumbar spine demonstrates a spondylolysis or pars defect on the right side at L5 (arrows). Note the intact pars at L4 (*). (Reproduced with permission from Chen MY, Pope TL, Ott DJ, eds. *Basic Radiology.* 2nd ed. New York: McGraw-Hill; 2011. Figure 12-12 A and B.)

Table 12-1 WILTSE CLASSIFICATION OF TYPES OF SPONDYLOLISTHESIS	
Type I Dysplastic/congenital	Congenital abnormalities of the upper sacrum or the arch of L5 permit the olisthesis (slip) to occur: • Type IA: dysplastic posterior elements and facets; usually associated with spina bifida • Type IB: dysplastic articular process with sagittal-oriented facet joints • Type IC: other congenital abnormalities, such as failure of formation or segmentations producing spondylolisthesis
Type II Isthmic	Lesion within the pars interarticularis: • Type IIA: lytic fatigue fracture • Type IIB: elongation (microfracture healed with elongation) • Type IIC: acute fracture secondary to trauma
Type III Degenerative	Long-standing intersegmental instability, such as within the apophyseal joints, permitting slippage.
Type IV Traumatic	Due to fractures in areas of the bony hook other than the pars interarticularis
Type V Pathological	Results from generalized or localized bone disease (*e.g.*, osteogenesis imperfecta, Paget's disease)

in women than men.[6] The classifications of spondylolisthesis by type[7] and severity[8] are described in Tables 12-1 and 12-2, respectively.

The pain associated with symptomatic spondylolisthesis can degrade motor control of the spine, leading to unbalanced loading of spinal structures.[9] Therefore, ensuring optimal motor control of the lumbopelvic region and entire kinetic chain is a priority. Optimizing functional core stability is one strategy to improve and maintain control of the spinal region. Core stability has been defined by Hodges[10] as the restoration or augmentation of the ability of the neuromuscular system to control and protect the spine from injury or reinjury. Core stability can be conceptualized as a product of trunk muscle capacity for control (strength and endurance) and the coordination and control of those same muscles to improve control of the lumbar spine and pelvis.[10] Deficits in motor control of the trunk have been associated not only with back pain but also with increased risk of lower extremity injury.[11]

Table 12-2 MEYERDING CLASSIFICATION OF SPONDYLOLISTHESIS SEVERITY[1]	
Grade	**Percentage of Vertebral Translation***
1	0%-25%
2	26%-50%
3	51%-75%
4	76%-100%
5	100%

*Calculated as the distance of translation divided by the A-P diameter of the inferior vertebral body × 100%
Reproduced with permission from Metz LN, Deviren V. Low-grade spondylolisthesis. Neurosurg Clin N Am. 2007; 18(2):237-248.

Physical Therapy Patient/Client Management

There are several potentially effective interventions for the patient with spondylolisthesis. Therapeutic exercises should be prescribed to optimize neuromuscular responsiveness and to alleviate soft tissue restrictions that would promote excessive lordosis.[12-14] Manual therapy is indicated to address identified mobility impairments above and below the area of the spondylolisthesis. Because this patient is experiencing only intermittent pain related to provocative activities, the routine use of modalities and medications is not an essential component of management. Other patients with this condition might present with a greater need for pain management and may benefit from select modalities and analgesic medications. It is important to note that patients with spondylolisthesis appear to have no greater disability from their back pain than the general public.[15] The implication of this finding is that clinicians should be wary of attributing *all* back pain in this population to the spondylolisthesis.

The primary goal for this patient and others of a similar age and activity level is to return to pain-free, unrestricted activity with minimal risk for further tissue trauma. This patient expressed interest in returning to football "as soon as possible." The therapist must ensure that the patient has realistic expectations about the prognosis and expected rehabilitation timeline. Education of the patient should also ensure that he has a thorough understanding of the requirements for returning to his sport. Because the patient's diagnostic category, type IIB, suggests tissue healing is complete, the primary determinant of readiness for return to play will be the patient's ability to demonstrate dynamic stability of the spine during loading conditions that simulate football.

Examination, Evaluation, and Diagnosis

Although the patient has received a full diagnostic examination by the orthopedist, the physical therapist must perform a thorough neuromusculoskeletal examination to confirm the patient's current status and guide the plan of care. While many individuals with this condition are asymptomatic, individuals presenting with type II spondylolisthesis usually report central low back pain of varying intensity. The pain is often described as dull and aching. Symptoms radiating to the buttocks and posterior thigh are not uncommon, although true radicular symptoms are more likely with degenerative spondylolisthesis (type III), because disc and facet degeneration often combine to narrow the neural foramina. Most often, patients report that their pain is aggravated by prolonged standing or walking and bending backward or twisting. The pain is often relieved by sitting or lying down with the hips and knees bent.

Physical examination starts with observation of posture. Although patients commonly present with an anterior tilt of the pelvis and increased lumbar lordosis, the patient in pain might present with decreased lordosis related to muscle guarding.[2] During gait, stride length might be shortened to decrease rotational stress to the spine or to accommodate tight hamstrings.[2] While any active spinal movement may be limited in this patient, spinal extension is most likely to recreate his pain. Similarly, passive extension and passive accessory movements of the spondylolytic L5/S1 segment (*e.g.*, posterior to anterior glides) are likely to provoke the patient's pain. The physical therapy examination must include muscle length testing with particular concern for tightness that can promote excessive lumbar lordosis (*e.g.*, iliopsoas, rectus femoris, tensor fascia lata). The therapist should evaluate whether the patient is able to activate deep trunk muscles (transversus abdominis and multifidi), and ask the patient to perform functional movement tests to identify patterns that suggest inadequate control of the kinetic chain.

The diagnosis of spondylolisthesis can be established with plain radiographs.[1] Oblique views aid in the identification of spondylolysis and flexion-extension films are used to measure instability. When radicular and other neurologic signs are present, MRI and CT myelogram assist in determining the site and degree of stenosis or impingement.[1]

Plan of Care and Interventions

Physical therapy interventions must address findings from the musculoskeletal examination. Interventions often include manual therapy and therapeutic exercise to address impaired joint kinematics, muscular tightness, muscular weakness, and deficient motor control. Most patients with spondylolisthesis benefit from therapeutic interventions to improve both *mobility* and dynamic *stability*.

Patients with spondylolisthesis often present with *decreased* mobility in the thoracic spine, hip, lumbar extensor muscles, and muscles that anteriorly tilt the pelvis. Because one objective for the person with symptomatic spondylolisthesis is to achieve dynamic stabilization of the lumbar spine, impaired mobility of the regions above (thoracic spine) and below (hip) has the potential to greatly limit functional mobility.[16] Optimizing thoracic and hip mobility might allow the patient to dynamically stabilize the lumbar spine. Manipulation, mobilization, stretching, and range of motion exercises are all potentially appropriate intervention options in the thoracic spine and hip regions. Because the spondylolisthesis increases the spinal extension moment, interventions are also aimed at reducing the tension of posterior lumbar structures. Spinal flexion exercises are normally indicated to decrease the load on posterior vertebral tissues.[17] Such exercises might reduce tension in lumbar extensor muscles and stretch passive and active structures of the posterior lumbar spine.[18] Examples of flexion exercises include: supine knees-to-chest, trunk curl-ups, and seated or quadruped lumbar flexion. Last, the physical therapist must **optimize length of the muscles that anteriorly tilt the pelvis**. Through their attachments to the pelvis, several muscles have the potential to exacerbate a spondylolisthesis by promoting an anterior tilt of the pelvis. Thus, **static and/or dynamic stretching of tight iliopsoas, rectus femoris, and tensor fascia lata muscles should be included in the exercise program.**[19]

Deficits in dynamic trunk stability have been associated with back pain,[11] and **strategies to improve spinal stabilization have been used to decrease pain and functional disability in patients with spondylolisthesis.**[12] Table 12-3 presents a three-phased approach, based on a training strategy by Smith *et al.*[20] that could be used to decrease pain and functional disability in patients with spondylolisthesis. The purpose of the

Table 12-3 PHASED EXERCISE APPROACH TO IMPROVING DYNAMIC STABILITY FOR ATHLETES WITH SPONDYLOLISTHESIS

Phase and Primary Focus	Exercise/Activity	Technique
Phase I Focus on developing kinesthetic awareness, foundational motor control, and endurance during slow-velocity, limited-excursion movements	Establish the neutral position of the pelvis ("neutral spine")	Perform this activity in various functional positions (supine, quadruped, seated, and standing). Exercise consists of isolated, rhythmic anterior and posterior tilting of the pelvis, with each set of repetitions stopping at a midpoint between anterior and posterior extremes of motion. Manual facilitation techniques from the therapist might be necessary to initiate isolated pelvic movement.
	Activation of the transversus abdominus (TrA) and multifidi muscles Activation of the TrA and multifidi should be confirmed with each new exercise added in Phase I. Once confirmed, the abdominal bracing strategy can be used to activate the core musculature.	As noted above for pelvic tilting, this activity should be performed in various functional positions. Transversus abdominus (TrA) may be activated by drawing the navel toward the spine and slightly upward. The patient or therapist may confirm TrA activation by palpating for tension just medial and inferior to the anterior-superior iliac spine. Multifidus activation is monitored by palpation (either by the patient or therapist) immediately lateral to the relevant lumbar spinous process as the patient attempts to "swell" the muscle into the palpating digit(s). Contractions of TrA and multifidi should be gentle and not disturb rhythmic breathing pattern. Observe for loss of pelvic neutral position, as this likely indicates that global trunk muscles are attempting to compensate for poor activation of deep stabilizers. Activation of pelvic floor muscles may facilitate coactivation of the TrA and multifidi. (Patient can be advised to contract as if stopping the flow of urine).
	Quadruped limb elevation progression	From quadruped position, establish neutral position of pelvis. Provide progressive challenges to this stable position by lifting and extending the limbs away from the trunk. Begin with single arm and leg lifts, then progress to reciprocal arm/leg lifts (Fig. 12-2). Do not elevate limbs beyond parallel with the spine. Stop the progression if the neutral position is not maintained.

(Continued)

Table 12-3 PHASED EXERCISE APPROACH TO IMPROVING DYNAMIC STABILITY FOR ATHLETES WITH SPONDYLOLISTHESIS (CONTINUED)

Phase and Primary Focus	Exercise/Activity	Technique
	Abdominal curl-ups	Begin in supine position with one leg straight and other flexed at the hip and knee with the pelvis and lumbar spine in a neutral position. Curl-up is performed by raising head and upper shoulders off floor. The motion takes place in the thoracic spine—*not* the lumbar or cervical region. To begin, the hands are placed under the lumbar region to monitor movement of the lumbar spine (Fig. 12-3A). Hold the curl-up for several seconds, then return smoothly to starting position and repeat as indicated. Progress exercise by using one or all of the following techniques: raising the elbows, placing the hands on the head (Fig. 12-3B), lifting the straight leg. Stop progression if neutral position is not maintained.
	Supine bridge	From supine, hooklying position (knees bent about 90°), gently squeeze gluteus maximus bilaterally. Slowly increase activation of this muscle until the hips rise a few inches from the floor. Ensure neutral position of the pelvis is maintained. Hold several sec, then return smoothly to starting position and repeat as indicated. To reduce tendency to extend the lumbar spine rather than the hip, consider fully flexing one hip and performing a single-leg support bridge.
	Side-bridge	Begin in modified sidelying with hips and knees flexed and upper body supported through forearm contact with the ground. Press through the forearm to establish protective stabilization of the shoulder girdle, and then gradually lift the pelvis from the ground. The pelvis should translate forward as it lifts so that sagittal plane alignment of knees, hips and shoulders is achieved. Stop elevation of hips when frontal plane alignment of spine and thighs is achieved. Hold several sec, and then return smoothly to starting position and repeat as indicated. Progress exercise by starting with the knees extended, with the foot of the top leg on the ground directly in front of the bottom leg (Fig. 12-4).
	Standing rotational resistance	Begin in standing with pelvis and lumbar spine in neutral and trunk muscles engaged with a gentle, bracing contraction. To train for control of rotational forces, begin with a cable or elastic cord positioned at chest level in the transverse plane. The handle attached to the resistance is initially held close to the chest (Fig. 12-5A). Perform exercise by slowly extending the elbows to increase transverse plane loading (Fig. 12-5B). Hold several seconds, and then return smoothly to starting position and repeat as indicated. Ensure stability is maintained in all planes of motion.

Phase II		
Progress to higher velocity, more dynamic multiplanar endurance, strength, power, and coordination challenges incorporating upper and lower extremity movements	Lunge progression	Begin by performing body-weight lunges in the cardinal planes. Ensure both lower extremity alignment and pelvis/lumbar spine stability throughout the movement. Progress the activity by adding a balanced load (e.g., weight vest, medicine ball) held at the center of the chest. Reduce the load and then position it away from the midline.
	Medicine ball throws	A medicine ball that bounces and a solid wall can be used to train reactive stability by performing progressively rapid, short-range throws and catches. Progress the load, speed, and volume of exercise as indicated. For the chest pass, begin about 6 feet from the wall in an athletic stance with the ball held close to the chest (Fig. 12-6A). Maintain the stance, neutral pelvis, and spine position as throws become progressively faster. For rotational passes, turn 90° away from the wall and assume athletic stance with the ball just lateral to outermost thigh, which bears most of the weight initially (Fig. 12-6B). Ensure sufficient hip/knee flexion, hip internal rotation, and vertical alignment of the ankle/knee/hip of the outer leg. The thoracic spine is also rotated away from the wall. Push off the outer leg and "unwind" the outside leg hip and thoracic spine in order to create the rotational force for the throw. The arms should act primarily as tethers to transfer the force created in the legs and thoracic spine.
	Multiplanar challenges using an exercise ball	An exercise ball can be used to create an unstable surface that challenges trunk motor control. From the plank position with legs supported on the ball (Fig. 12-7A), flex hips to draw the knees toward the chest (Fig. 12-7B). Do not allow the lumbar spine to drop into extension. From the plank position with the forearms supported on the ball, shift forearm pressure in all directions to include circular motions. With the upper back supported on the ball, slowly roll side to side (Fig. 12-7C) to engage rotational stabilizers.
	Lifting an asymmetrical load	Place an appropriate weight beside the patient at a height that permits optimal trunk and lower extremity alignment (Fig. 12-8A). Lift the weight while maintaining trunk stability (Fig. 12-8B). Observe for aberrant movement, primarily in the frontal plane.
	Asymmetrical push-press into split-squat	Start with an appropriate weight in one hand at shoulder level (Fig. 12-9A). Perform a push press by flexing slightly at the hips and knees, then quickly extend the hips and knees while guiding the weight overhead (Fig. 12-9B). Maintaining arm and trunk alignment, perform split squats or lunges (Fig. 12-9C). Key points of execution include: arm alignment perpendicular to the ground, maintenance of neutral lumbopelvic position, and frontal plane alignment of forward hip and knee.

(Continued)

Table 12-3 PHASED EXERCISE APPROACH TO IMPROVING DYNAMIC STABILITY FOR ATHLETES WITH SPONDYLOLISTHESIS (CONTINUED)

Phase and Primary Focus	Exercise/Activity	Technique
Phase III Activity-specific skill simulations, with emphasis on mastery of component motions that present the greatest challenge to neutral spine alignment. Listed are suggestions appropriate for a football lineman.	Sled push	First, match height of the handle to the requirements of the patient. After selecting an appropriate load, have patient demonstrate an athletic stance (flexed at hips and knees) with a neutral pelvis and core activation. Maintain the neutral pelvis, as force production for the sled push is achieved through powerful extension of the hips, knees, and ankles (Fig. 12-10).
	Isometric, axial loading	Use a barbell and weight rack hooks to create an isometric, axial load (Fig. 12-11). The barbell is placed under the hooks that are normally used to support the barbell on the rack. This simulates a common force as football lineman struggle for position. Ensure athlete maintains lumbopelvic neutral position throughout the application of force, generally in 3-4 second increments. As the athlete demonstrates proficiency, adjust rate of force application and degree of loading to simulate realistic conditions.
	Standing trunk rotation with unilateral "punch"	Cable or elastic resistance may be used to create resistance to combined leg/trunk/arm rotation, simulating a common movement in many sports. Most of the rotation for this exercise is produced at the hips and thoracic spine. Ensure that the pelvis and lumbar spine remain in neutral position (Fig. 12-12A). Observe for compensatory trunk movement in the sagittal and frontal planes as the athlete "punches" his arm forward (Fig. 12-12B).

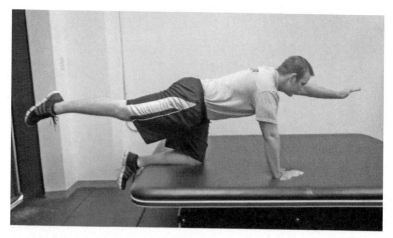

Figure 12-2. Quadruped limb elevation progression.

first phase (Phase I) is to develop kinesthetic awareness, provide foundational motor control, and improve endurance during slow-velocity, limited-excursion movements. Most activities are directed at the pelvis and lumbar spine. However, integration of activities involving the extremities should begin as soon as basic core stabilization is demonstrated.[21] A randomized, controlled trial by O'Sullivan *et al.*[12] studied the

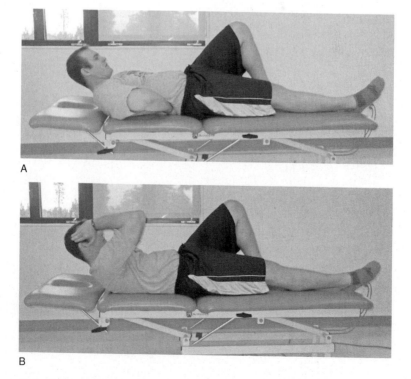

Figure 12-3. Abdominal curl-up. **A.** Elbow lift progression. **B.** Hands-on-head progression.

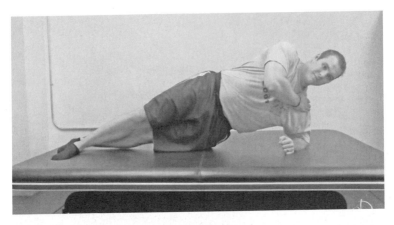

Figure 12-4. Side bridge.

effect of specific core training on patients with spondylolysis or spondylolisthesis. This study provided evidence to support the use of specific training for the deep abdominal muscles combined with coactivation of the lumbar multifidi. The results of this study, along with evidence supporting deep abdominal and lumbar multifidi

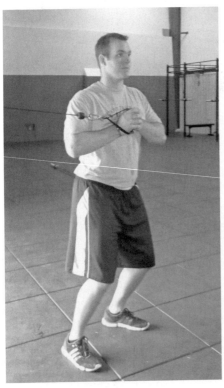
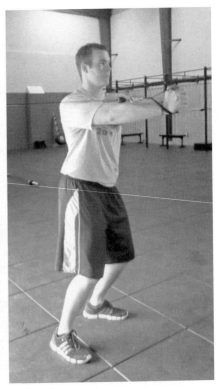

A   B

Figure 12-5. Standing rotational resistance. **A.** Starting position. **B.** Ending position.

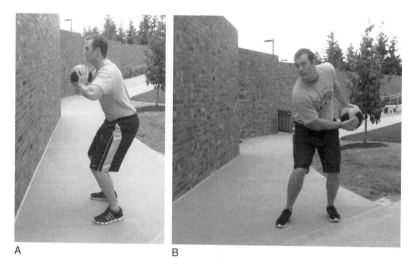

Figure 12-6. Medicine ball throws. **A.** Chest pass. **B.** Rotational pass.

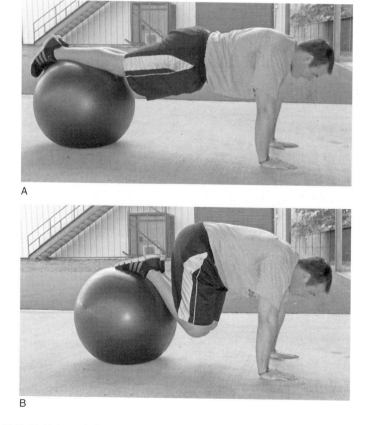

Figure 12-7. Multiplanar challenges with exercise ball. **A.** Plank. **B.** Plank with leg tucks. **C.** Twist.

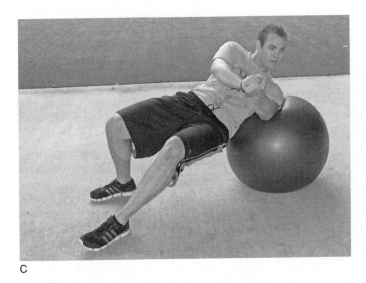

C

Figure 12-7. *(Continued)*

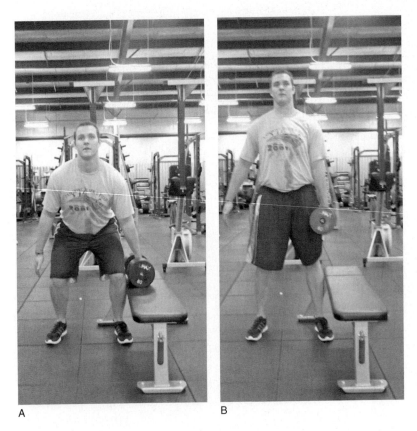

A

B

Figure 12-8. Asymmetrical lift. **A.** Starting position. **B.** Ending position.

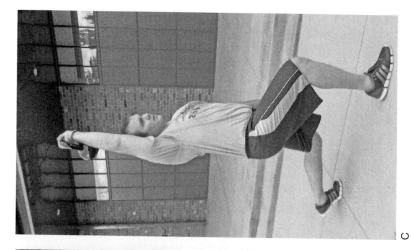

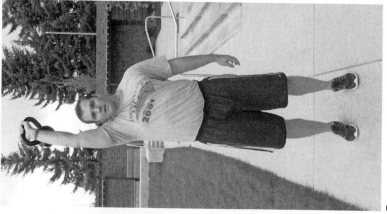

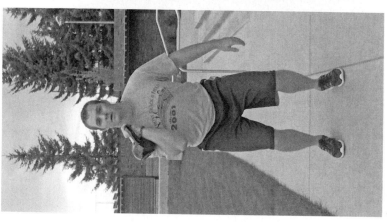

Figure 12-9. Asymmetrical push-press. **A.** Starting position. **B.** Ending position. **C.** Overhead split squat.

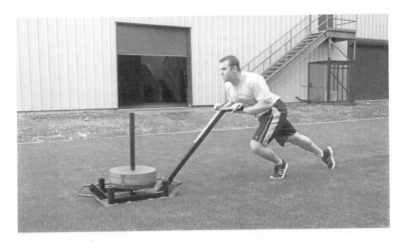

Figure 12-10. Sled push.

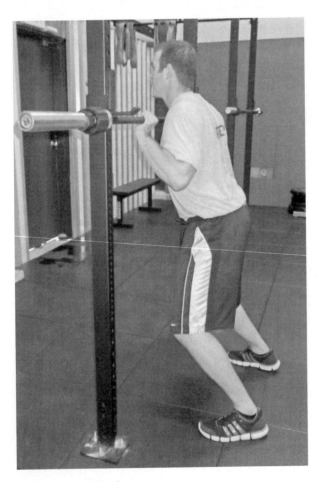

Figure 12-11. Isometric axial trunk loading.

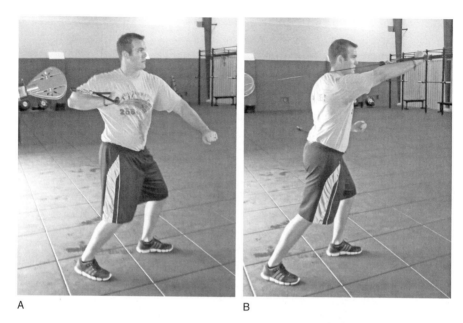

Figure 12-12. Standing trunk rotation. **A.** Starting position. **B.** Ending position with unilateral "punch."

activation training in the treatment of chronic low back pain,[10] has influenced many physical therapists to consider such training as the foundational approach to motor control for the patient with lumbar impairments. However, there remains controversy as to the *best* strategy for promoting motor control of the trunk. The common practice is for therapists to ensure that patients can successfully activate the transversus abdominis before initiating further training. Frequently, this is confirmed by the abdominal "drawing-in" maneuver in which the patient is instructed to draw the umbilicus toward the spine and upward, while the therapist palpates for transversus abdominis contractions medial and inferior to the anterior superior iliac spines. However, the strategy of having the patient successfully demonstrate bilateral activation of the transversus abdominis *before* initiation of any stabilization training has been called into question.[22-24] Evidence from Grenier and McGill[23] suggests that abdominal bracing (co-contraction of all abdominal and low back muscles) provides greater trunk stability than isolated activation of the transversus abdominis.

Given uncertainty in the literature about the optimal means for dynamically stabilizing the trunk, a reasonable middle ground might be as follows: early in the rehabilitation of a patient with low back impairments, establish the patient's ability to activate deep stabilizers such as the transversus abdominis and multifidi in static positions; then, as exercise and activities are progressed, emphasize alignment, coordination, and energy efficiency of movement rather than pre-activation of muscles that might or might not be a part of the optimal motor program for a given task. During Phase II of training to improve dynamic stability of the lumbar spine, progressive loads, speed, and excursion are introduced to challenge the newly gained lumbar stability. More complex, integrated movements are introduced based on the patient's proficiency with simple movements and his activity and sport requirements. The last phase of dynamic stability training includes activity-specific skill simulations, with emphasis on mastery of component motions that present the greatest challenge to neutral spine alignment. Factors to consider are occupational and sport-specific loads, acceleration, velocity, coordination, and endurance. Traditional training modes for a particular sport should be re-evaluated in light of the patient's unique impairments and risks. In the present case, the traditional practice of heavy-resistance squatting for football lineman should be reconsidered in light of evidence that such activity is associated with hyperextension of the lumbar spine, thus potentially exacerbating conditions such as spondylolysis and spondylolisthesis.[25]

Conservative care of athletes with spondylolisthesis is considered the first line of care and has been proven effective, with return-to-sport rates within a mean of 4.6 months.[26] Surgical interventions may be considered after 6 months of failed conservative management or progressive neurological deficit.[27] Although the young athlete described in this case did not present with pain-related fear of movement, the clinician might consider applying principles of cognitive functional therapy if such fear is noted.[28] Figures 12-2 to 12-12 show exercises commonly used in the rehabilitation of individuals with spondylolisthesis.

Evidence-Based Clinical Recommendations

SORT: Strength of Recommendation Taxonomy

A: Consistent, good-quality patient-oriented evidence
B: Inconsistent or limited-quality patient-oriented evidence
C: Consensus, disease-oriented evidence, usual practice, expert opinion, or case series

1. Spondylolisthesis and spondylolysis are the most common spinal injuries in young athletes, especially in those sports that require spinal extension and rotational forces. **Grade A**

2. Stretching tight muscles that anteriorly tilt the pelvis is an effective component of conservative care for spondylolisthesis. **Grade C**

3. Inclusion of specific exercises aimed to improve dynamic trunk stability are associated with less pain and better function for patients with spondylolisthesis. **Grade B**

COMPREHENSION QUESTIONS

12.1 Which pain-provoking activity is LEAST likely to raise suspicion of spondylolisthesis as an etiology of low back pain?

    A. A gymnastic floor routine

    B. Triathlon training

    C. Intensive practice of the tennis serve

    D. Intensive practice of the golf swing (driving)

12.2 Select the MOST appropriate exercise strategy for the rehabilitation of patients with spondylolisthesis.

    A. Flexion range of motion exercises; stretching tight muscles that promote anterior pelvic tilt; foundational motor control exercises for deep core stabilizers

    B. Extension range of motion exercises; stretching tight muscles that promote anterior pelvic tilt; activity-specific skill simulations with emphasis on mastery of component motions that present the greatest challenge to neutral spine alignment

    C. Flexion range of motion exercises; stretching tight muscles that promote anterior pelvic tilt; foundational motor control exercises for deep core stabilizers; progression to activity-specific skill simulations with emphasis on mastery of component motions that present the greatest challenge to neutral spine alignment

    D. Flexion range of motion exercises; stretching tight muscles that promote anterior pelvic tilt; progressive resistance exercise for all core muscles

12.3 Evidence suggests the following outcome for return-to-play following diagnosis of spondylolisthesis:

    A. Expected within 3 months of initiation of conservative care

    B. Unlikely with conservative care only

    C. Expected within 6 months of initiation of conservative care

    D. Expected at 12 to 14 months after initiation of conservative care

ANSWERS

12.1 **B.** Activities involving extension of the lumbar spine are most likely to provoke symptoms in the presence of spondylolisthesis.[2-4] When axial loads and rotation are added to extension, the forces on posterior vertebral structures are increased.[3] The components of triathlon training (crawl-stroke swim, bicycling, and running) have only modest extension moments and range of motion requirements. The other three activities listed have significant spinal extension and rotational components.

12.2 **C.** Range of motion exercises that promote flexion are better tolerated than extension.[17] Stretching is most effective when applied to muscles whose shortened length promotes anterior tilt of the pelvis. Activation of the deep stabilizers is often impaired in patients with low back pain.[9] Therefore, specific exercises to promote activation are indicated.[12] When consistent activation of the deep stabilizers has been achieved, progressing to activity-specific challenges allows the therapist to determine whether skills learned in previous simple exercises will transfer to goal-directed activities.[20,21]

12.3 **C.** A systematic review has established efficacy of conservative care for return-to-play at an average of 4.6 months.[26]

REFERENCES

1. Metz LN, Deviren V. Low-grade spondylolisthesis. *Neurosurg Clin N Am.* 2007;18:237-248.

2. Herman MJ, Pizzutillo PD, Cavalier R. Spondylolysis and spondylolisthesis in the child and adolescent athlete. *Orthop Clin N Am.* 2003;34:461-467.

3. Chosa E, Totoribe K, Tajima N. A biomechanical study of lumbar spondylolysis based on a three-dimensional finite element method. *J Orthop Res.* 2004;22:158-163.

4. O'Connor FG, d'Hemecourt PA, Nebzydoski M. Spondylolysis: a practical approach to an adolescent enigma. In: Seidenberg PH, Beutler AI, eds. *The Sports Medicine Resource Manual.* Philadelphia, PA: Saunders;2008:418-421.

5. Micheli LJ, Wood R. Back pain in young athletes. Significant differences from adults in causes and patterns. *Arch Pediatr Adolesc Med.* 1995;149:15-18.

6. Vibert BT, Sliva CD, Herkowitz HN. Treatment of instability and spondylolisthesis: surgical versus nonsurgical treatment. *Clin Orthop Relat Res.* 2006;443:222-227.

7. Wiltse LL, Newman PH, Macnab I. Classification of spondylolysis and spondylolisthesis. *Clin Orthop Relat Res.* 1976;117:23-29.

8. Meyerding HW. Spondylolisthesis: surgical treatment and results. *Surg Gynecol Obstet.* 1932; 54:371-377.

9. Hodges PW, Richardson CA. Relationship between limb movement speed and associated contraction of the trunk muscles. *Ergonomics.* 1997;40:1220-1230.

10. Hodges PW. Core stability exercise in chronic low back pain. *Orthop Clin N Am.* 2003;34:245-254.

11. Zazulak BT, Hewett TE, Reeves NP, et al. Deficits in neuromuscular control of the trunk predict knee injury risk: a prospective biomechanical-epidemiologic study. *Am J Sports Med.* 2007;35: 1123-1130.

12. O'Sullivan PB, Phyty GD, Twomey LT, Allison GT. Evaluation of specific stabilizing exercise in the treatment of chronic low back pain with radiologic diagnosis of spondylolysis or spondylolisthesis. *Spine.* 1997;22:2959-2967.

13. O'Sullivan PB. Lumbar segmental "instability": clinical presentation and specific stabilizing exercise management. *Man Ther.* 2000;5:2-12.

14. Macedo LG, Maher CG, Latimer J, McAuley JH. Motor control exercise for persistent, nonspecific low back pain: a systematic review. *Phys Ther.* 2009;89:9-25.

15. Frennered AK, Danielson BI, Nachemson AL. Natural history of symptomatic isthmic low-grade spondylolisthesis in children and adolescents: a seven-year follow-up study. *J Pediatr Orthop.* 1991;11:209-213.

16. Van Dillen LR, Bloom NJ, Gombatto SP, Susco TM. Hip rotation range of motion in people with and without low back pain who participate in rotation-related sports. *Phys Ther Sport.* 2008;9:72-81.

17. Sinaki M, Lutness MP, Ilstrup DM, et al. Lumbar spondylolisthesis: retrospective comparison and three-year follow-up of two conservative treatment programs. *Arch Phys Med Rehabil.* 1989;70:594-598.

18. Brotzman SB. Low back injuries. In: Brotzman SB, Wilk KE, eds. *Clinical Orthopaedic Rehabilitation.* Philadelphia, PA: Mosby; 2003:557-558.

19. Sampsell E. Rehabilitation of the spine following sports injury. *Clin Sports Med.* 2010;29:127-156.

20. Smith CE, Nyland J, Caudill P, et al. Dynamic trunk stabilization: a conceptual back injury prevention program for volleyball athletes. *J Orthop Sports Phys Ther.* 2008;38:703-720.

21. Kibler WB, Press J, Sciascia A. The role of core stability in athletic function. *Sports Med* 2006;36:189-198.

22. Allison GT, Morris SL, Lay B. Feedforward responses of transversus abdominis are directionally specific and act asymmetrically: implications for core stability theories. *J Orthop Sports Phys Ther.* 2008;38:228-237.

23. Grenier SG, McGill SM. Quantification of lumbar stability by using 2 different abdominal activation strategies. *Arch Phys Med Rehabil.* 2007;88:54-62.

24. Brown SH, Vera-Garcia FJ, McGill SM. Effects of abdominal muscle coactivation on the externally preloaded trunk: variations in motor control and its effect on spine stability. *Spine.* 2006;31:E387-E393.

25. Walsh JC, Quinlan JF, Stapleton R, et al. Three-dimensional motion analysis of the lumbar spine during "free squat" weight lift training. *Am J Sports Med.* 2007;35:927-932.

26. Grazina R, Andrade R, Lima Santos F, et al. Return to play after conservative and surgical treatment in athletes with spondylolysis: A systematic review. *Physical Therapy in Sport.* 2019;34-43.

27. Chung CC, Shimer AL. Lumbosacral Spondylolysis and Spondylolisthesis. *Clin Sports Med.* 2021;40:471-490.

28. Caneiro JP, Smith A, Rabey M, et al. Process of Change in Pain-Related Fear: Clinical Insights From a Single Case Report of Persistent Back Pain Managed With Cognitive Functional Therapy. *J Orthop Sports Phys Ther.* 2017;47(9):637-651.

Low Back Pain: Manipulation Intervention

Carl DeRosa
Brett Windsor

A 42-year-old first-generation American and university professor self-refers to physical therapy for evaluation and treatment of low back pain (LBP). He has had recurrent bouts of LBP over the past 12 years and for most of those episodes, the pain tends to resolve to his satisfaction, sometimes over a few days, but mostly over the course of a few weeks. On occasion, he has seen his family practice physician for episodes that did not resolve. Approximately 5 years ago, his doctor referred him to an orthopedic physician for further evaluation, but radiographs and magnetic resonance imaging of the lumbar spine and pelvis were unremarkable. In most instances, he was given nonsteroidal anti-inflammatory medication and a small booklet describing low back exercises. He feels that his LBP exacerbations now last longer, and the bouts seem more frequent. This most recent back pain episode began 7 days ago. He is a golfer, and his goal is to be able to walk a full 18 holes of play after a long morning of writing at his desk. He also does not want this episode to cause him to miss work as several of his past episodes have done.

▶ What are key questions to ask to further clarify the patient's complaints and provide direction for the examination?
▶ What are the most appropriate physical therapy interventions?
▶ What are key biopsychosocial factors driving the rehabilitation prognosis?

KEY DEFINITIONS

ACUTE, SUBACUTE, AND CHRONIC LOW BACK PAIN (LBP): Classic description of the course of LBP using a temporal guideline, with acute typically considered to last 0 to 4 weeks, subacute from 1 to 3 months, and chronic more than 3 months; most common back complaints are exacerbations of a recurrent back condition, which clouds the delineation between subacute conditions, chronic conditions, and chronic LBP syndrome.

CHRONIC LOW BACK PAIN SYNDROME (CLBP): Mixed pain syndrome that can include both nociceptive and neuropathic pain, but the psychosocial and behavioral aspects of pain exceed mechanical or chemical nociceptive influences; CLBP may be influenced by a patient's attitudes and beliefs, social determinants of health, psychological distress, and illness behavior.

MANIPULATION: Physical intervention intended to direct a specific force into a targeted region of the body (often a joint) identified by rate of force application and location within the range of motion (beginning, middle, or end of available range); distinction between mobilization and manipulation is typically related to *rate* of force application (*i.e.*, manipulation is a *high*-velocity thrust).

MULTIMODAL MANAGEMENT: Integrated multidisciplinary therapy with coordinated somatic and psychotherapeutic elements frequently used to treat CLBP[1]

PATIENT-CENTERED CARE: Practice of caring for patients by sharing power and responsibility, and developing a therapeutic alliance that integrates individual patient preferences, beliefs, needs, and values and ensures that patient's values guide clinical decisions

RADICULAR PAIN: Pain due to mechanical or chemical irritation of a damaged nerve root, which lowers the nerve root's threshold to mechanical stimulus (either tension or compression)

REFERRED PAIN: Pain felt at a distance from the actual anatomical source of involvement or injury; due to extensive innervation of spinal tissues, pain can be felt in the lower quarter due to involvement of low back tissues (or in the upper quarter due to involvement of cervical tissues), irrespective of involvement of the nerve roots in the region.

SEGMENTAL INSTABILITY: Displacement or aberrant motion between two bony segments that results when a force is applied; most types are translational motions due to applied shear loads; segmental instability is distinct from hypermobility.

Objectives

1. List key aspects of the history and physical examination that indicate a nonmusculoskeletal cause of the patient's symptoms.

2. Describe how to triage the person presenting with LBP and pain into the lower extremity into either a radicular pain category or a nonradicular pain category.

3. Describe the rationale for including manual therapy, specifically manipulation, in the management strategy for a person presenting with LBP.

4. Provide a rationale for the use of therapeutic exercise in conjunction with manipulation to optimize the prognosis for a person presenting with exacerbation of a recurrent low back condition.

5. Describe the role of education in improving the prognosis of this patient in relation to his functional goals.

Physical Therapy Considerations

Physical therapy considerations during management of the individual with a diagnosis of mechanical LBP:

▶ **General physical therapy plan of care/goals:** Shared decision-making around patient values, goals and preferences; educate to decrease fear characteristics and create a sense of freedom and decreased anxiety around movement; decrease pain in rapid and cost-effective manner; begin graded, active, spinal activity program and progress to therapeutic exercises focused on enhancing neuromuscular performance; long-term strengthening and endurance

▶ **Physical therapy interventions:** Spinal mobilization or manipulation to specific regions with primary intent of modulating pain; resistance exercises to increase strength and endurance (especially of spinal extensors, abdominals, and hip musculature) preferably in functional movement patterns; exercises to improve motor control and overall aerobic fitness; education regarding position, loads, and activities that have the potential to exacerbate condition as determined by the pathomechanics gleaned via the physical examination

▶ **Precautions during physical therapy:** Carefully consider the risk-benefit ratio regarding chosen pain modulation techniques; monitor that lower extremity pain symptoms do not extend distal to the knee; exercise overload must remain within the physiologic limits of patient's spinal condition

▶ **Complications interfering with physical therapy:** Psychosocial factors affecting prognosis including fear of movement and low expectation of recovery; exacerbation of pain following manipulation intervention; distal referral of symptoms as a result of manipulation or exercise regimen; patient dependency on passive manipulation interventions over active, self-management strategies

Understanding the Health Condition

LBP is the leading cause of years lost to disability worldwide and its impact is increasing as the population grows and ages, particularly in low- and middle-income countries.[2] All age groups are affected and LBP is generally positively correlated with sedentary occupations, smoking, obesity, and low socioeconomic status.[3] LBP is not as dependent on degenerative processes associated with aging as might be expected.

The prevalence of LBP appears to plateau at the sixth decade and then decline in the later decades of life.[4] Socioeconomic factors are also important to consider because they are recognized as potential risk factors for lumbar pain and disability, ultimately contributing to direct and indirect costs. A higher prevalence of LBP occurs in those with lower educational levels, unskilled laborers, and workers with physically demanding job responsibilities.[3] The total costs of LBP in the United States exceed $100 billion per year with two-thirds being indirect costs due to lost wages and reduced productivity.[5]

Systematic reviews of primary care studies show that 28% to 79% of people with acute LBP experience persistent or recurrent symptoms 12 months after their initial episode.[6] Therefore, the great majority of the costs of LBP are associated with management of the *chronic* disorder. This has significant influence on the goals of treatment and the physical therapist's approach toward management of the condition. Comprehensive care for the patient presenting with LBP includes attempts to manage the immediate clinical presentation. However, perhaps more importantly, management involves using interventions and appropriate patient education strategies to minimize the potential for the acute, simple LBP episode to evolve into a chronic pain syndrome. The physical therapist must recognize that most patients with nonsurgical LBP episodes are actually presenting with an exacerbation of a chronic back condition. Thus, the focus of intervention strategies is to help prevent recurrences, or at a minimum, provide information or strategies to help the patient self-manage a recurrent back problem.

Although a recent systematic review concluded it is not possible to accurately predict the risk of LBP recurrence, or to identify specific prognostic factors,[7] several factors contribute to recurrent back problems, including frequent exposure to awkward postures, longer time sitting (>5 hours per day), more than 2 previous LBP episodes,[8] and enhanced pronociceptive mechanisms and impaired anti-nociceptive mechanisms.[9] Physiological tissue changes due to aging and injury may also play a role in recurrence. Such changes decrease the ability of low back tissues to tolerate forces, especially forces that traverse the lumbopelvic region due to weightbearing and movement. When these forces exceed the physiological capacity of the tissues, pain can occur due to mechanical or chemical activation of the tissue nociceptive system.

In the low back (as in other areas of the musculoskeletal system), the mechanical loading capacity of tissues lowers as we age.[10] Because the low back is a hub of weightbearing, injuries can occur even with activities of daily living (ADLs). This lifetime accumulation of such injuries, coupled with normal aging and degenerative processes, renders the back susceptible to re-injury. For example, the spinal segment can be viewed similar to a three-legged stool, with the front leg of the stool representing the intervertebral disc, and the back two legs of the stool represented by the right and left apophyseal joints.[11] Apophyseal joint arthritis alone, or in combination with degeneration of the annulus fibrosus, results in an intervertebral segment that has less ability to tolerate forces such as tension, compression, and shear. The breakdown of these tissues can result in aberrant motion between vertebral segments,[12,13] resulting in segmental instability. Partial thickness degeneration of the facets of the apophyseal joints results in a segment that can no longer tolerate compressive and shear loading when compared to normal, healthy tissue.[14] When compression and shear loads exceed the physiological loading capacity of compromised tissue, discomfort or pain can result.[11]

Any structure within the spine that is innervated and provides afferent input to the central nervous system has the capacity to elicit pain.[15] The dura mater and nerve roots, apophyseal joints,[16] annulus fibrosus, bone, and ligaments all exhibit the capacity to generate pain when damaged.[15] Despite a reasonable understanding of tissue injury and innervation, identification of the *precise* anatomical structure responsible for a patient's episode of pain is not always possible.[2,3] In fact, in many low back conditions, the presence of abnormal imaging findings (radiographs, computerized tomography, magnetic resonance imaging) has no correlation to the presence or absence of clinical symptoms.[17-19] Thus, treatment of LBP using a pathoanatomical model of care is often futile and costly and can waste limited healthcare resources and harm patients.[2]

One of the few tissues in the spine that can be implicated with some degree of confidence as the patient's source of pain is the nerve root. When the nerve root is involved in the pain syndrome, a very distinct set of symptoms and/or signs emerge.[20] There are two nerve root conditions: nerve root compression and nerve root irritation. Nerve root compression can result in true neurologic signs such as muscle weakness, reflex changes, and/or clearly demarcated sensory disturbances. Nerve root irritation, which is often due to the chemical milieu that results from inflammation associated with intervertebral disc lesions, presents with a distinct set of symptoms (as opposed to signs). Symptoms of nerve root irritation include: leg pain greater than back pain, clearly demarcated region of lower extremity pain, pain often below the knee, a highly disturbing and distressing type of pain, reproduction of lower extremity pain with neural tension tests (especially positive straight leg raise [SLR]), and sharp peripheralizing pain with gentle spinal motions (*e.g.*, pain into the legs with slight active or passive lumbar flexion or rotation). Any direction of motion can result in peripheralization of true nerve root irritation. The hallmark is the remarkably small amount of motion necessary to elicit such a dramatic pain response.

Low back conditions that are nonradicular in nature (*i.e.*, not due to nerve root irritation or nerve root compression) present differently especially in regards to referral into the lower extremity. *Any* innervated tissue in the low back can refer pain into the lower extremity.[20] Nonradicular pain patterns typically present as conditions in which the pain in the low back is more aggravating and concerning to the patient than the discomfort referred to the lower extremity. In low back conditions that are nonradicular, the patient's description of lower extremity pain is neither as clearly demarcated over the lower extremity nor as disconcerting as true radicular pain. For the individual with nerve root (radicular) pain, the lower extremity pain is often the more problematic complaint than the pain in the low back. Therefore, an important goal of the examination is for the physical therapist to discern whether the LBP and leg pain that the patient presents with is radicular pain (*i.e.*, true nerve root problem) or nonradicular pain (*i.e.*, pain felt in the back and referred to the lower extremity due to injury to any innervated low back structure such as apophyseal or sacroiliac joints, muscle, ligament, fascia).

Physical Therapy Patient/Client Management

For the individual presenting with an exacerbation of a recurrent LBP problem, a multimodal management strategy that is achieved through a shared decision-making model should be used. The plan of care must integrate the patient's values and preferences to facilitate long-term self-efficacy in management.[21] Patient education around positive prognostic factors decreases fear and catastrophizing. Care begins with rapidly relieving pain, followed by progressing the patient toward an active exercise program to improve the strength and functional abilities of the trunk and extremities, and educating the patient in self-management strategies. Improving the health of the neuromuscular system after achieving pain relief is an essential component of management because the priority of therapeutic intervention should be to reduce injury recurrence or exacerbations and minimize the potential for the mechanical back pain problem to evolve into a chronic pain syndrome.[22-25]

Examination, Evaluation, and Diagnosis

The examination of a patient self-referred for LBP requires two initial triages. The first is to determine if the patient's pain is nonmechanical or mechanical in origin. Nonmechanical pain relevant to low back conditions is typically considered to be pain referred from pelvic or abdominal viscera, neoplasm, pain of vascular origin, or pain associated with other medical conditions. Nonmechanical pain is characterized by pain complaints not typically made worse with mechanical loading, positions, and movement. A systems review and questions regarding recent weight loss, fevers, past medical history, night pain, bowel or bladder disturbances, and recent surgeries are essential elements of the history and physical examination for the patient with LBP. Mechanical disorders are typically associated with some pain resolution with rest or relief from weightbearing and a pain pattern that can be correlated with activity, motion, or applied loads. Familiar pain can often be provoked with specific lumbopelvic motions, positions, or in response to specifically applied loads to the joints or soft tissues. In the absence of these phenomena, further medical evaluation is indicated. If there are no concerning features, the physical therapist can proceed as planned and monitor symptoms. If treatment proceeds as expected, there is no further cause for concern.[26]

The second triage is to ascertain whether the patient's pain complaint is radicular or nonradicular. Careful questioning regarding the pain pattern should be addressed early in the examination: "Is the back pain worse than the leg pain?" Or conversely, "Is the leg pain more disconcerting than the back pain?" Affirmative answers to these questions help the therapist determine if the condition is more likely nonradicular or radicular, respectively. In addition, a sickening quality to the pain, pain that is below the knee, and pain that is clearly demarcated in a dermatomal distribution are all strong indicators of radicular pain. A complaint of weakness in the lower extremity can also indicate a radicular disorder. If the history reveals suspicion of a radicular condition, confirmatory tests such as straight leg raising,[27] Slump testing,[28] myotome and reflex assessments, and dermatome screening must be done. A positive SLR combined with a positive Hancock Rule has been shown to suggest a radicular disorder.[29] The Hancock Rule is the presence of 3 of the following 4 factors: pain or sensory deficit in dermatomal region, reflex changes, or motor weakness in concordance with a specific nerve root.

Once the therapist has determined that the patient's condition is nonradicular in nature, the intent of the physical examination is not to precisely identify the anatomical structure considered to be at fault (a pathoanatomical model), but rather to determine the loads or positions that reproduce the patient's familiar pain (a pathomechanical model). Figure 13-1 shows several parts of the physical examination that uniquely place compressive and shear loads over the lumbar spine. Information gained from determining which positions and stresses reproduce the patient's symptoms can then be used to prescribe the activity and exercise interventions.

An acute episode of pain presents an opportunity to determine if spinal manipulation may be a beneficial intervention for the patient's LBP.[30] Key aspects of the history and the physical examination help determine whether regional lumbopelvic manipulation is likely to be effective.[31,32] Patients meeting certain criteria can experience significant changes in pain patterns and the perception of pain with the application of manipulation, advice to remain active, and a prescribed course of exercise.[33,34] Although these clinical prediction rules have limited application,[35,36] the criteria may be useful—particularly in otherwise healthy, young, active individuals with no comorbidities.[32-34] **Individuals considered most likely to benefit from a regional lumbopelvic manipulation** exhibit the following: duration of symptoms <16 days, no symptoms distal to the knee, lumbar hypomobility, at least one hip with >35° range of passive internal rotation, and a score <19 on the Fear Avoidance Belief Questionnaire (FABQ).[31] The probability of a successful outcome with lumbar manipulation increases from 45% to 95% with the presence of ≤4 of these examination findings.[31] The criteria presented in this clinical prediction rule (CPR) by Flynn *et al.* are most suggestive of nonradicular conditions that would benefit from the use of manipulation as an intervention. This illustrates why the second triage of determining whether the syndrome is radicular or nonradicular in nature is important.

After publication of the Flynn *et al.* CPR, a pragmatic rule was suggested to simplify the prediction of which patients with LBP would be likely to experience dramatic improvement in pain and perception of disability with regional lumbopelvic manipulation.[33] Two factors helped predict improvement: duration of symptoms <16 days and no symptoms distal to the knee. Subjects in this study had a moderate to large shift in probability of a successful outcome following a low back manipulation. Flynn *et al.*'s 2002 CPR has been further validated with two different manipulation techniques: the regional lumbopelvic manipulation and the rotary lumbopelvic manipulation.[34] Combining manipulation and stabilization exercises for patients meeting this CPR may be of even greater benefit, especially since one of the goals is to minimize LBP recurrences.[33]

For the current patient, his history contained 3 of the 5 factors (duration of symptoms 7 days, no pain below the knee, and FABQ score <19) predicting that he would benefit from manipulation, advice to remain active, and a prescribed course

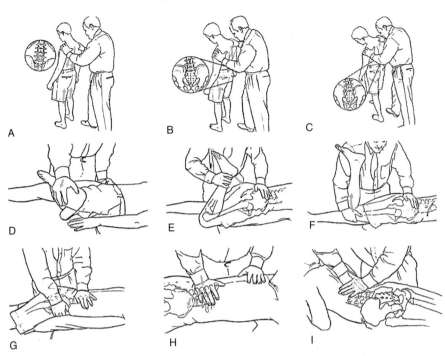

Figure 13-1. **A.** Overpressure in backward bending. The physical therapist manually retracts the scapulae to focus the extension force in the upper part of the lumbar spine. A gradual vertical force from above causes extension. **B.** Backward bending, sidebending to the left, and slight rotation to the right, with a superior-to-inferior overpressure applied to the right shoulder. **C.** Modification of standing examination to increase the extension, compression, and shear stresses in the left lumbosacral triangle by positioning the left lower extremity in extension, then having the patient backward bend and sidebend to the left. The examiner applies overpressure with the right hand. The patient's response to this end-range extension and compression is evaluated. **D.** The patient's left lower extremity is put into the FABER position (passive flexion, abduction, external rotation). As the examiner directs the femur toward the table, this stresses the left sacroiliac joint and produces a small rotary force to the lumbosacral junction. **E.** Passive knee flexion in prone is tested to assess the length of the rectus femoris. If this muscle is decreased in length, passive knee flexion can cause anterior torsional stress to the ilium that is transferred up to the lumbar spine as lumbosacral extension, which increases facet compression and shear stress. Anterior rotary movement of the pelvis before the knee reaches 90° of flexion is a positive sign. **F.** Prone passive femoral extension. The examiner lifts the femur beyond the point where the anterior thigh musculature and joint capsule become taut. This results in extension up through the remaining lumbar spine segments. **G.** Prone application of passive compressive and shear force to the pelvis and spine. The examiner pushes down with the top hand and up with the bottom hand until the two forces meet. A positive finding is reproduction of the familiar symptoms. **H.** Prone posterior-to-anterior rotary force imparted to the posterior superior iliac spine and right ilium. Intent is to determine if movement provokes familiar pain. **I.** Application of end-range stress to the lumbar spine in extension. The patient is asked to come up on his elbows. The examiner's index and middle fingers of one hand are placed on either side of the spinous process. The examiner's other hand is placed over the index and middle fingers to direct a force to the inferior articulating processes. (Reproduced with permission from Carl DeRosa, PT, PhD, FAPTA.)

of exercise. The physical examination will reveal whether the remaining two predictors are present (lumbar hypomobility and hip internal rotation range of motion). The physical examination starts with the patient in the standing position. Assessment includes: frontal and sagittal plane posture, active motion of the lumbar spine in forward bending, forward bending and side bending combined, backward bending, backward bending and side bending combined, overpressure in each of these directions, the effect of the pain pattern with these repeated motions, and gait analysis.

In the supine position, hip active and passive ROM can be assessed and various sacroiliac provocative stresses applied through the lever of the femur. Full flexion of the hips begins to flex the pelvis on the lumbar spine, which can then be compared to the results found with standing active flexion. SLR testing can be performed and lower extremity myotomes and reflexes effectively screened in this position.

In the prone position, hip ROM can be further assessed, in particular internal and external ROM.[37] Additional sacroiliac stresses can be applied, followed by posterior to anterior (PA) spring tests over the lumbar spine, which place a compressive force through the apophyseal joints and a shear stress between adjacent lumbar spinal segments. The response to compression and shear stresses over the lumbar spine should be compared to the results of the extension, and extension-side bending tests that were performed during the standing portion of the examination. Posterior to anterior forces over individual lumbar spinous processes, or bilaterally over the region of the lumbar transverse processes can be used to determine hypomobility, as well as to determine if such a compression and shear force applied to the lumbar spine reproduces the patient's familiar pain.

Plan of Care and Interventions

The physical therapist determined that the patient's LBP was of mechanical origin with a nonradicular component. The patient's primary complaint is pain and secondary complaints are related to loss of physical function and performance (concern about recurrences, fear of not being able to continue his work, unable to perform ADLs and recreational pursuits without fear of pain exacerbation). The patient's goals are to be able to walk and play 18 holes of recreational golf and to be able to continue his work without interruption.

Patient education is a critical piece of developing a therapeutic alliance between patient and physical therapist and facilitates the development of a shared-decision model of care.[21] Integrating patient values and preferences decreases fear responses, increases self-efficacy, and drives a long-term positive prognosis. Education should focus on the presence of positive prognostic factors (presentation belongs to a clear, classifiable form of lumbar pain; walking as an easing factor) and the absence of negative prognostic factors (deep leg symptoms, longer sick leave duration, clinically determined inflammation, more severe back and leg pain).[6] The physical therapist should clearly inform this patient that there is no reason why he should not make a full recovery and be able to achieve his goals. A thorough discussion with the patient about each of the proposed interventions and shared agreement about their application and prescription are indicated.

The history and physical exam suggest that the focus of intervention should be to rapidly relieve his pain and provide strategies to maximize his physical health (especially his overall strength) to minimize the likelihood of recurrences. With the age-related breakdown of the specialized tissues of the spine (e.g., intervertebral discs, apophyseal joints), the neuromuscular system becomes the primary means by which loads must be attenuated. Thus, attention to improving neuromuscular efficiency, especially of his trunk and hips, must be an important aspect of care.

Following discussion of the risks, benefits, and evidence for manual therapy, the patient stated a preference for spinal manipulation with the goal of achieving rapid pain relief. He then stated a desire to begin a series of active exercises designed around pain-free positions, in combination with a walking program to improve neuromuscular and cardiovascular endurance. The therapist performed a regional lumbopelvic manipulation with the patient in the supine position, and the patient experienced immediate pain relief. Success might also have been predicted if the therapist used a lumbar rotary-type manipulation.[34] For ease of understanding and reproducibility, the manipulation was documented in the manner suggested by Mintken et al.[38,39] This model outlines a documentation standard for manipulation techniques utilizing the following six descriptors: rate of force application, location in range of available movement, direction of force, target of force, relative structural movement, and patient position. Thus, the technique applied to this patient was documented as a high velocity, end range, left rotational force to the left ilium on the lumbar spine in supine (Fig. 13-2). Documentation in this manner allows the intervention to be clearly understood and potentially replicated, and avoids using biomechanical descriptions of manipulation techniques that have little evidence.

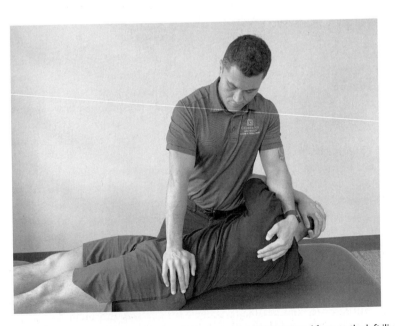

Figure 13-2. Manipulation technique: high velocity, end range, left rotational force to the left ilium on the lumbar spine in the supine position.

Following a successful manipulation intervention, a **series of dynamic exercises intended to improve trunk motor control and strength** is prescribed. The initial exercise prescription incorporates the results of the physical examination by determining pain-free positions and movements. Initial training should focus on strengthening the abdominal muscles, spine extensors, and hip musculature with the ultimate goal of progressing to functional movement patterns for the shoulder girdle and lower quarter using carefully applied controlled resistance. Such exercises can improve perceived disability in both the short- and long-term in patients with recurrent LBP.[33,40] The patient should be instructed to be aware of and avoid any peripheralization of pain during exercises or ADLs. The physical therapist must emphasize to the patient that the goal is *centralization* of pain (*i.e.*, pain felt in a more proximal location in response to repeated movements or sustained positions). The concept of centralizing pain should be utilized as a means to determine when to increase the frequency and intensity of his exercise program.[41] Carefully administered exercises that emphasize motor control are effective for nonspecific, nonradicular LBP. Motor control exercises for the spine include more than teaching a patient the "neutral" position of the spine. Instead, the physical therapist must incorporate the results of the physical examination to determine the motions and positions of the lumbar spine that have the least potential to exacerbate the pain pattern. With some patients, that may mean more of a flexion bias, whereas in others that may mean more of an extension bias. Results from the physical examination dictate the control of the spine necessary for pain-free activity. A systematic review of 14 randomized controlled trials concluded that motor control when used in isolation or in conjunction with additional interventions decreased LBP and disability.[42]

The importance of prescribing **progressive endurance exercises and dynamic exercises** is important when the goal is long-term, self-efficacy care. For this patient, the following exercises served as excellent strengthening stimuli for the trunk and hip musculature: air squats (squat exercises with close attention to form), squat thrusts (squats with an overhead press maneuver at the end), kettlebell swings that emphasize hip motion, dynamic plank exercises (plank position with alternating hip flexion), and standing pulley exercises that emphasize pulling motions, rowing motions, and hip rotary motions. Since this patient is a recreational golfer, lumbar rotation is especially important to monitor because this motion places excessive compressive loads to the lumbar apophyseal joints and tensile stresses to the annulus fibrosus. Rotation through the hips during the golf swing must be emphasized. Programs including the discussed exercises have a positive effect on patients who have recurrent exacerbations of a chronic back problem.[40,43-47]

Evidence-Based Clinical Recommendations

SORT: Strength of Recommendation Taxonomy

A: Consistent, good-quality patient-oriented evidence
B: Inconsistent or limited-quality patient-oriented evidence
C: Consensus, disease-oriented evidence, usual practice, expert opinion, or case series

1. To minimize recurrences and the potential for a mechanical back pain problem to evolve into a chronic pain syndrome, the management strategy for patients presenting with an exacerbation of recurrent low back pain should focus on rapid pain relief followed by strengthening exercises of the trunk and extremity musculature. **Grade A**

2. Lumbopelvic manipulation is effective for treating low back pain in individuals demonstrating specific history and physical exam criteria. **Grade A**

3. Spinal stabilization and progressive endurance exercises for the trunk and hip musculature are effective interventions to manage acute, subacute, or recurrent low back pain. **Grade B**

COMPREHENSION QUESTIONS

13.1 Which of the following pain characteristics is LEAST likely to be caused by nerve root irritation?

   A. Leg pain greater than back pain

   B. Pain in the lower extremity that is clearly demarcated as opposed to general aching

   C. Back pain that is made worse with lifting

   D. Pain below the knee

13.2 Manipulation can be considered an intervention of choice for a patient presenting with low back pain when:

   A. Pain is below the knee and made worse with spinal extension.

   B. Onset of symptoms is within a 2-week time period and generalized hypomobility can be determined with posterior to anterior spring testing of lumbar spine.

   C. More muscle spasm and guarding is detected on one side compared to the opposite side.

   D. Slump test and straight leg raise test are positive.

ANSWERS

13.1 **C.** Increased intradiscal pressure, which occurs during lifting when the spine is flexed, is associated with disc pathology. Leg pain greater than back pain (option A) and pain below the knee (option D) are typical indicators of nerve root pain. Pain in the lower extremity that is clearly demarcated suggests a specific referral pattern (e.g., dermatomal pattern) that could be due to irritation of a nerve root (option B).

13.2 **B.** Options A and C have no evidence-based correlation with the utilization of spinal manipulation. Positive Slump test and straight leg raise tests (option D) are more indicative of nerve root pathology, which can be a contraindication for manipulation—not an intervention of choice.

REFERENCES

1. Schega L, Kaps B, Broscheid KC, et al. Effects of a multimodal exercise intervention on physical and cognitive functions in patients with chronic low back pain (MultiMove): study protocol for a randomized controlled trial. *BMC Geriatr.* 2021;21(1):151.

2. Buchbinder R, van Tulder M, Öberg B, et al. Low back pain: a call for action. *Lancet.* 2018;391(10137): 2384-2388.

3. Hartvigsen J, Hancock MJ, Kongsted A, et al. What low back pain is and why we need to pay attention. *Lancet.* 2018;391(10137).

4. Papageorgiou AC, Macfarlane GJ, Thomas E, et al. Psychosocial factors in the workplace—do they predict new episodes of low back pain? Evidence from the South Manchester Back Pain Study. *Spine.* 1997;22:1137-1142.

5. Waterman BR, Belmont PJ Jr, Schoenfeld AJ. Low back pain in the United States: incidence and risk factors for presentation in the emergency setting. *Spine J.* 2012;12(1):63-70.

6. Ford J, Hahne A, Surkitt L, et al. The evolving case supporting individualized physiotherapy for low back pain. *J Clin Med.* 2019;8(9):1334.

7. da Silva T, Mills K, Brown BT, et al. Risk of recurrence of low back pain: a systematic review. *J Orthop Sports Phys Ther.* 2017;47(5):305-313.

8. da Silva T, Mills K, Brown BT, et al. Recurrence of low back pain is common: a prospective inception cohort study. *J Physiother.* 2019;65(3):159-165.

9. McPhee ME, Graven-Nielsen T. Recurrent low back pain patients demonstrate facilitated pronociceptive mechanisms when in pain, and impaired antinociceptive mechanisms with and without pain. *Pain.* 2019;160(12):2866-2876.

10. Leveille SG. Musculoskeletal aging. *Curr Opin Rheumatol.* 2004;16:114-118.

11. Gracovetsky S, Farfan H. The optimum spine. *Spine.* 1986; 11, 543-573.

12. Li W, Wang S, Xia Q, et al. Lumbar facet joint motion in patients with degenerative disc disease at affected and adjacent levels: an in vivo biomechanical study. *Spine* (Phila Pa 1976). 2011;36(10):E62 9-E637.

13. Yao Q, Wang S, Shin JH, et al. Lumbar facet joint motion in patients with degenerative spondylolisthesis. *J Spinal Disord Tech.* 2013;26(1):E19-E27.

14. Dunlop RB, Adams MA, Hutton WC. Disc space narrowing and facet joints. *J Bone Joint Surg Br.* 1984;66:706-710.

15. Peng B, Bogduk N, DePalma MJ, Ma K. Chronic spinal pain: pathophysiology, diagnosis, and treatment. *Pain Res Manag.* 2019:1729059.

16. MacVicar J, MacVicar AM, Bogduk N. The prevalence of "pure" lumbar zygapophysial joint pain in patients with chronic low back pain. *Pain Med.* 2021;22(1):41-48.

17. Wiesel SW, Tsourmas N, Feffer HL, et al. A study of computer-assisted tomography. I. The incidence of positive CAT scans in an asymptomatic group of patients. *Spine.* 1984;9: 549-551.

18. Boden SD, Davis DO, Din TS, et al. Abnormal magnetic-resonance scans of the lumbar spine in asymptomatic subjects. A prospective investigation. *J Bone Joint Surg Am.*1990;72:403-408.

19. Savage RA, Whitehouse GH, Roberts N. The relationship between the magnetic resonance imaging appearance of the lumbar spine and low back pain, age, and occupation in males. *Eur Spine J.* 1997;6:106-114.

20. Bogduk N. On the definitions and physiology of back pain, referred pain, and radicular pain. *Pain.* 2009;147(1-3):17-19.

21. Hoffmann TC, Lewis J, Maher CG. Shared decision-making should be an integral part of physiotherapy practice. *Physiotherapy.* 2020;107:43-49.

22. Airaksinen O, Brox JI, Cedraschi C, et al. COST B13 Working Group on Guidelines for Chronic Low Back Pain. Chapter 4. European guidelines for the management of chronic nonspecific low back pain. *Eur Spine J.* 2006;15 Suppl 2:S192-300.

23. Chou R, Qaseem A, Snow V, et al. Clinical Efficacy Assessment Subcommittee of the American College of Physicians; American Pain Society Low Back Pain Guidelines Panel. Diagnosis and treatment of low back pain: a joint clinical practice guideline from the American College of Physicians and the American Pain Society. *Ann Intern Med.* 2007;147:478-491.

24. Savigny P, Watson P, Underwood M. Guideline Development Group. Early management of persistent non-specific low back pain: summary of NICE guidance. *BMJ.* 2009;338:b1805.

25. Rainville J, Hartigan C, Martinez E, et al. Exercise as a treatment for chronic low back pain. *Spine J.* 2004;4:106-115.

26. Finucane LM, Downie A, Mercer C, et al. International framework for red flags for potential serious spinal pathologies. *J Orthop Sports Phys Ther.* 2020;50(7):350-372.

27. Camino Willhuber GO, Piuzzi NS. Straight Leg Raise Test. In: StatPearls. Treasure Island (FL): StatPearls Publishing; July 31, 2021.

28. Urban LM, MacNeil BJ. Diagnostic accuracy of the Slump test for identifying neuropathic pain in the lower limb. *J Orthop Sports Phys Ther.* 2015;45(8):596-603.

29. Petersen T, Laslett M, Juhl C. Clinical classification in low back pain: best-evidence diagnostic rules based on systematic reviews. *BMC Musculoskelet Disord.* 2017;18(1):188.

30. Ghasabmahaleh SH, Rezasoltani Z, Dadarkhah A, et al. Spinal manipulation for subacute and chronic lumbar radiculopathy: a randomized controlled trial. *Am J Med.* 2021;134(1):135-141.

31. Flynn T, Fritz J, Whitman J, et al. A clinical prediction rule for classifying patients with low back pain who demonstrate short-term improvement with spinal manipulation. *Spine.* 2002;27:2835-2843.

32. Childs JD, Fritz JM, Flynn TW, et al. A clinical prediction rule to identify patients with low back pain most likely to benefit from spinal manipulation: a validation study. *Ann Int Med.* 2004;141:920-928.

33. Fritz JM, Childs JD, Flynn TW. Pragmatic application of a clinical prediction rule in primary care to identify patients with low back pain with a good prognosis following a brief spinal manipulation intervention. *BMC Fam Prac.* 2005;6:29.

34. Cleland JA, Fritz JM, Kulig K, et al. Comparison of the effectiveness of three manual therapy techniques in a subgroup of patients with low back pain who satisfy a clinical prediction rule: a randomized clinical trial. *Spine.* 2009;34:2720-2729.

35. Walsh ME, French HP, Wallace E, et al. Existing validated clinical prediction rules for predicting response to physiotherapy interventions for musculoskeletal conditions have limited clinical value: A systematic review. *J Clin Epidemiol.* 2021;135:90-102.

36. Mitchell UH, Hurrell J. Clinical spinal instability: 10 years since the derivation of a clinical prediction rule. A narrative literature review. *J Back Musculoskelet Rehabil.* 2019;32(2):293-298.

37. Ellison JB, Rose SJ, Sahrmann SA. Patterns of hip rotation range of motion: a comparison between healthy subjects and patients with low back pain. *Phys Ther.*1990;70:537-541.

38. Mintken PE, DeRosa C, Little T, Smith B; American Academy of Orthopaedic Manual Physical Therapists. AAOMPT clinical guidelines: a model for standardizing manipulation terminology in physical therapy practice. *J Orthop Sports Phys Ther.* 2008;38:A1-6.

39. Mintken PE, DeRosa C, Little T, Smith B. A model for standardizing manipulation terminology in physical therapy practice. *J Man Manip Ther.* 2008;16:50-56.

40. Hayden JA, Ellis J, Ogilvie R, et al. Exercise therapy for chronic low back pain. *Cochrane Database Syst Rev.* 2021;9(9):CD009790.

41. Kilpikoski S, Airaksinen O, Kankaanpaa M, et al. Interexaminer reliability of low back pain assessment using the McKenzie method. *Spine.* 2002;27:E207-214.

42. Macedo LG, Maher CG, Latimer J, McAuley JH. Motor control exercise for persistent, nonspecific low back pain: a systematic review. *Phys Ther.* 2009;89:9-25.

43. Macedo LG, Smeets RJ, Maher CG, et al. Graded activity and graded exposure for persistent non-specific low back pain: a systematic review. *Phys Ther.* 2010;90:860-879.

44. Rainville J, Jouve CA, Hartigan C. Comparison of short- and long-term outcomes for aggressive spine rehabilitation delivered two versus three times per week. *Spine J*. 2002;2:402-407.

45. Smith C, Grimmer-Sommers K. The treatment effect of exercise programmes for chronic low back pain. *J Eval Clin Practice*. 2010;16:484-491.

46. Macedo LG, Saragiotto BT, Yamato TP, et al. (2016). Motor control exercise for acute non-specific low back pain. *Cochr database syst rev*. 2016;2:CD012085.

47. Niederer D, Mueller J. Sustainability effects of motor control stabilisation exercises on pain and function in chronic nonspecific low back pain patients: A systematic review with meta-analysis and meta-regression. *PloS one*. 2020;15(1):e0227423.

Low Back Pain: Mechanical Diagnosis and Therapy (McKenzie) Approach to Lumbar Disc Herniation

Jolene Bennett
Barbara J. Hoogenboom

CASE 14

A 36-year-old male construction worker self-referred to an outpatient physical therapy clinic with a complaint of low back pain and pain radiating from his posterior left hip down to his lateral foot. He first experienced pain 3 weeks ago while doing a home maintenance project. The onset of pain occurred when he attempted to lift an air conditioning unit. He reports that as he bent over to lift the unit, he experienced an intense, stabbing pain and immediately fell to the ground. He required assistance from his wife to walk back into the house. For the first 24 hours after the incident, he rested prone on the couch or bed. Over the past 3 days, he reports an improved tolerance to walking and standing for short periods. However, he rates his current pain 5 out of 10 on the numerical pain rating scale and he continues to experience radiating pain distal to his knee. Signs and symptoms are consistent with a lumbar herniated disc. His goal is to return to work as soon as possible.

- ▸ Based on the patient's suspected diagnosis, what do you anticipate may be the contributing factors to his condition?
- ▸ What examination signs may be associated with this diagnosis?
- ▸ What are the most appropriate physical therapy interventions?
- ▸ What are possible complications that may limit the effectiveness of physical therapy?
- ▸ How might interventions impact the movement system?

KEY DEFINITIONS

CENTRALIZATION: Phenomenon in which distal limb pain emanating from the spine is abolished in response to deliberate application of loading strategies; peripheral pain progressively retreats in a proximal direction, sometimes associated with simultaneous development or increase in proximal pain; centralization is described by McKenzie[1] to occur in the derangement syndrome.

DIRECTIONAL PREFERENCE/MECHANICAL DIAGNOSIS AND THERAPY: Preference for postures or movement in one direction (characteristic of the derangement syndrome). Postures or movements in one direction decrease, abolish, or centralize symptoms, whereas postures or movements in the opposite direction often worsen symptoms.[1]

LOADING STRATEGIES: Dynamic or static loads that are applied to preferentially stress particular structures; dynamic loads are repeated movements and static loads are sustained postures; significant loading strategies, postures, or repeated movements are those that alter symptoms.[1]

MOVEMENT SYSTEM: Represents a collection of systems (cardiovascular, pulmonary, endocrine, integumentary, nervous, and musculoskeletal) that interact to move the body and its component parts[2]

Objectives

1. Relate the anatomy of the lumbar disc and its mechanical response to specific directional movements of the spine.
2. Describe the McKenzie or Mechanical Diagnosis and Therapy (MDT) classification system.
3. Describe the MDT evaluation process and how objective findings define each syndrome into a classification system that determines a specific treatment approach.
4. Prescribe appropriate interventions for each phase of the condition—from acute injury to full restoration of function.
5. Describe the evidence for the efficacy of using the MDT approach in the treatment of lumbar spine disorders.
6. Describe how MDT interventions impact the movement system.

Physical Therapy Considerations

Physical therapy considerations during management of the individual with a diagnosis of a herniated lumbar disc:

▶ **General physical therapy plan of care/goals:** Decrease pain; centralize radicular pain; restore full trunk range of motion with no subsequent pain; return to full work duties

▶ **Physical therapy interventions:** Repeated movements with directional preference to centralize and eliminate pain in leg and lumbar spine; patient education for repeated movement exercises, posture, and body mechanics for activities of daily living and work tasks

▶ **Precautions during physical therapy:** Positioning and use of arms to provide repeated movements to lumbar spine: if upper extremities are unable to handle body weight during exercises, alternative positions may need to be used.

▶ **Complications interfering with physical therapy:** Irreducible derangement when peripheralization of symptoms (increase or worsening of distal symptoms) occurs in response to repeated movements or loading strategies.

Physical Therapy Patient/Client Management

The McKenzie system (also known as Mechanical Diagnosis and Therapy or MDT) is a classification system used for musculoskeletal injuries of the spine and extremities. **The McKenzie system consists of three distinct syndromes: derangement, dysfunction, and postural.** A patient's subjective history and response to active movements during the examination contribute to the classification of a syndrome and thus identify the specific treatment approach that should be taken. The physical examination consists of a series of loading stresses to the tissues of the spine or peripheral joints. Each syndrome presents with a unique set of responses to the loading tests. Correct identification of the syndrome helps the physical therapist define the proper mechanical treatment. A unique aspect of the MDT-based examination is that the patient performs several different movement patterns with the therapist noting the response to each direction of movement to help determine the syndrome classification.[1]

The derangement syndrome is most frequently observed.[1] As defined by Robin McKenzie, "internal derangement causes a disturbance in the normal resting position of the affected surfaces. Internal displacement of articular tissue of whatever origin will cause pain to remain constant until such time as the displacement is reduced. Internal displacement of articular tissue obstructs movements."[1] An example of a derangement syndrome is a knee meniscal tear that may cause a mechanical block that limits full knee function. The direction of mechanical forces across the knee changes the pain. An internal intervertebral disc displacement is also frequently classified as a derangement syndrome.

A "disc herniation" is a nonspecific term to indicate displaced disc material and/or a fissure or disruption in the annulus fibrosus of the disc. The intervertebral disc can be a source of mechanically generated pain via two avenues.[3] The presence of radial fissures within the annular wall disrupts the normal load-bearing properties of the annulus, which can cause disproportionate weightbearing distribution and stress on the outer innervated lamellae. Second, internal displacement of the disc material can also be a potential source of pain. The intervertebral disc is mobile and the position of disc material is influenced by postures—especially by *prolonged* spinal flexion or extension. Such conditions cause disc material displacement according to direction.[3-10] In the current patient, uneven loading of the intervertebral disc with a heavy loaded flexion position of the trunk may stimulate neurogenic pain.[6]

The McKenzie approach uses repeated movements in the sagittal plane to evaluate and treat the patient based on current symptom presentation. A derangement syndrome can be further labeled as reducible or irreducible based on the assumed integrity of the hydrostatic mechanism within the disc wall. If a herniation occurs in a disc in which the outer wall is intact, it is considered reducible and repeated movements may alleviate the mechanical stresses on the disc. If the herniation occurs in a disc in which the outer wall is *not* intact, the derangement is considered irreducible and repeated movements will not improve the pain or symptoms.[1]

The clinical presentation associated with a derangement syndrome includes the centralization of distal symptoms (*e.g.*, pain in the leg) and decreased pain during the application of therapeutic loading strategies. It is assumed that the pain associated with a derangement will change with induced directional movements as a result of the change within the intervertebral disc (due to varying positions of the spine). The pain may be present during the movement and at the end-range of movement. Lumbar flexion range of motion is frequently limited with a derangement, and this syndrome responds to extension-loading strategies. As the derangement is reduced with repeated extension motions, the patient's range of motion into flexion should improve and return to normal. McKenzie subclassifies the derangement syndrome into central symmetrical, unilateral asymmetrical symptoms *to* the knee, and unilateral asymmetrical symptoms *below* the knee. The reader is directed to Robin McKenzie's book titled *The Lumbar Spine Mechanical Diagnosis and Therapy* for further discussion of these subclassifications.[1]

The direction of disc herniation is also important because this directs the treatment approach. More than 50% of derangements appear to start centrally in the disc and approximately 25% start posterolaterally.[1] As the derangement extends into the dura and nerve root, over 50% of disc herniations displace posterolaterally and the other 25% displace posterocentrally. Since most derangements occur in the sagittal plane, lumbar flexion and extension are part of the mechanism of injury and also the avenue for repeated movement treatment. Less than 10% of disc derangements herniate directly laterally, which would require torsional or lateral forces to be a component of the treatment. The majority of derangements occur at the L4-L5 and L5-S1 levels.[1]

The term "centralization" is associated with the derangement syndrome and is referred to extensively in the literature when discussing disc herniations.[11-16] Centralization is the response to therapeutic loading strategies. With centralization, pain is progressively abolished in a distal to proximal direction with the symptoms diminishing in intensity with each progressive movement. For example, in the individual with pain distal to the low back (*i.e.*, radicular pain), successful treatment causes the pain to move from widespread distal locations to a more central location and then, ultimately the pain may be abolished.[1]

The dysfunction syndrome is characterized by pain caused by mechanical deformation of structurally impaired tissue and a limited range of motion in the affected direction. An example is adhesive capsulitis of the glenohumeral joint, which is a soft tissue restriction that limits range of motion. The patient reports pain primarily at the end-range of available motion. When the mechanical load is released, the pain disappears. Dysfunction syndrome is uncommon in the lumbar spine. Physical therapists using the MDT approach report its prevalence in less than 20% of individuals with lumbar pain.[1] The dysfunction syndrome may be in the flexion, extension, or side gliding direction and is named for the direction that is limited. For example, if flexion is limited, then the syndrome would be labeled a flexion dysfunction syndrome. The treatment for a dysfunction is to repeatedly stretch *into* the direction of limitation.

The postural syndrome is characterized by pain occurring only when normal tissue is deformed over a prolonged period of time (e.g., sitting in a slouched position for a long period of time). The postural syndrome is treated with postural correction exercises and patient education. Although this syndrome is rarely observed clinically, habitual abnormal postural loading may lead to a derangement or dysfunction syndrome.[1] Table 14-1 outlines the characteristics of the three syndromes defined by Robin McKenzie.

Through repeated movements, MDT facilitates specific loading patterns onto the musculoskeletal system that may optimize movement. Since the movement system represents a network of interdependent systems—musculoskeletal, cardiovascular, endocrine, pulmonary, nervous, and integumentary[2]—improvement in this system can have positive outcomes on the other systems and improve overall movement.

Examination, Evaluation, and Diagnosis

A key component of the McKenzie approach is the use of a structured history or subjective questioning format and follow-up with a consistent sequence of movement testing. It is imperative to test all planes of movement and repeat the movements sufficiently to get a consistent symptom response from the patient in reaction to each movement. The purpose of the examination is to evaluate the response of the patient's *chief* complaint (e.g., pain) to the movement patterns. Although the patient may describe a stretching sensation or other secondary response during directional movement testing, the physical therapist must differentiate between these secondary responses and those that are consistent with the patient's chief complaint.

The McKenzie evaluation process follows a specific examination and evaluative pathway. The key is to follow the same procedures for each patient to ensure consistency and thoroughness in all areas of the evaluation. Based on the patient's mechanism of injury and the characteristics of his pain, the physical therapist should be hypothesizing that he has a lumbar derangement. However, a complete repeated movement testing examination is required to confirm this hypothesis. The goal of the objective examination is to determine which positions and movements facilitate improvement in pain and function. The repeated movement testing applies mechanical stress to spinal tissues in different directions to reveal the mechanical or nonmechanical nature of the injury. The patient's responses to this testing allows the physical therapist to determine the particular syndrome and directional preference for treatment. During movement testing, the physical therapist needs to know the patient's baseline pain and if pain occurs during the movement and/or at the

Table 14-1 CHARACTERISTICS OF MECHANICAL DIAGNOSIS THERAPY SYNDROMES[1]

Characteristics of Patient and Clinical Presentation	Derangement	Dysfunction	Postural
Age (years)	Usually 20-55	Usually over 30, except following trauma or derangement	Usually under 30
Pain			
Constancy	Constant or intermittent	Intermittent	Intermittent
Location	Local and/or referred	Local (referred only with adherent nerve root)	Local
History			
Onset	Gradual or sudden	Gradual	Gradual
Reason	Often related to prolonged positions or repetitive movements	History of trauma	Sedentary lifestyle
Symptoms worse			
Type of load	Static/dynamic load at mid- or end-range	Static/dynamic loading at end-range	Static loading at end-range
Diurnal cycle	Worse in morning and evening	No diurnal cycle	Worse at end of day
Symptoms better	Opposite position of what causes pain	Positions that do not put shortened tissue at end-range	Change of position and when active

Examination findings associated with each syndrome	Acute deformity may be present Pain during movement Pain changes location and/or intensity Pain centralizes or peripheralizes Patient remains better or worse as a result of repeated loading or movements Rapid changes in pain and range of motion	Pain reported at end-range of motion only Pain stops shortly after removal of stretch Pain does not change location or intensity Patient remains no better and no worse as a result of repeated loading or movements	Movement does not produce pain Range of motion is normal Sustained end-range positions eventually produce local pain
Treatment	Correct the deformity Repeated movements in the direction that centralizes the pain Correct posture Patient education regarding prevention and self-management of symptoms	Repeated movements or stretches in the direction which produces end-range pain or limited motion Correct posture Patient education regarding prevention and self-management of symptoms	Correct posture Education on prevention

end-range of the movement. On returning to the starting position of the movement, the therapist needs to know how the movement affected the baseline pain and/or range of motion. Potential responses include: (1) increase, decrease, or no effect on baseline pain during directional movement; (2) centralization, peripheralization, or no effect on baseline pain during or after loading; (3) pain abolished as a result of the loading; (4) better, worse, or no effect on pain after loading; (5) presence or absence of pain at end-range during loading; (6) increase, decrease, or no effect on range of motion after loading (mechanical response); and (7) pain worse/not worse or better/not better after loading (pain response).[1] Table 14-2 summarizes the potential responses to repeated movement testing to determine whether the patient has a dysfunction or derangement syndrome.

The main differences between the dysfunction and derangement syndromes are whether pain is present only at the end-range of motion and whether there is a change in range of motion after loading the tissue by repeated movements. Dysfunction syndromes generally present with no pain unless the tissue is loaded at end-range and when the tissue is unloaded, the pain resolves quickly. In contrast, the **derangement syndrome presents with a directional preference and loading into this direction decreases and centralizes the pain.** The key is to determine *which* repeated movement in the sagittal plane (flexion or extension) centralizes the distal pain. With a derangement, repeated movements produce a mechanical response and increase the range of motion. If the patient presents with a lateral trunk shift, the physical therapist should test lateral side gliding range of motion in both directions to determine if a lateral component is involved in the mechanical blocking of lumbar range of motion. If a lateral component is suspected and confirmed, that component must be treated *prior* to performing repeated sagittal movements. Testing for a lateral component is performed in the standing position with the patient's feet shoulder-width apart. To perform a right-side gliding motion, the patient moves his hips to the left while his trunk remains in neutral. The physical therapist may assist with this motion by placing one hand on the left shoulder and the opposite hand on the right iliac crest and applying force toward the midline. The shoulders should remain parallel to the ground. Because this movement pattern is a difficult concept for many patients to understand, demonstration by the physical therapist and tactile guides for the movement are often needed for proper execution. The movement is a side glide and not a side bending movement. The physical therapist asks the patient to perform one repetition of the side gliding movement and notes the response to the movement. As the patient performs repeated movements, symptom response and range of motion limitations are noted. If restrictions and symptoms are noted, the treatment sequence should start with determining the directional preference and follow with repeated movements to centralize the distal symptoms.[1]

Based on the repeated movement testing performed on the patient in this case study, the physical therapist identified that he presented with a derangement syndrome with an extension direction preference. The MDT approach to examination requires that the physical therapist not be hesitant to ask the patient to perform repeated movements even if he experiences pain during movement and at the end-range of motion. It is important to get the patient to the available end-range on each repeated movement and monitor symptom behavior such as centralization.

Table 14-2 SPINAL PHYSICAL EXAMINATION USING REPEATED MOVEMENT TESTING

	Dysfunction				Derangement			
Physical Test	Pain During	Centralization or Peripheralization	End-Range Pain	ROM Response	Pain During	Centralization or Peripheralization	End-Range Pain	ROM Response
Flexion in standing	No	No effect	Yes—with every repetition	No effect	Increase	Peripheralization	Yes	No effect
Extension in standing	No	No effect	No	No effect	Decrease	Centralization	Yes	Increased extension/ increased flexion
Flexion in supine	No	No effect	Yes—with every repetition	No effect	Increase	Peripheralization	Yes	No effect
Extension in prone	No	No effect	No	No effect	Decrease	Centralization	Yes	Increased extension/ increased flexion

Plan of Care and Interventions

According to McKenzie, passive or "chemical" treatments (*e.g.*, electrical stimulation, ultrasound, ice) will not decrease pain that is caused by a mechanical deformation.[1] In addition, no mechanical treatment such as mobilization or repeated movements will totally resolve pain arising from a majority of chemical stresses (*e.g.*, inflammation). These principles are the basis for the McKenzie approach to treating any type of musculoskeletal pain with repeated movements.[3]

The degree of chemical and mechanical pain present with each injury must be determined during the examination and subsequent evaluation.[1] Characteristics of chemical pain include: constancy, appearance shortly after injury, presence of cardinal signs of inflammation, lasting pain aggravation by all repeated movements, and pain that is not responsive to any movement (*i.e.*, movement does not reduce, abolish, or centralize pain). In contrast, mechanical pain is characterized by: intermittency; persistent reduction, abolition or centralization of pain induced by repeated movements; and, a directional preference in which one direction of movement decreases the pain while the opposite direction increases the pain. This patient presented with both chemical and mechanical pain and over the past 3 days, the pain had begun to subside. This is indicated by his improved tolerance to walking and standing for short periods of time.

The McKenzie treatment approach is tailored to each of the three stages of healing.[1] The first stage of inflammation lasts a maximum of 1 week, if treated promptly and correctly. The most important treatment principle during this phase is to minimize inflammation by chemical means and eliminate mechanical stresses with proper body positioning and/or movements within pain-free range of motion. For the current patient with a disc injury at L4-5, chemical treatment includes ice. Proper positioning or movements includes lying prone with progression to prone on elbows static lying for 5-minute intervals, or as tolerated. Aggressive repeated movements applied during the inflammation stage may delay healing.[1] At 2 to 4 weeks postinjury, the patient enters the repair stage. In this phase, repeated stress should be applied to spinal tissues and more specifically to the disc to facilitate tissue repair along functional stress lines and to increase the tensile strength of healing tissues. The patient should move into the edge of stiffness, but the movements should not cause lasting pain after completion. For this patient, the treatment included progression from prone lying to prone press-ups (Fig. 14-1) with the goal of regaining full available trunk extension. During this stage, the patient should be in control of the force production at the end-range of movement (Fig. 14-2). The area should not be over-stressed, which can cause a new onset of inflammation and delay recovery. The final stage of healing is remodeling, which starts approximately 5 weeks after injury. At this stage, regular stresses sufficient to provide tension without damage must be applied so that collagen elongates and strengthens. More force may be necessary to create such stresses—these may include physical therapist-provided overpressure (Fig. 14-3), mobilization (Fig. 14-4), or manipulation, if centralization and symptoms are not totally resolved. Return to full range of motion in all directions is the goal. By optimizing movement of neuromusculoskeletal structures through repeated movements, the patient may be better able to move the entire body. Table 14-3 outlines sample interventions for this patient during each stage of healing.

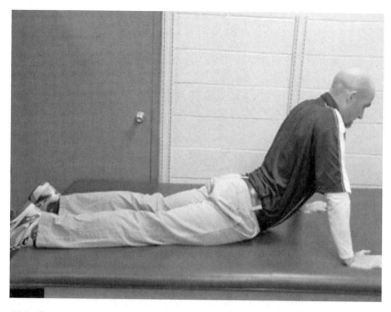

Figure 14-1. Dynamic patient-generated forces: lumbar extension at end-range.

To determine which syndrome the patient presents with, dynamic movements are used more often than static postures. Once the syndrome has been identified, then dynamic or repeated movements are used to treat the syndrome. The general guideline for the number of movements is 10 to 15 repetitions per set. The number

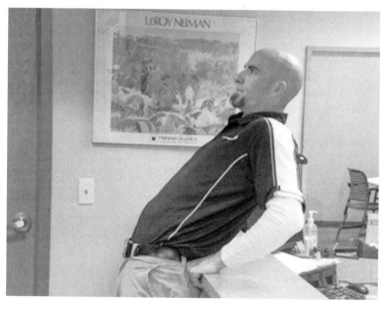

Figure 14-2. Dynamic patient-generated forces: lumbar extension at end-range with use of counter-top for overpressure.

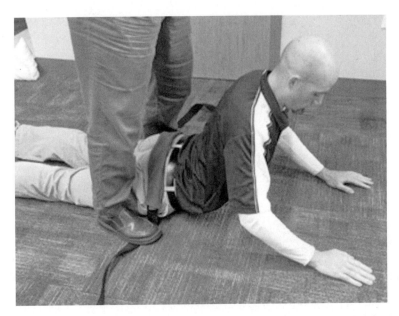

Figure 14-3. Dynamic patient-generated forces: lumbar extension at end-range with belt fixation for overpressure.

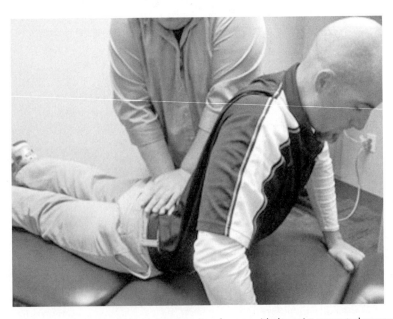

Figure 14-4. Dynamic motion: lumbar extension at end-range with therapist-generated overpressure mobilization.

Table 14-3 INTERVENTIONS ACCORDING TO STAGES OF HEALING		
Injury and Inflammation (Week 1)	Repair and Healing (Weeks 2-4)	Remodeling (Week 5 and beyond)
Relative rest Prone lying Prone on elbows: static positioning in mid-range with progression to end-range position	Unweighted position in prone and progress to weightbearing in standing Prone press-ups Patient moves in mid-range Patient moves to end-range (Fig. 14-1) Patient moves to end-range with patient-applied overpressure (Fig. 14-2)	Prone position: patient moves to end-range with physical therapist-provided overpressure using a belt for fixation (Fig. 14-3) Physical therapist-provided mobilization (Fig. 14-4) or manipulation

of sets used for treatment depends on symptom acuity and usually varies from 2 to 4 sets per exercise session. A minimum of 4 to 5 exercise sessions per day is necessary to produce a clinical change in symptoms. The repeated movements should include a brief relaxation time between each repetition and the patient should try to make the movements as passive as possible. In this case, the therapist advised the patient to relax his buttock and lumbar muscles, using only his upper extremities to allow full trunk extension in the prone position.[1] The main guide to the number of repetitions and frequency of exercise is how the patient tolerates the physical loading and the symptom response.

The **efficacy of the MDT approach** has been tested as a clinical approach to treating low back pain (LBP). Petersen *et al.*[11] conducted a randomized controlled trial comparing manipulation and patient education to a McKenzie-based treatment program and patient education. The sample included 350 adults with LBP of more than 6 weeks duration and centralization or peripheralization of symptoms. The manipulation group received thrust and non-thrust manipulations along with trigger point massage, whereas the MDT group was treated with repeated movements with directional preference. Compared to the manipulation group, the MDT group showed significant improvement in level of disability (measured by the 23-item modified Roland Morris Disability Questionnaire) at 2- and 12-month follow-up.[11]

The efficacy of key assessment and treatment components of the McKenzie approach—centralization and directional preference—has been tested in several trials. In a prospective cohort of 584 adults with nonspecific LBP that centralized, did not centralize, or could not be classified, Werneke *et al.*[12] found that the overall prevalence of directional preference and centralization was 60% and 41%, respectively. These classifications were investigated to determine if classifications predicted functional status and pain intensity at discharge from care. Subjects with directional preference *and* centralization on initial evaluation reported significantly better functional status and less pain at the end of care than subjects classified as having directional preference without centralization and subjects that were classified as having no directional preference and no centralization.

Long *et al.*[13] evaluated directional preference of adults with varying acuity of LBP. Of the 312 subjects, 74% had a directional preference: 83% responded to extension, 7% responded to flexion, and 10% were identified as lateral responders.

Subjects identified as having a directional preference were then randomized into subgroups: directional exercises matching each patient's directional preference, directional exercises opposite the patient's directional preference, or nondirectional exercises. After 2 weeks (3-6 visits), the directional exercise group that performed exercise matched to their directional preference experienced significant reduction in pain, pain medication use, and disability measures compared to the other treatment groups. One-third of the nonmatching exercise group dropped out from the study because their symptoms were either not improving or were worsening. In a follow-up study, Long et al.[14] investigated factors that predicted favorable outcomes when patients were grouped according to presence or absence of directional preference. The results revealed that patients who performed exercises in the same direction as was determined to be appropriate in their initial evaluation had a 7.8 times greater likelihood of a good outcome (defined as a minimal reduction of 30% on the Roland-Morris Disability Questionnaire) at 2 weeks than subjects whose rehabilitation program was not matched to their directional preference. In a 2004 systematic review of 6 randomized/quasi-randomized controlled studies, Clare et al.[15] concluded that the reviewed studies suggested that the MDT approach was more effective than comparison treatments consisting of medications, educational booklet, and strengthening at short-term follow-up (less than 3 months).

In 2018, Garcia et al.[17] investigated the effect of MDT in 148 adults with chronic LBP. Subjects were randomly placed in the MDT or the comparison group (5 minutes of detuned pulsed ultrasound and 25 minutes of detuned short-wave diathermy). Each group received 10 treatment sessions over 5 weeks. Clinical outcomes were assessed at the end of 5 weeks, and at 3, 6, and 12 months after randomization. At 12 months, the MDT group had greater mean improvements in pain intensity than the comparison group, though the difference was likely not clinically significant because the confidence intervals crossed zero. No significant between-group differences were found for other outcome measures (e.g., disability), or at other timepoints.

In 2019, Namnaqani et al.[18] published a systematic review and meta-analysis of 5 studies examining the effectiveness of the McKenzie method compared to manual therapy for chronic LBP (pain duration 7 days to >6 weeks). The authors concluded that the McKenzie method was better than manual therapy at short-term pain reduction and long-term improvement in patient function. Although most of the studies were of good quality (PEDro score 8 out of 11), the majority did not have therapist blinding.

In a meta-analysis of 11 articles, Lam et al.[19] examined the effectiveness of MDT for improving pain and disability in adults with either *acute* or *chronic* LBP. These authors concluded that although there is moderate to high-quality evidence that MDT is not superior to other rehabilitation approaches for reducing pain and disability in *acute* LBP, there is moderate to high-quality evidence that MDT is superior to other rehabilitation approaches for reducing pain and disability in individuals with *chronic* LBP.

In contrast, a 2021 systematic review and meta-analysis of 11 studies investigating the effectiveness of the MDT method in adults with nonspecific *chronic* LBP concluded that there was low to moderate evidence that MDT was no more effective than other active or passive physical therapy treatments in improving disability or reducing pain.[20] Notably however, some studies did not classify participants according to the MDT system and treating clinicians were not MDT-trained.

Evidence-Based Clinical Recommendations

SORT: Strength of Recommendation Taxonomy

A: Consistent, good-quality patient-oriented evidence
B: Inconsistent or limited-quality patient-oriented evidence
C: Consensus, disease-oriented evidence, usual practice, expert opinion, or case series

1. The McKenzie classification system of three distinct syndromes (derangement, dysfunction, postural) for musculoskeletal injuries of the spine and extremities outlines a systematic approach to direct patient examination and potential treatment strategies. **Grade B**

2. When the McKenzie approach determines directional preference at initial evaluation and matches repeated movement exercises with the same directional preference, pain intensity and disability are reduced for those with chronic LBP. **Grade A**

3. The McKenzie treatment approach is effective at decreasing pain and improving function in adults with chronic LBP compared to manipulation, manual therapy, strengthening exercises, medication, and educational booklets. **Grade B**

COMPREHENSION QUESTIONS

14.1 The derangement syndrome consists of all of the following characteristics, EXCEPT:

   A. Reproduction of pain only at the end-range of motion

   B. Reproduction of pain at the mid-range and at the end-range of motion

   C. A directional preference is demonstrated in response to repeated movements

   D. Centralization of distal symptoms occurs in response to repeated movements

14.2 Key factors of mechanical pain consist of all of the following characteristics, EXCEPT:

   A. Centralization of distal symptoms with repeated movements

   B. Directional preference to repeated movements

   C. Intermittent pain

   D. Constant pain

14.3 Which of the following statements is NOT true regarding the MDT evaluation?

A. The evaluation process follows a very specific pathway.

B. The evaluation tests only the response to movement and baseline pain is not important.

C. It is imperative to test all planes of movement.

D. Potential responses to repeated movements include increase, decrease, or no effect on baseline pain during or after loading.

ANSWERS

14.1 **A.** The dysfunction syndrome is the only syndrome that has pain only at the end-range of motion.

14.2 **D.** Constant pain is not a feature of mechanical pain. Mechanical pain will be diminished or abolished when mechanical load is removed from the painful structure.

14.3 **B.** Baseline pain is the key to determining if repeated movements are making an impact on the patient's pain, by using specific evaluative pathways and consistent potential responses.

REFERENCES

1. McKenzie R, May S. *The Lumbar Spine: Mechanical Diagnosis and Therapy.* Waikanae, New Zealand: Spinal Publications; 2003.

2. American Physical Therapy Association. White Paper - Physical Therapist Practice and the Movement System. Alexandria VA: American Physical Therapy Association; 2015.

3. Bogduk N. *Clinical Anatomy of the Lumbar Spine and Sacrum.* 3rd ed. New York, NY: Churchill Livingstone; 1997.

4. Bogduk N. The anatomy and physiology of nociception. In: Crosbie J, McConnell J, eds. *Key Issues in Musculoskeletal Physiotherapy.* Oxford: Butterworth-Heineman; 1993.

5. Bogduk N. Innervation, pain patterns, and mechanism of pain production. In: Twomey LT, Taylor JR, eds. *Physical Therapy of the Low Back.* New York, NY: Churchill Livingstone; 1994.

6. Schnebel BE, Simmons JW, Chowning J, Davidson R. A digitizing technique for the study of movement of intradiscal dye in response to flexion and extension of the lumbar spine. *Spine.* 1988;13:309-312.

7. Beattie PF, Brooks WM, Rothstein JM, et al. Effect of lordosis on the position of the nucleus pulposus in supine subjects. A study using magnetic resonance imaging. *Spine.*1994;19:2096-2102.

8. Fennell AJ, Jones AP, Hukins DW. Migration of the nucleus pulposus within the intervertebral disc during flexion and extension of the spine. *Spine.* 1996;21:2753-2757.

9. Brault JS, Driscoll DM, Laako LL, et al. Quantification of lumbar intradiscal deformation during flexion and extension, by mathematical analysis of magnetic resonance imaging pixel intensity profiles. *Spine.* 1997;22:2066-2072.

10. Edmondston SJ, Song S, Bricknell RV, et al. MRI evaluation of lumbar spine flexion and extension in asymptomatic individuals. *Man Ther.* 2000;5:158-164.

11. Petersen T, Larsen K, Nordsteen J, et al. The McKenzie method compared with manipulation when used adjunctive to information and advice in LBP patients presenting with centralization or peripheralization: a randomized controlled trial. *Spine.* 2011;36:1999-2010.

12. Werneke MW, Hart DL, Cutrone G, et al. Association between directional preference and centralization in patients with low back pain. *J Orthop Sports Phys Ther.* 2011;41:22-31.

13. Long A, Donelson R, Fung T. Does it matter which exercise? A randomized control trial of exercise for low back pain. *Spine.* 2004;29:2593-2602.

14. Long A, May S, Fung T. The comparative prognostic value of directional preference and centralization: a useful tool for front-line clinicians? *J Man Manip Ther.* 2008;16:248-254.

15. Clare HA, Adams R, Maher CG. A systematic review of efficacy of McKenzie therapy for spinal pain. *Aust J Physiother.* 2004;50:209-216.

16. Browder DA, Childs JD, Cleland JA, Fritz JM. Effectiveness of an extension-oriented treatment approach in a subgroup of subjects with low back pain: a randomized clinical trial. *Phys Ther.* 2007;87:1608-1618.

17. Garcia AN, Costa LDCM, Hancock MJ, et al. McKenzie method of Mechanical Diagnosis and Therapy was slightly more effective than placebo for pain, but not for disability, in patients with chronic nonspecific low back pain: a randomised placebo-controlled trial with short- and longer-term follow-up. *Br J Sports Med.* 2018;52(9):594-600.

18. Namnaqani FI, Mashabi AS, Yaseen KM, Alshehri MA. The effectiveness of McKenzie method compared to manual therapy for treating chronic low back pain: a systematic review. *J Musculoskelet Neuronal Interact.* 2019;19(4):492-499.

19. Lam OT, Strenger DM, Chan-Fee M, et al. Effectiveness of the McKenzie Method of Mechanical Diagnosis and Therapy for treating low back pain: literature review with meta-analysis. *J Orthop Sports Phys Ther.* 2018;48(6):476-490.

20. Sanchis-Sánchez E, Lluch-Girbés E, Guillart-Castells P, et al. Effectiveness of mechanical diagnosis and therapy in patients with non-specific chronic low back pain: a literature review with meta-analysis. *Braz J Phys Ther.* 2021;25(2):117-134.

Evaluation and Treatment of Low Back Pain in the Primary Care Setting

Daniel Jenkins
Jeff Houck
Li-Zandre Philbrook
Dan Kang

CASE 15

A 30-year-old homemaker presents to her primary care provider (PCP) in a rural family medicine clinic with low back pain (LBP). The PCP requested a "warm hand-off" consultation from an onsite physical therapist. After receiving a brief history from the PCP, the therapist initiates a physical therapy evaluation. The patient shared that the pain started 3 days ago approximately 30 minutes after she lifted an air conditioner. Since then, she has been lying in bed, taking 200 mg ibuprofen twice per day, and using a hot pack intermittently. The patient is concerned that her spine "may be severely damaged." She rates her pain as a consistent 8 out of 10 on the numerical pain rating scale, and is "experiencing tightness and muscle spasming." The patient scored 3/12 on the STarT MSK tool. On the Patient Reported Outcome Measurement Information System (PROMIS), she scored 23 and 37 for physical function and self-efficacy, respectively. On the Patient Acceptable Symptom State (PASS), she responded "no" to the question: "considering your current low back function, pain and activity level, do you feel your current state is satisfactory?" The patient denied prior history of LBP, cancer, fever, saddle paresthesia, difficulty urinating, or fecal incontinence. The PCP has asked the therapist to assess the etiology of the patient's LBP and determine if imaging studies are indicated. The physical therapist determines that the patient's presentation is consistent with a lumbar strain injury and that medical imaging is not warranted.

The patient's main concerns are to know "what is wrong with her back" and how long the pain will persist. She does not participate in any regular exercise.

▶ What examination signs may be associated with this diagnosis?
▶ What considerations are used to determine if diagnostic imaging studies are warranted for this patient?
▶ How can care be directed for both an ideal patient outcome and efficient utilization of therapy service?
▶ Based on the patient's presentation, would she benefit from a referral to traditional outpatient physical therapy, or does she need medical care outside the scope of physical therapy?

KEY DEFINITIONS

COGNITIVE-BEHAVIORAL THERAPY (CBT): Effective psychological intervention for pain;[1,2] the premise is that cognitive and behavioral factors, including a person's thoughts, beliefs, and actions, play a key role in the development and/or maintenance of chronic pain.

FEAR-AVOIDANCE: Model of chronic pain describing how individuals experiencing pain may continue to avoid certain activities or behaviors due to fear of potential tissue damage[3,4]

NONSPECIFIC LOW BACK PAIN: Acute or chronic low back pain with no relevant specific pathoanatomical cause[5]

PATIENT ACCEPTABLE SYMPTOM STATE (PASS): Highest threshold of symptoms beyond which patients consider themselves well; the most widely used anchoring question to identify the PASS cut-off point is: "Taking into account all the activities you have during your daily life, your level of pain, and also your functional impairment, do you consider that your current state is satisfactory?"[6]

PATIENT-REPORTED OUTCOMES MEASUREMENT INFORMATION SYSTEM (PROMIS™): Publicly available system of reliable and valid measures of patient-reported health status for physical, mental, and social well-being; contains item banks to measure health symptoms and health-related quality of life that are relevant to many chronic diseases. For this case, physical function and self-efficacy of symptom management scales were used.[7,8]

SELF-EFFICACY: Individual's belief in their capacity to execute behaviors necessary to achieve specific performance by exerting control over motivation, behavior, and social environment[9,10]

STarT MSK TOOL: 10-item tool with good predictive and discriminative ability for prognostic stratification of individuals with the 5 most common musculoskeletal (MSK) pain presentations in primary care (back, neck, shoulder, knee, and multisite pain); score places patients into low, medium, and high risk for a poor outcome and predicts potential development of chronic pain over 6 months.[11-13] Goal of its use is to ensure that patients with common MSK conditions receive appropriate treatment at the earliest opportunity.

WARM HAND-OFF CONSULTATION: Collaboration between PCP and another on-site healthcare provider; once the PCP deems the need for skilled physical therapy intervention or evaluation, he/she transfers care over to the physical therapist in front of the patient.[14]

Objectives

1. Describe a brief low back pain consultation by a physical therapist embedded in the primary care setting and the collaboration between physical therapist and primary care provider.

2. Identify red flags that indicate referral to other healthcare providers and/or necessitate additional testing or ordering of diagnostic imaging studies.

3. Select appropriate physical examination tests and measures to assess a patient presenting with acute low back pain in the primary care setting.

4. Describe appropriate self-reported outcome measures for individuals with acute low back pain and how they impact clinical decision-making.

Physical Therapy Considerations

Physical therapy considerations during the examination and treatment of an individual in a primary care setting with a diagnosis of acute LBP:

▶ **General physical therapy plan of care/goals:** Screen for medical pathology; rule out indications for further medical screening; triage patients and determine appropriate treatment pathway: one-time treatment followed by self-management; traditional outpatient physical therapy; recommendation to PCP for specialty referral (e.g., neurosurgery, orthopedics, physiatry); provide education regarding typical outcomes and management of LBP

▶ **Physical therapy interventions:** Patient education in self-care/home management; discussion of typical outcomes associated with acute LBP; prescription of flexibility exercises; prescription of resistance exercises to increase low back and lower extremity muscle strength; communication with PCP regarding recommended clinical pathway as indicated by exam findings and patient preference

▶ **Precautions during physical therapy:** Address precautions or contraindications for flexibility or resistance exercises; screen for referral for further management outside the scope of physical therapy

▶ **Complications interfering with physical therapy:** In the primary care setting, the physical therapist travels from room to room to consult with each patient. Due to the (potential) volume of patient visits, there are times when the therapist is unable to meet the patient as a result of time and space constraints. As appropriate, patients are referred to traditional outpatient physical therapy clinics.

Understanding the Health Condition

Eighty percent of adults in the United States frequently experience LBP, which is the leading cause of disability worldwide.[15,16] In 2016, healthcare spending for low back and neck pain led all other conditions—totaling $134.5 billion.[17] Up to 90% of LBP is considered nonspecific (i.e., cannot be attributed to a pathoanatomical source[5,18]). Fewer than 1% of patients presenting to primary care with LBP have a specific serious spinal condition such as a fracture, cancer, infection, cauda equina syndrome, or inflammatory disorder.[19,20] Because of the low incidence of serious spinal pathology in individuals with LBP, **imaging of the lumbar spine is not warranted for patients with acute or subacute LBP unless there is the presence of red flags.**[21-24]

The inability to provide a pathoanatomic etiology for most individuals with LBP in conjunction with our newer understanding of pain mechanisms[25] suggests that the most appropriate diagnosis for the patient in the current case is "nonspecific LBP." Nonspecific LBP may be treated with several different movement-based therapies that have similar beneficial effects on pain and function.[2] To lower costs and prevent overutilization of health services, no medical imaging was recommended in this case.[26,27]

PCPs can use a range of treatment options to manage individuals with acute LBP. The American Academy of Family Practice (AAFP), an organization founded to promote and maintain high-quality standards for family medicine physicians, recommends over-the-counter and/or prescription nonsteroidal anti-inflammatory drugs (NSAIDs), skeletal muscle relaxants, and acetaminophen as first-line medications for acute LBP.[28] Although the **AAFP recommends *against* opioid prescription for acute episodes of LBP**,[29] 30% of patients with chronic LBP are prescribed opioids in family practice settings and a large number of patients with LBP receive care that is inconsistent with evidence-based clinical practice guidelines.[30] In the United States, prescriptions for opioids to treat LBP grew substantially from 2000 to 2010.[31,32] In 2011, 28.5% of patients with new-onset LBP filled prescriptions for opioids.[33] A national survey showed a 660% increase in expenditure for opioids prescribed for spine problems from 1997 to 2006 due to both increased utilization and medication cost.[34] From 1999 to 2010, the proportion of visits to ambulatory physician practices for back and neck pain that resulted in prescription of opioids also increased from 19% to 29%.[35] While PCPs have the option to refer patients with LBP for outpatient physical therapy, only 7% to 20% of patients actually receive physical therapy.[36]

Some PCPs overuse imaging studies for acute and chronic LBP, resulting in unnecessary radiation exposure and increased costs to patients and the American healthcare system.[37] Early use of imaging for individuals with acute LBP is *not* associated with improved clinical outcomes and analysis indicates that patients who receive early imaging have substantially higher average medical costs in their first year after diagnosis.[38] More conservative use of imaging is associated with lower costs for managing acute nonspecific LBP.[39]

Physical Therapy Patient/Client Management

In a primary care setting, physical therapists are expected to contribute to the clinical decision-making process in ways not traditionally observed in outpatient physical therapy practice. Collaboration between PCPs and physical therapists in primary care can support care concordant with practice guidelines and such team approaches have been shown to improve health outcomes.[40] In the primary care setting, physical therapists also have an opportunity to offer conservative MSK treatment at the patient's initial medical appointment. This is advantageous because early treatment may help reduce symptoms, restore function, reduce the fear of movement (*i.e.*, fear avoidance) prevent *chronic* LBP (*e.g.*, see Case 13: Low Back Pain: Manipulation Intervention), and reduce total healthcare expenditures.[41,42] In addition to providing recommendations to both the patient and PCP for managing MSK conditions, the physical therapist screens the patient for "red flags" (Table 15-1).[20,43-45] If present, the therapists collaborates further with the PCP about the potential need for imaging and further medical management (*i.e.*, referral to medical specialist in neurology, orthopedics, or rheumatology). Finally, physical therapists can provide reassurance and education to the patient and recommend referral to outpatient physical therapy, if indicated. Due to their training and expertise in management of MSK pathologies, physical therapists are often effective at determining patient motivation to actively participate in a treatment plan, which plays a key role in determining if a patient will benefit from formal physical therapy. This information can help inform the PCP as to whether physical therapy, or another treatment option, is best practice for a specific patient's needs.[46]

Examination, Evaluation, and Diagnosis

In the primary care setting, consultations occur as the need arises (*i.e.*, when the PCP determines that a particular patient may benefit from a physical therapist consultation). Patient visits are brief, usually only 15 to 20 minutes. In most cases, the PCP provides the therapist the reason for the consultation and any concerns. For example, the PCP may prompt the physical therapist in this case with the following query: "Would this 30-year-old female with acute LBP and sciatica benefit from an MRI?"

The physical therapy visit is generally initiated with open-ended questions and the therapist should avoid interrupting to ensure the patient has an opportunity to tell their full story.[47] Careful listening skills directed at the patient's biggest concerns are crucial in ensuring a productive visit.[48] After the patient interview, the

Table 15-1 RED FLAGS THAT WARRANT REFERRAL TO MEDICAL PROVIDER[20,43-45]
History of cancer
Unexpected weight loss or gain
Saddle paresthesia
Bowel and bladder changes
Progressive nonmechanical pain
Failure to improve after one month
Older age (>50 y)
Prolonged glucocorticoid use
Severe trauma
Contusions or abrasions
Fever (>100°F)
Central spine tenderness
Widespread neurological symptoms (*e.g.*, motor weakness, sensation loss at lower extremities or groin)
History of cancer, with additional symptoms such as unexpected weight loss, failure to improve after 1 month of conservative therapy, duration of symptoms over 1 month and age over 50 years all increase the likelihood of the back pain being related to malignancy.

STaRT MSK Tool and PROMIS are administered by the physical therapist and completed by the patient in the examination room. The STaRT MSK Tool uses a scoring system to predict whether a patient is at low risk (0-3), medium risk (4-8), or high risk (>9) of persistent symptoms.[11,13] Patients deemed at low risk are appropriate for reassurance and self-management (*i.e.*, "wait and see" approach), whereas those deemed at medium risk are appropriate for medications and physical therapy.[13] Patients whose scores indicate that they are at high risk of persistent symptoms are appropriate for specialty referral (*e.g.*, orthopedist, behavioral health specialist, or spine specialist).[13]

The PROMIS physical function and self-efficacy subscales are especially useful in the primary care setting because they provide insight into the patient's *perception* of their physical ability as well as their ability to manage symptoms.[7,8] The PROMIS physical function subscale is referenced to the United States adult population where a score of 50 is average and 10 points in either direction is a single standard deviation. The PROMIS self-efficacy of symptom management subscale is referenced to American adults with *chronic* diseases where a score of 50 is the average of others suffering from chronic conditions and 10 is a single standard deviation.[10] A patient with low scores on the self-efficacy subscale, yet high scores on the physical function subscale suggests lack of confidence in managing symptoms more than poor functional ability.[8] Based on this information from the PROMIS, the physical therapist may choose a one-time intervention consisting of education/reassurance (*i.e.*, persuasion), prescription of performance of safe movements that challenge patients beliefs (*i.e.*, exposure), and/or active listening approaches in response to negative fears/beliefs (*i.e.*, self-regulation) with no follow-up required.[42]

The physical exam and treatment portion of the primary care visit vary depending on the information obtained from the interview and patient-reported outcomes. The essential goal of the physical exam is to determine how to move forward based on the patient's needs. The exam is typically concise, and may consist of myotome and dermatome testing, palpation, and a functional measure such as the 30-second-sit-to-stand test. The 30-second-sit-to-stand test is often selected as a brief assessment of lower extremity and lumbar spine strength and endurance, as well as pain during a functional movement.[49]

Table 15-1 lists **several red flags that must be ruled out when assessing a patient with LBP.** Of these, spinal fracture, malignancy, and infection are the most likely differential diagnoses in this setting.[43,50] Between 1% and 4% of patients presenting to primary care with acute LBP will have a spinal fracture.[50] A systematic review by Downie *et al.*[43] examined the diagnostic accuracy of using red flags to screen patients who present with LBP in primary, secondary, or tertiary care for the presence of malignancy or fracture. They found that patients who present with a *single* red flag for fracture have a 10% to 33% probability of fracture, while the presence of *multiple* red flags increases the probability of fracture to between 42% and 90%.[43] In addition, individuals seen in a primary care setting with a history of cancer and new LBP had a 7% of a *new* malignancy.[43] Therefore, although the probability is low, because of the serious consequences of fractures or malignancy, the presence of any red flag warrants consultation with the PCP and may require imaging.

This is especially important when several red flags are present. Although red flags have relatively low prevalence in primary care, their presence can indicate serious consequences so screening for them is imperative.[20]

Plan of Care and Interventions

Developing a plan of care in the primary care setting requires rapid synthesis of patient preferences, exam findings, and patient-reported outcome measures. The PROMIS outcome measures provide an informative way for clinical decision-making in primary care. Although interpretation of these person-centered outcomes continues to evolve, the negligible floor and ceiling effects and rapid administration (~3-4 minutes) make them ideal for primary care. Table 15-2 provides guidelines for clinical decision-making based on the two PROMIS outcomes, the STarT MSK tool, and the PASS score. A "no concerns" level of concern is associated with PROMIS outcomes that are above known thresholds for a PASS state[8] and STarT MSK Tool that indicates the patient is at low risk of persistent symptoms. A "few concerns" level of concern is when 1 or 2 of these outcomes are below the PASS threshold, whereas a "some concerns" level of concern is when all of the outcomes are below PASS. The distinction between "few concerns" and "some concerns" is that with few concerns, the physical therapist can *initiate* treatment (e.g., manual therapy, therapeutic exercise prescription) and institute "watchful waiting." Watchful waiting means that the therapist closely monitors the patient's condition while providing physical therapy treatments. If the patient's symptoms worsen, or do not respond to treatment as would be expected for the diagnosis, then the therapist refers the patient back to the primary provider. "Some concerns" indicates that there needs to be further investigation of the patient's clinical presentation and a referral to other providers. Within the category of "some concerns," the distinction between urgency or emergency depends on the *timing* of the specific pathology. For example, concerns for potential spinal fracture or spinal malignancy indicate an urgent referral, but that referral may not occur the same day. In contrast, concern for cauda equina syndrome is an example of an emergency referral that requires a same-day consultation.

Table 15-2 **CLINICAL DECISION-MAKING BASED ON LEVELS OF CONCERN**[8,10,11,13,20,43-45]		
No Concerns	**Few Concerns** *Contradictory findings (some are positive/some negative):*	**Some Concerns** **(Urgency or Emergency)** *Several of the following are positive:*
• Self-efficacy >45 • Physical function >40 • PASS "Yes" • STarT MSK Tool ≤3, indicating low risk of chronicity • Red flags negative	• Self-efficacy <45 • Physical function <40 • PASS "No" • STarT MSK Tool: 4-8, indicating medium risk of chronicity • Red flags negative	• Self-efficacy <45 • Physical function <40 • PASS "No" • STarT MSK Tool: 4-8, indicating medium risk of chronicity • Red flags could be positive

In the current case, the patient scored very low on the physical function and self-efficacy scales: 23 and 37, respectively. A PROMIS physical function score of 23 is 2.7 standard deviations below average, classified as a severe loss of physical function. This low level of perceived physical function is associated with much difficulty walking one block on flat ground and running errands and shopping. A PROMIS self-efficacy of symptom management score of 37 is 1.3 standard deviations below average of others with chronic conditions. This low score is associated with a response of "not confident" in managing symptoms during daily activities and in the ability to keep symptoms from interfering with personal care. Thus, although the patient's score on the physical function subscale indicated that she may benefit from formal physical therapy, her low self-efficacy symptom management score indicated that confidence was low, which likely impacts her perceptions of physical ability. The patient's score on the StarT MSK Tool classified her at low risk of developing a chronic condition and based on the data from Hill et al.,[11] self-management would be recommended. The patient also answered "no" to the PASS question; this question is used to obtain the patient's opinion regarding a desire for further treatment.[51,52]

The physical therapist integrated results from the STarT MSK, PROMIS, and PASS and had a discussion with the patient about whether she would consider formal physical therapy. The patient declined further physical therapy due to limited time. Therefore, the physical therapist reasoned that an improvement in self-efficacy might be achieved in the current visit to help the patient self-manage. The physical therapist spent the remainder of the visit (about 10 minutes) educating and reassuring the patient that the risk of serious damage to her spine was quite low, especially given the lack of red flags and history of LBP.[2] The therapist shared the results of the PROMIS and STarT MSK Tool and discussed their interpretation. The patient was relieved to know that for a majority of individuals with LBP, the pain resolves within 6 weeks[5] and that activity would not damage her spine.

The therapist provided the patient with a gentle flexibility program consisting of supine and seated lumbar range of motion exercises and recommendation to gradually return to her previous level of activity.[2,53] The therapist encouraged her to contact her PCP for further management if she did not experience any improvement over the next 6 weeks. The physical therapist waited in the hallway for the PCP to become available. The physical therapist discussed the findings and recommendations, including a recommendation *against* imaging. This recommendation was based on the fact that this was the patient's first episode of LBP with duration of less than 6 weeks, and the absence of red flags.[21-24,54] Since the patient did not have availability or time to commit to formal physical therapy, the physical therapist and PCP decided not to place a referral for PT.

Evidence-Based Clinical Recommendations

SORT: Strength of Recommendation Taxonomy

A: Consistent, good-quality patient-oriented evidence
B: Inconsistent or limited-quality patient-oriented evidence
C: Consensus, disease-oriented evidence, usual practice, expert opinion

1. Medical imaging should not be ordered for individuals with acute or subacute LBP, unless there is the presence of red flags. **Grade A**

2. Opioid prescription is not recommended as a first-line intervention for patients with acute LBP. **Grade A**

3. Red flags should be assessed for every patient presenting with acute LBP. **Grade A**

COMPREHENSION QUESTIONS

15.1 Which medical imaging test should be ordered for a patient with acute low back pain (<6 weeks) and no red flags?

 A. Magnetic resonance imaging (MRI) without contrast

 B. Anterior-posterior and lateral plain radiographs

 C. Computed tomography (CT) scan

 D. None of the above

15.2 Which of the following patient interview findings would indicate the presence of a red flag?

 A. Patient recently tripped over a concrete bench.

 B. Patient lost 25 lb in the last 6 weeks with no change in diet or activity level.

 C. Patient is 72 years old.

 D. All of the above.

15.3 Which of the following patients presenting to a primary care clinic with acute low back pain would be MOST likely to benefit from formal physical therapy?

 A. High self-efficacy score on PROMIS and high STarT MSK score

 B. High self-efficacy score on PROMIS and low STarT MSK score

 C. Low self-efficacy score on PROMIS and high STarT MSK score

 D. Low self-efficacy score on PROMIS and low STarT MSK score

ANSWERS

15.1 **D.** 90% of acute low back pain has no specific pathoanatomical cause and in the absence of red flags, no imaging is indicated.[21-24]

15.2 **D.** All of the above—recent trauma, unexplained weight loss, and older age are all red flags that require further imaging and medical work-up.[42]

15.3. **C.** Individuals that have high MSK tool scores indicate that they are at higher risk for developing chronic pain and may be more likely to benefit from formal physical therapy and other behavioral and/or mental health resources. Low self-efficacy indicates need for patient education and other interventions aimed at promoting self-management.[11,12]

REFERENCES

1. Williams ACC, Fisher E, Hearn L, Eccleston C. Psychological therapies for the management of chronic pain (excluding headache) in adults. *Cochrane Database Syst Rev*. 2020;8:CD007407.

2. O'Sullivan PB, Caneiro JP, O'Keeffe M, et al. Cognitive functional therapy: an integrated behavioral approach for the targeted management of disabling low back pain. *Phys Ther*. 2018;98:408-423.

3. Crombez G, Eccleston C, Van Damme S, et al. Fear-avoidance model of chronic pain: the next generation. *Clin J Pain*. 2012;28:475-483.

4. Trinderup JS, Fisker A, Juhl CB, Petersen T. Fear avoidance beliefs as a predictor for long-term sick leave, disability and pain in patients with chronic low back pain. *BMC Musculoskelet Disord*. 2018;19:431.

5. Maher C, Underwood M, Buchbinder R. Non-specific low back pain. *Lancet*. 2017;389:736-747.

6. Kvien TK, Heiberg T, Hagen KB. Minimal clinically important improvement/difference (MCII/MCID) and patient acceptable symptom state (PASS): what do these concepts mean? *Ann Rheum Dis*. 2007;66 Suppl 3:iii40-iii41.

7. Cella D, Riley W, Stone A, et al, PROMIS Cooperative Group. The Patient-Reported Outcomes Measurement Information System (PROMIS) developed and tested its first wave of adult self-reported health outcome item banks: 2005-2008. *J Clin Epidemiol*. 2010;63:1179-1194.

8. Houck J, Kang D, Cuddeford T. Do clinical criteria based on PROMIS outcomes identify acceptable symptoms and function for patients with musculoskeletal problems. *Musculoskelet Sci Pract*. 2021;55:102423.

9. Bandura A. Self-efficacy: toward a unifying theory of behavioral change. *Psychol Review*. 1977;84:191-215.

10. Gruber-Baldini AL, Velozo C, Romero S, Shulman LM. Validation of the PROMIS® measures of self-efficacy for managing chronic conditions. *Qual Life Res*. 2017;26:1915-1924.

11. Hill J, Garvin S, Chen Y, et al. Computer-based stratified primary care for musculoskeletal consultations compared with usual care: study protocol for the STarT MSK cluster randomized controlled trial. *JMIR Res Protoc*. 2020;9:e17939.

12. Hill JC, Garvin S, Chen Y, et al. Stratified primary care versus non-stratified care for musculoskeletal pain: findings from the STarT MSK feasibility and pilot cluster randomized controlled trial. *BMC Fam Pract*. 2020;21:30.

13. Dunn KM, Campbell P, Lewis M, et al. Refinement and validation of a tool for stratifying patients with musculoskeletal pain. *Eur J Pain*. 2021;25:2081-2093.

14. Sanderson D, Braganza S, Philips K, et al. Increasing warm handoffs: optimizing community based referrals in primary care using qi methodology. *J Prim Care Community Health*. 2021;12:215013211023883.

15. Jordan KP, Kadam UT, Hayward R, et al. Annual consultation prevalence of regional musculoskeletal problems in primary care: an observational study. *BMC Musculoskelet Disord*. 2010;11:144.

16. Atlas SJ, Deyo RA. Evaluating and managing acute low back pain in the primary care setting. *J Gen Intern Med*. 2001;16:120-131.

17. Dieleman JL, Cao J, Chapin A, et al. US health care spending by payer and health condition. 1996-2016. *JAMA*. 2020;323:863-884.

18. McCarthy CJ, Roberts C, Gittins M, Oldham JA. A process of subgroup identification in non-specific low back pain using a standard clinical examination and cluster analysis. *Physiother Res Int*. 2012;17:92-100.

19. Henschke N, Maher CG, Refshauge KM, et al. Prevalence of and screening for serious spinal pathology in patients presenting to primary care settings with acute low back pain. *Arthritis Rheum*. 2009;60:3072-3080.

20. Finucane LM, Downie A, Mercer C, et al. International Framework for Red Flags for Potential Serious Spinal Pathologies. *J Orthop Sports Phys Ther*. 2020;50:7:350-372.

21. Hall AM, Aubrey-Bassler K, Thorne B, Maher CG. Do not routinely offer imaging for uncompli- cated low back pain. *BMJ.* 2021;372:n291.

22. Chou R, Fu R, Carrino JA, Deyo RA. Imaging strategies for low-back pain: systematic review and meta-analysis. *Lancet.* 373:463-472.

23. Chou R, Deyo RA, Jarvik JG. Appropriate use of lumbar imaging for evaluation of low back pain. *Radiol Clin North Am.* 2012;50:569-585.

24. Chou R, Qaseem A, Snow V, et al. Clinical Efficacy Assessment Subcommittee of the American College of Physicians; American College of Physicians; American Pain Society Low Back Pain Guidelines Panel. Diagnosis and treatment of low back pain: a joint clinical practice guideline from the American College of Physicians and the American Pain Society. *Ann Intern Med.* 2007;147: 478-491.

25. Chimenti RL, Frey-Law LA, Sluka KA. A mechanism-based approach to physical therapist man- agement of pain. *Phys Ther.* 2018;98:302-314.

26. Casazza BA. Diagnosis and treatment of acute low back pain. *Am Fam Physician.* 2012;85:343-350.

27. Garber AM, Azad TD, Dixit A, et al. Medicare savings from conservative management of low back pain. *Am J Manag Care.* 2018;24:e332-e337.

28. Qaseem A, McLean RM, O'Gurek D, et al. Nonpharmacologic and pharmacologic management of acute pain from non-low back, musculoskeletal injuries in adults: a clinical guideline from the American College of Physicians and American Academy of Family Physicians. *Ann Intern Med.* 2020;173:739-748.

29. Deyo RA, Von Korff M, Duhrkoop D. Opioids for low back pain. *BMJ.* 2015;350:g6380.

30. Deyo RA, Mirza SK, Turner JA, Martin BI. Overtreating chronic back pain: time to back off? *J Am Board Fam Med.* 2009;22:62-68.

31. Hudson TJ, Edlund MJ, Steffick DE, et al. Epidemiology of regular prescribed opioid use: results from a national, population-based survey. *J Pain Symptom Manage.* 2008;36:280-288.

32. Boudreau D, Von Korff M, Rutter CM, et al. Trends in long-term opioid therapy for chronic non- cancer pain. *Pharmacoepidemiol Drug Saf.* 2009;18:1166-1175.

33. Raad M, Pakpoor J, Harris AB, et al. Opioid prescriptions for new low back pain: trends and vari- ability by state. *J Am Board Fam Med.* 2020;33:138-142.

34. Martin BI, Turner JA, Mirza SK, et al. Trends in health care expenditures, utilization, and health status among US adults with spine problems, 1997-2006. *Spine.* 2009;34:2077-2084.

35. Mafi JN, McCarthy EP, Davis RB, Landon BE. Worsening trends in the management and treatment of back pain. *JAMA Intern Med.* 2013;173:1573-1581.

36. Fritz JM, Childs JD, Wainner RS, Flynn TW. Primary care referral of patients with low back pain to physical therapy: impact on future health care utilization and costs. *Spine.* 2012;37:2114-2121.

37. Fritz JM, Brennan GP, Hunter SJ. Physical therapy or advanced imaging as first management strat- egy following a new consultation for low back pain in primary care: associations with future health care utilization and charges. *Health Serv Res.* 2015;50:1927-1940.

38. Graves JM, Fulton-Kehoe D, Jarvik JG, Franklin GM. Early imaging for acute low back pain: one- year health and disability outcomes among Washington State workers. *Spine.* 2012;37:1617-1627.

39. Andersen JC. Is immediate imaging important in managing low back pain? *J Athl Train.* 2011;46:99-102.

40. Wranik WD, Price S, Haydt SM, et al. Implications of interprofessional primary care team charac- teristics for health services and patient health outcomes: A systematic review with narrative synthe- sis. *Health Policy.* 2019;123:550-563.

41. Lentz TA, Goode AP, Thigpen CA, George SZ. Value-based care for musculoskeletal pain: are physical therapists ready to deliver? *Phys Ther.* 2020;100:621-632.

42. Traeger AC, Lee H, Hübscher M, et al. Effect of intensive patient education vs placebo patient edu- cation on outcomes in patients with acute low back pain: a randomized clinical trial. *JAMA Neurol.* 2019;76(2):161-169.

43. Downie A, Williams CM, Henschke N, et al. Red flags to screen for malignancy and fracture in patients with low back pain: systematic review. *BMJ.* 2013;347:f7095.

44. Shaw B, Kinsella R, Henschke N, et al. Back pain "red flags": which are most predictive of serious pathology in the Emergency Department? *Eur Spine J.* 2020;29:1870-1878.

45. Yusuf M, Finucane L, Selfe J. Red flags for the early detection of spinal infection in back pain patients. *BMC Musculoskelet Disord.* 2019;20(606).

46. Ross M, Adams K, Engle K, et al. The knowledge of low back pain management between physical therapists and family practice physicians. *J Man Manip Ther.* 2018;26:264-271.

47. Takemura Y, Sakurai Y, Yokoya S, et al. Open-ended questions: are they really beneficial for gathering medical information from patients? *Tohoku J Exp Med.* 2005;206:151-154.

48. Pinto RZ, Ferreira ML, Oliveira VC, et al. Patient-centered communication is associated with positive therapeutic alliance: a systematic review. *J Physiother.* 2012;58:77-87.

49. Jones CJ, Rikli RE, Beam WC. A 30-s chair-stand test as a measure of lower body strength in community-residing older adults. *Res Q Exerc Sport.* 1999;70:113-119.

50. Williams CM, Henschke N, Maher CG, et al. Red flags to screen for vertebral fracture in patients presenting with low-back pain. *Cochrane Database Syst Rev.* 2013;(1):CD008643.

51. Daste C, Abdoul H, Foissac F, et al. Patient acceptable symptom state for patient-reported outcomes in people with non-specific chronic low back pain. *Ann Phys Rehabil Med.* 2022;65:101451.

52. Tubach F, Dougados M, Falissard B, et al. Feeling good rather than feeling better matters more to patients. *Arthritis Rheum.* 2006;55:526-530.

53. Saraceni N, Kent P, Ng L, et al. To lex or not to flex? Is there a relationship between lumbar spine flexion during lifting and low back pain? A systematic review with meta-analysis. *J Orthop Sports Phys Ther.* 2020;50:121-130.

54. Johnson SM, Shah LM. Imaging of acute low back pain. *Radiol Clin North Am.* 2019;57:397-413.

Slipped Capital Femoral Epiphysis

Michael D. Ross
Kristi Greene Kelch

An 11-year-old female with a history of progressively worsening right knee pain for the past 5 months was referred to physical therapy. The patient has a body mass index of 24 kg/m^2 and her previous medical history is unremarkable. When she was evaluated by the physical therapist, the patient presented with an antalgic gait pattern with the right lower extremity in a slight externally rotated position. Her knee examination was unremarkable and testing did not reproduce her chief complaint of knee pain. However, the patient experienced anterolateral hip pain during examination of her right hip. Right hip flexion and internal rotation range of motion were limited both actively and passively and these motions reproduced her hip and knee pain. Based on the history and physical examination findings, the physical therapist was concerned about a possible slipped capital femoral epiphysis.

▶ What examination signs may be associated with the diagnosis of a slipped capital femoral epiphysis?
▶ What are the examination priorities?
▶ Based on the patient's suspected diagnosis, what do you anticipate may be the contributing factors to her condition?
▶ What are the most appropriate physical therapy interventions?
▶ What is her rehabilitation prognosis?

KEY DEFINITIONS

IN SITU SURGICAL FIXATION: Standard treatment for a slipped capital femoral epiphysis in which a screw is placed through the physis and epiphysis to prevent further progression of the slip

KLEIN LINE: Method to assess for a slipped capital femoral epiphysis on the anterior to posterior hip radiograph by drawing a line along the superior border of the femoral neck; in a normal hip, the Klein line intersects a portion of the femoral epiphysis; in the individual with a slipped capital femoral epiphysis, the Klein line is level with or lateral to the epiphysis

SLIPPED CAPITAL FEMORAL EPIPHYSIS: Posterior and inferior displacement of the proximal femoral epiphysis (femoral head) on the metaphysis (femoral neck) through the proximal femoral physis (growth plate)

STABLE SLIPPED CAPITAL FEMORAL EPIPHYSIS: Slip classification in terms of mechanical stability in which the individual is able to bear weight with or without crutches but may walk with an antalgic gait

UNSTABLE SLIPPED CAPITAL FEMORAL EPIPHYSIS: Slip classification in terms of mechanical stability in which the slip is too painful and unstable to allow the individual to bear weight even with crutches

Objectives

1. Describe slipped capital femoral epiphysis and identify risk factors associated with this condition.

2. Identify appropriate diagnostic imaging that should be completed to rule in or rule out slipped capital femoral epiphysis.

3. Describe the most appropriate physical therapy interventions for a patient with a slipped capital femoral epiphysis.

4. Determine the prognosis for an individual with a slipped capital femoral epiphysis.

Physical Therapy Considerations

Physical therapy considerations during management of the individual with a suspected diagnosis of slipped capital femoral epiphysis:

▶ **General physical therapy plan of care/goals:** Prevent slip progression; avoid complications such as osteonecrosis and chondrolysis

▶ **Physical therapy interventions:** Patient education regarding functional anatomy and injury pathomechanics; instruct patient in a nonweightbearing gait pattern on affected lower extremity; referral for radiographs; if radiographs confirm diagnosis of slipped capital femoral epiphysis, an urgent referral to an orthopedic surgeon should be placed so appropriate surgical options can be considered in a timely manner.

▶ **Precautions during physical therapy:** Avoid weightbearing on affected lower extremity

▶ **Complications interfering with physical therapy:** Slip progression, osteonecrosis, chondrolysis, development of a contralateral slipped capital femoral epiphysis

Understanding the Health Condition

Slipped capital femoral epiphysis (SCFE) occurs when there is posterior and inferior displacement of the proximal femoral epiphysis (femoral head) on the metaphysis (femoral neck).[1,2] The slip occurs through the proximal femoral physis (growth plate), usually as a result of chronic microfractures through the physis due to physiologic loading from rapid growth during adolescence.[3] SCFE may be either idiopathic or atypical (*i.e.*, associated with renal failure, radiation therapy, or endocrine disorders).[4]

In the United States, the incidence of SCFE for children between the ages 8 and 15 years is 10.80 cases per 100,000 children, with a predominance in boys (65%) versus girls.[5] Mean age at the time of diagnosis is 11.2 and 12.0 years for girls and boys, respectively.[5] Polynesian, African American, and Hispanic American children are more commonly affected than Caucasian children.[5]

Although the etiology is typically multifactorial, the ultimate result is increased shear stresses across a weakened physis.[6] Anatomic risk factors for SCFE include femoral neck retroversion, a reduced femoral neck-shaft angle, increased obliquity of the physis, and weakening of the perichondrial ring complex.[7] Biomechanical and biochemical factors are also important contributors to the development of an SCFE. Increased body mass increases the shear forces across the physis, potentially leading to weakening and eventual displacement of the femoral epiphysis on the metaphysis. The majority of affected individuals are ≥95th percentile for body mass index for their age (BMI-for-age).[8] The current patient has a BMI of 24, placing her BMI-for-age at the 95th percentile,[6] which may have been a contributing factor in the development of her SCFE. Individuals with an SCFE of one extremity are at increased risk of a contralateral SCFE as bilateral involvement may be seen in 20% to 80% of patients.[9] SCFE is occasionally associated with endocrine or metabolic disorders (*e.g.*, hypothyroidism, hyperthyroidism, growth hormone deficiency, hypogonadism, panhypopituitarism, renal disease).[2] Therefore, individuals who do not fit the typical profile for SCFE (*e.g.*, younger in age, low to normal BMI-for-age)[10] should be referred for evaluation for endocrine or metabolic disorders.[4,11]

SCFE is most commonly classified as either mechanically stable or unstable, with approximately 90% of cases classified as stable.[10,12] Individuals with a stable SCFE are able to bear weight with or without crutches, but may walk with an antalgic gait.[10] A patient with a stable SCFE is usually a male in early adolescence with a brief history of pain that is insidious in onset and poorly localized, and it can affect the hip, groin, thigh, or knee regions.[10] An individual with an unstable SCFE is not able to bear weight even with crutches because the slip is too painful and unstable.[10] Classification of SCFE in terms of mechanical stability is important since individuals with a stable SCFE have a better prognosis for achieving improved outcomes with fewer complications compared to those with an unstable SCFE.[5,10] All patients with suspected SCFE require urgent referral to an orthopedic surgeon. Because of the increased risk of osteonecrosis, patients with an unstable SCFE require an *emergent* referral to an orthopedic surgeon. Early diagnosis of an SCFE is associated with an improved prognosis.[13] Delays in diagnosis and continued weightbearing can lead to progression of the SCFE and further deformity, delayed surgical intervention, as well as complications such as osteonecrosis, chondrolysis, femoroacetabular impingement secondary to proximal femoral deformity, and early onset of osteoarthritis.[2,13,14]

Physical Therapy Patient/Client Management

If there is concern for an SCFE based on patient history and physical examination findings, the physical therapist should educate the patient on functional anatomy and injury pathomechanics. Since weightbearing should be avoided,[10] the physical therapist should train the patient in a nonweightbearing gait pattern on the affected lower extremity. The patient should also be referred for radiographs and if diagnosis of SCFE is confirmed, an urgent referral to an orthopedic surgeon should be placed to ensure appropriate surgical options can be considered in a timely manner.[14] The primary goal for most injured individuals is to return to pain-free activity as quickly and as safely as possible after surgery in a manner that does not overload the healing tissues.

Examination, Evaluation, and Diagnosis

The most common symptom for the young person with an SCFE is pain usually localized to the hip or groin regions, or less commonly, in the distal thigh and knee regions.[1,14,15] Patients with SCFE who present with knee pain experience significantly longer diagnostic delay than those with hip pain.[13] The most common differential diagnoses for hip pain in younger individuals include: apophyseal avulsion fractures of the hip and pelvis; hip apophysitis; groin strain; transient synovitis; stress fractures of the femoral neck or pelvis; Legg-Calve-Perthes disease, and septic arthritis.[16] Pain associated with an SCFE is worse with activity and patients usually report an inability to perform athletic activities. When a patient presents primarily with distal thigh and knee pain, the physical therapist may overlook SCFE as a cause and instead focus the examination and treatment on the primary area of symptoms.[15] This can delay identification of the etiology of the patient's symptoms and lead to further progression of the SCFE, and potentially an adverse outcome. Therefore, in young patients with a primary complaint of distal thigh and knee pain, the hip should always be thoroughly examined.

In most cases, the pain associated with an SCFE develops insidiously and progressively worsens over the course of several weeks without a clear mechanism of injury.[10,17] In this case, the patient may present with an antalgic gait (*i.e.,* stable SCFE) and the lower extremity may be held in a position of abduction and external rotation (Fig. 16-1).[18] In less than 10% of cases, pain associated with SCFE is severe and associated with a traumatic incident such as a fall.[2] In this case, the patient may not be able to bear weight on the involved lower extremity even with the use of crutches because of severe pain and instability (*i.e.,* unstable SCFE).

For hip range of motion (ROM) assessment, the physical therapist compares the findings of the involved hip with the uninvolved hip. **Limited and painful internal rotation and flexion at the hip are common findings with an SCFE.**[2] If the patient is able to flex the hip beyond 90°, it may move into obligatory external rotation as the prominent femoral neck contacts the acetabulum (due to posterior and inferior displacement of the proximal femoral epiphysis).[2] Examination of the knee is often normal, even if the chief complaint is pain referred to the distal thigh or knee.[15]

The **diagnosis of an SCFE should be considered in any patient between the ages of 8 and 15 years with a primary complaint of hip, groin, thigh, and knee pain who**

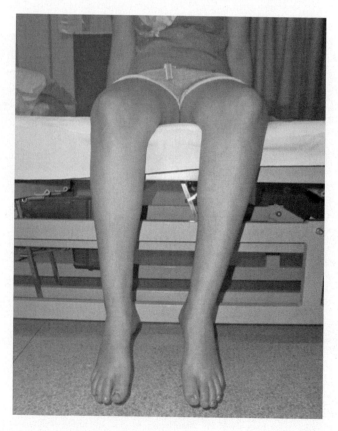

Figure 16-1. 11-year-old female with a left-sided slipped capital femoral epiphysis. Note the left hip is positioned in slight abduction and external rotation.

presents with an antalgic gait.[16] Bilateral anterior to posterior and lateral view radiographs (lateral frog-leg views for a stable SCFE; cross-table lateral views for an unstable SCFE to minimize patient discomfort and the risk of further slip progression) **allow for comparison between extremities and are crucial in establishing the diagnosis of an SCFE.**[1,14,18] When ordering radiographs, it is critical that the radiologist is informed that an SCFE is suspected so it can be properly confirmed or ruled out. Since there is an increased risk of bilateral SCFE at initial presentation,[6,9] it is important to note that symmetric appearance of the physes does not necessarily mean both are normal.

On the anterior to posterior radiographic view, the Klein line can be used to assess for an SCFE by drawing a line along the superior border of the femoral neck.[1] In a normal hip joint, the Klein line intersects a portion of the femoral epiphysis; with an SCFE, the Klein line is level with, or lateral to, the epiphysis. Anterior to posterior (Fig. 16-2) and lateral frog-leg view (Fig. 16-3) radiographs of the current patient[19] demonstrate the Klein line positioned slightly lateral to the femoral epiphysis and proximal femoral osteopenia and widening of the physis. The osteopenia correlates well with the patient's 5-month history of right knee pain and likely limited weightbearing on the right lower extremity. The widening

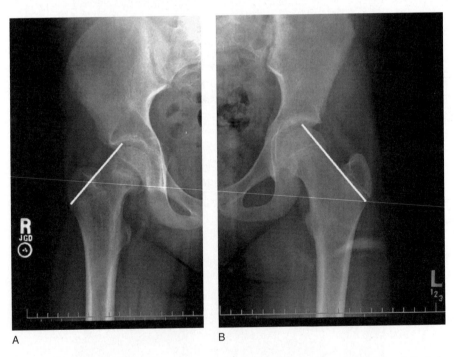

A   B

Figure 16-2. Anterior to posterior hip radiographs of an 11-year-old female with history and physical examination findings concerning for a slipped capital femoral epiphysis. **A.** The patient's involved right hip with Klein line positioned slightly lateral to the femoral epiphysis, consistent with a slipped capital femoral epiphysis. Proximal femoral osteopenia and widening of the physis are also seen. **B.** The patient's uninvolved left hip with Klein line intersecting the femoral epiphysis. (Reproduced with permission from Michael D. Ross.)

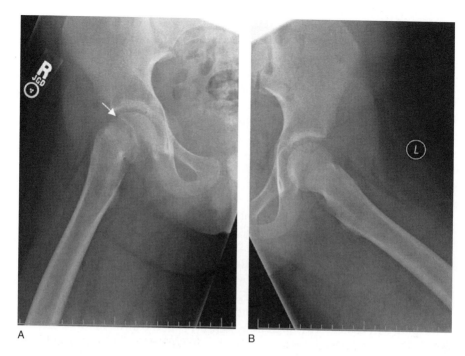

Figure 16-3. Lateral frog-leg radiographs of an 11-year-old female with history and physical examination findings concerning for a slipped capital femoral epiphysis. **A.** The patient's involved right hip demonstrated inferior displacement of the femoral epiphysis consistent with a slipped capital femoral epiphysis (arrow). **B.** The patient's uninvolved left hip. (Reproduced with permission from Michael D. Ross.)

of the physis may be seen in the early stages of the disorder before posterior and inferior displacement of the proximal femoral epiphysis is observed.

In a patient with normal or inconclusive radiographs with a high index of suspicion of an SCFE, a bone scan or magnetic resonance imaging (MRI) may be helpful in confirming the diagnosis. At the "pre-slip" stage, the bone scan may demonstrate increased uptake at the proximal aspect of the femoral neck and MRI may demonstrate abnormalities in the physis.

Plan of Care and Interventions

Diagnosing an SCFE can be challenging and clinicians may initially overlook the diagnosis, especially when patients present with vague symptoms that may appear unrelated to the hip.[19-21] Prognosis for the patient with an SCFE often depends on how quickly the diagnosis is made because this influences the timing of appropriate surgical interventions.[20,21] Unfortunately, diagnostic delay is common.[22] According to Perry et al.,[13] the majority of patients (75.4%) had multiple contacts with primary care providers where they displayed relevant symptoms before a diagnosis was firmly established. Furthermore, in a retrospective chart review of 149 patients with a diagnosis of a stable SCFE who had undergone screw stabilization, the mean time from the first physician visit to diagnosis was 94 days in patients seen by a non-orthopedic provider compared with a mean of 2.9 days in patients seen by an orthopedic provider. In this study, 75% of patients with SCFE initially saw non-orthopedic providers. Thus, the vast majority of patients with an SCFE could experience diagnostic delay.[23] Patients who initially presented with a chief complaint of knee pain (approximately one-third) were less likely to be diagnosed in a timely fashion than those with complaints of hip pain or gait abnormalities.[23] Delays in diagnosis can lead to osteonecrosis and chondrolysis, femoroacetabular impingement secondary to proximal femoral deformity, as well as early-onset hip osteoarthritis.[24,25] Therefore, it is particularly important that non-orthopedic providers are educated regarding clinical presentation and appropriate evaluation and management of SCFE, including when to order radiographs and refer to an orthopedic surgeon, as they are most likely to encounter patients with hip, groin, thigh, and knee pain that could be related to an undiagnosed SCFE.[23] There is also potential benefit in educating at-risk children, their families and caregivers, school nurses, and coaches about SCFE to assist in decreasing diagnostic delay.[22,23]

Once diagnosed, the typical management of a patient with an SCFE is preventing progression of the slip through surgical stabilization of the physis.[1,26] Due to the risk of slip progression, the patient with an SCFE should be referred to an orthopedic surgeon and remain nonweightbearing on the involved lower extremity until surgery. Since surgery is the primary treatment, there is little evidence on conservative treatment approaches, including physical therapy.[2,16] The **surgical treatment approach for a mild to moderate stable slip is *in situ* fixation of the epiphysis.** Under fluoroscopic guidance, this surgical approach involves inserting 1 or 2 cannulated hip screws perpendicular to the physis. This approach usually provides adequate fixation (Fig. 16-4)[1,21,26-29] and allows the epiphyseal plate to be stabilized

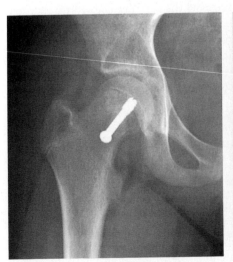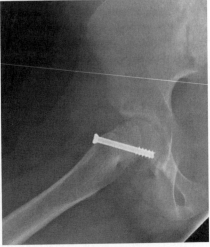

Figure 16-4. Anterior to posterior (left image) and lateral frog-leg (right image) radiographs of an 11-year-old female's right hip following *in situ* fixation of a slipped capital femoral epiphysis. (Reproduced with permission from Michael D. Ross.)

without further slippage with the goal of early closure of the physis. This technique is effective with low rates of recurrence and complications.[21,27]

An unstable SCFE is a more severe injury than a stable SCFE.[16] There is some controversy regarding the specifics of the surgery including timing of surgical intervention, need for preoperative traction, importance of realigning the epiphysis, and whether prophylactic pinning of the contralateral hip is indicated.[14,27] Nonetheless, the treatment for an unstable SCFE must consider the blood supply to the femoral head because the rate of osteonecrosis following surgical intervention was reported as high as 47% in 1993, though more recent studies have reported a rate of 24%.[29] The surgical treatment approach for an unstable slip has commonly entailed decompression of the hip joint (to reduce intra-articular pressure) with gentle closed reduction, depending on the degree of the deformity and fixation with 1 or 2 screws.[2] Others have advocated for urgent open reduction and stabilization of the slip through various surgical methods, a strategy that may be associated with less osteonecrosis in comparison to other interventions.[30,31]

Patients are typically toe-touch weightbearing (non-weightbearing for an unstable SCFE) for the first 6 weeks following surgery. Careful radiographic and clinical monitoring is necessary to ensure that appropriate closure of the proximal femoral physis occurs without progression of the slip.[2] Patients are allowed to gradually return to full weightbearing and normal daily activities after 6 weeks (although this timeframe may be longer for patients with an unstable SCFE), but athletic activities are usually restricted until the physis has closed. After closure of the physis, patients may eventually progress to athletic activities.[32]

Although there is **limited research for rehabilitation after surgery for SCFE**, physical therapists can play an important role. For the patient referred following surgery, the physical therapist should address findings from the musculoskeletal examination while adhering to precautions associated with the surgery.[33] As the patient progresses with rehabilitation activities, any increase in pain or decrease in hip ROM should be communicated to the orthopedic surgeon because these could be early signs of osteonecrosis. Alternatively, it could indicate that the patient is progressing too quickly, which could potentially delay closure of the physis.

It is imperative that the patient and family are properly educated regarding functional anatomy, injury pathomechanics, and activity restrictions/modifications. These are important factors that often assist with patient adherence to the rehabilitation plan of care and weightbearing and activity restrictions. In the early stages of rehabilitation, the main goals are to reduce joint inflammation, protect the surgical site, facilitate synergistic muscle activation and ROM, and ensure that patients adhere to weightbearing and activity restrictions. Once the patient is able to bear weight, appropriate assistive devices should be used as needed to ensure the patient can demonstrate a non-antalgic heel-to-toe gait pattern. Ambulatory aids may be discarded once the patient has a normal pain-free gait and can perform a straight leg raise into abduction without any pain. The next phase of rehabilitation involves resistance exercises to increase strength and endurance of the core and lower extremity musculature, facilitation of neuromuscular control within functional movement patterns, stretching exercises to increase ROM, and aerobic conditioning. The final phase of rehabilitation must ensure that the patient has adequate functional power for return to athletic or daily activities through an appropriate functional exercise progression. The timeframe for return to play is variable and set by the orthopedic surgeon.

It is critical that the patient's overall health is monitored in an interdisciplinary fashion, particularly with respect to appropriate management of medical comorbidities and lifestyle modifications to help the patient achieve and maintain a healthy body weight. The majority of affected individuals are ≥95th percentile BMI-for-age at the time of diagnosis.[8] Furthermore, in the years following surgical management of SCFE, patients' mean BMI increased to 10.2 kg/m^2, and self-reported health is generally poor, with higher rates of diabetes, obesity, and hypertension compared with that of age-matched peers from the general population.[34,35] Individuals with an SCFE also have a higher lifetime risk of hypothyroidism, as well as a higher risk of all-cause mortality compared with individuals without SCFE.[36] These findings highlight the lifetime comorbidity burden of patients who develop an SCFE during their childhood years. Thus, appropriate counseling for patients and their families with regard to the complications of obesity and other medical comorbidities is key and should be a part of the routine management of patients with an SCFE.[34-36]

Evidence-Based Clinical Recommendations

SORT: Strength of Recommendation Taxonomy

A: Consistent, good-quality patient-oriented evidence
B: Inconsistent or limited-quality patient-oriented evidence
C: Consensus, disease-oriented evidence, usual practice, expert opinion, or case series

1. Physical examination of individuals with an SCFE typically reveals an antalgic gait, decreased internal rotation of the hip, and obligatory external rotation as the hip flexes beyond 90°. **Grade C**

2. Physical therapists should consider the diagnosis of SCFE when a young individual presents with an antalgic gait and groin, hip, thigh, or knee pain. **Grade C**

3. When history and physical examination findings are concerning for an SCFE, conventional radiography should include anterior to posterior and lateral views of the hips (lateral frog-leg views for a stable SCFE; cross-table lateral views for an unstable SCFE). **Grade C**

4. The standard treatment of a stable SCFE is *in situ* fixation with a single screw. **Grade C**

5. Rehabilitation for a person with a SCFE includes a comprehensive management plan that includes joint protection of the surgical site (to prevent delayed physis closure or hardware failure), pain-free ambulation, aerobic conditioning, neuromuscular control, strengthening, and performance enhancement through an appropriate functional exercise progression. **Grade C**

COMPREHENSION QUESTIONS

16.1 A physical therapist is evaluating a 12-year-old boy who has moderate groin and knee pain. The patient is able to bear weight, but has an antalgic gait. Hip internal rotation is limited and painful, and when the hip is passively flexed, it abducts and externally rotates. Which of the following diagnostic imaging modalities would be initially indicated to assess for a slipped capital femoral epiphysis?

 A. Anterior to posterior and cross-table lateral view radiographs

 B. Anterior to posterior and lateral frog-leg view radiographs

 C. Bone scan

 D. Magnetic resonance imaging

16.2 Which of the following is the MOST appropriate treatment for a patient with a stable slipped capital femoral epiphysis?

 A. Core decompression

 B. Curettage and bone grafting

 C. *In situ* screw fixation

 D. Total hip arthroplasty

16.3 Which of the following is NOT an anatomic risk factor for a slipped capital femoral epiphysis?

 A. Femoral neck anteversion

 B. Increased obliquity of the physis

 C. Reduced femoral neck-shaft angle

 D. Weakening of the perichondrial ring complex

ANSWERS

16.1 **B.** Since this patient is able to bear weight, he would be classified as potentially having a stable slipped capital femoral epiphysis. Therefore, the appropriate imaging would include anterior to posterior and lateral frog-leg view radiographs. Anterior to posterior and cross-table lateral view radiographs (option A) would be indicated for an unstable SCFE (*i.e.*, the patient would not be able to bear weight). Bone scan and magnetic resonance imaging are not indicated as initial imaging modalities for patients with an SCFE (options C and D). These latter modalities would be useful for a patient with normal or inconclusive radiographs with a high index of suspicion of an SCFE.

16.2 **C.** The standard treatment of stable SCFE is *in situ* fixation with a single cannulated hip screw.

16.3 **A.** Femoral neck retroversion, rather than anteversion, is an anatomic risk factor for a slipped capital femoral epiphysis.

REFERENCES

1. Aronsson DD, Loder RT, Breur GJ, Weinstein SL. Slipped capital femoral epiphysis: current concepts. *J Am Acad Orthop Surg*. 2006;14:666-679.

2. Gholve PA, Cameron DB, Millis MB. Slipped capital femoral epiphysis update. *Curr Opin Pediatr*. 2009;21:39-45.

3. Harris WR. The endocrine basis for the slipping of the femoral head. *J Bone Joint Surg Br*. 1950;32:5-10.

4. Chung CH, Ko KR, Kim JH, Shim JS. Clinical and radiographic characteristics of atypical slipped capital femoral epiphysis. *J Pediatr Orthop*. 2019;39:e742-e749.

5. Loder RT, Skopelja EN. The epidemiology and demographics of slipped capital femoral epiphysis. *ISRN Orthop*. 2011;2011:486512.

6. Aversano MW, Moazzaz P, Scaduto AA, Otsuka NY. Association between body mass index-for-age and slipped capital femoral epiphysis: the long-term risk for subsequent slip in patients followed until physeal closure. *J Child Orthop*. 2016;10:209-213.

7. Cohen M, Gelberman RH, Griffin PP, et al. Slipped capital femoral epiphysis: assessment of epiphyseal displacement and angulation. *J Pediatr Orthop*. 1986;6:259-264.

8. Manoff EM, Banffy MB, Winell JJ. Relationship between body mass index and slipped capital femoral epiphysis. *J Pediatr Orthop*. 2005;25:744-746.

9. Riad J, Bajelidze G, Gabos PG. Bilateral slipped capital femoral epiphysis: predictive factors for contralateral slip. *J Pediatr Orthop*. 2007;27:411-414.

10. Aprato A, Conti A, Bertolo F, Massè A. Slipped capital femoral epiphysis: current management strategies. *Orthop Res Rev*. 2019;11:47-54.

11. Papavasiliou KA, Kirkos JM, Kapetanos GA, Pournaras J. Potential influence of hormones in the development of slipped capital femoral epiphysis: a preliminary study. *J Pediatr Orthop B*. 2007;16:1-5.

12. Loder RT, Starnes T, Dikos G, Aronsson DD. Demographic predictors of severity of stable slipped capital femoral epiphyses. *J Bone Joint Surg Am*. 2006;88:97-105.

13. Perry DC, Metcalfe D, Costa ML, Van Staa T. A nationwide cohort study of slipped capital femoral epiphysis. *Arch Dis Child*. 2017;102:1132-1136.

14. Peck DM, Voss LM, Voss TM. Slipped capital femoral epiphysis: diagnosis and management. *Am Fam Physician*. 2017;95:779-784.

15. Matava MJ, Patton CM, Luhmann S, et al. Knee pain as the initial symptom of slipped capital femoral epiphysis: an analysis of initial presentation and treatment. *J Pediatr Orthop*. 1999;19:455-460.

16. Peck D. Slipped capital femoral epiphysis: diagnosis and management. *Am Fam Physician*. 2010;82:259-262.

17. Otani T, Kawaguchi Y, Marumo K. Diagnosis and treatment of slipped capital femoral epiphysis: Recent trends to note. *J Orthop Sci*. 2018;23:220-228.

18. Houghton KM. Review for the generalist: evaluation of pediatric hip pain. *Pediatr Rheum Online J*. 2009;7:10.

19. Greene KA, Ross MD. Slipped capital femoral epiphysis in a patient referred to physical therapy for knee pain. *J Orthop Sports Phys Ther*. 2008;38:26.

20. Rahme D, Comley A, Foster B, Cundy P. Consequences of diagnostic delays in slipped capital femoral epiphysis. *J Pediatr Orthop B*. 2006;15:93-97.

21. Katz DA. Slipped capital femoral epiphysis: the importance of early diagnosis. *Pediatr Ann*. 2006;35:102-111.

22. Schur MD, Andras LM, Broom AM, et al. Continuing delay in the diagnosis of slipped capital femoral epiphysis. *J Pediatr*. 2016;177:250-254.

23. Hosseinzadeh P, Iwinski HJ, Salava J, Oeffinger D. Delay in the diagnosis of stable slipped capital femoral epiphysis. *J Pediatr Orthop.* 2017;37:e19-e22.

24. Kocher MS, Bishop JA, Weed B, et al. Delay in diagnosis of slipped capital femoral epiphysis. *Pediatrics.* 2004;113:e322-e325.

25. Green DW, Reynolds RA, Khan SN, Tolo V. The delay in diagnosis of slipped capital femoral epiphysis: a review of 102 patients. *HSS J.* 2005;1:103-106.

26. Givon U, Bowen JR. Chronic slipped capital femoral epiphysis: treatment by pinning in-situ. *J Pediatr Orthop B.* 1999;8:216-222.

27. Kalogrianitis S, Tan CK, Kemp GJ, et al. Does unstable slipped capital femoral epiphysis require urgent stabilization? *J Pediatr Orthop B.* 2007;16:6-9.

28. Morrissy RT. Slipped capital femoral epiphysis-natural history, etiology, and treatment. *Instr Course Lect.* 1980;29:81-86.

29. Daley E, Zaltz I. Strategies to avoid osteonecrosis in unstable slipped capital femoral epiphysis: a critical analysis review. *JBJS Rev.* 2019;7(4):e7.

30. Alshryda S, Tsang K, Chytas A, et al. Evidence-based treatment for unstable slipped upper femoral epiphysis: systematic review and exploratory patient level analysis. *Surgeon.* 2018;16:46-54.

31. Loder RT. Slipped capital femoral epiphysis: a spectrum of surgical care and changes over time. *J Child Orthop.* 2017;11:154-159.

32. Loder RT. Slipped capital femoral epiphysis. *Am Fam Physician.* 1998;57:2135-2142, 2148-2150.

33. Spencer-Gardner L, Eischen JJ, Levy BA, et al. A comprehensive five-phase rehabilitation programme after hip arthroscopy for femoroacetabular impingement. *Knee Surg Sports Traumatol Arthrosc.* 2014;22:848-859.

34. Escott BG, De La Rocha A, Jo CH, et al. Patient-reported health outcomes after in situ percutaneous fixation for slipped capital femoral epiphysis: an average twenty-year follow-up study. *J Bone Joint Surg Am.* 2015;97:1929-1934.

35. Taussig MD, Powell KP, Cole HA, et al. Prevalence of hypertension in pediatric tibia vara and slipped capital femoral epiphysis. *J Pediatr Orthop.* 2016;36:877-883.

36. Hailer YD. Fate of patients with slipped capital femoral epiphysis (SCFE) in later life: risk of obesity, hypothyroidism, and death in 2,564 patients with SCFE compared with 25,638 controls. *Acta Orthop.* 2020;91:457-463.

Hip Osteoarthritis

Paul Reuteman

CASE 17

A 58-year-old male self-referred to outpatient physical therapy with a primary complaint of right anterolateral hip pain. The pain intensity and progression of his functional limitations prompted him to seek medical attention. Diagnostic imaging was performed that revealed signs of hip osteoarthritis (Fig. 17-1). His primary care physician referred him to an orthopedic surgeon to discuss surgical options. However, the patient decided on a conservative route and scheduled a consultation with a physical therapist. He describes experiencing intermittent hip pain that is aggravated by squatting, ascending stairs, and rotating his hip during weightbearing activities. He has not been able to engage in his usual cardiovascular conditioning program or strength training due to pain. His goal is to return to his previous level of function during his activities of daily living and resume his cardiovascular and strength training program at his local fitness club.

▶ Based on the patient's diagnosis, what are the contributing factors to his condition?
▶ What examination signs and priorities are associated with hip osteoarthritis?
▶ What are the functional limitations and contextual factors of the patient?
▶ What are the most appropriate physical therapy interventions for a person with hip osteoarthritis?

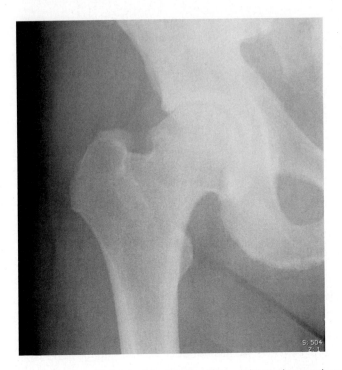

Figure 17-1. Anteroposterior radiograph of the right hip showing sclerotic changes, decreased joint space and an osteophyte on the superior joint margin.

KEY DEFINITIONS

IMPAIRMENT-BASED PHYSICAL THERAPY: Physical therapy interventions addressing modifiable musculoskeletal impairments that are associated with decreased function and/or increased activity-related pain; the decision to use specific interventions is based on continual assessment of the patient's impairments and how these are affected by each intervention; as the status of the patient changes, the plan of care is modified

JOINT MOBILIZATION: Passive movement directed at joint structures with the aim of achieving a therapeutic effect (increased joint motion and/or decreased pain); a high velocity, low amplitude thrust maneuver is type of mobilization technique also known as a joint manipulation

Objectives

1. Utilize evidence and clinical practice guidelines for the examination and treatment of individuals with hip osteoarthritis.

2. Prescribe appropriate manual therapy and joint range of motion activities for a person with hip osteoarthritis.

3. Prescribe appropriate therapeutic resistance and stretching exercises for a person with hip osteoarthritis.

Physical Therapy Considerations

Physical therapy considerations during the management of an individual with a diagnosis of hip osteoarthritis:

▶ **General physical therapy plan of care/goals:** Improve joint mobility and range of motion, decrease pain; increase function, strength, tolerance to daily activities; prevent or minimize loss of aerobic fitness capacity

▶ **Physical therapy interventions:** Patient education regarding functional anatomy and pathomechanics; manual therapy to lumbopelvic region and hip joint to decrease pain and improve motion; resistance exercises to increase strength and endurance of the trunk and lower extremity muscles; aerobic exercises to increase cardiovascular conditioning; primary prevention of further joint damage

▶ **Precautions during physical therapy interventions:** Monitor vital signs; monitor symptom reproduction during treatment; address activities that are contraindicated for patients with hip osteoarthritis

Understanding the Health Condition

Hip pain associated with osteoarthritis (OA) is one of the most common causes of hip pain in older adults.[1,2] OA of the hip joint is a clinical syndrome with signs and symptoms associated with defective integrity of the articular cartilage and changes in the underlying bone and at the joint margins.[3] The condition is associated with pain, loss of mobility and strength, impaired function, and decreased quality of life. The cause of OA is multifactorial and several risk factors have been identified. Age appears to be the most common predisposing factor as the condition mostly affects those 50 years of age and older.[1] Limitations in hip motion, specifically internal rotation and flexion, and loss of function that requires motion in those directions (*i.e.*, squatting) is associated with hip OA.[4]

In the medical community, radiographs remain the gold standard for the diagnosis of hip OA. The Kellgren Lawrence scale has defined 4 grades of hip OA based on joint space narrowing, sclerotic changes of subchondral bone, and the presence of osteophytes.[5] **Clinical criteria have also been established by the American College of Rheumatology to assist clinicians in identifying patients presenting with hip OA.**[6] From these original criteria, patients are classified as having hip OA if they report experiencing hip pain, their age is >50 years, and they present with either of the following two clusters of findings: (1) hip passive internal rotation (IR) <15° and hip flexion ≤115°; or, (2) hip IR >15° but accompanied by pain and duration of morning stiffness of the hip <60 minutes.[6] Updated criteria for the diagnosis of hip OA for individuals over 50 years of age include: moderate anterior or lateral hip pain during weightbearing activities; morning stiffness <1 hour after wakening; passive hip IR <24° or IR and hip flexion 15° less than the nonpainful side; and/or, increased hip pain associated with passive hip IR.[1]

Total hip arthroplasty (THA) is typically the intervention of choice for patients with hip OA. The number of THA procedures performed in the management of hip

OA continues to grow. In 2010, the prevalence of THA in the total United States population was 0.83%. This increased with age reaching 5.26% for individuals older than 80 years.[7] From 1969 to 2009, the rate of THA procedures on younger individuals (up to 49 years of age) increased more than 7-fold with almost a doubling between the 1997-2000 and 2005-2008 time period.[8] The dramatic increase in THA procedures likely reflects both an increased vigilance in hip OA diagnosis and recommendations for earlier surgical intervention. A predictable consequence of THAs being performed in younger individuals is the increased likelihood that an individual will "outlive" the lifespan of the prosthesis, thus requiring THA revision surgery and rehabilitation.[9]

In recent years, several authors have advocated for conservative management with supervised physical therapy as an alternative to surgery to prevent or delay the impact of disability associated with hip OA.[1,10-12] Physical therapy appears to offer the most appropriate multimodal approach combining aerobic and strengthening exercises with directed manual therapy techniques that enhance function and decrease pain.

The current patient presented with radiographic-confirmed hip OA and exhibited range of motion (ROM) deficits and functional limitations that met the OA classification identified by clinical guidelines. Because the patient met these criteria, surgical intervention was recommended by his physician. However, the patient made a personal choice to pursue physical therapy in hopes of avoiding surgery.

Physical Therapy Patient/Client Management

Appropriate conservative management of hip OA requires a multimodal approach. Physical therapy interventions of directed manual therapy techniques should be combined with exercises to improve function and decrease pain. Educating the patient on mind-body principles and how to modify activity to prevent or reduce pain is also critical. It is important to encourage the patient to find activities that enhance general conditioning without placing undue stress at the hip that may result in increased pain. The primary physical therapy goal for most individuals is to enhance function, decrease frequency and intensity of pain during daily activities, and prolong or avoid surgery. Due to the heterogeneity of individuals with hip OA, management models must be tailored to the patient's current impairments, anticipated goals, and how the patient responds to each intervention.

Examination, Evaluation, and Diagnosis

The examination of a patient with hip pain starts with taking a thorough history of the patient's primary complaints and general medical history along with a discussion about the goals for rehabilitation. Individuals presenting with hip pain due to OA most commonly complain of pain in the anterior groin and thigh and potentially pain referral into the buttock, knee, and lower extremity distal to the knee.[13] Weightbearing activities, especially those that involve twisting on the involved extremity and deep squatting are usually painful. At times, prolonged sitting may be painful, especially if the hip is flexed >90°. Frequently, pain is more common in the early morning or after long periods of inactivity.[1]

A disease-specific health-related quality of life questionnaire should be administered to assess the patient's perceived level of disability. The Western Ontario and McMaster Universities Osteoarthritis (WOMAC) Index[14] and the Harris Hip Score (HHS)[15] are two outcome assessments recommended for patients with hip OA. The HHS is a reliable and valid instrument that has been frequently used in studies that assess effectiveness of conservative management of hip OA.[16]

The physical therapist must perform a complete musculoskeletal examination to identify the impairments associated with the patient's health condition. Table 17-1 outlines the components of the examination of an individual with

Table 17-1 GAIT, MOTION ASSESSMENT, AND SPECIAL TESTS ASSOCIATED WITH HIP OSTEOARTHRITIS		
Clinical Assessment	**Patient Position**	**Measurements/Observations**
Observational gait assessment	The patient is asked to ambulate on a level surface.	Compensated or non-compensated Trendelenburg gait is indicative of hip abductor weakness.
Active and passive hip internal rotation (Fig. 17-2)	Patient may either be prone or sitting on the edge of the table. The patient is asked to internally rotate the hip as the therapist measures IR. Therapist prevents any compensations at the pelvis.	The number of degrees the tibia moves from the neutral vertical position is measured with an inclinometer. Motion is assessed passively to determine end feel. ROM is compared bilaterally.
FABER test (Patrick Test) (Fig. 17-3)	Patient lies supine with the symptomatic lower extremity crossed over the opposite leg so that the lateral aspect of the ankle rests proximal to the patella (if possible). Therapist stabilizes the opposite pelvis as the therapist lowers the patient's knee toward the table.	The amount the tibia (on the symptomatic lower extremity) moves from the neutral vertical position is measured with an inclinometer. Motion is compared bilaterally. Pain provocation is also documented.
Scour test (Fig. 17-4)	Patient lies supine. Therapist passively flexes the hip beyond 90° flexion and applies a vertical compressive force to the femur. The therapist moves the femur from abduction to adduction.	Painful range is documented.
Squat test (Fig. 17-5)	Patient is standing and is asked to squat, lowering his hips to his heels. He is asked to squat as low as possible prior to experiencing pain.	The amount the tibia moves from the neutral vertical position is measured with an inclinometer.
6-minute walk test	Patient is asked to cover as much distance while walking in a 6-minute time period.	Physical therapist monitors blood pressure, heart rate, and rate of perceived exertion (RPE) and any hip signs or symptoms before, during, and after the testing.

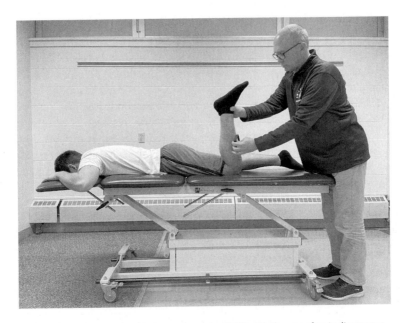

Figure 17-2. Therapist measuring hip internal rotation ROM with the use of an inclinometer.

hip OA. Assessment of impairments serves as a baseline for subsequent visits to identify if improvements are being made.

Initial observational gait assessment may reveal either a compensated or non-compensated Trendelenburg gait. These gait patterns signify weakness of the ipsilateral hip abductors.[16,17]

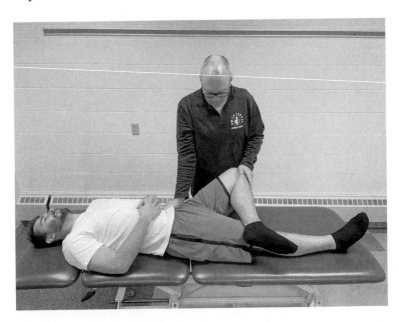

Figure 17-3. Therapist performing the FABER test.

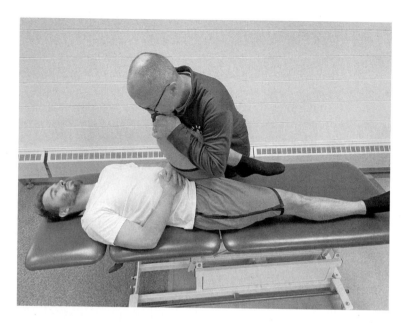

Figure 17-4. Therapist performing the scour test.

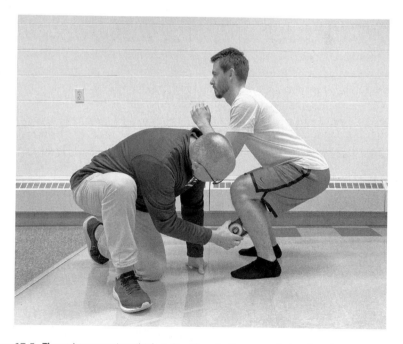

Figure 17-5. Therapist measuring tibial angle with an inclinometer during the squat test.

There is a strong correlation between hip OA and hip ROM deficits.[1,4] Limitations in hip flexion and IR are especially prevalent due to tightness of the joint capsule that is associated with hip OA. Measuring hip IR ROM is easier and more standardized than measuring hip flexion ROM. Measurements of hip IR ROM have been found to be reliable with the patient in either a prone or supine position.[18] True assessment of hip joint mobility is difficult due to the general stability associated with the hip joint. Assessing end feel during the application of overpressure at end-range motions is valuable to determine capsular restrictions. A tight capsular end feel is an indication for specific manual therapy techniques to enhance hip capsule flexibility.[19]

Manual muscle testing is performed to assess strength deficits of the hip with specific attention directed at hip abduction, external rotation, and extension since the muscles that perform these actions are commonly weak in the presence of hip OA.[20]

Special tests have been described that may identify joint restrictions or reproduce pain in a patient with hip OA. These include the FABER test,[1,21] the scour test,[1,21] and the squat test.[21] Little research exists on the diagnostic value of these tests; however, the results of these tests may be valuable to determine if a change has been achieved after a physical therapy intervention to further clarify if that intervention will benefit the patient.

Finally, a six-minute walk test[22] should be performed to assess the patient's baseline fitness level. In addition, the physical therapist can calculate the patient's gait speed from this self-paced walk because gait speed is a prognostic variable for rehabilitation.

To establish an accurate prognosis for a patient with hip OA, multiple variables must be considered. Wright et al.[23] determined 5 baseline variables that may be used as prognostic indicators to identify patients likely to have a *favorable* response to physical therapy intervention for primary hip OA. The variables were: (1) presence of unilateral pain; (2) age ≤58 years; (3) self-reported pain ≥6/10 on a 0 to10 numeric pain rating scale; (4) a 40-meter self-paced walk test time of ≤25.9 seconds; and, (5) duration of symptoms ≤1 year. Having 3 or more of the 5 variables increased the post-test probability of success with physical therapy intervention to 99%. Failure of having any one of the 5 variables decreased the post-test probability of responding favorably to physical therapy intervention from 32% to <1% (negative likelihood ratio = 0.00, 95% confidence interval = 0.00-0.70).[23] The current patient exhibited 4 out of 5 variables, therefore, he was considered to have a favorable prognosis for conservative care.

Plan of Care and Interventions

Intervention should include an impairment-based approach. Patient education, manual therapy techniques, muscle and joint capsule stretching, and prescription of exercises to improve hip muscle strength and endurance and general conditioning are recommended. The decision to use specific interventions is based on the continual re-assessment of the patient's impairments and how these impairments are affected by the intervention. As the status of the patient changes, the treatment is modified.

An important consideration in managing hip pain is educating the patient on ways to reduce muscle-generated hip joint forces during ambulation. If pain is limiting the patient from walking in the community or for exercise, the therapist should explain the biomechanical rationale for using a cane or walking stick on the uninvolved side and carrying items on the involved side. These techniques are based primarily on reducing the magnitude of hip abductor muscle forces during walking.[24] In simple terms, by using these techniques, the patient decreases loading to the hip joint, which results in less stress to the joint. Educating the patient on these concepts may decrease hip joint pain, normalize gait pattern, and increase walking tolerance.

The inclusion of manual therapy techniques in the plan of care enhances outcomes for patients with hip OA.[1,25-28] Two recent evidence-based practice guidelines advocate for the use of manual therapy in conjunction with education and therapeutic exercise.[1,25] In a case series of 27 patients (median age 52 ± 7.5 years), physical therapists performed manual therapy that included 5 different hip joint mobilization techniques (long axis distraction, internal rotation with distraction, caudal glides, posterior-anterior glides, and anterior and posterior hip stretching) followed by prescribed exercise deemed appropriate by the treating physical therapist.[26] Subjects attended 10 sessions over an 8-week period. At the end of treatment, there was a median increase of 28° in hip flexion and 10° in hip IR; the median improvement on the Harris Hip Score was 20 points; and, mean decrease in pain was 2.3 points (on 0-10-point scale). Even at the 29-week follow up, statistically significant improvements were maintained in the Harris Hip Score and hip ROM.[26]

In a larger randomized clinical trial of patients with hip OA, one group received manual therapy plus exercise prescription and another received only exercise prescription over 5 weeks. The inclusion of manual therapy to address mobility of both the lumbo-pelvic region and the hip joint improved treatment outcomes as assessed by the Harris Hip Score, walking speed, pain, and hip flexion ROM. At 5 weeks after completion of physical therapy, effect sizes favoring the manual therapy plus exercise group were greatest for the Harris Hip Score (mean between-group difference 11.2, 95% CI: 6.1, 16.3) and hip flexion ROM (mean between-group difference 16.0°, 95% CI: 8.1, 22.6). Similar results were noted at a 9-month follow-up.[27]

Recommended joint mobilization techniques for managing hip OA include, but are not limited to: long axis joint traction with a high velocity-low amplitude thrust to address general hip capsule mobility; lateral distraction with internal rotation motion to improve pain-free IR motion; anterior-posterior (AP) joint mobilizations to address posterior capsule mobility; and, posterior-anterior (PA) joint mobilizations to address anterior capsule mobility (Figs. 17-6 to 17-9). Following any joint mobilization technique, it is advisable to instruct the patient in exercises to use and maintain the newly gained motion. Common stretching exercises include those directed at anterior hip or hip flexors; medial hip or hip adductors; and posterior hip or piriformis (Figs. 17-10 to 17-12). Using mobilization straps with movement in various positions may also improve pain-free motion of the hip (Figs. 17-13 and 17-14).

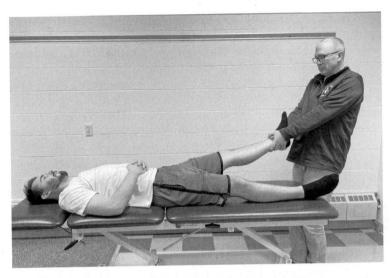

Figure 17-6. Therapist performing long axis traction with high-velocity, low-amplitude thrust.

A 2019 systematic review and meta-analysis has shown that a variety of therapeutic exercises improve multiple outcomes in individuals with hip OA.[29] **Aerobic exercise and mind-body exercise, such as tai-chi and yoga, may be best for reducing pain and improving function. Strengthening and flexibility/skill exercises may be used to improve multiple outcomes including pain and quality of life.**[29] Some examples of skill exercises include squatting, lateral stepping, and balance training to simulate activities the patient wishes to participate in at home or recreationally. **Strengthening**

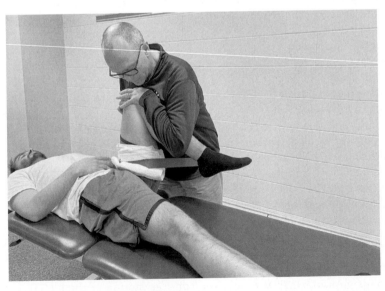

Figure 17-7. Therapist performing lateral distraction with internal rotation joint mobilization.

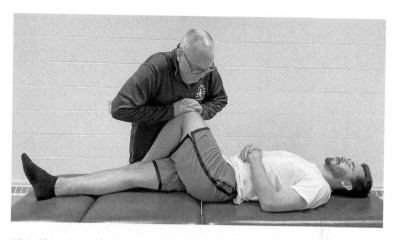

Figure 17-8. Therapist performing anterior-posterior (AP) joint mobilization.

exercises that target the hip abductors, hip extensors, and hip external rotators are commonly emphasized. Exercises are progressed from a nonweightbearing position to a weightbearing position, as tolerated. Initial exercises include sidelying hip abduction/external rotation and supine bridging activities. Based on electromyography (EMG) data, progression to single limb activity such as single-limb squats and deadlifts achieve optimal recruitment of the hip muscles.[30] Strengthening exercises should be modified as necessary to avoid symptom provocation and improve patient tolerance. Aside from the positive effect of aerobic exercise on pain and function, any achieved excess weight loss will also reduce stress on the hip joint.

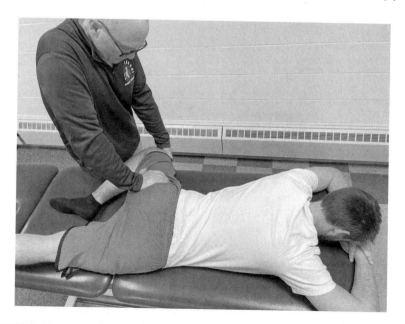

Figure 17-9. Therapist performing posterior-anterior (PA) joint mobilization.

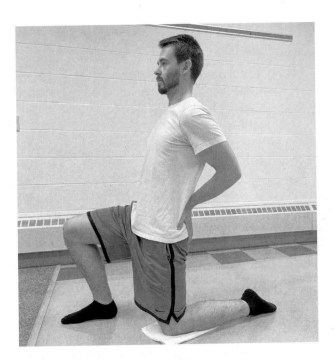

Figure 17-10. Patient performing left anterior hip/hip flexor stretch.

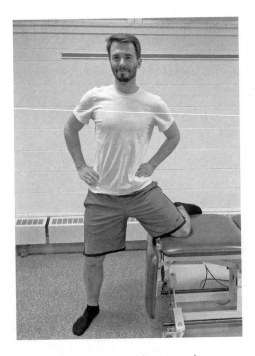

Figure 17-11. Patient performing left medial hip/adductor stretch.

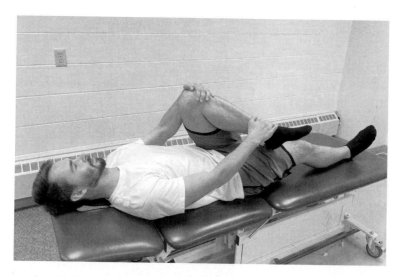

Figure 17-12. Patient performing left posterior hip/piriformis stretch.

A structured stationary cycling or walking program focusing on duration, intensity, and frequency has been recommended for individuals with hip OA, especially for adults ≥60 years old. In a large systematic review and meta-analysis, data suggest that exercise training for this age group has a significant benefit not only for physical function, but also for cognitive function.[31]

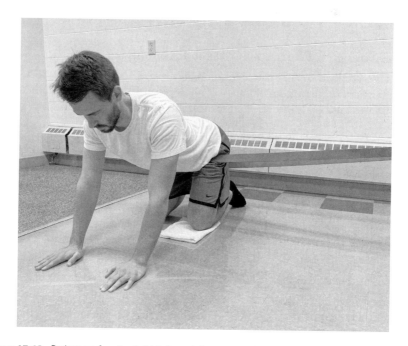

Figure 17-13. Patient performing left hip lateral distraction self-mobilization with band.

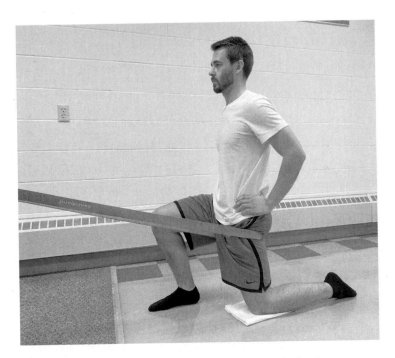

Figure 17 14. Patient performing left hip anterior self-mobilization with band.

Evidence-Based Clinical Recommendations

SORT: Strength of Recommendation Taxonomy

A: Consistent, good-quality patient-oriented evidence
B: Inconsistent or limited-quality patient-oriented evidence
C: Consensus, disease-oriented evidence, usual practice, expert opinion, or case series

1. Hip OA can be diagnosed with clusters of signs or symptoms outlined by the American College of Rheumatology. **Grade A**

2. Education and implementation of joint protection strategies (*e.g.*, ambulation with a cane in the hand opposite the involved hip) is effective in managing symptoms associated with hip OA. **Grade B**

3. Manual therapy techniques addressed at the lumbo-pelvic and hip joint improve hip pain and short- and long-term function in individuals with hip OA. **Grade A**

4. Exercise interventions focusing on stretching and strengthening of muscles surrounding the hip improve hip strength and tolerance to activity in individuals with hip OA. **Grade A**

5. Aerobic exercise reduces pain and increases function in individuals with hip OA. **Grade A**

COMPREHENSION QUESTIONS

17.1 Which of the following sets of motion deficits are most commonly associated with hip OA?

A. Hip abduction, hip flexion

B. Hip internal rotation, hip extension

C. Hip flexion, hip external rotation

D. Hip abduction, hip internal rotation

17.2 Which of the following statements is MOST accurate regarding the use of manual therapy in the treatment of hip OA?

A. Manual therapy improves pain but does not have any effect on hip range of motion.

B. Manual therapy has a short-term effect on patient outcomes but has no effect in the long term (6-9 months following discharge from physical therapy).

C. Manual therapy has both short- and long-term effects on patient outcomes (6-9 months following discharge from physical therapy).

D. Manual therapy has no positive effect on patients with hip OA.

ANSWERS

17.1 **B.** Current recommendations for clinicians classifying adults >50 years in the category of hip OA include moderate anterior or lateral hip pain during weightbearing activities, morning stiffness <1 hour after wakening; hip IR <24° or internal rotation and hip flexion 15° less than the nonpainful side; and/or increased hip pain associated with passive hip internal rotation.[1]

17.2 **C.** Hoeksma and colleagues[27] published a randomized clinical trial comparing manual therapy and exercise versus exercise alone in patients with hip OA. Outcomes including the Harris Hip Score, walking speed, pain, and range of motion showed significant improvement at 5 weeks after initiating treatment and at a 9-month follow-up.

REFERENCES

1. Cibulka MT, Bloom NJ, Enseki KR, et al. Hip pain and mobility deficits—hip osteoarthritis: revision 2017: Clinical practice guidelines linked to the international classification of functioning, disability and health from the orthopaedic section of the American Physical Therapy Association. *J Orthop Sports Phys Ther.* 2017;47:A1-A37.

2. Kim C, Linsenmeyer KD, Vlad SC, et al. Prevalence of radiographic and symptomatic hip osteoarthritis in an urban United States community: the Framingham osteoarthritis study. *Arthritis Rheum.* 2014;66:3013-3017.

3. Teichtahl AJ, Wang Y, Smith S, et al. Structural changes of hip osteoarthritis using magnetic resonance imaging. *Arthritis Res Ther.* 2014;16:1-9.

4. Holla J, Steultjens M, van der Leeden M, et al. Determinants of range of joint motion in patients with early symptomatic osteoarthritis of the hip and/or knee: an exploratory study in the CHECK cohort. *Osteoarthritis Cart.* 2011;19:411-419.

5. Kellgren JH, Lawrence JS. Radiological assessment of osteo-arthrosis. *Ann Rheum Dis.* 1957;16:494-502.

6. Altman RD, Alarcon G, Appelrouth D, et al. The American College of Rheumatology criteria for the classification and reporting of osteoarthritis of the hip. *Arthritis Rheum.* 1991;34:505-514.

7. Kremers H, Larson D, Crowson C, et al. Prevalence of total hip and knee replacement in the United States. *JBJS.* 2015;97:1386.

8. Singh JA, Vessely MB, Harmsen WS, et al. A population-based study of trends in the use of total hip and total knee arthroplasty, 1969-2008. *Mayo Clin Proc.* 2010;85:898-904.

9. Schwartz AM, Farley KX, Guild GN, Bradbury TL. Projections and epidemiology of revision hip and knee arthroplasty in the United States to 2030. *J Arthroplasty.* 2020;35:S79-S85.

10. Skou ST, Roos EM. Physical therapy for patients with knee and hip osteoarthritis: supervised, active treatment is current best practice. *Clin Exp Rheumatol.* 2019;37:112-117.

11. Holden MA, Button K, Collins NJ, et al. Guidance for implementing best practice therapeutic exercise for patients with knee and hip osteoarthritis: what does the current evidence base tell us? *Arthritis Care Res.* 2021;73:1746-1753.

12. Wainner RS, Whitman JM. First-line interventions for hip pain: is it surgery, drugs or us? *J Orthop Sports Phys Ther.* 2007;37:511-513.

13. Lesher JM, Dreyfuss P, Hager N, et al. Hip joint pain referral patterns: a descriptive study. *Pain Med.* 2008;9:22-25.

14. Bellamy N, Buchanan WW, Goldsmith CH, et al. Validation study of WOMAC: a health status instrument for measuring clinically important patient relevant outcomes to antirheumatic drug therapy in patients with osteoarthritis of the hip or knee. *J Rheumatol.* 1988;15:1833-1844.

15. Harris WH. Traumatic arthritis of the hip after dislocation and acetabular fractures: treatment by mold arthroplasty. An end-result study using a new method of result evaluation. *J Bone Joint Surg Am.* 1969;51:737-755.

16. Hoeksma HL, Van Den Ende CH, Ronday HK, et al. Comparison of the responsiveness of the Harris Hip Score with generic measures for hip function in osteoarthritis of the hip. *Ann Rheum Dis.* 2003;62:935-938.

17. Neumann DA. An electromyographic study of the hip abductor muscles as subjects with a hip prosthesis walked with different methods of using a cane and carrying a load. *Phys Ther.* 1999;79:1174-1176.

18. Simoneau GG, Hoenig KJ, Lepley JE, Papanek PE. Influence of hip position and gender on active hip internal and external rotation. *J Orthop Sports Phys Ther.* 1998;28:158-164.

19. Cyriax JH, Coldham M. *Textbook of Orthopaedic Medicine.* 11th ed. Bailliere Tindall, 1984.

20. Loureiro A, Mills PM, Barrett RS. Muscle weakness in hip osteoarthritis: a systematic review. *Arthritis Care Res.* 2013;65:340-352.

21. Cliborne AV, Wainner RS, Rhon DI, et al. Clinical hip tests and a functional squat test in patients with knee osteoarthritis: reliability, prevalence of positive findings, and short-term response to hip mobilization. *J Orthop Sports Phys Ther.* 2004;34:676-685.

22. Enright PL, Sherrill DL. Reference equations for the six-minute walk in healthy adults. *Am J Respir Crit Care Med.* 1998;158:1384-1387.

23. Wright AA, Cook CE, Flynn TW, et al. Predictors of response to physical therapy intervention in patients with primary hip osteoarthritis. *Phys Ther.* 2011;91:510-524.

24. Neumann DA. Biomechanical analysis of selected principles of hip joint protection. *Arthritis Care Res.* 1989;2:146-155.

25. Peter WF, Jansen MJ, Hurkmans EJ, et al, Guideline Steering Committee – Hip and Knee Osteoarthritis. Physiotherapy in hip and knee osteoarthritis: development of a practice guideline concerning initial assessment, treatment and evaluation. *Acta Rheumatol Port.* 2011;36:268-281.

26. Hando BR, Gill NW, Walker MJ, Garber M. Short- and long-term clinical outcomes following a standardized protocol of orthopedic manual physical therapy and exercise in individuals with osteoarthritis of the hip: a case series. *J Man Manip Ther.* 2012;20:192-200.

27. Hoeksma HL, Dekker J, Ronday HK, et al. Comparison of manual therapy and exercise therapy in osteoarthritis of the hip: a randomized clinical trial. *Arthritis Care Res.* 2004;51:722-729.

28. Poulsen E, Hartvigsen J, Christensen HW, et al. Patient education with or without manual therapy compared to a control group in patients with osteoarthritis of the hip. A proof-of-principle three-arm parallel group randomized clinical trial. *Osteoarthritis Cartilage.* 2013;21:1494-1503.

29. Goh SL, Persson MSM, Stocks J, et al. Relative efficacy of different exercises for pain, function, performance and quality of life in knee and hip osteoarthritis: systematic review and network meta-analysis. *Sports Med.* 2019;49:743-761.

30. DiStefano LJ, Blackburn JT, Marshall SW, Padua DA. Gluteal muscle activation during common therapeutic exercises. *J Ortho Sports Phys Ther.* 2009;39:532-540.

31. Falck RS, Davis JC, Best JR, et al. Impact of exercise training on physical and cognitive function among older adults: a systematic review and meta-analysis. *Neurobiol Aging.* 2019;79:119-130.

Femoroacetabular Impingement Syndrome

Erik P. Meira

A 24-year-old recreational soccer player is referred to physical therapy by a general practitioner with a diagnosis of "hip pain." The patient reports that she has had left hip pain which has been progressively increasing over the past 4 years. She reports the primary location of pain is in the front of the hip with an occasional "piercing sensation deep inside." She cannot recall a specific injury, although her pain worsened 2 months ago during a soccer game when her hip went into extreme flexion. She now has pain, especially when lifting her leg to get out of bed or out of a car. In addition to an intensification of her hip pain, she now notices a "catching" sensation as she moves her hip around. She has been unable to play soccer for 2 months and there has been no improvement in her symptoms. Based on the patient's history, the physical therapist suspects femoroacetabular impingement syndrome with possible acetabular labral tear.

▶ What examination signs may be associated with this suspected diagnosis?
▶ What are the most appropriate examination tests?
▶ What is her rehabilitation prognosis?
▶ What are possible complications that may limit the effectiveness of physical therapy?

KEY DEFINITIONS

ACETABULAR LABRUM: Fibrocartilaginous ring around the rim of the acetabulum that can become damaged during femoroacetabular impingement; often the source of pain in symptomatic patients with femoroacetabular impingement[1,2]

CAM IMPINGEMENT: Femoroacetabular impingement caused by a cam or egg-shaped deformity of the femoral head

COMBINATION IMPINGEMENT: Femoroacetabular impingement caused by a combination of cam and pincer impingements

FEMOROACETABULAR IMPINGEMENT SYNDROME (FAIS): Painful condition in which the femoral head and/or neck makes above-average contact with the acetabulum

PINCER IMPINGEMENT: Femoroacetabular impingement caused by a retroverted acetabulum that creates above-average anterior coverage of the femoral head

Objectives

1. Describe femoroacetabular impingement syndrome and identify potential risk factors associated with this diagnosis.
2. Describe the clinical examination for the patient with suspected FAIS, including special tests and their associated diagnostic accuracy.
3. Prescribe appropriate joint range of motion and/or strengthening exercises for a patient with FAIS.
4. Provide appropriate medical referral for the patient with suspected FAIS.

Physical Therapy Considerations

Physical therapy considerations during management of the individual with a suspected diagnosis of femoroacetabular impingement syndrome:

▶ **General physical therapy plan of care/goals:** Decrease pain; increase lower quadrant strength; increase hip range of motion as necessary and tolerated; prevent or minimize loss of aerobic fitness capacity

▶ **Physical therapy interventions:** Patient education regarding functional anatomy and injury pathomechanics; modalities and manual therapy to decrease pain; resistance exercises to increase core muscular endurance and to increase strength of lower extremity muscles; gentle stretching as tolerated to increase the range of motion as necessary; aerobic exercise program

▶ **Precautions during physical therapy:** Monitor vital signs; address precautions or contraindications for exercise, based on patient's pre-existing condition(s); avoid activities/positions that exacerbate symptoms

▶ **Differential diagnoses:** Extra-articular pathology such as external coxa saltans, internal coxa saltans, iliopsoas strain, athletic pubalgia, or stress fracture

Understanding the Health Condition

Femoroacetabular impingement syndrome (FAIS) is a condition in which there is an incongruence of the femoral head with the acetabulum (femoroacetabular impingement or FAI), leading to increased contact between these two bones at the end ranges of hip motion with associated hip pain. FAI generally presents as a cam impingement, pincer impingement, or a combination of the two. In a cam impingement, the femoral head has an aspherical shape like that of a cam or an egg (Fig. 18-1). As the femoral head articulates in the acetabulum, a cam-shaped femoral head can apply increased stress at the edges of the joint. In a pincer impingement, it is the shape of the acetabulum that causes the impingement. In this case, the acetabulum is relatively retroverted, which can cause the anterior wall of the acetabulum to cover an increased amount of the femoral head (Fig. 18-2). As the hip joint articulates, the femoral neck makes contact with the acetabular rim earlier in the range of motion, which can cause increased stress to the joint that can damage the acetabular labrum, the articular cartilage, or both. This damage can result in the pain that causes the patient to seek medical services.[1,2]

The incidence of FAI in the general population is relatively high. A recent systematic review has shown that roughly 23% of asymptomatic individuals and 55% of asymptomatic *athletes* have cam morphology.[3] FAI usually affects people

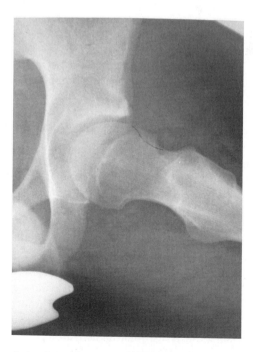

Figure 18-1. Radiograph showing a cam- or egg-shaped femoral head. The portion of the bone inside the darkened line represents a normal shape of the femoral head. (Reproduced with permission from Mark B. Wagner, MD.)

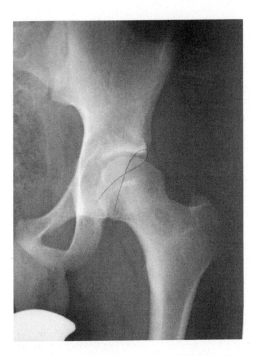

Figure 18-2. Pincer impingement with crossover sign on an anteroposterior radiograph. The darkened line demonstrates the "crossing over" of **A** (anterior rim of acetabulum) and **B** (posterior rim of acetabulum). (Reproduced with permission from Mark B. Wagner, MD.)

between 20 and 40 years of age. Cam impingement is more common in males, whereas pincer impingement is slightly more common in females. In one study of 200 asymptomatic adults, 14% had at least one hip with cam morphology and 79% of those were males.[4] A retrospective study reported close to 30% of asymptomatic males have evidence of a cam deformity.[5] In a radiographic database of over 4000 individuals, pincer deformity was seen in 19% of asymptomatic females and 15% of asymptomatic males.[6]

A study of 39 asymptomatic collegiate and professional hockey players reported that 64% had abnormal magnetic resonance imaging findings.[7] A follow-up study 4 years later with the same cohort was unable to show a higher rate of hip pain in those with abnormal initial findings.[8] Because hip pathologies are common, it is essential to determine whether a patient's pain is caused by FAI, or the associated damage to the acetabular labrum and/or articular cartilage.

Over time, FAI may damage the hip joint through repetitive contact between the two incongruent joint surfaces. Since many sports require extensive hip mobility, individuals with FAI often become symptomatic through repeated athletic activities.[1,2] Because the individual with FAI experiences pain with deep squatting and end-range internal and external rotation activities, these motions should be avoided when FAI is suspected.[1,2] Athletes often mistake their limited comfortable hip range of motion as an indication of poor flexibility and try to resolve the problem through stretching. This can exacerbate the pain and potentially cause more irritation to the joint.[1,2] It is common for patients to present with increasing pain over time that becomes significantly exacerbated and intolerable after one "final" event.[1,2]

Pain originating from a source in the hip usually refers to the anterior hip and into the groin.[1] Since patients who have hip joint pathology frequently have guarding and irritation in the hip flexors and adductors, it can be difficult to differentiate between muscle and joint pathology. Studies have shown the incidence of asymptomatic labral tears to be as high as 68% in the general population.[3] Therefore, radiographic evidence of FAI and even damage to the acetabular labrum *without* the presence of pain should not be corrected.[9] However, in symptomatic patients, **arthroscopic surgical correction of FAI is very effective for reducing pain and increasing function.**[10]

Physical Therapy Patient/Client Management

A primary role for the physical therapist is in differentially diagnosing the etiology of hip pain. If FAIS is the suspected diagnosis, it is appropriate to involve an orthopedic surgeon for assistance with case management and further diagnostic imaging. Because FAIS is a condition involving the shape of the bone, therapy interventions cannot alter its underlying cause. Instead, interventions focus on managing pain and improving function. Increasing strength and teaching the patient to avoid painful positions may be enough to allow them to return to desired activities. Low-level evidence supports nonoperative management in reducing pain and increasing function, but stronger evidence supports the benefits of surgical correction of FAI.[10]

Examination, Evaluation, and Diagnosis

The physical therapist must take a thorough patient history. The patient with suspected FAIS often complains of pain *deep* in the anterior hip. The pain often increases with activities that create resistance to the iliopsoas muscle group such as raising the leg to get out of bed or a car because this increases the stress on the hip joint and the anterior-superior labrum. The patient may also complain of mechanical signs such as a sporadic "catching" in the joint with subsequent pain. The pain often improves with rest. However, the pain may return when more athletic activities are resumed.[2,9]

On deep palpation, the supine patient may present with tenderness in the anterior hip. Resisted straight leg raise is often painful because it places increased load to the iliopsoas and anterior joint.[2,9] The FABER (femoral abduction external rotation) position (Fig. 18-3) is often restricted and uncomfortable when compared to the uninvolved side. In the person with FAIS, the FADIR (flexion-adduction-internal-rotation) test is often painful because this test positions the hip into combined end-range flexion, adduction, and internal rotation (Fig. 18-4) that recreates the abnormal contact in FAI and can reproduce the patient's symptoms.[1] Table 18-1 lists **seven special tests for intra-articular hip joint pathology.** The reported diagnostic accuracy of each test was based on comparison to the criterion

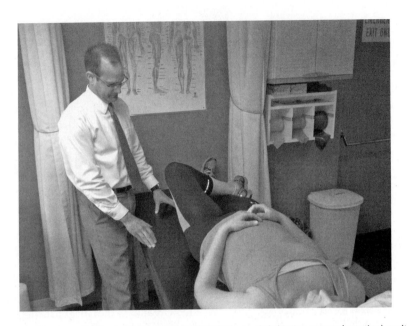

Figure 18-3. Patient's left lower extremity in the FABER (femoral abduction external rotation) position. This position is often restricted and uncomfortable when compared to the uninvolved side.

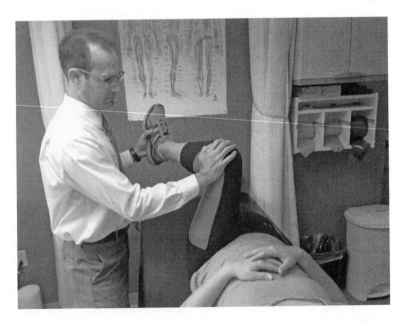

Figure 18-4. Therapist performing FADIR test on the left lower extremity. Placement of the hip into combined end-range flexion, adduction, and internal rotation recreates the contact in FAI and reproduces the patient's symptoms.

Table 18-1   SPECIAL TESTS FOR INTRA-ARTICULAR HIP JOINT PATHOLOGY WITH REPORTED SENSITIVITY AND SPECIFICITY[9]

Signs/Symptoms	Sensitivity (%)	Specificity (%)
+ Groin pain	59	14
+ Catching	63	54
+ Pinching pain in sitting	48	54
− Lateral thigh pain	78	36
+ FABER	60	18
+ Impingement	78	10
− Trochanteric tenderness	57	45

"+" indicates that pain is present or elicited; "−" indicates that pain is absent.
Reproduced with permission from Martin RL, Irrgang JJ, Sekiya JK. The diagnostic accuracy of a clinical examination in determining intra-articular hip pain for potential hip arthroscopy candidates. Arthroscopy. 2008;24(9):1013-1018.

standard of >50% pain relief with an intra-articular anesthetic injection.[9] None of these special tests have good diagnostic accuracy. In particular, none of the tests is useful to identify intra-articular structures as the cause of a patient's hip pain. The especially low specificity means that many individuals *without* intra-articular pathology would be falsely diagnosed with intra-articular hip pathology with these tests.

If the physical therapist suspects FAIS and/or a possible acetabular labral tear after completing the evaluation, the therapist might refer the patient to a physician for radiographic evaluation. Radiographs can show the presence of FAI and whether the impingement is caused by a cam or pincer deformity. Confirmation of an acetabular labral tear can be achieved via a magnetic resonance arthrogram with gadolinium contrast followed by an injection of an anesthetic such as lidocaine into the hip joint.[1,9] A significant reduction in symptoms after the anesthetic injection indicates a higher likelihood that the pain is coming from the joint itself and not surrounding tissues.[9]

Plan of Care and Interventions

Patients with confirmed and painful FAI may respond to conservative management.[10] Since range of motion limitations may be restricted by bony morphology, attempts to increase flexibility and range of motion should be performed with caution. Focus should be placed on increasing muscular strength and coordination while avoiding positions that exacerbate pain such as end-range hip flexion, internal rotation, and abduction. A recent systematic review examining interventions for FAIS found that nonoperative management such as physical therapy may be effective, but the quality of the studies was not high enough to draw stronger conclusions.[10] Some authors suggest that controlling functional knee valgus by emphasizing hip and lumbopelvic stabilization may reduce symptoms caused by an acetabular labral tear, but it is also possible that temporary avoidance of painful positions while building overall lower quarter strength is the driver of the positive effects. If a patient is unable to improve symptoms and be functional in sport or activities of daily living, surgical correction has been shown to be effective.[10]

Evidence-Based Clinical Recommendations

SORT: Strength of Recommendation Taxonomy

A: Consistent, good-quality patient-oriented evidence
B: Inconsistent or limited-quality patient-oriented evidence
C: Consensus, disease-oriented evidence, usual practice, expert opinion, or case series

1. Surgical correction is effective for decreasing pain and increasing function in individuals with femoroacetabular impingement syndrome. **Grade A**

2. Special diagnostic tests for intra-articular hip pathology have better sensitivity than specificity, but have poor overall diagnostic accuracy. **Grade B**

3. A treatment program consisting of therapeutic strengthening exercises while avoiding painful positions may be effective for reducing pain in individuals with hip labral injuries associated with FAIS. **Grade C**

COMPREHENSION QUESTIONS

18.1 Muscles around the hip may become irritated and exacerbate pre-existing hip pathology. Activation of which muscle consistently reproduces pain associated with a torn acetabular labrum?

    A. Adductor magnus

    B. Iliopsoas

    C. Gluteus medius

    D. Piriformis

18.2 A patient presents to an outpatient physical therapist with signs and symptoms of FAI with an acetabular labral tear. What is the MOST accurate way to indicate that their symptoms are likely coming from the hip joint and not surrounding soft tissue?

    A. Clinical examination

    B. Plain radiographs

    C. Magnetic resonance arthrogram with gadolinium

    D. Injection of an anesthetic into the joint that causes temporary reduction of pain

ANSWERS

18.1 **B.** Pain often increases with activities that create resistance to the iliopsoas muscle group such as raising the leg to get out of bed or a car because this increases the stress to the hip joint and the anterior-superior labrum.

18.2 **D.** The clinical examination (history and physical examination) is critical for the physical therapist to narrow down the differential diagnoses; however, the special tests have poor accuracy to diagnose intra-articular hip pathology (option A). Imaging studies (plain radiographs or magnetic resonance arthrogram with gadolinium) may demonstrate the presence of FAI. However, studies have demonstrated that *asymptomatic* subjects may present with cam or pincer deformities (options B and C).

REFERENCES

1. Griffin DR, Dickenson EJ, O'Donnell J, et al. The Warwick Agreement on femoroacetabular impingement syndrome (FAI syndrome): an international consensus statement. *Br J Sports Med.* 2016;50(19):1169-1176.

2. Philippon MJ, Stubbs AJ, Schenker ML, et al. Arthroscopic management of femoroacetabular impingement: osteoplasty technique and literature review. *Am J Sports Med.* 2007;35:1571-1580.

3. Frank JM, Harris JD, Erickson BJ, et al. Prevalence of femoroacetabular impingement imaging findings in asymptomatic volunteers: a systematic review. *Arthroscopy.* 2015;31:1199-1204.

4. Hack K, Di Primio G, Rakhra K, Beaule PE. Prevalence of cam-type femoroacetabular impingement morphology in asymptomatic volunteers. *J Bone Joint Surg.* 2010;92:2436-2444.

5. Jung KA, Restrepo C, Hellman M, et al. The prevalence of cam-type femoroacetabular deformity in asymptomatic adults. *J Bone Joint Surg Br.* 2011;93:1303-1307.

6. Gosvig KK, Jacobsen S, Sonne-Holm S, et al. Prevalence of malformations of the hip joint and their relationship to sex, groin pain, and risk of osteoarthritis: a population-based survey. *J Bone Joint Surg.* 2010;92:1162-1169.

7. Silvis ML, Mosher TJ, Smetana BS, et al. High prevalence of pelvic and hip magnetic resonance imaging findings in asymptomatic collegiate and professional hockey players. *Am J Sports Med.* 2011;39:715-721.

8. Gallo RA, Silvis ML, Smetana B, et al. Asymptomatic hip/groin pathology identified on magnetic resonance imaging of professional hockey players: outcomes and playing status at 4 years' follow-up. *Arthroscopy.* 2014 Oct;30(10):1222-1228.

9. Martin RL, Irrgang JJ, Sekiya JK. The diagnostic accuracy of a clinical examination in determining intra-articular hip pain for potential hip arthroscopy candidates. *Arthroscopy.* 2008;24:1013-1018.

10. Kemp JL, Mosler AB, Hart H, et al. Improving function in people with hip-related pain: a systematic review and meta-analysis of physiotherapist-led interventions for hip-related pain. *Br J Sports Med.* 2020;54:1382-1394.

Iliotibial Band Syndrome

Jason Brumitt

CASE 19

A 32-year-old recreational runner self-referred to an outpatient physical therapy clinic with a complaint of right lateral knee pain. He first experienced pain 6 weeks ago. Two weeks prior to symptom onset, he initiated a marathon-training program. His symptoms have gradually worsened; now, he is no longer able to run due to the immediate onset of the same pain. The patient's medical history is otherwise unremarkable. Signs and symptoms are consistent with iliotibial band syndrome (ITBS). His goal is to return to training for the upcoming marathon.

▶ Based on the patient's suspected diagnosis, what do you anticipate may be the contributing factors to his condition?
▶ What examination signs may be associated with this diagnosis?
▶ What are the most appropriate physical therapy interventions?

KEY DEFINITIONS

CORE STABILITY: Ability of muscles within the "core" region (abdomen, lumbar spine, pelvis, and hips) to protect (*i.e.*, stabilize) the lumbar spine from potentially injurious forces and to create and/or transfer forces between anatomical segments during functional movements

ILIOTIBIAL BAND SYNDROME: Overuse injury primarily experienced by distance runners, marked by lateral knee or lateral hip pain

TRIGGER POINT: Taut band of contracted muscle fibers within a skeletal muscle that may cause pain, decrease range of motion, and may be associated with muscular weakness[1]

Objectives

1. Describe iliotibial band syndrome and identify potential risk factors associated with this diagnosis.
2. Prescribe appropriate joint range of motion and/or muscular flexibility exercises for a person with iliotibial band syndrome.
3. Prescribe appropriate resistance exercises during each stage of healing for a person with iliotibial band syndrome.

Physical Therapy Considerations

Physical therapy considerations during management of the individual with a diagnosis of ITBS:

▶ **General physical therapy plan of care/goals:** Decrease pain; increase muscular flexibility and/or joint range of motion; increase lower quadrant strength; prevent or minimize loss of aerobic fitness capacity

▶ **Physical therapy interventions:** Patient education regarding functional anatomy and injury pathomechanics; modalities and manual therapy to decrease pain; muscular flexibility exercises; resistance exercises to increase muscular endurance capacity of the core and to increase strength of lower extremity muscles; aerobic exercise program; orthotic fabrication

▶ **Precautions during physical therapy:** Monitor vital signs; address precautions or contraindications for exercise, based on patient's pre-existing condition(s)

Understanding the Health Condition

The iliotibial band (ITB) is a thickening of the thigh's tensor fascia latae that is categorized as dense, regular connective tissue.[2,3] The ITB functions during the stance phase of gait to provide stability at the hip joint, resist femoral internal rotation and hip adduction, and to limit tibial internal rotation and anterior translation.[4] Proximally, the ITB originates from the anterolateral iliac tubercle of the iliac crest, envelops the tensor fasciae latae (TFL) muscle, and receives tendinous attachments from the gluteus maximus muscle before extending distally to attach to the lateral patella, the lateral patellar retinaculum, and Gerdy's (lateral tibial) tubercle (Fig. 19-1).[2,5]

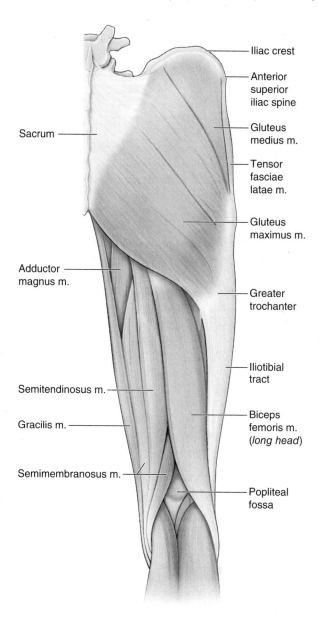

Figure 19-1. Posterior view of hip and leg, showing tensor fasciae latae muscle and its inferior thickened extension as the iliotibial tract (band). (Reproduced with permission from Morton DA, Foreman KB, Albertine KH, eds. The Big Picture: Gross Anatomy. 2nd ed; New York: McGraw-Hill; 2011.)

Table 19-1 DISTAL BANDS AND BONY ATTACHMENTS OF THE ITB	
Broad band	Patella
	Patellar tendon
	Quadriceps tendon
Broad and dense band	Deep fascia
	Gerdy's tubercle
Thin band	Fibular head
	Deep fascia
	Biceps femoris muscle and tendon

Whiteside et al.[5] have identified three distal bands of the ITB: a broad band, a broad and dense central band, and a thin band (Table 19-1). The distal anatomy of the ITB likely helps increase stability on the lateral aspect of the knee.[5]

ITBS is an overuse injury experienced primarily by distance runners.[6] ITBS has also been reported in other athletes (*e.g.*, cyclists) and active individuals (*e.g.*, hikers).[7] The primary symptom associated with ITBS is lateral knee pain.[6-8] Initial symptoms may be mild, with pain experienced at some point during one's run (or activity). If the condition worsens, pain may prevent the individual from training and pain may be present even when at rest.

The onset of the syndrome was originally thought to result from repetitive friction stress, especially to the posterior portion of the distal ITB as it crosses the lateral femoral epicondyle.[4,6-11] It was hypothesized that the ITB slides anterior to the lateral femoral epicondyle during knee extension and posterior to the lateral femoral epicondyle during knee flexion.[6,8] Repetitive movement of the ITB over the lateral femoral epicondyle was believed to inflame a bursa and/or the tract itself.[4,10] This "movement" of the ITB across the lateral femoral epicondyle occurs at approximately 30° of knee flexion (referred to as the impingement zone).[6,8] The precise structures that are actually impinged between the ITB and the femoral epicondyle have been debated.[2,8] Anatomical studies suggest that innervated fat and connective tissue are compressed between the ITB and the epicondyle.[2,3] Fairclough et al.[2] have suggested that the ITB does not truly slide across the epicondyle. Based on their study of 15 human cadavers (anatomical and microscopic analysis) and six asymptomatic subjects (magnetic resonance imaging), different fibers of the ITB are tensed throughout the range of knee flexion and extension. Instead of an anterior-posterior *slide* creating friction leading to ITBS, they propose that pain onset is due to *compression* of the fat between the ITB and the femur.[2]

ITBS may be the result of extrinsic and/or intrinsic risk factors. **Extrinsic factors that have been proposed to contribute to the onset of ITBS** include poor footwear, increasing weekly training distances too quickly, running too many miles in general, and running downhill.[6,9,12] **Potential intrinsic risk factors** include hip adduction and knee internal rotation when running, weakness in the hip abductors, muscular imbalance around the hip, and muscular tightness in the lower extremity.[6,9-15]

Physical Therapy Patient/Client Management

There may be one or more appropriate interventions based on the patient's presentation. Physical therapy interventions include modalities, soft tissue mobilization, therapeutic exercise, footwear evaluation, running evaluation, and/or orthotics.[6,8,14] Some patients may benefit from prescription nonsteroidal anti-inflammatory drugs (NSAIDs) or combinations of glucocorticoid injections.[7,9] In recalcitrant cases, the patient may require a surgical consult with an orthopedic physician.[9,16,17] The primary goal for most injured athletes/individuals is to return to pain-free sport or activity as quickly and safely as possible in a manner that does not overload the healing tissues.

Examination, Evaluation, and Diagnosis

Individuals presenting with symptoms consistent with ITBS are likely to be distance runners.[6] The injured distance runner describes pain at the lateral knee when running. In some cases, pain may also be present at rest. During the history portion of the examination, the physical therapist asks the patient questions regarding their medical history. In addition, the physical therapist inquires about the patient's specific training habits, including types of surfaces the individual trains on (*e.g.*, flat terrain or hills) and which positions or activities reproduce symptoms when not running. For example, an individual with ITBS may report running on a track in only one direction or running on the crown of a road. The patient may experience pain running downhill, descending stairs, walking, or sitting with the injured leg flexed.[6]

A comprehensive musculoskeletal examination must be conducted to rule out other potential sources of lateral knee pain, including lateral collateral ligament sprain, meniscal injury, or patellofemoral pain. Musculoskeletal findings consistent with ITBS include pain with palpation to the distal ITB near the lateral femoral epicondyle, pain with palpation to trigger points in the ITB, TFL, biceps femoris, and/or the vastus lateralis, lack of muscular flexibility in the involved lower extremity, and asymmetrical lower extremity strength.[6,18,19] Proximally, the muscles of the hip and thigh may present with asymmetrical tightness between the involved and uninvolved side. Wang *et al.*[20] found that distance runners were significantly less flexible than healthy controls in their gastrocnemius, soleus, and hamstring muscles. In addition, hamstring muscles in the runner's dominant leg were significantly less flexible than the hamstrings in the nondominant leg. Patients with ITBS often present with positive findings during the Noble Compression test (Fig. 19-2) or the Ober test (Fig. 19-3; Table 19-2).[6,9] The performance of manual muscle tests is critical to assess the strength of the hip and thigh muscles.[18,21] Fredericson *et al.*[18] identified hip abductor weakness on the involved side of 24 injured distance runners with ITBS (10 females, mean age 27 years). Niemuth *et al.*[21] assessed hip strength in 30 recreational runners with a unilateral lower extremity overuse injury. Injured runners (30% of whom presented with ITBS) had significantly weaker hip abductor and flexor strength compared to their uninvolved leg.

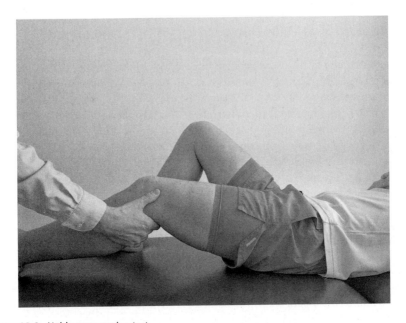

Figure 19-2. Noble compression test.

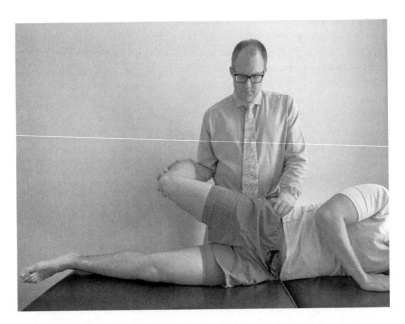

Figure 19-3. Ober test.

Table 19-2 FLEXIBILITY AND SPECIAL TESTS ASSOCIATED WITH ITBS

Tests	Patient Position	Findings
Thomas test	Patient sits at the edge of treatment table. Therapist assists patient into supine position or patient lies supine independently. Patient brings both knees to the chest. The leg to be tested is released and allowed to extend toward the table.	Asymmetrical hip extension is a positive sign of tight hip flexors (iliopsoas).
Passive straight leg raise	Patient lies supine on treatment table. The therapist passively elevates the straight leg to the point of either increased muscular tension or loss of a neutral pelvic position.	Hamstring tightness is noted with either an asymmetry between lower extremities or a general lack of flexibility.
Noble compression test (Fig. 19-2)	Patient lies supine. Therapist passively flexes knee to approximately 90°. Therapist applies pressure to distal ITB near the femoral epicondyle and passively extends patient's knee.	Report of pain at ~30° of knee flexion is a positive sign.
Ober test (Fig. 19-3)	Patient assumes sidelying position on the unaffected lower extremity. Therapist passively flexes the top knee to 90°. The therapist's proximal hand (one closest to hip) stabilizes the pelvis while the distal hand abducts and extends the hip.	An inability of the hip to adduct toward the table suggests tightness in the tensor fasciae latae/iliotibial band.

Plan of Care and Interventions

Physical therapy interventions must address findings from the musculoskeletal examination. To help reduce pain in the acute phase, modalities may be beneficial. To address muscular tightness and weakness, therapeutic exercises are prescribed.[4,6,8,18,19,22,23]

A standardized 6-week (1 session per week) treatment program consisting of rest, NSAIDs, and physical therapy interventions statistically improved hip abductor strength and successfully enabled a majority (22 of 24) of injured runners with ITBS to return to running.[18] In this study, Fredericson et al.[18] performed **phonophoresis** (parameters not presented) for up to two sessions. Patients were also prescribed two stretching and two strengthening exercises. The stretching exercises (a supine ITB stretch using a rope and a standing ITB stretch) were performed 3 times per day with each stretch held for 15 seconds each. Two strengthening exercises—the sidelying hip abduction and the standing pelvic drop—were progressed from an initial dosing of one set of 15 repetitions, with the patient adding 5 repetitions per day, to a goal of performing 3 sets of 30 repetitions.

Fredericson et al.[6,8,18,19,23] have spent years investigating the most effective ITBS interventions, resulting in precise treatment recommendations that reflect an appreciation for the different phases of tissue healing. During the acute phase, it is recommended that patients rest and avoid pain-provoking activities. Modalities are also introduced to decrease pain and inflammation. To reduce inflammation, oral NSAIDs are recommended. For patients experiencing intense pain, glucocorticoid injection was also recommended.[8] During the subacute phase of healing, **stretching**

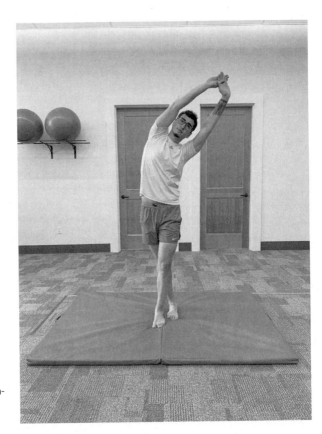

Figure 19-4. Patient performing standing ITB stretch for the right lower extremity.

exercises to address muscular inflexibility should be initiated. Fredericson *et al.*[23] reported that the position that creates the most effective stretch is the standing ITB position with overhead arm extension (Fig. 19-4). It is important to highlight that stretching exercises intended for the ITB are likely only improving flexibility of the TFL and adjacent muscles and not directly increasing the length of the band.[24,25] In addition to the classic "ITB" stretching exercises, some individuals have reported improved flexibility and decreased pain during and after performing the ITB **foam roll exercise**[7] (Fig. 19-5). While the effectiveness of this foam roll exercise in increasing muscular flexibility is untested, the pain reduction reported by some patients may be due to the pressure applied to trigger points in the TFL or ITB.[8]

Strengthening exercises should also be introduced during the subacute phase.[6,8,18,19] The hip abductors (especially gluteus medius) have been identified as dysfunctional in individuals diagnosed with ITBS.[6,8,18] The gluteus medius (along with gluteus minimus and TFL muscles) maintain pelvic stability during gait and eccentrically contract to resist adduction moments at the hip. Weakness in the hip abductors allows increased hip adduction and knee internal rotation, factors that may contribute to the onset of ITBS.[15] Lower extremity strengthening is progressed from open kinetic chain positions that emphasize concentric muscular contractions (*e.g.*, sidelying hip abduction, pelvic drop exercise) to closed kinetic chain positions emphasizing eccentric muscular contractions (Table 19-3).[6,8]

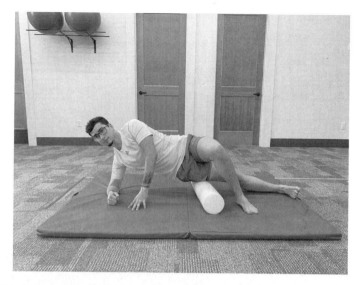

Figure 19-5. Patient performing foam roll exercise. The patient is positioned with involved right ITB on a foam roll, with the uninvolved lower extremity flexed and externally rotated to allow him to place the foot to the front of the involved leg. Both upper extremities are positioned to assist balance.

Table 19-3	ECCENTRIC EXERCISES FOR ITBS	
Eccentric Exercise	**Starting Position**	**Exercise Technique**
Modified matrix exercise	Have the patient stand with lower extremities positioned shoulder width apart. The involved leg (right leg) is externally rotated with the foot oriented in the 3 o'clock position. The uninvolved left leg is positioned with the foot pointing in the 12 o'clock direction (Fig. 19-6A).	Instruct the patient to perform an abdominal bracing contraction prior to initiating the exercise. The movement is performed by having the patient rotate his hips toward the uninvolved (left) leg, transferring weight from the involved (right) to the uninvolved leg. As the weight-shifting occurs, the involved hip is lowered. Simultaneously, the patient reaches his upper extremity on the involved hip side across his body toward the uninvolved mid-thigh region (Fig. 19-6B). Patient returns to the start position and repeats.
Wallbangers	Have the patient stand with the involved lower extremity (right) positioned 6-12 inches from a wall (Fig. 19-7A).	Have patient flex shoulders to 90° and rotate pelvis away from the wall (Fig. 19-8). As the patient rotates the anterior pelvis away from the wall, he should flex his knees and lower the involved hip (right) toward the wall (Fig. 19-7B). When the involved hip contacts ("bangs") against the wall, the patient returns to the start position (Fig. 19-7A).
Frontal plane lunges	Have the patient start in a standing position.	The first lunge position is performed by placing the uninvolved lower extremity (left) to the side (Fig. 19-8A). The second lunge position is performed with the patient reaching the upper extremities toward the uninvolved side (Fig. 19-8B). The third lunge is performed by reaching the upper extremities toward the weightbearing leg (Fig. 19-8C).

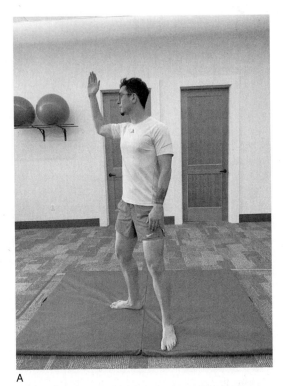

A

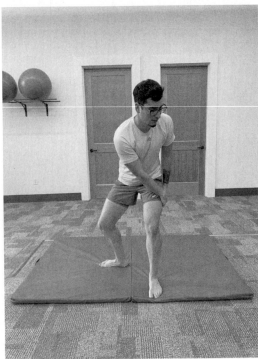

Figure 19-6. Modified matrix exercise. **A.** Starting position. **B.** Ending position.

B

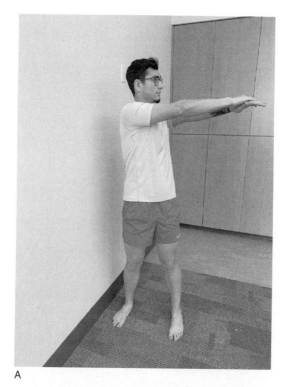

A

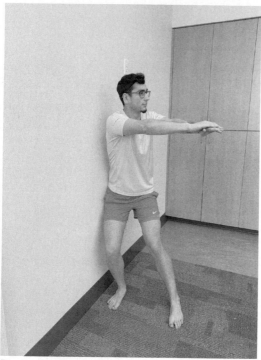

B

Figure 19-7. Wallbangers exercise.
A. Starting position. **B.** Ending
position.

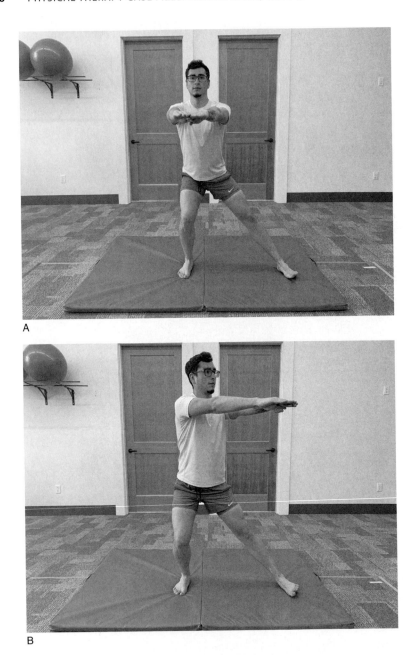

Figure 19-8. Frontal plane lunges. **A**, frontal plane lunge on involved right side. **B**, with reach toward the uninvolved left side. **C**, with reach toward involved right side.

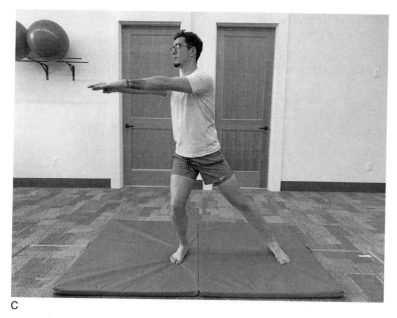

C

Figure 19-8. *(Continued)*

Fredericson *et al.*[6,8] recommended that each eccentric exercise be performed bilaterally for 2 to 3 sets of 5 to 8 repetitions progressing to sets of 15 repetitions.

In the acute and subacute healing phases, therapeutic interventions are aimed at resolving pain and inflammations with rest, anti-inflammatories, modalities, and therapeutic exercise to strengthen weak muscles and stretch tight muscles. As acute symptoms resolve, the goal for many patients is to return to sport participation. Evaluating the patient's training habits and lower extremity biomechanics during sport is warranted. If these skills are outside of the treating therapist's current skill set, referral to a professional coach or to a physical therapist that specializes in correcting biomechanical faults is warranted.

Evidence-Based Clinical Recommendations

SORT: Strength of Recommendation Taxonomy

A: Consistent, good-quality patient-oriented evidence
B: Inconsistent or limited-quality patient-oriented evidence
C: Consensus, disease-oriented evidence, usual practice, expert opinion, or case series

1. Extrinsic risk factors are associated with the onset of iliotibial band syndrome. **Grade C**

2. Intrinsic risk factors are associated with the onset of iliotibial band syndrome. **Grade B**

3. The use of phonophoresis decreases pain associated with ITBS. **Grade C**

4. Stretching and strengthening therapeutic exercises decrease pain and/or restore function in patients with ITBS. **Grade B**

5. Rolling the iliotibial band over a foam roll decreases pain and increases flexibility in patients with ITBS. **Grade C**

COMPREHENSION QUESTIONS

19.1 An outpatient physical therapist examines a distance runner suffering from ITBS in the right lower extremity. The patient presents with right hip abductor weakness. Which of the following lower extremity biomechanical dysfunctions will result from hip abduction weakness?

A. Hip abduction, knee external rotation

B. Hip abduction, knee internal rotation

C. Hip adduction, knee external rotation

D. Hip adduction, knee internal rotation

19.2 The pain associated with ITBS may not be due to repetitive friction, but rather due to compression of soft tissue. Which of the following soft tissue structures is compressed between the distal ITB and the femoral epicondyle?

A. ITB bursae

B. Lateral patellar ligament

C. Fat

D. Vastus lateralis

ANSWERS

19.1 **D.** The hip abductors are responsible for stabilizing the pelvis and eccentrically contracting to resist hip adduction. Weakness in the hip abductors (*e.g.*, gluteus medius) allows for increased hip adduction and knee internal rotation. In a prospective study of potential risk factors for ITBS, Noehren et al.[15] found that recreational runners with increased peak adduction at the hip and internal rotation at the knee were at an increased risk for ITBS.

19.2 **C.** A recent anatomical investigation by Fairclough et al.[2] identified innervated fat and connective tissue that, if compressed between the ITB and the femoral epicondyle, may contribute to the onset of ITBS.

REFERENCES

1. Simons DG, Travell JG, Simons LS. *Travell and Simons' Myofascial Pain and Dysfunction: The Trigger Point Manual. Volume 1: Upper Half of Body.* 2nd ed. Baltimore, MD: Williams & Wilkins;1999.

2. Fairclough J, Hayashi K, Toumi H, et al. The functional anatomy of the iliotibial band during flexion and extension of the knee: implications for understanding iliotibial band syndrome. *J Anat.* 2006;208:309-316.

3. Fairclough J, Hayashi K, Toumi H, et al. Is iliotibial band syndrome really a friction syndrome? *J Sci Med Sport*. 2007;10:74-76.

4. Geisler PR. Current clinical concepts: synthesizing the available evidence for improved clinical outcomes in iliotibial band impingement syndrome. *J Athl Train*. 2021;56:805-815.

5. Whiteside LA, Roy ME. Anatomy, function, and surgical access of the iliotibial band in total knee arthroplasty. *J Bone Joint Surg Am*. 2009;91:101-106.

6. Fredericson M, Wolf C. Iliotibial band syndrome in runners: innovations in treatment. *Sports Med*. 2005;35:451-459.

7. Cosca DD, Navazio F. Common problems in endurance athletes. *Am Fam Physician*. 2007;76:237-244.

8. Fredericson M, Weir A. Practical management of iliotibial band friction syndrome in runners. *Clin J Sports Med*. 2006;16:261-268.

9. Beals RK. The iliotibial tract: a review. *Curr Orthop Pract*. 2009;20:87-91.

10. Renne JW. The iliotibial band friction syndrome. *J Bone Joint Surg Am*. 1975;57:1110-1111.

11. Kaplan EB. The iliotibial tract: clinical and morphological significance. *J Bone Joint Surg Am*. 1958;40:817-832.

12. Messier SP, Legault C, Schoenlank CR, et al. Risk factors and mechanisms of 3nee injury in runners. *Med Sci Sports Exerc*. 2008;40:1873-1879.

13. Richards DP, Alan Barber F, Troop RL. Iliotibial band z-lengthening. *Arthroscopy*. 2003;19:326-329.

14. Strakowski JA, Jamil T. Management of common running injuries. *Phys Med Rehabil Clin N Am*. 2006;17:537-552.

15. Noehren B, Davis I, Hamill J. ASB clinical biomechanics award winner 2006 prospective study of the biomechanical factors associated with iliotibial band syndrome. *Clin Biomech*. 2007;22:951-956.

16. Michels F, Jambou S, Allard M, et al. An arthroscopic technique to treat the iliotibial band syndrome. *Knee Surg Sports Traumatol Arthrosc*. 2009;17:233-236.

17. Barber FA, Boothby MH, Troop RL. Z-plasty lengthening for iliotibial band friction syndrome. *J Knee Surg*. 2007;20:281-284.

18. Fredericson M, Cookingham CL, Chaudhari AM, et al. Hip abductor weakness in distance runners with iliotibial band syndrome. *Clin J Sports Med*. 2000;10:169-175.

19. Baker RL, Fredericson M. Iliotibial band syndrome in runners. Biomechanical implications and exercise interventions. *Phys Med Rehabil Clin N Am*. 2016;27:53-77.

20. Wang SS, Whitney SL, Burdett RG, Janosky JE. Lower extremity muscular flexibility in long distance runners. *J Orthop Sports Phys Ther*. 1993;17:102-107.

21. Niemuth PE, Johnson RJ, Myers MJ, Thieman TJ. Hip muscle weakness and overuse injuries in recreational runners. *Clin J Sports Med*. 2005;15:14-21.

22. Beers A, Ryan M, Kasubuchi Z, et al. Effects of multi-modal physiotherapy, including hip abductor strengthening, in patients with iliotibial band friction syndrome. *Physiother Can*. 2008;60:180-188.

23. Fredericson M, White JJ, Macmahon JM, Andriacchi TP. Quantitative analysis of the relative effectiveness of 3 iliotibial band stretches. *Arch Phys Med Rehabil*. 2002;83:589-592.

24. Falvey EC, Clark RA, Franklyn-Miller A, et al. Iliotibial band syndrome: an examination of the evidence behind a number of treatment options. *Scand J Med Sci Sports*. 2010;20:580-587.

25. Seeber GH, Wilhelm MP, Sizer PS Jr, et al. The tensile behaviors of the iliotibial band – a cadaveric investigation. *Int J Sports Phys Ther*. 2020;15:451-459.

Patellofemoral Pain

Robert C. Manske

A 16-year-old female competitive volleyball player with a 2-year history of intermittent anterior right knee pain and swelling is referred to physical therapy for evaluation and treatment. Six weeks ago, she had a fat pad debridement surgery and has been going to physical therapy sessions at another outpatient physical therapy facility. Each time she returns to volleyball, her pain and swelling return. Each of the activities required for volleyball (running, cutting, jumping, pivoting) increases her pain. During the 2 years prior to surgery, her pain was isolated to the medial aspect of her knee. Since surgery, she has pain on both sides of the knee. In the last 4 weeks, her pain and swelling is similar to what she experienced prior to surgery. With either an increase in practice or game frequency, the anterior knee pain increases to 8/10 from a baseline of 1/10 on a visual analog scale. With a couple of days of rest, the pain and swelling are eliminated. She has tried multiple treatments (*e.g.*, ice, heat, compression, over-the-counter nonsteroidal anti-inflammatories), which have provided symptomatic relief for a short duration and are only effective if she is not playing volleyball. For the last 6 weeks, her physical therapy sessions have primarily focused on knee-strengthening exercises, but her pain and swelling have not been effectively reduced. Her goal is to return to volleyball symptom-free now that the season has started. Her physician has not placed any restrictions on her activity.

▸ Based on her health condition, what do you anticipate are contributors to activity limitations?
▸ What are the examination priorities?
▸ What are the most appropriate physical therapy interventions?
▸ What precautions should be taken during physical therapy interventions?

KEY DEFINITIONS

FAT PAD: Area of highly vascularized adipose tissue directly beneath the patellar ligament that can become a source of anterior knee pain; its role is thought to help lubricate and cushion the patellar ligament from stress.

LATERAL BUTTRESS EFFECT: Effect of the higher lateral patellar trochlea on the anterior surface of the distal femur; the higher lateral trochlea resists the natural lateral translation of the patella during knee flexion and extension.

PATELLOFEMORAL PAIN: Also known as anterior knee pain; one of the most common forms of chronic pain in or around the anterior knee and usually has insidious onset

REGIONAL INTERDEPENDENCE: Theory that dysfunction either proximal, distal, or both from the knee joint may cause localized pain in and around the anterior knee

SCREW-HOME MECHANISM: Obligate lateral tibial rotation that occurs during the last few degrees of knee extension as the tibia glides along the longer medial femoral condyle

Objectives

1. Describe patellofemoral pain.
2. Describe examination tests, including diagnostic imaging, that are used in the differential diagnosis of nontraumatic knee injuries.
3. Identify methods to assess for regional interdependence.
4. Describe common muscle weaknesses that may contribute to patellofemoral pain.
5. Select appropriate treatment interventions for the individual with patellofemoral pain.
6. Prescribe exercises to treat patellofemoral pain that may be caused by sources other thans the knee.

Physical Therapy Considerations

Physical therapy considerations during management of the individual with patellofemoral pain:

▶ **General physical therapy plan of care/goals:** Decrease pain; increase flexibility; increase lower quadrant strength; prevent or minimize loss of aerobic fitness capacity

▶ **Physical therapy interventions:** Patient education regarding functional anatomy and injury pathomechanics; modalities and manual therapy to decrease pain; flexibility exercises; resistance exercises to increase endurance of core muscles and to increase strength of lower extremity muscles around the hip; aerobic exercise program; home exercise program with emphasis on strengthening symptomatic lower extremity in positions that do not allow compensatory patterns

▶ **Precautions during physical therapy:** Monitor vital signs; address precautions or contraindications for exercise, based on patient's pre-existing condition(s)

Understanding the Health Condition

Patellofemoral pain (PFP), also known as anterior knee pain, is one of the most common chronic knee musculoskeletal conditions in relatively active adolescents and adults. The incidence of PFP ranges from 9% to 15% in active young populations,[1-5] and up to 22.7% in the general population annually.[6] Recent evidence has concurred with the historical perspective that **PFP occurs most often in females.**[7-9] PFP is usually a diffuse anterior knee pain that is aggravated with activities that increase compressive forces across the knee. These types of activities include ascending and descending stairs, squatting, and prolonged sitting.[10-13]

Physical therapy has historically been recommended in clinical practice guidelines for those with PFP.[14,15] Timing of therapy likely plays a role in decreasing unnecessary imaging, pharmacological management, or prolonged treatments as has been shown for some musculoskeletal spinal conditions.[16-18] Recently, it has been shown that individuals with PFP that received therapy within the first 30 days of their diagnosis were less likely to receive additional medical care including radiographs, advanced imaging, medications, and glucocorticoid injections.[19]

To better understand PFP, a basic review of normal patellofemoral anatomy is needed. The patella is a large sesamoid bone embedded within the tendon of the quadriceps muscles. The bone is shaped like an inverted triangle with the apex directed inferior and the base superior. Both the superior and inferior aspects are roughened for the attachments of the quadriceps and the patellar ligament, respectively. The anterior surface of the patella is convex in each direction, while the posterior surface has two slightly concave regions called facets. The posterior surface is covered with articular cartilage 5 to 7 mm thick in the mid-patellar region and narrowing to less than 1 mm thick along its periphery.[20-23] The lateral portion of the patella in the area of the lateral facet has increased bone mineral density, indicating provision of more bony support and possible stress shielding.[24] Within the distal portion of the femur is the femoral sulcus, or patellar or trochlear groove. This groove is a ridge that articulates with the posterior portion of the patella. Normally, the lateral trochlear facet of the patella is higher than the medial. A common form of PFP comes from patellar instability. This occurs when the patella cannot maintain a stable location on the anterior knee and the patient has symptoms of the knee "giving way." This may be caused by a trochlear dysplasia in which the lateral facet is not of optimal height. This anatomic variation leads to a decreased lateral buttress effect, meaning that with active quadriceps contractions, the patella translates laterally instead of directly within the patellar groove.

Although the patella acts as a bony shield along the anterior knee, its other more important function is to guide the quadriceps tendon and increase the moment arm for the quadriceps muscle. Because the tendon of the quadriceps inserts onto the patella, the moment arm of the muscle is located at a further distance from the axis of knee motion. A longer moment arm facilitates knee extension by increasing the distance of the extensor mechanism from the center of the knee joint. This extensor moment arm appears to provide the greatest quadriceps torque at roughly 20° to 60° of knee flexion.[25,26] This range of motion is also the range in which the greatest amount of patellofemoral compressive force occurs. As knee flexion motion increases during weightbearing, compressive forces increase as the angle between the femur and tibia becomes more acute and the lever arm between the two increases. Contact forces on the posterior patella are 0.5 to 1.5 times one's body weight with walking, 3 times body weight with stairs, and up to 8 times body weight with squatting.[25-28]

Physical Therapy Patient/Client Management

For most individuals with PFP, a nonsurgical approach is advocated because it usually decreases pain and allows return to prior functional levels.[4,29-32] Recent evidence shows an association between PFP and altered lower extremity kinematics caused by proximal and/or distal influences.[5,13,33-47] This proximal or distal influence is commonly referred to as regional interdependence, meaning that PFP may be caused by etiology *outside* of the knee itself. For example, patellofemoral tracking abnormalities could be caused by weakness in proximal hip musculature,[14,48] knee muscles,[49,50] or from structural abnormalities at the foot and ankle. In addition, individuals with PFP appear to have decreased rates of force development and power.[51,52]

Examination, Evaluation, and Diagnosis

The clinical examination begins with a review of the patient's current symptoms. For the person with PFP, this begins with observation of the knee and gait analysis. The patient reports that her anterior knee pain is approximately 2-3/10 on the VAS (0 = no pain and 10 = worst pain possible) today. Her pain can increase to 8/10 during and after playing volleyball. She also reports that the skin around her knee turns bluish following volleyball practice or competition, although during the examination the skin is observed to be normal in color and texture. She has several incision sites from her prior fat pad debridement that are well healed with no signs of redness or infection. Although no gait deviations were observed today, it is not uncommon to see excessive foot pronation during weight acceptance to mid-stance phase of gait. In patients with significant proximal hip weakness, a Trendelenburg gait pattern with contralateral hip drop during the swing-through phase and a trunk lean toward the weak side (abductor lurch) during stance phase may be observed.

Her knee range of motion (ROM) is not quite symmetrical. On the left, she has 7°-0°-155°, while on the right (symptomatic), she has 2°-0°-155°. This notation means that on her *uninvolved* side, her knee ROM is from 7° of hyperextension to 155° of flexion, while on her *symptomatic* side, she has a 5° deficit of knee hyperextension. The therapist noted that she also has approximately 50% loss of passive and active external tibial rotation (measured with the knee in 90° of knee flexion). This decreased tibial rotation may be why she has lost some terminal knee extension due to the obligate external tibial rotation required during the screw-home mechanism at the tibiofemoral joint.

Her lower extremity strength was nearly normal on the uninvolved left side with quadriceps and hamstrings graded at 5/5 and hip abductors, extensors, and lateral rotators graded 4⁺/5. On the right side, quadriceps and hamstrings were graded 5/5, but the hip abductors, extensors, and lateral rotators were graded 4/5. Though the overall strength in her hip musculature was normal or good, she exhibited abnormal motor control patterns when she was asked to perform a functional test of hip strength. With both the step-down test,[53,54] and the right single-leg squat, she demonstrated a dramatic amount of valgus collapse with concomitant hip adduction and tibial abduction (Fig. 20-1). In adults, the step-down test highlights differences between those with PFP and controls.[55] Crossley et al.[56] have found that poor performance on the single-leg squat task indicates functional hip abductor muscle weakness. To enable clinicians to record clear objective data, they made recommendations on what constitutes a poor single-leg squat (Table 20-1). When this patient was asked to perform the single-leg squat task on the uninvolved side, these patterns did not occur. The patient also reported pain with a new provocation test, in which pain is assessed during a 45-second hold of a single-leg squat

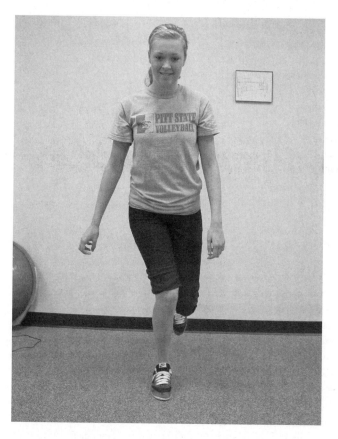

Figure 20-1. Knee valgus collapse with single-leg squat.

Table 20-1   POSSIBLE COMPENSATORY PATTERNS DURING SINGLE-LEG SQUAT

Trunk/Posture	Pelvis	Hip	Knee
Lateral deviation/shift	Shunt or lateral deviation	Adduction	Valgus
Rotation	Rotation	Femoral internal rotation	Knee not over foot
Lateral flexion	Tilt		
Forward flexion			

position in 60° knee flexion.[57] In adolescents, the 45-second anterior knee pain provocation test can adequately discriminate anterior knee pain and can also be used to demonstrate improvements in self-reported knee pain. [57]

To complete a thorough neurologic screen, sensation and reflexes should be tested. The patient had normal sensation to light and deep touch along lower extremity dermatomes bilaterally. Patellar and Achilles deep tendon reflexes were normal and symmetrical (2/3 bilaterally). Deep tendon reflexes were graded as 0 = no reflex or absent; 1/3 = hypotonic reflex; 2/3 = normal reflex; and 3/3 = hypertonic reflex.[58]

It is important for physical therapists to understand basics of musculoskeletal imaging of the knee. For evaluation of most knee injuries, the anteroposterior (AP) and lateral radiographic views are most frequently ordered.[58] In the younger active population, radiographs are ordered to rule out serious pathology such as a tumor or accessory ossification centers. When evaluating the AP view, the clinician should note: the presence of fracture(s), diminished joint space, epiphyseal damage, lipping, loose bodies, alterations in bone texture, abnormal calcifications, ossification, tumors, accessory ossification centers, varus or valgus deformity, patellar position, patella alta or baja, and asymmetry of femoral condyles.[59,60] The lateral view is usually performed with the patient sidelying with slight knee flexion (about 45°). This view allows determination of normal patellar position and the ratio of patellar length to patellar height (to determine patella alta or baja). An axial (or skyline) view is a 30° tangential view, which is ordered if there is suspicion of patellar problems such as dysplasia or subluxation.[61,62]

Plan of Care and Interventions

For the individual with PFP, there are multiple interventions, with varying levels of evidence supporting their efficacy. The treatment for PFP depends on the signs and symptoms found during the clinical examination. The current patient already had surgical intervention for her current complaint and had been treated by several physical therapists. However, none of these interventions allowed her to play volleyball pain-free.

Since the patient was unable to perform single-limb exercises without her right lower extremity falling into valgus collapse, the first exercises prescribed were in supine and in standing with bilateral weightbearing. These initial exercises were chosen to strengthen the hip musculature because she was not able to perform single-limb exercises correctly at this time. Furthermore, evidence continues to support that **strengthening for *both* the hip and quadriceps muscles is more effective than a therapeutic exercise program targeting only the quadriceps.**[63-66] Therapeutic

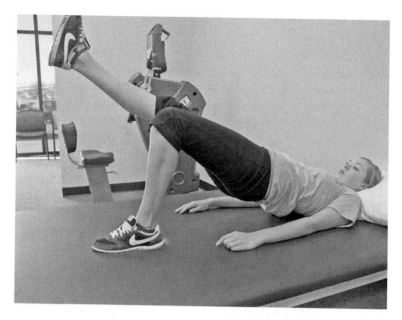

Figure 20-2. Single-leg bridge.

exercises to strengthen the gluteus maximus and medius were first performed with bilateral bridging and then progressed to a bridge with single limb support (Fig. 20-2). A sidelying clam exercise was done to strengthen the gluteus medius and external hip rotators (Fig. 20-3). Resistance tubing around the knees can

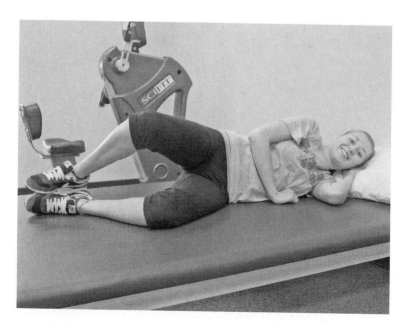

Figure 20-3. Sidelying clam exercise.

be added to increase difficulty. Prone hip extension and sidelying hip abduction exercises were performed to strengthen the gluteus muscles.

Standing exercises are the next appropriate progression. Isometric hip abduction can be performed with the patient's affected extremity against the wall. The patient is asked to contract the core muscles (*e.g.*, perform an abdominal bracing contraction) for stabilization while contracting the gluteus medius. No pelvic movement should occur during this fatiguing exercise because its purpose is to promote *endurance* of the hip musculature. Isotonic exercises facilitate greater gluteus medius activity, especially if performed in single limb stance. Even *greater* gluteus medius activity can be elicited by placing a load in the contralateral hand to that of the stance limb during exercises.[67,68] This can be done by having the patient stand on the symptomatic leg while holding a weight or applying some form of resistance in the opposite arm. Distefano et al.[69] have shown high electromyographic activity in the gluteus medius during lateral band walking, single-limb squat, and the single-limb deadlift. These exercises can be incorporated as soon as the patient is able to tolerate higher-level exercises without exacerbation of symptoms or demonstration of compensatory patterns.

Once strength of the gluteus muscles and external hip rotators improves to 5/5 on manual muscle testing, the patient can be progressed to sports-specific activities like jumping and hopping. Several weeks after initiation of jumping and hopping drills, the patient was formally discharged with a home exercise program of hip and trunk strengthening to maintain the strength and endurance gained during rehabilitation.

Manual therapy techniques can also be performed to gain the lost external tibial rotation identified during the initial examination. For this patient, three sessions of external tibial rotation glides of passive overpressure were needed to gain lost motion (Fig. 20-4). Anterior tibiofemoral glides were also performed to restore to 7° of knee hyperextension.

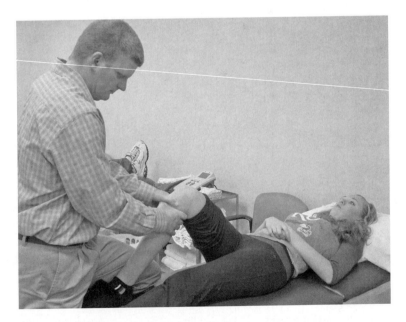

Figure 20-4. Tibial external rotation joint mobilization.

Evidence-Based Clinical Recommendations

SORT: Strength of Recommendation Taxonomy

A: Consistent, good-quality patient-oriented evidence
B: Inconsistent or limited-quality patient-oriented evidence
C: Consensus, disease-oriented evidence, usual practice, expert opinion, or case series

1. Patellofemoral pain is often associated with decreased hip strength in young, active females. **Grade B**

2. Physical therapy interventions decrease pain and disability in the majority of individuals with patellofemoral pain. **Grade B**

3. Strengthening exercises for the gluteus maximus and medius muscles, combined with exercises targeting the muscles of the knee, decrease patellofemoral pain. **Grade A**

COMPREHENSION QUESTIONS

20.1 A patient comes to a physical therapist with a 6-month history of patellofemoral pain. Patellar tendinopathy has been ruled out by the referring physician. She complains of pain with squatting and descending stairs. Despite her pain, she continues to play volleyball and jog for cardiovascular conditioning. What is the MOST appropriate physical therapy intervention that should be done first for this patient?

    A. Increasing quadriceps strength

    B. Increasing quadriceps flexibility

    C. Relative rest

    D. Plyometric jump training

20.2 During examination of dynamic movement patterns of a single-leg squat and step-down test, the physical therapist notices the patient's lower extremity falls into a valgus collapse on the involved side. Which of the following muscle groups is NOT likely to have functional weakness?

    A. Hip flexors

    B. Hip extensors

    C. Hip external rotators

    D. Hip abductors

ANSWERS

20.1 **C.** The patient is already dealing with a chronic painful condition that she has not allowed to adequately heal. The first goal is to encourage relative rest to decrease the overuse that is occurring at the knee. Plyometric jump training would be far too aggressive for this stage of rehabilitation (option D). Without further examination, the physical therapist would be unable to ascertain yet if she needs strengthening or flexibility training (options A and B).

20.3 **A.** Although Tyler *et al.*[47] found the hip flexors to be significantly weak in a population of those with patellofemoral pain, this appears to be a relatively rare finding. In most instances, hip abductors, external rotators, and extensors are weak.

REFERENCES

1. Hetsroni I, Finestone A, Milgrom C, et al. A prospective biomechanical study of the association between foot pronation and the incidence of anterior knee pain among military recruits. *J Bone Joint Surg Br.* 2006;88:905-908.
2. Milgrom C, Finestone A, Eldad A, Shlamkovitch N. Patellofemoral pain caused by overactivity. A prospective study of risk factors in infantry recruits. *J Bone Joint Surg Am.* 1991;73:1041-1043.
3. Schwellnus MP, Jordaan G, Noakes TD. Prevention of common overuse injuries by the use of shock absorbing insoles. A prospective study. *Am J Sports Med.* 1990;18:636-641.
4. Wills AK, Ramasamy A, Ewins DJ, Etherington J. The incidence and occupational outcome of overuse anterior knee pain during army recruit training. *J R Army Med Corps.* 2004;150:264-269.
5. Witvrouw E, Lysens R, Bellemans J, et al. Intrinsic risk factors for the development of anterior knee pain in an athletic population. A two-year prospective study. *Am J Sports Med.* 2000;28:480-489.
6. Smith BE, Selfe J, Thacker D, et al. Incidence and prevalence of patellofemoral pain: A systematic review and meta-analysis. *PLoS One.* 2018;13:e0190892.
7. Boling M, Padua D, Marshall S, et al. Gender differences in the incidence and prevalence of patellofemoral pain syndrome. *Scan J Med Sci Sports.* 2010;20:725-730.
8. DeHaven KE, Lintner DM. Athletic injuries: comparison by age, sport, and gender. *Am J Sports Med.* 1986;14:218-224.
9. Taunton JE, Ryan MB, Clement DB, et al. A retrospective case-control analysis of 2002 running injuries. *Br J Sports Med.* 2002;36:95-101.
10. Barton CJ, Webster KE, Menz HB. Evaluation of the scope and quality of systematic reviews on nonpharmacological conservative treatment for patellofemoral pain syndrome. *J Orthop Sports Phys Ther.* 2008;38:529-541.
11. Bohannon RW. Effect of electrical stimulation to the vastus medialis muscle in a patient with chronically dislocating patella. A case report. *Phys Ther.* 1983;63:1445-1447.
12. Powers CM. Rehabilitation of patellofemoral joint disorders: a critical review. *J Orthop Sports Phys Ther.* 1998;28:345-354.
13. Wilson T, Carter N, Thomas G. A multicenter, single-masked study of medial, neutral, and lateral patellar taping in individuals with patellofemoral pain syndrome. *J Orthop Sports Ther.* 2003;33:437-448.
14. Willy RW, Hoglund LT, Barton CJ, et al. Patellofemoral pain: clinical practice guidelines linked to the international classification of functioning, disability, and health from the academy of

Orthopaedic Physical Therapy of the American Physical Therapy Association. *J Orthop Sports Phys Ther.* 2019;49:CPG1-95.

15. Crossley KM, van Middelkoop M, Callaghan MH, et al. 2016 patellofemoral pain consensus statement from the 4th International patellofemoral pain research retreat, Manchester. Part 2: recommended physical interventions (exercise, taping, bracing, foot orthoses and combined interventions). *Br J Sports Med.* 2016;50(14):844-852.

16. Horn ME, Fritz JM. Timing of physical therapy consultation on 1-year healthcare utilization and costs in patients seeking care for neck pain: a retrospective cohort. *BMC Health Serv Res.* 2018;18:887.

17. Ojha HA, Wyrsta NJ, Davenport TE, et al. Timing of physical therapy initiation for nonsurgical management of musculoskeletal disorders and effects on patient outcomes a systematic review. *J Orthop Sports Phys Ther.* 2016;46:56-70.

18. Arnold E, La Barroie J, DaSilva L, et al. The effect of timing of physical therapy for acute low back pain on health services utilization: a systematic review. *Arch Phys Med Rehabil.* 2019;100:1324-1338.

19. Young JL, Snodgrass SJ, Cleland JA, Rhon DI. Timing of physical therapy for individuals with patellofemoral pain and the influence on healthcare use, costs and recurrence rates: an observational study. *BMC Health Services Res.* 2021;21:751.

20. Fulkerson JP. *Disorders of the Patellofemoral Joint.* 3rd ed. Baltimore, MD: Williams & Wilkins;1997.

21. Fulkerson JP. Diagnosis and treatment of patients with patellofemoral pain. *Am J Sports Med.* 2002;30:447-456.

22. Grelsamer RP, Weinstein CH. Applied biomechanics of the patella. *Clin Orthop Rel Res.* 2001;389:9-14.

23. Heegaard J, Leyvraz PF, Curnier A, et al. The biomechanics of the human patella during passive knee flexion. *J Biomech.* 1995;28:1265-1279.

24. Leppala J, Kannus P, Natri A, et al. Bone mineral density in the chronic patellofemoral pain syndrome. *Calcif Tissue Int.* 1998;62:548-553.

25. Huberti HH, Hayes WC. Patellofemoral contact pressures. The incidence of q-angle and tendofemoral contact. *J Bone Joint Surg.* 1984;66:715-724.

26. Huberti HH, Hayes WC, Stone JL, Shybut GT. Force ratios in the quadriceps tendon and ligamentum patella. *J Orthop Res.* 1984;21:49-54.

27. Perry EC, Strother RT. Patellalgia. *Phys Sports Med.* 1985;13:43-59.

28. Reilly DT, Martens M. Experimental analysis of the quadriceps muscle force and patello-femoral joint reaction force for various activities. *Acta Orthop Scan.* 1972;43:126-137.

29. Manske RC, Davies GJ. A nonsurgical approach to examination and treatment of the patellofemoral joint, part I: examination of the patellofemoral joint. *Crit Rev Phys Rehabil Med.* 2003;15:141-166.

30. Manske RC, Davies GJ. A nonsurgical approach to examination and treatment of the patellofemoral joint, part 2: pathology and nonsurgical treatment of the patellofemoral joint. *Crit Rev Phys Rehabil Med.* 2003;15:253-294.

31. Thomee R. A comprehensive treatment approach for patellofemoral pain syndrome in young women. *Phys Ther.* 1997;77:1690-1703.

32. Wilk KE, Davies GJ, Mangine RE, Malone TR. Patellofemoral disorders: a classification system and clinical guidelines for nonoperative rehabilitation. *J Orthop Sports Phys Ther.* 1998;28:307-322.

33. Bolgla LA, Malone TR, Umberger BR, Uhl TL. Hip strength and hip and knee kinematics during stair descent in females with and without patellofemoral pain syndrome. *J Orthop Sports Phys Ther.* 2008;38:12-18.

34. Cichanowski HR, Schmitt JS, Johnson RJ, Niemuth PE. Hip strength in collegiate female athletes with patellofemoral pain. *Med Sci Sports Exer.* 2007;39:1227-1232.

35. Dierks TA, Manal KT, Hamill J, Davis IS. Proximal and distal influences on hip and knee kinematics in runners with patellofemoral pain during a prolonged run. *J Orthop Sports Phys Ther.* 2008;38:448-456.

36. Fukuda TY, Rossetto FM, Magalhaes E, et al. Short-term effects of hip abductors and lateral rotators strengthening in females with patellofemoral pain syndrome: a randomized controlled trial. *J Orthop Sports Phys Ther.* 2010;40:736-742.

37. Ireland ML, Willson JD, Ballantyne BT, Davis IM. Hip strength in females with and without patellofemoral pain. *J Orthop Sports Phys Ther.* 2003;33:671-676.

38. Leetun DT, Ireland ML, Willson JD, et al. Core stability measures as risk factors for lower extremity injury in athletes. *Med Sci Sports Exerc.* 2004;36:926-934.

39. Lewis CL, Sahrmann SA, Moran DW. Anterior hip joint force increases with hip extension, decreased gluteal force, or decreased iliopsoas force. *J Biomech.* 2007;40:3725-3731.

40. Magalhaes E, Fukuda TY, Sacramento SN, et al. A comparison of hip strength between sedentary females with and without patellofemoral pain syndrome. *J Orthop Sports Phys Ther.* 2010;40: 641-647.

41. Mascal CL, Landel R, Powers C. Management of patellofemoral pain targeting hip, pelvis, and trunk muscle function: 2 case reports. *J Orthop Sports Phys Ther.* 2003;33:642-660.

42. Nakagawa TH, Muniz TB, Baldon Rde M, et al. The effect of additional strengthening of hip abductor and lateral rotator muscles in patellofemoral pain syndrome: a randomized controlled pilot study. *Clin Rehabil.* 2008;22:1051-1060.

43. Piva SR, Goodnite EA, Childs JD. Strength around the hip and flexibility of soft tissue in individuals with and without patellofemoral pain syndrome. *J Orthop Sports Phys Ther.* 2005; 35:793-801.

44. Prins MR, van der Wurff P. Females with patellofemoral pain syndrome have weak hip muscles: a systematic review. *Aust J Physiother.* 2009;55:9-15.

45. Robinson RL, Nee RJ. Analysis of hip strength in females seeking physical therapy treatment for unilateral patellofemoral pain syndrome. *J Orthop Sports Phys Ther.* 2007;37:232-238.

46. Souza RB, Powers CM. Predictors of hip internal rotation during running: an evaluation of hip strength and femoral structure in women with and without patellofemoral pain. *Am J Sports Med.* 2009;37:579-587.

47. Tyler TF, Nicholas SJ, Mullaney MH, McHugh MP. The role of hip muscle function in the treatment of patellofemoral pain syndrome. *Am J Sports Med.* 2006;34:630-636.

48. Rathleff MS, Rathleff CR, Crossley KM, Barton CJ. Is hip strength a risk factor for patellofemoral pain? A systematic review and meta-analysis. *Br J Sports Med.* 2014;48:1088.

49. Duffey MJ, Martin DF, Cannon DW, et al. Etiologic factors associated with anterior knee pain in distance runners. *Med Sci Sports Exerc.* 2000;32:1825-1832.

50. Kaya D, Citaker S, Kerimoglu U, et al. Women with patellofemoral pain syndrome have quadriceps femoris volume and strength deficiency. *Knee Surg Sports Traumatol Arthrosc.* 2011;19:242-247.

51. Nunes GS, Barton CJ, Serrao FV. Impaired knee muscle capacity is correlated to impaired sagittal kinematics during jump landing in females with patellofemoral pain. *J Strength Cond Res.* 2022;36(5):1264-1270.

52. Nunes GS, de Oliveira Silva D, Crossley KM, et al. People with patellofemoral pain have impaired functional performance, that is correlated to hip muscle capacity. *Phys Ther Sport.* 2019;40:85-90.

53. Aminaka N, Gribble PA. Patellar taping, patellofemoral pain syndrome, lower extremity kinematics, and dynamic postural control. *J Athl Train.* 2008;43:21-28.

54. Goto S, Aminaka N, Gribble PA. Lower-extremity muscle activity, kinematics, and dynamic postural control in individuals with patellofemoral pain. *J Sports Rehabil.* 2018;27:505-512.

55. Ophey MH, Bosch K, Khalfallah FZ, et al. The decline step-down test measuring maximum pain-free flexion angle: a reliable and valid performance test in patients with patellofemoral pain. *Phys Ther Sport.* 2019;36:43-50.

56. Crossley KM, Zhang WJ, Schache AG, et al. Performance on the single-leg squat task indicates hip abductor muscle function. *Am J Sports Med.* 2011;39:866-873.

57. Rathleff MS, Holden S, Krommes K, et al. The 45-second anterior knee pain provocation test: a quick test of knee pain and sporting function in 10-14-year-old adolescents with patellofemoral pain. *Phys Ther Sport*. 2022;53:28-33.

58. Magee DJ, Manske RC. *Orthopedic Physical Assessment*. 7th ed. Saunders. St. Louis, MO: Saunders Elsevier;2021:51.

59. Carson WG, Jr, James SL, Larson RL, et al. Patellofemoral disorders: physical and radiographic evaluation. I. Physical examination. *Clin Orthop*. 1984;185:178-186.

60. Merchant AC. Extensor mechanism injuries: Classification and diagnosis. In: Scott WN, ed. *Ligament and Extensor Mechanism Injuries of the Knee: Diagnosis and Treatment*. St. Louis: Mosby, 1991.

61. Beaconsfield T, Pintore E, Maffulli N, Petri GJ. Radiographic measurements in patellofemoral disorders. A review. *Clin Orthop Relat Res*. 1994:308:18-28.

62. Murray TF, Dupont JY, Fulkerson JP. Axial and lateral radiographs in evaluating patellofemoral malalignment. *Am J Sports Med*. 1999;27:580-584.

63. Lack S, Barton C, Sohan O, et al. Proximal muscle rehabilitation is effective for patellofemoral pain: a systematic review with meta-analysis. *Br J Sports Med*. 2015;49:1365-1376.

64. Nascimento LR, Teixeira-Salmalea LF, Souza RB, Resender RA. Hip and knee strengthening is more effective than knee strengthening alone for reducing pain and improving activity in individuals with patellofemoral pain: a systematic review with meta-analysis. *J Orthop Sports Phys Ther*. 2018;48:19-31.

65. Collins NJ, Barton CJ, Van Middlekoop M, et al. 2018 Consensus statement on exercise therapy and physical interventions (orthoses, taping and manual therapy) to treat patellofemoral pain: recommendations from the 5th International Patellofemoral Pain Research Retreat, Gold Coast, Australia, 2017. *Br J Sports Med*. 2018; 52:1170-1178.

66. Willy RW, Hoglund LT, Barton CJ, et al. Patellofemoral pain. *J Orthop Sport Phys Ther*. 2019;49:CPG1-CPG95.

67. Hodges PW, Richardson CA. Contraction of the abdominal muscles associated with movement of the lower limb. *Phys Ther*. 1997;77:132-142.

68. Neumann DA, Cook TM. Effect of load and carrying position of the electromyographic activity of the gluteus medius muscle during walking. *Phys Ther*. 1985;65:305-311.

69. Distefano LJ, Blackburn JT, Marshall SW, Padua DA. Gluteal muscle activation during common therapeutic exercises. *J Orthop Sports Phys Ther*. 2009;39:532-540.

Patellofemoral Pain: Blood Flow Restriction Training

Johnny Owens
Jason Brumitt

CASE 21

A 24-year-old female was referred to physical therapy with a 4-month history of anterior knee pain. She first noted pain when climbing stairs at work. Now, she experiences pain when squatting and after prolonged sitting. By the end of a workday, she describes her pain as a 7/10 on the numerical pain rating scale (NPRS). She reported no known cause for her symptoms. She has used ice and over-the-counter nonsteroidal anti-inflammatories, which have provided temporary pain relief. The patient is not currently participating in an exercise program. In college, she played softball for a National Collegiate Athletic Association Division II institution. However, since graduation and gaining full-time employment, she reports having limited time to exercise. Her goal is to become symptom-free and to initiate a regular physical activity program.

▶ What symptoms are associated with this diagnosis?
▶ What are the most appropriate physical therapy interventions?
▶ What precautions should be taken during physical therapy interventions?

KEY DEFINITIONS

BLOOD FLOW RESTRICTION (BFR) TRAINING: Also known as occlusion training; BFR utilizes a tourniquet system to occlude blood flow in one or more extremities during exercise.

HYPOXIA: Physiologic state in which there is not enough oxygen available to meet tissue requirements

LIMB OCCLUSION PRESSURE (LOP): Pressure (in mmHg) required to occlude arterial blood flow into an extremity; in BFR training, a LOP of 60% to 80% is currently recommended for rehabilitating lower extremity injuries.

MOTOR UNIT: Single alpha motor neuron and all of the skeletal muscle fibers that it innervates

ONE REPETITION MAXIMUM TEST (one repetition max or 1RM): Testing procedure to determine the maximum weight that a person can lift for one repetition

PATELLOFEMORAL PAIN: Musculoskeletal condition marked by anterior knee pain that is provoked by squatting, climbing stairs, and sitting for prolonged periods of time

SIZE PRINCIPLE: Recruitment of motor units that occurs in response to the intensity of skeletal muscle contraction. Physiologically, lower threshold motor units that innervate slow-twitch (type I) muscle fibers are recruited first. These motor units produce low force, but are fatigue-resistant. As force production increases, higher threshold motor units that innervate fast-twitch (type II) muscle fibers are recruited. These units produce significant force, but fatigue more readily.

Objectives

1. Evaluate strength of the lower extremity using 1-repetition maximum.
2. Describe the potential benefits associated with BFR training.
3. Describe the physiological mechanisms associated with BFR training.
4. Prescribe a therapeutic exercise program, including the use of BFR training for an individual with patellofemoral pain.

Physical Therapy Considerations

Physical therapy considerations during management of the individual with patellofemoral pain:

▶ **General physical therapy plan of care/goals:** Decrease pain; increase muscular flexibility; increase muscular strength of the core region and lower extremities; increase aerobic fitness capacity

► **Physical therapy interventions:** Aerobic exercise program; therapeutic exercises to improve muscular flexibility; therapeutic exercise to increase muscular strength of the core region and lower extremities; utilization of BFR training; patient education for self-management of symptoms

► **Complications interfering with physical therapy:** Intolerance to pressure produced by the tourniquet or production of muscle metabolites that occurs with BFR exercise; fear avoidance traits; poor adherence due to delayed-onset muscle soreness (DOMS)

Understanding the Health Condition

A description of patellofemoral joint anatomy and the pathomechanics associated with patellofemoral pain are presented in Case 20.

Blood flow restriction (BFR) training (or BFR therapy) utilizes a tourniquet system (Fig. 21-1) with the pressure cuff attached to the proximal portion of an extremity to occlude blood flow during exercise.[1,2] The use of BFR training allows a person to train at a lower load while experiencing the benefits (*i.e.,* increased

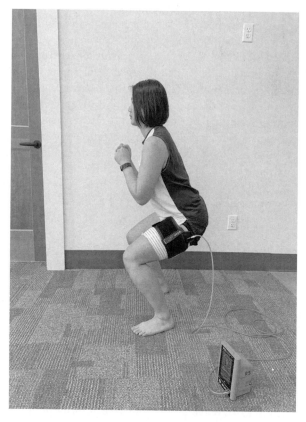

Figure 21-1. Squat with blood flow restriction applied unilaterally to the proximal thigh.

strength and muscle hypertrophy) associated with training at heavier loads.[1,3] BFR training is potentially advantageous for patients who are unable to train with higher loads due to injury, symptom reproduction, or postoperative restrictions.

In the United States, the use of BFR training was initially popularized in military settings to increase muscular strength and size in service members suffering high-energy injuries in combat.[4-6] The successful outcomes observed in these patients led military medical providers to use this technique with other patient populations.[7-9] While the use of BFR in non-military populations is relatively new, the concept and techniques have been reported for decades.[3,10,11] In fact, the first published use of tourniquets with the intention of limb-induced hypoxia for rehabilitation was published in 1937.[12] Proposed physiological mechanisms for hypoxia-induced muscle strength and hypertrophy adaptations associated with BFR include muscle metabolite accumulation, recruitment of high threshold motor units, enhanced gene expression, upregulation of anabolic signaling, and myocyte swelling.[13-23]

Normally, performance of an exercise at a lower percentage of an individual's 1-repetition max (1RM; e.g., 20%-30%) preferentially recruits lower threshold motor units, unless the exercise involves a very large number of repetitions taken to failure. When lifting a weight at a higher percentage of 1RM, higher threshold motor units are recruited. However, many patients may be unable to tolerate or may be restricted from lifting these heavier loads during rehabilitation. The hypoxic environment created by BFR combined with low-load exercise results in an accumulation of muscle metabolites (e.g., lactate) as a byproduct of anaerobic metabolism.[21-23] Lactate inhibits the nearby muscle fibers, which results in increased muscle fiber recruitment and more rapid muscle fatigue. As the individual continues to exercise the limb at a low intensity with the application of BFR, additional motor units are recruited, including those that innervate type II muscle fibers.[24-27] Downstream effects of this hypoxia-induced metabolite response include upregulation of anabolic factors such as growth hormone (GH) and insulin-like growth factor (IGF-1).[19,27-30] Although not directly responsible for muscle growth and hypertrophy, GH may play a secondary permissive role in its ability to enhance collagen synthesis.[31] In contrast, IGF-1 directly upregulates muscle mass by transporting and binding satellite cells (precursors to skeletal muscle fibers) to the resident muscle fibers.[32]

During immobilization or reduced activity, key changes occur in skeletal muscle that result in rapid loss of muscle mass. Muscle protein synthesis is downregulated which is partially responsible for disuse atrophy.[33] In an acute trial, Fujita et al.[29] reported that training at 20% 1RM with BFR increased muscle protein synthesis in healthy untrained males (mean age 32 years) compared to those who trained without BFR. Increases in muscle protein synthesis were also observed in older adults who trained with BFR, whereas those in the non-BFR cohort failed to experience a significant increase.[14,34,35] Reduced activity and injury can also upregulate the gene myostatin (MSTN), which is a negative regulator of muscle mass.[33,36] In healthy and clinical populations, BFR with low-load exercise downregulated MSTN.[18] Last, the application of BFR reduces venous return, resulting in venous congestion that produces a plasma fluid shift from outside to inside the muscle fibers.

This swelling effect may spare muscle mass during periods of disuse via both anabolic and catabolic mechanisms.[37] Although these physiologic mechanisms have been observed in individuals training with BFR, the exact mechanism or the contributions of each to increases in muscle quantity and quality have not been completely elucidated.

Physical Therapy Patient/Client Management

A thorough musculoskeletal examination of the knee including manual muscle tests, goniometric measurements for the hip and thigh, muscular flexibility tests, neurologic screen (*i.e.*, dermatomes, myotomes, and reflex testing), special testing, and palpation must be conducted. Many individuals with PFPS are unable to tolerate training with heavier loads, especially for the knee extensors, but may tolerate and benefit from performing low-load resistance exercises with the addition of BFR.

Examination, Evaluation, and Diagnosis

The examination priorities for individuals with patellofemoral pain are discussed in Case 20. The diagnosis of patellofemoral pain (previously called patellofemoral pain syndrome; PFPS) is indicated if pain is experienced behind the patella (*i.e.*, retropatellar) or adjacent to the patella (*i.e.*, peripatellar) during functional activities like climbing stairs or squatting or when sitting for extended periods, and if no other diagnosis accounts for the pain.[38] When utilizing BFR, the training load is based on a percentage of the individual's 1RM. Although some people can tolerate 1RM testing, most patients cannot due to symptom reproduction or postoperative restrictions. An estimation of 1RM can be made based on the number of repetitions that an individual can perform at a lighter weight. The National Strength and Conditioning Association has published 1RM and training load tables.[39] A variety of prediction equations for estimating 1RM are available, but the therapist should select an equation specific to the patient's requirements. For example, the therapist should not use an equation for a bench press if the goal is to determine 1RM for a squat.[40]

Although adverse events to BFR are rare and the application of vascular occlusion is generally well tolerated, certain populations may not tolerate the pressure produced by the tourniquet. Furthermore, the production of muscle metabolites associated with BFR exercise may be an uncomfortable sensation similar to strenuous exercise. In individuals unaccustomed to exercise or in those that demonstrate fear avoidance traits, BFR may not be tolerated. Last, although muscle damage from BFR training is thought to be minimal, the requisite high volume of repetitions in combination with a build-up of metabolites can lead to DOMS that may interfere with adherence. A thorough discussion of the risks and benefits of BFR must be discussed with the patient before engaging in this intervention. Prior to initiating a rehabilitation program utilizing BFR, the physical therapist must rule out the presence of contraindications for its application (Table 21-1).

Table 21-1 CONTRAINDICATIONS FOR BLOOD FLOW RESTRICTION TRAINING[41,42]
Venous thromboembolism
Impaired circulation or peripheral vascular compromise
Previous revascularization of the extremity
Extremities with dialysis access
Acidosis
Sickle cell anemia
Extremity infection
Tumor distal to the tourniquet
Medications and dietary supplements known to increase clotting risk
Open fracture
Increased intracranial pressure
Open soft tissue injuries
Post-traumatic lengthy hand reconstructions
Severe crushing injuries
Hypertensive crisis (systolic blood pressure >180 mmHg and/or diastolic blood pressure >120 mmHg)
Elbow surgery (with concomitant excess swelling)
Skin grafts that have not completely healed
Secondary or delayed procedures after immobilization
Vascular grafting
Lymphectomies
Cancer

Plan of Care and Interventions

Numerous treatments for PFPS have been described. There are varying degrees of efficacy reported for therapeutic exercise, patellar taping, bracing, foot orthoses, modalities, dry needling, biofeedback, and manual therapy.[38,43] Currently, bracing, modalities, and biofeedback are *not* recommended.[38] In 2019, the American Academy of Orthopaedic Physical Therapy (AAOPT) produced a clinical practice guideline (CPG) recommending that physical therapists prescribe therapeutic exercise (Grade A), with the addition of patellofemoral taping techniques, patella mobilization, and foot orthoses for some patients.[38] The AAOPT's CPG also notes that therapists could use BFR training for those individuals unable to perform exercise with higher loads due to pain.[38] The AAOPT gave BFR training a Grade F (*i.e.*, expert opinion), which reflected the available evidence at that time.

Therapeutic exercise interventions—either open or closed kinetic chain (OKC or CKC)—reduce pain and improve function in individuals with patellofemoral pain.[44-48] For patients unable to tolerate heavier loading that may be required to strengthen the knee extensors, the application of BFR to the affected lower extremity during the lifting of very low loads (*e.g.*, 20%-30% 1RM) may permit initiation of the therapeutic exercises. Then, as symptoms improve, the physical therapist can transition to exercises with heavier loads.

Several studies have demonstrated that low-intensity training performed with BFR is superior to low-intensity training without BFR (and may be as effective as high-intensity training) with respect to increasing strength and cross-sectional area (CSA) of the thigh. Improvements in strength and CSA are observed in patients, untrained individuals, and athletes.[49,50] **Three studies in particular deserve closer attention with respect to strength and CSA increases that can occur in muscles *distal* to the cuff: the quadriceps and hamstrings.** In patients after knee arthroscopy, Tennent et al.[51] reported significantly greater improvements in thigh girth, thigh strength (quadriceps and hamstrings), and time to ascend stairs compared to those who did not perform rehabilitation with BFR. Subjects in both groups participated in the same postoperative protocol; however, those in the BFR group performed three additional exercises with blood flow occluded in the involved extremity. Ferraz et al.[52] randomized 48 women with knee osteoarthritis to either a lower-intensity training group with BFR or without BFR (training at 30% 1RM) or to a higher-intensity training group (training at 80% 1RM). Load and training volume were increased progressively during the 12-week training period. Those in the lower-intensity training groups initially performed 4 sets of 15 repetitions at 20% 1RM, with limb occlusion pressure (LOP) set to 70% in the BFR group. Training load was increased to 30% 1RM at week 2 and by week 5 they performed 5 sets of each exercise. Subjects in the higher-intensity training group performed 4 sets of 10 repetitions of each exercise at 50% 1RM. By week 2, the training intensity was set at 80% 1RM and by week 5, they were performing 5 sets of 10 repetitions per exercise. Every 4 weeks, 1RM was reassessed and training loads were adjusted based on test performance. Bilateral leg press and knee extension exercises were performed by all subjects twice per week over the 12-week training period. Those in the lower-intensity BFR group and the higher-intensity group experienced significant gains in leg press strength, knee extension strength, and CSA.[52] Last, Takarada et al.[53] randomized 18 young male athletes to one of three groups: low intensity exercise with or without BFR and a BFR group without exercise. The exercise groups performed seated bilateral knee extension (90°-0°) twice per week for 8 weeks at approximately 20% 1RM. Five sets were performed to failure (mean repetitions per set 16.8 ± 2.1). The limb occlusion groups had tourniquets applied bilaterally with a mean pressure of 218 ± 8.1 mmHg (similar pressure for the occlusion group that did not perform exercise). Significant increases in isometric and isokinetic strength was observed in the BFR group, but no changes were observed in the other two groups. In the BFR training group, there was also a significant increase in knee extensor muscle CSA.

Strength gains *proximal* to cuff application have also been demonstrated. Bowman et al.[54] randomized untrained individuals to a BFR or a non-BFR group. Subjects performed 4 exercises bilaterally: straight leg raise, sidelying hip abduction, long-arc quadriceps extension (Fig. 21-2), and standing hamstring curl. Subjects performed exercises twice per week for 8 weeks with a training load of 30% 1RM. Four sets of each exercise were performed (repetitions: 30/15/15/15) with those

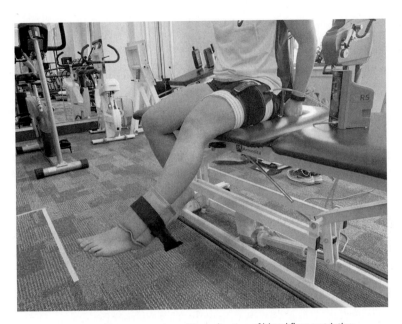

Figure 21-2. Long arc quadriceps extension with application of blood flow restriction.

in the BFR group only having one of their legs occluded (around the proximal thigh). The authors found significant increases in thigh and leg circumference, knee extension torque and power, hip abduction and extension strength, plantarflexion strength, and total number of single-level heel raises in the BFR-trained limbs versus the non-BFR trained limbs in the control group. In support of potential proximal changes, Abe et al.[13] demonstrated improvements in squat strength and gluteus maximus CSA in subjects who performed low-load BFR squat and hamstring curls, with the cuff positioned around the proximal thigh. Work-matched controls did not demonstrate improvement. The demonstrated *proximal* strength gain is highly relevant in this case because the inclusion of exercises to strengthen hip muscles is well recognized as an important component of a therapeutic exercise program for patients with patellofemoral pain.[38,43,55-57]

To date, three studies have investigated the benefits of BFR for individuals with patellofemoral pain. Giles et al.[58] randomized 79 males and females with PFPS to a BFR group (mean age 28.5 years) or a non-BFR group (mean age 26.7 years). Both groups performed a 5-minute bicycle warm-up followed by a leg press performed from 0° to 60° knee flexion (Fig. 21-3) and leg extension performed from 90° to 45°. Four sets of multiple repetitions (30/15/15/15) were performed at 30% 1RM with LOP set to 60% in the BFR group. After the 8-week training program, both groups improved quadriceps strength, pain scores, and Kujala Anterior Knee Pain Scale scores. However, the **BFR group experienced a 93% greater reduction in pain with ADLs compared to the non-BFR group.** In addition, a subgroup analysis of subjects that had pain during resisted knee extension testing revealed that only the BFR group significantly increased their baseline quadriceps strength. From this, BFR

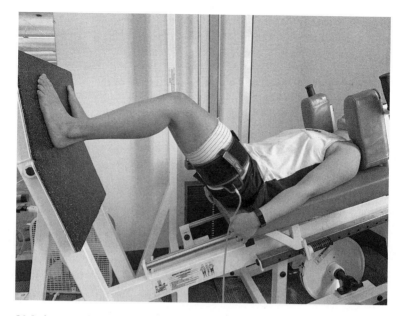

Figure 21-3. Leg press (0°-60°) with single-limb application of blood flow restriction.

may be more appropriate in patients who present with painful knee extension on clinical exam where standard quadriceps strengthening is not tolerated.[58]

Korakakis *et al.*[59] randomized 40 adult males with anterior knee pain (*i.e.*, patellofemoral pain) to a BFR or a non-BFR training group. Their goal was to determine if **exercise with BFR (LOP set to 80%) created a greater hypoalgesic response compared to exercise alone.** The training program consisted of one session performing 4 sets of multiple repetitions (30/15/15/15) of the 90°-0° knee extension exercise. The BFR group experienced significantly greater improvements in pain reduction immediately after exercise and 45 minutes later. In contrast, the non-BFR group experienced a significant decrease in pain in only one of the testing positions and only during the post-exercise period (*i.e.*, 45 minutes after exercise). The pain reduction response after the application of BFR may be the result of an upregulation of endogenous opioids.[60] If so, this may be an additional benefit beyond increases in muscle strength and hypertrophy.

Constantinou *et al.*[61] randomized adults (18-40 years old) with patellofemoral pain to either BFR and exercise (experimental group) or to exercise only (comparison group). The comparison group performed open and closed kinetic chain exercises to strengthen the quadriceps, hamstrings, and the abductors, extensors, and external rotators of the hip. Each exercise was performed for 3 sets of 10 repetitions at 70% of 1RM.[61] This exercise program was performed 3 times per week for 4 weeks with each session lasting 45 minutes. The experimental group performed the same number and frequency of sessions, except that each session lasted 60 minutes. The experimental group performed open and closed kinetic chain exercises to strengthen the quadriceps, hip extensors, and hip abductors. Four sets of each exercise were performed (30 repetitions for the first set followed by 3 sets of 15 repetitions) at 30% of 1RM. LOP was set at 70%. The occlusion pressure was maintained during exercise and the rest period between sets; however, the cuff was deflated for a 2-minute period between each exercise.[61] Both groups also performed stretching exercises for the quadriceps, hamstrings, gastrocnemius-soleus complex, and the iliotibial band (3 repetitions per stretch; 30-second holds per stretch).[61] Both groups experienced significant improvements in pain, kinesiophobia, catastrophizing, and isometric strength of the knee extensors, hip abductors, and hip extensors at the end of treatment and at the 2-month follow-up. However, only the **experimental group experienced significantly greater reductions in *worst* pain immediately following the 4-week study.** The experimental group had significantly greater gains in knee extensor isometric strength than the comparison group at the 2-month follow-up.[61]

There is no established ideal exercise protocol using BFR for individuals with PFPS. A program should consist of multiple exercises that may be OKC or CKC (depending on symptom provocation) that target muscles distal (*i.e.*, thigh) and proximal (*i.e.*, hip) to cuff application.[43,47,48,54-57] Recommended dosing and training volume include performance of exercise with BFR for multiple sets and repetitions (*i.e.*, 4 sets and 30/15/15/15 reps) at a load of 20% to 30% 1RM, and a LOP set at 60% to 80%.

Evidence-Based Clinical Recommendations

SORT: Strength of Recommendation Taxonomy

A: Consistent, good-quality patient-oriented evidence
B: Inconsistent or limited-quality patient-oriented evidence
C: Consensus, disease-oriented evidence, usual practice, expert opinion, or case series

1. In untrained individuals, performing lower extremity exercises with blood flow restriction (BFR) increases strength of the thigh and the hip muscles greater than training without BFR. **Grade A**

2. For individuals with patellofemoral pain, an exercise program performed with BFR significantly reduces pain immediately after exercise, worst pain (after 4 weeks of training), and during ADLs (after 8 weeks of training) compared to those who performed the exercise without BFR. **Grade B**

COMPREHENSION QUESTIONS

21.1 When applying blood flow restriction to the lower extremity, the limb occlusion pressure should be set at what percentage of full occlusion?

   A. 30%

   B. 50%

   C. 60% to 80%

   D. 100%

21.2 Which of the following would NOT be a contraindication for blood flow restriction training?

A. Hypertensive crisis (*e.g.*, 180/130)

B   Stage 1 hypertension (*e.g.*, 135/89)

C. Cancer

D. Open fracture

ANSWERS

21.1 **C.** A LOP of 60% to 80% is recommended when applying BFR to a lower extremity. This range has been associated with increased strength and/or increases in muscular cross-sectional area.[42,54,58,59]

21.2 **B.**

REFERENCES

1. Anderson AB, Owens JG, Patterson SD, et al. Blood flow restriction therapy: from development to applications. *Sports Med Arthrosc Rev.* 2019;27:119-123.

2. Jessee MB, Mattocks KT, Buckner SL, et al. Mechanisms of blood flow restriction: the new testament. *Tech Orthop.* 2018;33:72-79.

3. Kouzaki M, Youshihisa T, Fukunaga T. Efficacy of tourniquet ischemia for strength training with low resistance. *Eur J Appl Physiol Occup Physiol.* 1998;77:189-191.

4. Blair JA, Eisenstein ED, Pierrie SN, et al. Lower extremity limb salvage: lessons learned from 14 years at war. *J Orthop Trauma.* 2016;30 (Suppl 3):S11-S15.

5. Hylden C, Burns T, Stinner D, Owens J. Blood flow strengthening as a rehabilitation modality: a case series. *J Spec Oper Med.* 2015;15(1):50-56.

6. Wilken JM, Roy CW, Shaffer SW. Physical performance limitations after severe lower extremity trauma in military service members. *J Orthop Trauma.* 2018;32:183-189.

7. Cancio J, Rhee P. Blood flow restriction therapy after non-operative management of distal radius fracture: a randomized controlled pilot study. *J Hand Ther.* 2018;31:161.

8. Tennent DJ, Hylden CM, Johnson AE, et al. Blood flow restriction training after knee arthroscopy: a randomized pilot study. *Clin J Sport Med.* 2017;27:245-252.

9. Yow BG, Tennent DJ, Dowd TC, et al. Blood flow restriction training after Achilles tendon rupture. *J Foot Ankle Surg.* 2018;57:635-638.

10. Eiken O, Bjurstedt H. Dynamic exercise in man as influenced by experimental restriction of blood flow in the working muscles. *Acta Physiol Scand.* 1987;131:339-345.

11. Sato Y. The history and future of KAATSU training. *Int J KAATSU Training Res.* 2005;1:1-5.

12. Alam M, Smirk FH. Observations in man upon a blood pressure raising reflex arising from the voluntary muscles. *J Physiol.* 1937;89:372-383.

13. Abe T, Yasuda T, Midorikawa T, et al. Skeletal muscle size and circulating IGF-1 are increased after two weeks of twice daily "KAATSU" resistance training. *Int J Kaatsu Train Res.* 2005;1:6-12.

14. Fry CS, Glynn EL, Drummond MJ, et al. Blood flow restriction exercise stimulates mTORC1 signaling and muscle protein synthesis in older men. *J Appl Physiol.* 2010;108:1199-1209.

15. Gunderman DM, Walker DK, Reidy PT, et al. Activation of mTROC1 signaling and protein synthesis in human muscle following blood flow restriction exercise is inhibited by rapamycin. *Am J Physiol Endocrinol Metab.* 2014;306: E1198-E1204.

16. Loenneke JP, Abe T, Wilson JM, et al. Blood flow restriction: how does it work? *Front Physiol.* 2012;3:392.

17. Loenneke JP, Fahs CA, Thiebaud RS, et al. The acute muscle swelling effects of blood flow restriction. *Acta Physiol Hung.* 2012;99:400-410.

18. Laurentino GC, Ugrinowitsch C, Roschel H, et al. Strength training with blood flow restriction diminishes myostatin gene expression. *Med Sci Sports Exerc.* 2012;44:406-412.

19. Madarame H, Sasaki K, Ishii N. Endocrine responses to upper- and lower-limb resistance exercises with blood flow restriction. *Acta Physiol Hung.* 2010;97:192-200.

20. Pierce JR, Clark BC, Ploutz-Synder LL, Kanaley JA. Growth hormone and muscle function responses to skeletal muscle ischemia. *J Appl Physiol.* 2006;101:1588-1595.

21. Poton R, Polito MD. Hemodynamic response to resistance exercise with and without blood flow restriction in healthy subjects. *Clin Physiol Funct Imaging.* 2016;36:231-236.

22. Takarada Y, Nakamura Y, Aruga S, et al. Rapid increase in plasma growth hormone after low-intensity resistance exercise with vascular occlusion. *J Appl Physiol.* 2000;88:61-65.

23. Scott BR, Loenneke JP, Slattery KM, Dascombe BJ. Exercise with blood flow restriction: an updated evidence-based approach for enhanced muscular development. *Sports Med.* 2015;45:313-325.

24. Miller KS, Garland SJ, Ivanova T, Ohtsuki T. Motor-unit behavior in humans during fatiguing arm movements. *J Neurophysiol.* 1996;75:1629-1636.

25. Moritani T, Sherman WM, Shibata M, et al. Oxygen availability and motor unit activity in humans. *Eur J Appl Occup Physiol.* 1992;64:552-556.

26. Sundberg CJ. Exercise and training during graded leg ischaemia in healthy man with special reference to effects on skeletal muscle. *Acta Physiol Scand Suppl.* 1994;615:1-50.

27. Yasuda T, Abe T, Brechue WF, et al. Venous blood gas and metabolite response to low-intensity muscle contractions with external limb compression. *Metabolism.* 2010;59:1510-1519.

28. Madarame H, Neya M, Ochi E, et al. Cross-transfer effects of resistance training with blood flow restriction. *Med Sci Sports Exerc.* 2008;40:258-263.

29. Fujita S, Abe T, Drummond MJ, et al. Blood flow restriction during low-intensity resistance exercise increases S6K1 phosphorylation and muscle protein synthesis. *J Appl Physiol.* 2007;103:903-910.

30. Takano H, Morita T, Iida H, et al. Hemodynamic and hormonal responses to a short-term low-intensity resistance exercise with the reduction of muscle blood flow. *Eur J Appl Physiol.* 2005; 95:65-73.

31. Doessing S, Heinemeier KM, Holm L, et al. Growth hormone stimulates the collagen synthesis in human tendon and skeletal muscle without affecting myofibrillar protein synthesis. *J Physiol.* 588(Pt 2):341-351.

32. Nielsen JL, Aagaard P, Bech RD, et al. Proliferation of myogenic stem cells in human skeletal muscle in response to low-load resistance training with blood flow restriction. *J Physiol.* 2012;590:4351-4361.

33. Shad BJ, Thompson JL, Holwerda AM, et al. One week of step reduction lowers myofibrillar protein synthesis rates in young men. *Med Sci Sports Exerc.* 2019;51:2125-2134.

34. Kumar V, Selby A, Rankin D, et al. Age-related differences in the dose-response relationship of muscle protein synthesis to resistance exercise in young and old men. *J Physiol.* 2009;587:211-217.

35. Sheffield-Moore M, Paddon-Jones D, Patel R, et al. Mixed muscle and hepatic derived plasma protein metabolism is differentially regulated in older and younger men following resistance exercise. *Am J Physiol Endocrinol Metab.* 2005;288:E922-929.

36. Peck BD, Brightwell CR, Johnson DL, et al. Anterior cruciate ligament tear promotes skeletal muscle myostatin expression, fibrogenic cell expansion, and a decline in muscle quality. *Am J Sports Med.* 2019;47:1385-1395.

37. Kakehi S, Tamura Y, Kubota A, et al. Effects of blood flow restriction on muscle size and gene expression inn muscle during immobilization: a pilot study. *Physiol Rep.* 2020;8:e14516.

38. Willy RW, Hoglund LT, Barton CJ, et al. Patellofemoral Pain. *J Orthop Sports Phys Ther.* 2019;49:CPG1-CPG95.

39. Baechle TR, Earle RW, Wathen D. Chapter 15: Resistance Training. In: Baechle TR, Earle RW, eds. *Essentials of Strength Training and Conditioning.* 4th ed. Human Kinetics;2016:394.

40. LeSuer DA, McCormick JH, Mayhew JL, et al. The accuracy of prediction equations for estimating 1-RM performance in the bench press, squat, and deadlift. *J Strength Cond Res.* 1997;11:211-213.

41. Lorenz DS, Bailey L, Wilk KE, et al. Blood flow restriction training. *J Athl Train.* 2021;56:937-944.

42. Owens J. *Blood Flow Restriction Rehabilitation.* Owens Recovery Science, Inc; 2016.

43. Hott A, Brox JL, Pripp AH, et al. Effectiveness of isolated hip exercise, knee exercise, or free physical activity for patellofemoral pain: a randomized controlled trial. *Am J Sports Med.* 2019;47:1312-1322.

44. Collins NJ, Barton CJ, van Middelkoop M, et al. 2018 Consensus statement on exercise therapy and physical interventions (orthoses, taping and manual therapy) to treat patellofemoral pain: recommendations from the 5th International Patellofemoral Pain Research Retreat, Gold Coast, Australia, 2017. *Br J Sports Med.* 2018;52:1170-1178.

45. Ferber R, Bolgla L, Earl-Boehm JE, et al. Strengthening of the hip and core versus knee muscles for the treatment of patellofemoral pain: a multicenter randomized controlled trial. *J Athl Train.* 2015;50:366-377.

46. Ismail MM, Gamaledein MH, Hassa KA. Closed kinetic chain exercises with or without additional hip strengthening exercises in management of patellofemoral pain syndrome: a randomized controlled trial. *Eur J Phys Rehabil Med.* 2013;49:687-698.

47. Witvrouw E, Lysens R, Bellemans J, et al. Open versus closed kinetic chain exercises for patellofemoral pain. A prospective, randomized study. *Am J Sports Med.* 2000;28:687-694.

48. Witvrouw E, Danneels L, Van Tiggelen D, et al. Open versus closed kinetic chain exercises inn patellofemoral pain: a 5-year prospective randomized study. *Am J Sports Med.* 2004;32:1122-1130.

49. Hughes L, Paton B, Rosenblatt B, et al. Blood flow restriction training in clinical musculoskeletal rehabilitation: a systematic review and meta-analysis. *Br J Sports Med.* 2017;51:1003-1011.

50. Luebbers PE, Fry AC, Kriley LM, Butler MS. The effects of a 7-week practical blood flow restriction program on well-trained collegiate athletes. *J Strength Cond Res.* 2014;28:2270-2280.

51. Tennent DJ, Hylden CM, Johnson AE, et al. Blood flow restriction training after knee arthroscopy: a randomized controlled pilot study. *Clin J Sport Med.* 2017;27:245-252.

52. Ferraz RB, Gualano B, Rodrigues R, et al. Benefits of resistance training with blood flow restriction in knee osteoarthritis. *Med Sci Sports Exerc.* 2018;50:897-905.

53. Takarada Y, Tsuruta T, Ishii N. Cooperative effects of exercise and occlusive stimuli on muscular function in low-intensity resistance exercise with moderate vascular occlusion. *Jpn J Physiol.* 2004;54:585-592.

54. Bowman EN. Proximal, distal, and contralateral effects of blood flow restriction training on the lower extremities: a randomized controlled trial. *Sports Health.* 2019;11:149-156.

55. Mascal CL, Landel R, Powers C. Management of patellofemoral pain targeting hip, pelvis, and trunk muscle function: 2 case reports. *J Orthop Sports Phys Ther.* 2003;33:642-660.

56. Willy RW, Meira EP. Current concepts in biomechanical interventions for patellofemoral pain. *Int J Sports Phys Ther.* 2016;11:87-890.

57. Meira EP, Brumitt J. Influence of the hip on patients with patellofemoral pain syndrome: a systematic review. *Sports Health.* 2011;3:455-465.

58. Giles L, Webster E, McClelland J, Cook JL. Quadriceps strengthening with and without blood flow restriction in the treatment of patellofemoral pain: a double-blind randomised trial. *Br J Sports Med.* 201;51:1688-1694.

59. Korakakis V, Whiteley R, Giakas G. Low load resistance training with blood flow restriction decreases anterior knee pain more than resistance training alone. A pilot randomised controlled trial. *Phys Ther Sport.* 2018;34:121-128.

60. Hughes L, Patterson SD. The effect of blood flow restriction exercise on exercise-induced hypoalgesia and endogenous opioid and endocannabinoid mechanisms of pain modulation. *J Appl Physiol.* 2020;128:914-924.

61. Constantinou A, Mamais I, Papathanasiou G, et al. Comparing hip and knee focused exercises versus hip and knee focused exercises with the use of blood flow restriction training in adults with patellofemoral pain: a randomized controlled trial. *Eur J Phys Rehabil Med.* 2022;58:225-235.

Patellar Tendinopathy

Luke T. O'Brien
Thomas J. Olson
Marcey Keefer Hutchison

CASE 22

A 17-year-old basketball player has been referred to physical therapy by his family physician for evaluation and treatment of anterior knee pain. His pain had been intermittent over the past summer. However, since the start of the fall season, the pain has increased in severity and become constant. Pain is now limiting his ability to practice and play, as well as his ability to negotiate stairs and stand after long periods of sitting. His coach told him that he has "jumper's knee" and that he should "get a knee strap and he should be fine." Plain film images revealed no bony abnormalities, though his tibial and femoral epiphyseal plates are almost completely ossified. The patient's medical history is otherwise unremarkable. Signs and symptoms are consistent with patellar tendinopathy. The patient hopes to finish the basketball season and be ready to compete in an all-star game in the spring.

▶ Based on the patient's symptoms and history, what are the most appropriate examination tests to help confirm the diagnosis of patellar tendinopathy?

▶ What are the most appropriate physical therapy interventions?

▶ What is his rehabilitation prognosis?

KEY DEFINITIONS

APOPTOSIS: Programmed cell death in response to specific stimuli

ECCENTRIC CONTRACTION: Controlled lengthening of a muscle as it responds to an external force greater than the contractile force it is exerting

MUCOID DEGENERATION: Deterioration of collagen fibers into a nonfunctional gelatinous or mucus-like substance

NEOVASCULARIZATION: Formation of new microvascular networks within a tissue that does not normally contain blood vessels, or contains blood vessels of a different type within a tissue

PROTEOGLYCANS: Mucopolysaccharides bound to protein chains in the extracellular matrix of connective tissue

TENDINITIS: Acute inflammation of a tendon, typically affecting its bony insertion; a type of tendinopathy[1]

TENDINOPATHY: Clinical term that encompasses all overuse conditions that affect a tendon (proximally, distally, or midsubstance) in the presence or absence of an inflammatory response; includes tendinosis[2]

TENDINOSIS: Chronic degeneration and a failed healing response within a tendon, but without the presence of characteristic inflammatory markers; a type of tendinopathy[3]

Objectives

1. Explain the distinctions between tendinitis, tendinosis, and tendinopathy.
2. Describe the pathophysiology that contributes to the development of patellar tendinosis.
3. Describe the differential diagnoses for patellar tendinopathy.
4. Prescribe the most appropriate strengthening interventions for patellar tendinopathy based on examination findings.
5. Describe treatment options for individuals with patellar tendinopathy that have failed to improve with conservative management.

Physical Therapy Considerations

Physical therapy considerations during management of the individual with a diagnosis of patellar tendinopathy:

▶ **General physical therapy plan of care/goals:** Decrease pain and increase function; increase lower extremity strength; prevent or minimize loss of aerobic fitness

▶ **Physical therapy interventions:** Patient education regarding functional anatomy and pathophysiology; modalities and manual therapy to decrease pain; management of training volume; incorporation of heavy load or eccentric-focused resistance exercises to promote tendon remodeling; resistance exercises to increase lower extremity stability and strength; aerobic exercise program; patellar tendon straps or unloading tape

▶ **Precautions during physical therapy:** Monitor vital signs; address precautions or contraindications for exercise based on patient's pre-existing condition

▶ **Complications interfering with physical therapy:** Therapist and patient understanding that pain during therapeutic exercise is an accepted part of treating chronic patellar tendinopathy

Understanding the Health Condition

Jumper's knee, incorrectly referred to as patellar tendinitis, was first described in the early 1970s as an overuse syndrome of the knee characterized by pain at the junction of the inferior pole of the patella and the proximal patellar tendon.[4] Although "jumper's knee" seemed to be an acceptable common name for this condition, labeling it "tendinitis" is misleading because the suffix "-itis" refers to an inflammatory process. However, the pathophysiology and pathoanatomy associated with protracted patellar tendon symptoms suggest the presence of little, if any, inflammation. As a result, the clinical condition should be referred to as tendinopathy and the degenerative process described as tendinosis.[3,5,6] Throughout this patient case, the terms will be used in this fashion. Patellar tendinopathy is typically diagnosed in athletes who participate in sports requiring aggressive knee extension and/or repetitive eccentric knee flexion.[3,4] Pain most often occurs over the inferior pole of the patella[7] and interferes with normal training and competition in one of every five elite athletes.[8] Male athletes experience patellar tendinopathy symptoms more frequently than their female counterparts.[8] This latter characteristic may be helpful in differential diagnosis because more general types of anterior knee pain, like patellofemoral pain, is more common in female athletes. The incidence of jumper's knee has been estimated as high as 30% to 50% in basketball and volleyball where jumping is common, but it is also common among soccer players and cross-country runners due to the demands of cutting, rapid acceleration/deceleration, and repetitive impact absorption on the quadriceps.[7-10] Though patellar tendinopathy is most often described as an overuse injury, a single direct trauma can also lead to tendon pathology with the same clinical presentation.[4,11,12]

The patellar tendon is a continuation of the quadriceps tendon. It aids in force transmission from the quadriceps musculature to the bones of the lower extremity, resulting in movement of the hip and knee joints (Fig. 22-1). Though often referred to as the patellar ligament due to its bone-to-bone attachments, the histological appearance and function of the structure is tendinous and therefore, it should be referred to as the patellar tendon.[2] Generally, a tendon is composed primarily of type I collagen fibers arranged hierarchically into bundles called fascicles that are surrounded by connective tissue sheaths. The fascicles are then grouped and surrounded superficially by a two-layered membrane referred to as the paratenon. In addition to collagen, the tendon contains extracellular matrix and tenocytes. The extracellular matrix, or ground substance, is a viscous proteoglycan-rich material

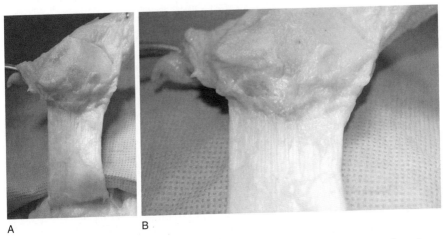

A   B

Figure 22-1. A. Posterior patellar tendon showing average length, with origin at the patella and insertion at the tibial tuberosity. **B.** Posterior aspect of normal patellar tendon. Note absence of fibers over the posterior surface and presence of crescent-shaped fiber alignment with the shortest fibers at the apex of the inferior patellar pole.

that provides support for the collagen fibers and regulates maturation. Tenocytes are flat, elongated cells found in small numbers in the tendon. Tenocytes control the synthesis of ground substance and collagen.[3,13]

Basso et al.[6] investigated the normal cellular structure of the patellar tendon in almost two dozen human cadaveric knees. They demonstrated that fascicles attach to the distal two-thirds of the patella in a crescent-shaped fashion, with the largest concentration found anteriorly. The anterior fascicles are longer than those that attach posteriorly. The blood supply of the patellar tendon originates from the genicular arteries and the anterior tibial artery, and it typically terminates in a network of small arterioles from the paratenon through the deeper connective tissue sheaths.[2,13] Sensory and sympathetic nerve fibers terminate in the paratenon.[3] Under light microscope, a healthy patellar tendon appears shiny, white, and reflective. It consists of densely packed parallel collagen bundles, minimally visible ground substance, and a thin distribution of tenocytes.[5] In contrast, in an individual **with patellar tendinopathy, the tendon appears quite different.** When viewed macroscopically following surgical excision and under a polarized light microscope, there is a loss of reflectivity and the tissue along the posterior proximal origin adjacent to the inferior patellar pole appears yellow and disorganized.[2,5,12] This appearance is known as "mucoid degeneration."[5,12,14] Collagen bundles appear separated due to infiltration of abnormal ground substance and there is microtearing and necrosis of the collagen fibers themselves.[2,5,13,15,16] Changes in tenocyte nuclei and apoptosis are evident and fibroblast infiltration and neovascularization are observed.[2,5,8,13,14,16] Conspicuously absent are the white blood cells (e.g., neutrophils, macrophages) associated with inflammation. Although a brief period of tendinitis cannot be ruled out during the early phases of a tendon overuse injury, by the time patients are symptomatic and seeking treatment, their condition may be a chronic state of tendinosis.[13] By understanding the cellular differences between tendinitis and tendinosis, the physical therapist can appreciate the need to prescribe appropriate interventions to address the degenerative changes associated with tendinosis.

The exact pathogenesis of patellar tendinopathy is unclear, though it is likely a combination of mechanical and biochemical factors that lead to degeneration.[6,8,14,17] Degeneration seems to most commonly affect the posterior fascicles of the patellar tendon. This may be related to the fascicles' crescent alignment both coronally and longitudinally around the inferior patella.[8] The posterior fascicles are typically shorter than those attached anteriorly, and as the patellar tendon elongates during quadriceps muscle contraction and knee flexion, the shorter posterior fascicles are subject to greater strain.[6] Excessive or repeated loading may exceed a tendon's ability to repair itself. Lian and colleagues[8] demonstrated increased tenocyte apoptosis in the patellar tendons of athletes diagnosed with jumper's knee compared to controls without a history of patellar tendinopathy. In animal models, Zhang and Wang[14] found that the concentration of the common inflammatory mediator prostaglandin E2 (PGE2) increases in response to repetitive mechanical loading. When they exposed tendon stem cells to increased concentrations of PGE2 *in vitro*, stem cell production decreased and cell differentiation was altered. The result was an increased production of adipocytes and osteoclasts rather than tenocytes. Thus, repetitive mechanical stress that induces localized increases in PGE2 may decrease the pool of tenocytes available for the tendon repair required by initial overuse of the extensor mechanism.[14] In addition, the neovascularization associated with patellar tendinosis is accompanied by an increased proliferation of substance P-receptive sensory nerve fibers in the tendon itself, not just in the paratenon.[16,17] Increased substance P concentration and nociceptive activity from the tendon increase the perception of pain and may suppress the synthesis of growth factors and inhibit tendon repair.[16,17] Together, these processes contribute to degeneration of the patellar tendon.

The specific combination of risk factors that predispose an athlete to develop patellar tendinopathy are unknown. Identified intrinsic factors include male sex, quadriceps weakness, and decreased quadriceps and hamstring flexibility.[2,3,16,18,19] Extrinsic risk factors include increased training volume and/or intensity, increased ground reaction forces due to activity or training surface, and poor landing mechanics.[2,3,16,18] When examining an athlete with anterior knee pain, these factors must be considered and investigated to assist in the diagnosis of patellar tendinopathy.

Physical Therapy Patient/Client Management

Traditional interventions for patellar tendinosis emphasized reducing inflammation—based on the inaccurate assumption that the condition was a tendinitis. Not surprisingly, common interventions like ultrasound, cross-friction massage, cryotherapy, oral nonsteroidal anti-inflammatories (NSAIDs), and steroidal anti-inflammatory injections have not proven to be effective.[2,4,12,13,20-22] It has been suggested that the use of NSAIDs and glucocorticoid injections are contraindicated because they may exacerbate patellar tendinopathy by masking symptoms which allows the person to continue activity that can cause additional tendon damage, or by increasing cellular degeneration and weakening the tendon.[2,3,13,20,22] Based on the growing body of evidence indicating that patellar tendinopathy is a failed healing response, the cornerstone of the initial plan of care should be interventions addressing the quadriceps muscle and patellar tendon unit, such as activity modification and strengthening.

Examination, Evaluation, and Diagnosis

During the acute and subacute phases, patients who demonstrate symptoms consistent with patellar tendinopathy typically complain of anterior knee pain worsened by athletic activity. As the condition progresses, pain may be experienced during activities of daily living such as stair negotiation and walking downhill. Since numerous pathologies cause anterior knee pain, a thorough history is extremely valuable in developing differential diagnoses. Table 22-1 presents specific components of the patient's history that should be elucidated during the subjective examination.[23,24]

A thorough physical assessment, including diagnostic ultrasound examination of the tendon, is essential to confirm a patellar tendinopathy diagnosis. Since the patellar tendon shares a close anatomical relationship with other potential sources of anterior knee pain, the physical therapist must carefully examine the surrounding

Table 22-1 CONTENT OF QUESTIONS THAT SHOULD BE INCLUDED IN SUBJECTIVE EXAMINATION	
Question Content	Clinical Relevance
History of previous knee surgery	Scarring of the anterior interval and fat pad can cause anterior knee pain[23]
History of patella instability	Disruption of the medial patellofemoral ligament may alter patellofemoral biomechanics
Mechanism of injury	Patellar tendinosis is commonly an overuse injury; however, it may also be the result of a direct blow to the patella tendon[11]
Vocation	Some occupations may predispose the patella tendon to excessive loads (*e.g.*, ski patrol)
Previous injury	Prior injuries to the knee, as well as to the hip and ankle (which may affect biomechanics)
Prior treatments	Athletes that have failed to improve with an eccentric loading program will have a different course of treatment compared to those that failed to improve with use of NSAIDs.
Provocative movements and activities	Identifying painful movement patterns is helpful in the diagnosis and development of training modification plans.
Load, volume, intensity, and duration	Important training variables manipulated incorrectly can overload a tendon resulting in the development of a tendinopathy.[24]

bone and soft tissues to rule out other conditions. Differential diagnoses include patellofemoral pain, patella instability, avulsion fracture, Sinding-Larsen-Johansson syndrome, Osgood-Schlatter disease, anterior interval scarring, fat pad entrapment, meniscal tear, patellar tendon tear, and infrapatellar plica.

Objective findings from four different patient examination positions (supine, seated, seated figure four, and prone) can assist in developing an accurate diagnosis of patellar tendinopathy. In supine, observation of obvious differences in symmetry of the quadriceps musculature may provide clues to the chronicity and severity of the condition. It is also a position in which gross observations, such as a prominent tibial tubercle, can be made to determine the presence of other contributing conditions. With the patient in a seated position, the physical therapist can view the knee from directly above to assess patella tilt and patellar tendon alignment. Figure 22-2 shows a patient seated with the knee in a nonweightbearing position, hanging over

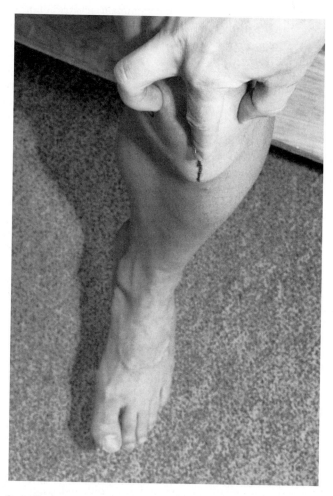

Figure 22-2. Seated knee exam position for observing patellar tendon alignment and the tibial tuberosity. Note the hypertrophied tibial tuberosity secondary to Osgood-Schlatter disease.

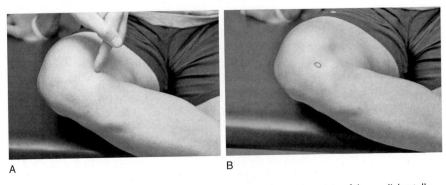

A   B

Figure 22-3. Figure four knee exam position. **A.** Therapist palpates the origin of the medial patellofemoral ligament. **B.** Circle drawn on knee identifies the anterior horn of the medial meniscus.

the edge of the treatment table. In a neutral alignment, a vertical line drawn down the middle of the patellar tendon should bisect the second and third toes. Since the tendon is placed on tension, this is a good position to palpate for tendon defects associated with a patellar tendon tear or rupture. Tibial tuberosity tenderness, with reproduction of the patient's symptoms may indicate Osgood-Schlatter disease. The seated figure four position involves the patient placing the ankle of the limb being examined over the thigh of the opposite leg, which places the limb into maximal external rotation (Fig. 22-3). In this position, the medial collateral ligament shifts posteriorly, exposing the medial meniscus, making it an excellent position to palpate the medial meniscal and the retinacular ligaments. Beginning on the medial side of the knee joint and moving from posterior to anterior, the physical therapist palpates the medial collateral ligament, the medial patellofemoral ligament (Fig. 22-3A), the anterior horn of the medial meniscus (Fig. 22-3B), and the patellar tendon. The lateral joint can then be examined in a similar posterior to anterior order. Tenderness to palpation of structures other than the patellar tendon should direct the therapist to consider competing differential diagnoses. Last, the physical therapist has the patient lie prone with the involved knee hanging over the edge of the treatment table (Fig. 22-4). The compression provided by the edge of the treatment table inhibits the quadriceps, which allows the therapist to assess the anterior knee without unconscious protective guarding. In this prone position, the therapist first assesses patellar excursion and apprehension. Then, by placing fingers on the medial and lateral sides of the patellar tendon and moving inferiorly, the physical therapist can assess the infrapatellar fat pad for size, tenderness, and sagittal mobility (Fig. 22-5). Movement of the fat pad can further be assessed by passively flexing the knee to 90°. The fat pat should be "sucked in" or disappear from underneath the therapist's fingers.[23] Last, the therapist palpates the patellar tendon for thickening and tenderness—signs consistent with patellar tendinopathy. Patients typically report the greatest degree of pain to palpation at the insertion of the tendon to the inferior pole of the patella.[25] However, in jumping athletes (*e.g.*, volleyball players, basketball players, high jumpers), mild tenderness to palpation is considered normal.[25] Thus, the presence of pain with palpation to the tendon should not be used as the *only* test to diagnose patellar tendinopathy; as an isolated clinical test, pain on palpation has poor sensitivity (56%) and specificity (47%).[25]

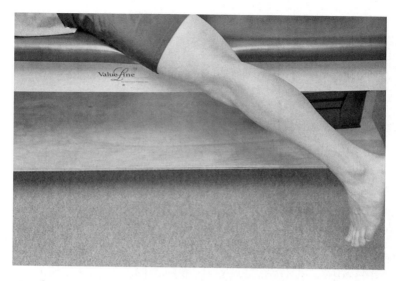

Figure 22-4. Prone exam position with limb over edge of treatment table to eliminate quadriceps guarding.

There are few special tests specific to patellar tendinopathy. One test is the flexion-extension sign, performed with the patient in supine. With the knee extended, the therapist palpates the point of maximal tendon tenderness, and then passively flexes the knee to 90°. A significant *reduction* in tenderness in the flexed position is considered a positive test and indicative of patellar tendinopathy.[26] Although the flexion-extension sign lacks published diagnostic accuracy, cadaveric dissection has shown that pressure applied anteriorly at 90° of knee flexion does not deform the deep fibers of the patellar tendon.[26] In flexion, the tensioned anterior fibers shield the posterior fibers—providing an anatomic rationale for decreased tenderness in the flexed position. The definitive diagnosis of patellar tendinopathy has primarily been based on physical examination. While MRI and ultrasonography can confirm

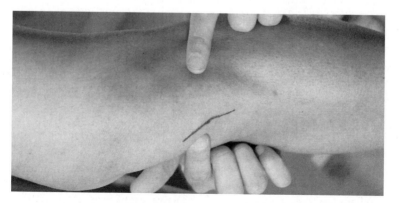

Figure 22-5. With the patient in the prone exam position, the therapist palpates the medial and lateral border of the infrapatellar fat pad.

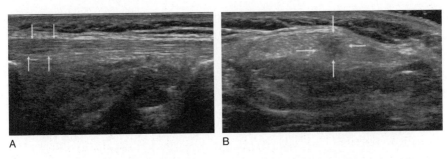

Figure 22-6. A. Patellar tendon with hypoechoic region (longitudinal view). **B.** Patellar tendon with hypoechoic region (cross-sectional view). Arrows are identifying areas of hypoechogenicity.

patellar tendinosis, the physical therapist should keep in mind that the presence of abnormal anatomical structures on imaging does not necessarily mean that the tendon is the source of the pain.[19,27] In contrast, if the physical therapist has access and the expertise to perform diagnostic ultrasound, ultrasound imaging of the symptomatic patellar tendon can confirm the diagnosis of tendinopathy.[28-30] To evaluate the patellar tendon, the patient is in the supine position with knees flexed to approximately 110°. Images should be collected transverse to the tendon and longitudinally from the distal pole of the patella to the tibial tuberosity. The transverse images should be captured at three points: proximally (near the apex of the patella), at the midpoint of the tendon, and at the distal end near the tibial tuberosity. Figure 22-6 shows sonographic images of an abnormal tendon, evident by a hypoechoic region and/or a thickening of the tendon compared to the uninvolved side.[31-33] For best diagnostic accuracy, a positive clinical examination is confirmed with positive imaging results.[19,27]

Outcome measures are useful to assess clinical outcomes or progression toward therapy goals. The Victorian Institute of Sport Assessment Patellar Tendinopathy Questionnaire (VISA-P) is a reliable outcome measure designed to measure clinical outcomes of patients with patellar tendionopathy.[34] It is an 8-item questionnaire assessing symptoms, function, and the ability to play sports. The VISA-P is scored form 0 to 100, with 100 representing unrestricted, pain-free performance. It is typically administered at the initial evaluation to establish a baseline, at 6-week reassessment intervals, and at discharge.[28]

Plan of Care and Interventions

The use of eccentric exercises for the treatment of patellar tendinopathy stems from literature that supports eccentric training in Achilles tendiopathy.[35] While it is still uncertain exactly how eccentric exercise influences tendons, it is proposed that eccentric loading stimulates collagen fiber cross-linkage formation and helps tendon remodeling, which overcomes the failed healing response that is the hallmark of tendinopathy.[36]

A number of studies have assessed **the effectiveness of eccentric exercise in treating patellar tendinopathy**. Purdam *et al.*[37] investigated the effects of two different eccentric training programs on 17 subjects with painful patellar tendinopathy. One group of 9 subjects performed unilateral squats in the standard foot flat position, while the second group of 8 subjects performed the same exercise on a 25° decline board. Both groups performed 3 sets of 15 repetitions twice daily for 12 weeks. Pain during performance was expected and allowed. When a subject was able to perform the prescribed number of repetitions without pain, load was increased via a weighted backpack to achieve painful training. The decline board training group experienced significantly decreased pain at 12-week and 15-month follow-ups compared to baseline. In contrast, the standard foot-flat position training group reported no significant pain improvement between baseline and 12-week follow-up.

Jonsson et al.[38] compared the effectiveness of an eccentric training program to a concentric training program in 15 athletes with painful patellar tendinopathy. Eccentric and concentric loading were performed using training parameters described by Purdam et al.[37] and all subjects were instructed to stop sporting activity for the first 6 weeks. At 12 weeks, the eccentric training group reported significantly decreased pain ratings and increased VISA-P outcome scores compared to the concentric training group.

Visnes et al.[39] assessed the effectiveness of eccentric exercise in 29 elite male and female volleyball players between 19 and 35 years old that continued with regular training and competitions. The exercise group performed eccentric unilateral squats (3 sets of 15 repetitions, twice daily) on a 25° decline board. Loaded backpacks were added when unilateral squat pain decreased. The control group continued their regular training, but did not perform the eccentric exercise program. No differences in VISA-P scores were identified at 6-week or 6-month follow-ups in either group. Lack of improvement in the athletes that performed the eccentric exercise program suggests that there may be a dose-response to tendon loading. Conventional exercises may not place enough load on the tendon to stimulate remodeling (as occurs with concentric squats or with foot-flat eccentric squats as performed in Purdam et al.[37]), but too *much* load may result in increased tendon soreness (which may have occurred in Visnes et al.[39]).

Heavy and slow resistance training has shown promise in patellar tendinopathy management. A randomized controlled trial showed that heavy and slow resistance training was *as effective* as eccentric training and *more effective* than glucocorticoid injections.[40] While resistance programs are effective at reducing patellar tendon symptoms in the medium- to long-term, these exercises are also painful and may be difficult for athletes to perform during their competitive season.[39] However, integration of isometric exercise may help athletes adhere to performance of painful tendinopathy interventions within a competitive season. Isometric exercise has been shown to induce analgesia and improve maximum voluntary isometric contraction. Investigating volleyball players with patellar tendinopathy, Rio et al.[41] showed that performance of 5 repetitions of 45-second isometric contractions at 60° knee flexion reduced patellar tendon pain for at least 45 minutes. Athletes may use isometric contractions immediately before a competition to reduce pain during competition. Further, clinicians may prescribe isometric contractions immediately prior to patients performing patellar tendon-targeted strength programs to reduce the pain and associated muscle inhibition during the performance of those programs.

Table 22-2 TWO DIFFERENT STRENGTH TRAINING PROTOCOLS FOR TREATMENT OF PATELLAR TENDINOPATHY

Training Type	Exercise	Frequency	Load	Pain
Eccentric loading training[33]	Single leg squat on 25°decline board (Fig. 23-7)	Twice daily, 7 days/wk for 12 wk	3 sets of 15 reps; load in backpack increased so that exercise is always performed with discomfort	Expected
Heavy slow resistance training[36]	1. Bilateral leg press 2. Squat 3. Sled hack squat	3 times/wk for 12 wk 2-3 minutes rest between sets	Wk 1: 4 sets of 15 reps of progressively increasing fraction of the repetition maximum (RM) Wk 2-3: 12 RM Wk 4-5: 10 RM Wk 6-8: 8 RM Wk 9-12: 6 RM	Acceptable, but pain not to increase 24 h after cessation of training

Table 22-2 shows sample strength training protocols for treating patellar tendinopathy. Figure 22-7 shows single-leg decline squats on the involved knee from the starting (Fig. 22-7A) to the ending position (Fig. 22-7B).

Strengthening programs are designed to positively influence tendon remodeling to address the degenerative changes associated with tendinopathy. Excessive training *volume* has been identified as a key element in the development of athletic-related patellar tendinopathy.[26] Therefore, the physical therapist should modify and monitor the training volume that contributed to the development of the condition. One suggestion is to identify the training threshold (time, load, *etc.*) when symptoms first occur. Training volume should then be set below this established symptomatic threshold, with incremental increases in volume made at regular intervals. While pain during the performance of an exercise is expected, an increase in baseline tendon pain 24 hours following a loading activity may indicate tendon overload. In this situation, load should be reduced to a previously tolerated load volume.

Many nonexercise interventions have been used in the management of patellar tendinosis. Unloading tape or patellar tendon straps are hypothesized to limit strain on the patellar tendon.[42] While some clinical reports suggest these devices may be useful in decreasing symptoms, limited evidence exists to support this practice.[43]

Injection therapies are being used more frequently as adjunctive treatments for tendinopathy. Dry needling is a type of injection therapy that involves repeatedly passing a needle (ranging in size from 0.20 × 40 mm to 0.30 × 60 mm) through an abnormal tendon with the goal of stimulating an inflammatory response to promote normal tendon repair.[20] Due to the technique's invasive nature, its inclusion as a component of physical therapy practice varies by individual state regulatory boards. As of 2022, 37 states and the District of Columbia have affirmed that dry needling should be included in the physical therapist scope of practice.[44] However, the American Physical Therapy Association's description of dry needling

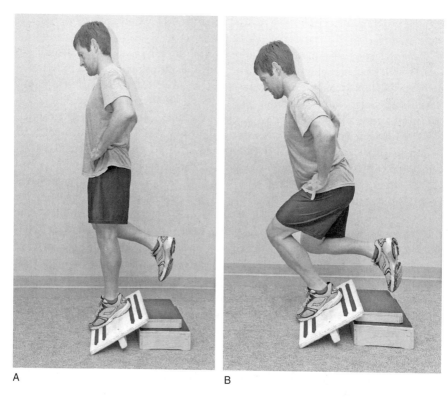

A   B

Figure 22-7. A. Start position for single leg squat on 25° decline board. **B.** Final position single leg squat on 25° decline board.

emphasizes its use to address myofascial pain by releasing or inactivating trigger points.[44] The use of dry needling in isolation or in conjunction with another injection therapy to promote tendon healing should be approved and supervised by a licensed physician. James *et al.*[45] reported that dry needling combined with an injection of autologous blood at the site of the tendinosis and a standardized protocol of eccentric strengthening[37] and lower extremity stretching exercises (performed up to 6 months by some patients) resulted in an 86% improvement in VISA-P scores (mean follow-up 14.8 months). At follow-up, sonographic imaging was performed on approximately one-half of the patients. A majority of tendons demonstrated reductions in hypoechoic area and tendon thickness, indicating improvements in tendon health. Unfortunately, the use of simultaneous therapies in this study makes it impossible to identify which technique or combination of techniques contributed to the reported improvements. However, one other study has shown that dry needling combined with autologous blood injection demonstrated decreased pain and increased function in individuals with recalcitrant tendinopathy.[46] Connell *et al.*[47] found that ultrasound-guided dry needling alone resulted in positive outcomes for two-thirds of 35 patients with lateral epicondylalgia. Further studies are warranted to determine if a multimodal treatment program consisting of dry needling and autologous blood injection at the site of the tendinosis combined with an eccentric exercise program is more effective than an eccentric exercise program alone in treating tendinopathy.

Other injection therapies that require referral to a physician have shown promise in treating patellar tendinopathy. These include ultrasound-guided injection of polidocanol (a sclerosing agent) into areas of concentrated neovascularization along the dorsal patellar tendon[48] and injection of protein-rich plasma followed by eccentric strengthening.[20] Prolotherapy, in which a pharmacologically inert substance like dextrose is injected into the area of tendinosis, is also being investigated.[49]

The use of extracorporeal shockwave therapy (ESWT) has been explored as an adjunctive treatment for degenerative tendons. ESWT is a noninvasive technique used by physiotherapists in Europe and Asia[50-51] and by physicians in the United States. ESWT uses acoustic waves to generate high-stress forces in the target tissue. The waves are generated electrohydraulically, electromagnetically, or piezoelectrically and are thought to stimulate a tissue's own repair processes.[51-53] The extracorporeal shockwave is characterized by high pressure-almost 1000 times greater than that produced by an ultrasound wave.[51,53] As a result, the procedure may provoke pain, which can be lessened by a local anesthetic, if necessary. How ESWT affects a degenerative tendon is not well understood, but hypotheses include reduced concentration of substance P-positive nerve fibers and increased blood flow to promote tissue regeneration.[42,52,53] The evidence regarding the efficacy of ESWT on patellar tendinopathy is mixed. In a systematic review, van Leeuwen et al.[54] concluded that ESWT is effective for patellar tendinopathy, but cautions that the methodological quality of existing studies is variable, with most studies using small sample populations with short-term follow-ups. A recent blinded, randomized controlled trial by Zwerver et al.[55] indicated that ESWT applied over symptomatic patellar tendons during a competitive season provided no benefit over placebo in the treatment of 18- to 35-year-old volleyball, basketball, and handball athletes.[55]

It is widely accepted that nonsurgical care is the first treatment option for patellar tendinopathy. However, only 50% of patients with severe cases may be able to return to pain-free activity after a rehabilitation program.[20] In cases where 6 months of conservative management (e.g., eccentric exercise) has failed to eliminate symptoms and restore unrestricted function, referral for **surgical intervention** may be warranted.[7] Several different techniques have been proposed to address intractable patellar tendinopathy—from open or arthroscopic debridement of the proximal tendon to drilling and excision of the inferior pole of the patella. Approximately 80% of postoperative patients are able to return to their previous or lower level of athletic participation with minimal to no symptoms in 4 to 6 months.[7,56,57] Pascarella et al.[57] promote the initiation of rehabilitation the day following surgery with a progressive range of motion emphasis for the first 2 weeks. This includes the use of a continuous passive motion machine for 4 hours per day for the first week. Isometric quadriceps exercises are advocated during this immediate postoperative phase, along with a transition from partial to full weightbearing. Aquatic therapy and low-resistance closed kinetic chain exercises are introduced in the third postoperative week and resistance loads are increased based on symptom-free activity. A running progression is allowed beginning the sixth postoperative week, with a return to sports-specific training anticipated at 12 weeks.[57] Further details regarding postoperative rehabilitation are limited, but early mobilization seems to produce improved clinical outcomes.[56]

Evidence-Based Clinical Recommendations

SORT: Strength of Recommendation Taxonomy

A: Consistent, good-quality patient-oriented evidence
B: Inconsistent or limited-quality patient-oriented evidence
C: Consensus, disease-oriented evidence, usual practice, expert opinion, or case series

1. Jumper's knee is a patellar tendinosis characterized by tendon degeneration rather than a cellular inflammatory response. **Grade A**

2. Eccentric strength training decreases pain and restores function in athletes with patellar tendinopathy. **Grade B**

3. Injection therapies decrease symptoms associated with patellar tendinopathy. **Grade B**

4. Surgical intervention is an effective treatment option for athletes with refractory patellar tendinopathy. **Grade A**

COMPREHENSION QUESTIONS

22.1 Which of the following training prescriptions has been shown to be effective in the treatment of patellar tendinopathy?

    A. Decline squat, 3 sets × 15 repetitions, once per day for 6 weeks, with pain-free performance

    B. Decline squat, 3 sets × 15 repetitions, once per day for 12 weeks, with pain-allowed performance

    C. Decline squat, 3 sets × 10 repetitions, twice per day for 6 weeks, with pain-allowed performance

    D. Decline squat, 3 sets × 15 repetitions, twice per day for 12 weeks, with pain-allowed performance

22.2 Which of the following does NOT accurately describe the tendon pathology associated with symptoms described as patellar tendinosis?

    A. Mucoid degeneration

    B. Increased concentration of macrophages

    C. Tenocyte proliferation and apoptosis

    D. Disorganized orientation of collagen fibers

ANSWERS

22.1 **D.** Purdam et al.[37] compared the effectiveness of eccentric quadriceps strengthening in a foot-flat position using a decline board. Their results indicated that the performance of decline squats (allowing pain during performance) twice daily for 12 weeks was superior to other test conditions in reducing pain and increasing functional level.

22.2 **B.** Pathology associated with a tendinosis can be described as mucoid degeneration (option A).[5,12,14] The gross appearance is characterized as yellow and disorganized. Microscopically, collagen bundles appear separated secondary to an increased infiltration of abnormal ground substance and there is microtearing and necrosis of collagen fibers (option D).[2,5,13,15,16] Changes in tenocyte nuclei and apoptosis are appreciated and fibroblast infiltration and neovascularization are observed (option C). Inflammatory cells like neutrophils and macrophages are absent.[2,5,13,14,16]

REFERENCES

1. *The American Heritage Medical Dictionary*. Boston, MA: Houghton Mifflin Company; 2007.
2. Peers KH, Lysens RJ. Patellar tendinopathy in athletes: current diagnostic and therapeutic recommendations. *Sports Med*. 2005;35:71-87.
3. Tan SC, Chan O. Achilles and patellar tendinopathy: current understanding of pathophysiology and management. *Disabil Rehabil*. 2008;30:1608-1615.
4. Blazina ME, Kerlan RK, Jobe FW, et al. Jumper's knee. *Orthop Clin North Am*. 1973;4:665-678.
5. Khan KM, Cook JL, Bonar F, et al. Histopathology of common tendinopathies. Update and implications for clinical management. *Sports Med*. 1999;27:393-408.
6. Basso O, Johnson DP, Amis AA. The anatomy of the patellar tendon. *Knee Surg Sports Traumatol Arthrosc*. 2001;9:2-5.
7. Cucurulo T, Louis ML, Thaunat M, Franceschi JP. Surgical treatment of patellar tendinopathy in athletes. A retrospective multicentric study. *Orthop Traumatol Surg Res*. 2009;95:S78-S84.
8. Lian OB, Engebretsen, Bahr R. Prevalence of jumper's knee among elite athletes from different sports: a cross-sectional study. *Am J Sports Med*. 2005;33:561-567.
9. Santander J, Zarba E, Iraporda H, Puleo S. Can arthroscopically assisted treatment of chronic patellar tendinopathy reduce pain and restore function? *Clin Orthop Relat Res*. 2012;470:993-997.
10. Visnes H, Bahr R. The evolution of eccentric training as treatment for patellar tendinopathy (jumper's knee): a critical review of exercise programmes. *Br J Sports Med*. 2007;41:217-223.
11. Garau G, Rittweger J, Mallarias P, et al. Traumatic patellar tendinopathy. *Disabil Rehabil*. 2008; 30:1616-1620.
12. Roels J, Martens M, Mulier JC, Burssens A. Patellar tendinitis: (jumper's knee). *Am J Sports Med*. 1978;6:362-368.
13. Pecina M, Bojanic I, Ivkovic A, et al. Patellar tendinopathy: histopathological examination and follow-up of surgical treatment. *Acta Chir Orthop Traumatol Cech*. 2010;77:277-283.
14. Zhang J, Wang JH. Production of PGE(2) increases in tendons subjected to repetitive mechanical loading and induces differentiation of tendon stem cells in non-tenocytes. *J Orthop Res*. 2010;28:198-203.
15. Parkinson J, Samiric T, Ilic MZ, et al. Change in proteoglycan metabolism is a characteristic of human patellar tendinopathy. *Arthritis Rheum*. 2010;62:3028-3035.

16. Lian ø, Dahl J, Ackermann PW, et al. Pronociceptive and antinociceptive neuromediators in patellar tendinopathy. *Am J Sports Med*. 2006; 34:1801-1808.

17. Khan KM, Cook JL, Maffulli N, Kannus P. Where is the pain coming from in tendinopathy? It may be biochemical, not only structural, in origin. *Br J Sports Med*. 2000;34:81-83.

18. Scott A, Ashe MC. Common tendinopathies in upper and lower extremities. *Curr Sports Med Rep*. 2006;5:233-241.

19. Cook JL, Kiss ZS, Khan KM, et al. Anthropometry, physical performance, and ultrasound patellar tendon abnormality in elite junior basketball players: a cross-sectional study. *Br J Sports Med*. 2004;38:206-209.

20. Volpi P, Quaglia A, Schoenhuber H, et al. Growth factors in the management of sport-induced tendinopathies: results after 24 months from treatment. A pilot study. *J Sports Med Phys Fitness*. 2010;50:494-500.

21. Stasinopoulos D, Stasinopoulos I. Comparison of effects of exercise programme, pulsed ultrasound and transverse friction in the treatment of chronic patellar tendinopathy. *Clin Rehabil*. 2004;18:347-352.

22. Speed CA. Fortnightly review: corticosteroid injections in tendon lesions. *BMJ*. 2001;323:382-386.

23. Feagin JA, Steadman JR. *The Crucial Principles in Care of the Knee*. Philadelphia, PA: Lippincott Williams & Wilkins; 2008.

24. Cook JL, Purdam C. Is compressive load a factor in the development of tendinopathy? *Br J Sports Med*. 2012;46:163-168.

25. Cook JL, Kahn KM, Kiss ZS, et al. Reproducibility and clinical utility of tendon palpation to detect patellar tendinopathy in young basketball players. Victorian Institute of Sport Tendon Study Group. *Br J Sports Med*. 2001;35:65-69.

26. Rath E, Schwarzkopf R, Richmond JC. Clinical signs and anatomic correlation of patellar tendinitis. *Indian J Orthop*. 2010;44:435-437.

27. Warden SJ, Kiss ZS, Malara FA, et al. Comparative accuracy of magnetic resonance imaging and ultrasonography in confirming clinically diagnosed patellar tendinopathy. *Am J Sports Med*. 2007; 35:427-436

28. Cook JL, Khan KM, Kiss ZS, et al. Prospective imaging study of asymptomatic patellar tendinopathy in elite junior basketball players. *J Ultrasound Med*. 2000;19(7):473-479.

29. Malliaras P, Cook J, Purdam C, Rio E. Patellar tendinopathy: clinical diagnosis, load management, and advice for challenging case presentations. *J Orthop Sports Phys Ther*. 2015;45(11):887-898.

30. Mendonca Lde M, Ocarino JM, Bittencourt NF, et al. The accuracy of the VISA-P questionnaire, single-leg decline squat, and tendon pain history to identify patellar tendon abnormalities in adult athletes. *J Orthop Sports Phys Ther*. 2016;46(8):673-680.

31. Black J, Cook J, Kiss ZS, Smith M. Intertester reliability of sonography in patellar tendinopathy. *J Ultrasound Med*. 2004;23(5):671-675.

32. Gellhorn AC, Carlson MJ. Inter-rater, intra-rater, and inter-machine reliability of quantitative ultrasound measurements of the patellar tendon. *Ultrasound Med Biol*. 2013;39(5):791-796.

33. Del Bano-Aledo ME, Martinez-Paya JJ, Rios-Diaz J, et al. Ultrasound measures of tendon thickness: intra-rater, inter-rater, and inter-machine reliability. *Muscles Ligaments Tendons J*. 2017;7(1):92-99.

34. Visentini PJ, Kahn KM, Cook JL, et al. The VISA score: an index of severity of symptoms in patients with jumper's knee (patellar tendinosis). Victorian Institute of Sport Tendon Study Group. *J Sci Med Sport*. 1998;1:22-28.

35. Woodley BL, Newsham-West RJ, Baxter GD. Chronic tendinopathy: effectiveness of eccentric exercise. *Br J Sports Med*. 2007;41:188-199.

36. Jeffery R, Cronin J, Bressel E. Eccentric strengthening: clinical applications to Achilles tendinopathy. *NZ J Sports Med*. 2005;35:71-87.

37. Purdam CR, Jonsson P, Alfredson H, et al. A pilot study of the eccentric decline squat in the management of painful chronic patellar tendinopathy. *Br J Sports Med*. 2004;38:395-397.

38. Jonsson P, Alfredson H. Superior results with eccentric compared to concentric quadriceps training in patients with jumper's knee: a prospective randomised study. *Br J Sports Med*. 2005;39:847-850.

39. Visnes H, Hoksrud A, Cook J, Bahr R. No effect of eccentric training on jumper's knee in volleyball players during the competitive season: a randomized clinical trial. *Clin J Sport Med*. 2005;15:227-234.

40. Kongsgaard M, Kovanen V, Aagaard P, et al. Corticosteroid injections, eccentric decline squat training and heavy slow resistance training in patellar tendinopathy. *Scan J Med Sci Sports*. 2009;19:790-802.

41. Rio E, Kidgell D, Purdam C, et al. Isometric exercise induces analgesia and reduces inhibition in patellar tendinopathy. *Br J Sports Med*. 2015;49:1277-1283.

42. Wang CJ, Ko JY, Chan YS, et al. Extracorporeal shockwave therapy for chronic patellar tendinopathy. *Am J Sports Med*. 2007;35:972-978.

43. Struijs PA, Smidt N, Arola H, et al. Orthotic devices for the treatment of tennis elbow: a systematic review. *Br J Gen Pract*. 2001;51:924-929.

44. American Physical Therapy Association. State laws and regulations governing dry needling performed by PTs. Available at: https://www.apta.org/patient-care/interventions/dry-needling/laws-by-state. Accessed August 31, 2022.

45. James SL, Ali K, Pocock C, et al. Ultrasound-guided dry needling and autologous blood injection for patellar tendinosis. *Br J Sports Med*. 2007;41:518-522.

46. Suresh SP, Ali KE, Jones H, Connell DA. Medial epicondylitis: is ultrasound guided autologous blood injection an effective treatment? *Br J Sports Med*. 2006;40:935-939.

47. Connell DA, Ali KE, Ahmad M, et al. Ultrasound-guided autologous blood injection for tennis elbow. *Skeletal Radiol*. 2006;35:371-377.

48. Hoksrud A, Öhberg L, Alfredson H, Bahr R. Ultrasound-guided sclerosis of neovessels in painful chronic patellar tendinopathy: a randomized controlled trial. *Am J Sports Med*. 2006;34:1738-1747.

49. Ryan M, Wong A, Rabago D, et al. Ultrasound-guided injections of hyperosmolar dextrose for overuse patellar tendinopathy: a pilot study. *Br J Sports Med*. 2011;45:972-977.

50. Engebretsen K, Grotle M, Bautz-Holter E, et al. Supervised exercises compared with radial extracorporeal shock-wave therapy for subacromial shoulder pain: 1-year results of a single-blind randomized controlled trial. *Phys Ther*. 2011;91:37-47.

51. Cheing GL, Chang H. Extracorporeal shock wave therapy. *J Orthop Sports Phys Ther*. 2003;33:337-343.

52. Berta L, Fazzari A, Ficco AM, et al. Extracorporeal shock waves enhance normal fibroblast proliferation in vitro and activate mRNA expression for TGF-beta1 and for collagen types I and III. *Acta Orthop*. 2009;80:612-617.

53. Wang CJ. Extracorporeal shockwave therapy in musculoskeletal disorders. *J Orthop Surg Res*. 2012;7:11.

54. van Leeuwen MT, Zwerver J, van den Akker-Scheek I. Extracorporeal shockwave therapy for patellar tendinopathy: a review of the literature. *Br J Sports Med*. 2009;43:163-168.

55. Zwerver J, Hartgens F, Verhagen E, et al. No effect of extracorporeal shockwave therapy on patellar tendinopathy in jumping athletes during the competitive season: a randomized clinical trial. *Am J Sports Med*. 2011;39:1191-1199.

56. Kaeding CC, Pedroza AD, Powers BC. Surgical treatment of chronic patellar tendinosis: a systematic review. *Clin Orthop Relat Res*. 2007;455:102-106.

57. Pascarella A, Alam M, Pascarella F, et al. Arthroscopic management of chronic patellar tendinopathy. *Am J Sports Med*. 2011;39:1975-1983.

Anterior Cruciate Ligament (ACL) Sprain: Diagnosis

Mark V. Paterno

CASE 23

A 17-year-old competitive female athlete reported injuring her knee in a soccer game. On the field, she attempted to execute a cutting maneuver when an opponent collided with her trunk and threw her off balance. She felt a "pop" in her right knee and an immediate sensation of her knee "giving way." She was unable to continue playing and was removed from the game. On the sideline, the physical therapist working at the game observed significant effusion in the suprapatellar region. The patient reports difficulty bearing weight on the right lower extremity due to pain and lack of muscle control.

▶ Based on the patient's suspected diagnosis, what do you anticipate may be the contributing factors to her condition?

▶ What examination signs may be associated with this diagnosis?

KEY DEFINITIONS

FUNCTIONAL INSTABILITY: Sensation of "giving way" due to excessive motion and/or translation within the knee joint or inadequate neuromuscular stability within the lower extremity

MECHANICAL INSTABILITY: Increase in translation of the knee joint due to ligamentous insufficiency

Objectives

1. Describe the anatomic structure and function of the anterior cruciate ligament (ACL).
2. Identify potential secondary injuries that may occur at the time of an ACL injury and how these could affect rehabilitation prognosis.
3. Describe clinical tests with acceptable diagnostic accuracy to identify ACL laxity.

Physical Therapy Considerations

Physical therapy considerations during examination of the individual with suspected acute anterior cruciate ligament insufficiency:

▶ **General physical therapy plan of care/goals:** Decrease pain and effusion; increase muscular strength; increase lower quadrant strength; improve functional stability; prevent or minimize loss of aerobic fitness capacity

▶ **Physical therapy tests and measures:** Lachman test, pivot shift examination

▶ **Differential diagnoses:** Patellar dislocation, osteochondral injury

Understanding the Health Condition

Acute injury to the anterior cruciate ligament (ACL) is common in pivoting and cutting activities. As many as 200,000 to 300,000 ACL injuries occur each year in the United States.[1,2] A thorough clinical assessment and diagnosis is critical for early treatment plan development.

The primary role of the ACL is to create stability in the knee joint. The ACL attaches distally in the knee joint on the tibial plateau, anterior to the medial tibial spine.[3,4] The ACL ascends in a posterior lateral direction to its femoral attachment along the posterior inner surface of the lateral femoral condyle (Fig. 23-1).[3,4] Functionally, the ACL comprises two functional bundles that provide mechanical stability through a full arc of motion.[1] The anterior medial bundle (AMB) is taut in a flexed position, while the posterior lateral bundle (PLB) tends to be taut in full extension.[2] Some authors discuss a third intermediate bundle whose

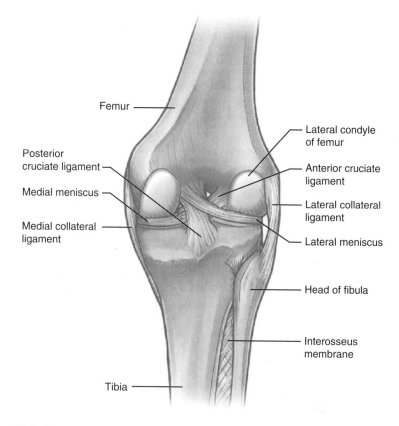

Figure 23-1. Posterior view of the lower extremity showing the attachment of the anterior cruciate ligament along the posterior inner surface of the lateral femoral condyle. (Reproduced with permission from Morton DA, Foreman KB, Albertine KH, eds. *The Big Picture: Gross Anatomy.* New York, NY: McGraw-Hill; 2011. Figure 36-5B)

functional contribution is significantly less than the AMB and PLB.[2] Together, these bundles assist to create mechanical stability in the knee. Primarily, the ACL provides restraint to anterior tibial translation and assists in rotatory stability in the knee.[3] Injury to the ACL can result in excessive anterior translation of the tibia on the femur, often described as mechanical instability. As a result of several concurrent factors including excessive translation in the knee joint, deficits in neuromuscular control of the knee, and altered proprioception, the patient may experience episodes of giving way in the knee described as functional instability.

Treatment planning after ACL injury can follow a surgical or nonsurgical route. Surgical ACL reconstruction is often recommended in an attempt to restore normal anatomy and allow the patient to return to pivoting and cutting activities.[4] Nonoperative management is discussed in Case 24. The decision to manage operatively versus nonoperatively may be influenced by the presence of secondary pathology at the time of injury. Injury to the secondary stabilizers of the knee (*e.g.,* collateral ligaments and menisci) may result in additional instability.[5] Injury to the menisci or articular cartilage may raise concern about progressive joint surface breakdown in the presence of a joint with excessive translation.[6,7] These additional pathologies may increase the likelihood of surgical management.

Short-term and long-term outcomes after ACL injury are variable. Although many patients are able to return to prior levels of function following ACL injury, issues with residual functional instability, pain, and a high incidence of repeat injuries have been reported.[8,9] Recent evidence has shown that the percentage of athletes who return to prior levels of function may be less than initially reported.[10-12] With respect to long-term outcomes after ACL injury, current evidence suggests **injury to the ACL can result in a high incidence of osteoarthritis (OA) in as few as 10 years after the index injury.**[9,13,14] These reports suggested that the incidence of OA was similar with both operative and nonoperative management of ACL injury. These limitations with both short- and long-term outcomes after ACL injury highlight the need to implement and improve injury prevention programs and postinjury management to improve outcomes for these patients.

Examination, Evaluation, and Diagnosis

Clinical assessment of potential ACL injury has evolved. Early clinical assessment of the knee focused on quantifying the amount of anterior-posterior (AP) translation in the knee as a means to assess ACL integrity. The first examination to quantify this AP translation was the anterior drawer (Fig. 23-2). This examination requires the therapist to pull the tibial plateau anteriorly while the patient's involved knee is in 90° of knee flexion and 45° of hip flexion.[15] The anterior drawer has two major limitations. First, the testing position allows increased stability from the secondary

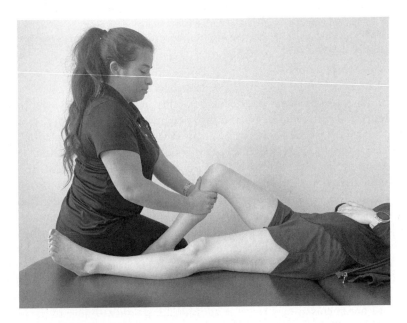

Figure 23-2. Anterior drawer test.

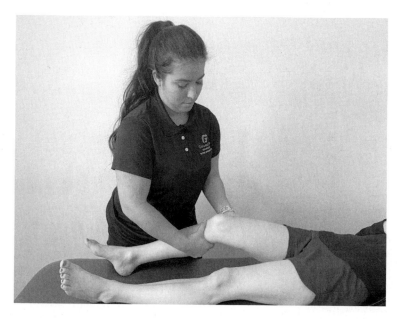

Figure 23-3. Lachman test.

restraints of the knee such as the collateral ligaments and the menisci.[3] Second, the hamstrings have a mechanical advantage to resist anterior translation at 90° of knee flexion, potentially decreasing anterior translation during the examination. The **Lachman test** (Fig. 23-3) also evaluates anterior translation, but this assessment is performed with the knee in 20° to 30° of flexion. At this angle of knee flexion, the secondary restraints of the knee are lax and the ACL serves as the primary restraint to AP translation with little contribution from supporting structures.[3]

The **pivot shift** examination is a third clinical test to assess knee stability in the presence of suspected ACL pathology. The pivot shift examination goes beyond a simple assessment of AP translation and attempts to reproduce the "giving way" mechanism. With the patient supine, the physical therapist keeps the involved knee internally rotated and moves the knee from flexion to full extension while applying a valgus stress (Fig. 23-4). This maneuver stresses the knee in AP, medial-lateral, and rotational planes. In an ACL-deficient knee, this maneuver results in a sudden reduction of a previously anteriorly subluxed lateral compartment of the knee as a result of the iliotibial band becoming taut, which simulates the "giving way" mechanism.[15,16] Unlike the anterior drawer and the Lachman test, the pivot shift test is strongly associated with functional outcome after ACL reconstruction (*e.g.,* "giving way," activity limitation, sports participation).[17] Biomechanical evidence suggests that the pivot shift examination may be better than simple assessments of AP translation to detect restoration of normal knee kinematics after ACL reconstruction. A frequently reported limitation of the pivot shift examination is the technical difficulty to perform the test as well as the patient's potential inability to relax during the examination. If a patient is hesitant to experience the **giving-way**

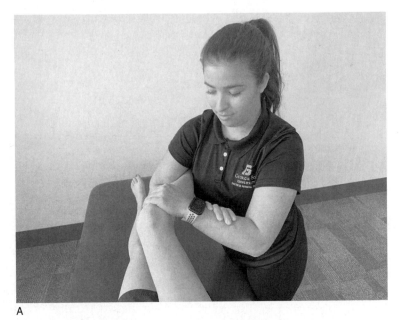

A

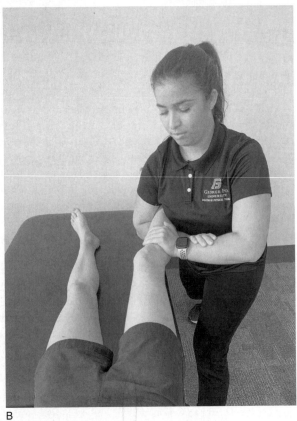

B

Figure 23-4. Pivot shift test. **A**, starting position. **B**, end position.

phenomenon reproduced by the pivot shift examination, she may recruit neuromuscular stabilizers to guard against this sensation, which significantly decreases the diagnostic accuracy of the examination.

A meta-analysis of 28 studies reported the diagnostic accuracy of clinical tests for assessment of ACL injury compared to the gold standards of arthroscopy, arthrotomy, or MRI.[15] Benjaminse et al.[15] reported the Lachman test was the most accurate test to determine ACL insufficiency with a pooled specificity of 94% and a pooled sensitivity of 85%. The pivot shift examination had even better specificity (98%), but inadequate sensitivity (24%). Finally, the anterior drawer had good specificity (91%) and sensitivity (92%) in individuals with chronic ACL insufficiency, but *not* in those with acute ACL injuries. The poor sensitivity of the pivot shift examination may be due to the technical difficulty of the examination as well as issues with patient relaxation during the examination. The reported poor diagnostic accuracy with the anterior drawer examination after acute disruption of the ACL may also be attributed to a patient's inability to relax the hamstrings to allow the therapist to appreciate the true AP translation.

Plan of Care and Interventions

If an ACL injury is suspected, the patient should be referred to an orthopedic physician while physical therapy treatment is continued. The physical therapy plan of care and interventions for nonoperative management of ACL injury are discussed in Case 24.

Evidence-Based Clinical Recommendations

SORT: Strength of Recommendation Taxonomy

A: Consistent, good-quality patient-oriented evidence
B: Inconsistent or limited-quality patient-oriented evidence
C: Consensus, disease-oriented evidence, usual practice, expert opinion, or case series

1. Injury to the ACL often leads to a long-term outcome of osteoarthritis. **Grade B**

2. Lachman test is the most sensitive and specific clinical assessment to identify ACL instability in patients with both acute and chronic ACL insufficiency. **Grade A**

3. The pivot shift test has high specificity, but low sensitivity to diagnose ACL ruptures. **Grade A**

4. History of a noncontact, pivoting/twisting mechanism to the knee in conjunction with patient reports of "popping," "giving way," and immediate effusion are consistent with a potential ACL injury. **Grade C**

COMPREHENSION QUESTIONS

23.1 Which of the following accurately describes the sensitivity and specificity of the Lachman test to diagnose acute anterior cruciate ligament (ACL) rupture?

  A. High sensitivity and high specificity

  B. Low sensitivity and high specificity

  C. Low sensitivity and low specificity

  D. High sensitivity and low specificity

23.2 Which clinical test has the highest diagnostic accuracy for a *chronic* ACL injury versus an *acute* ACL injury?

  A. Lachman

  B. Anterior drawer

  C. Pivot shift

  D. None of the above

ANSWERS

23.1 **A.** The Lachman test is both highly sensitive (85%) and specific (94%) to assess acute ACL rupture.[15]

23.2 **B.** The anterior drawer is the clinical test that has the highest sensitivity (92%) and specificity (91%) for diagnosis of ACL instability in individuals with chronic ACL injuries.[15]

REFERENCES

 1. Duthon VB, Barea C, Abrassart S, et al. Anatomy of the anterior cruciate ligament. *Knee Surg Sports Traumatol Arthrosc.* 2006;14:204-213.

 2. Hollis JM, Takai S, Adams DJ, et al. The effects of knee motion and external loading on the length of the anterior cruciate ligament (ACL): a kinematic study. *J Biomech Eng.* 1991;113:208-214.

 3. Butler DL, Noyes FR, Grood ES. Ligamentous restraints to anterior-posterior drawer in the human knee. A biomechanical study. *J Bone Joint Surg Am.* 1980;62:259-270.

 4. Linko E, Harilainen A, Malmivaara A, Seitsalo S. Surgical versus conservative interventions for anterior cruciate ligament ruptures in adults. *Cochrane Database Syst Rev.* 2005;(2):CD001356.

 5. Petrigliano FA, Musahl V, Suero EM, et al. Effect of meniscal loss on knee stability after single-bundle anterior cruciate ligament reconstruction. *Knee Surg Sports Traumatol Arthrosc.* 2011;19 Suppl 1:86-93.

 6. Dunn WR, Spindler KP, Amendola A, et al. Which preoperative factors, including bone bruise, are associated with knee pain/symptoms at index anterior cruciate ligament reconstruction (ACLR)? A Multicenter Orthopaedic Outcomes Network (MOON) ACLR Cohort Study. *Am J Sports Med.* 2010;38:1778-1787.

 7. Theologis AA, Kuo D, Cheng J, et al. Evaluation of bone bruises and associated cartilage in anterior cruciate ligament-injured and reconstructed knees using quantitative t(1rho) magnetic resonance imaging: 1-year cohort study. *Arthroscopy.* 2011;27:65-76.

8. Paterno MV, Schmitt LC, Ford KR, et al. Biomechanical measures during landing and postural stability predict second anterior cruciate ligament injury after anterior cruciate ligament reconstruction and return to sport. *Am J Sports Med.* 2010;38:1968-1978.

9. Spindler KP, Wright RW. Clinical practice. Anterior cruciate ligament tear. *N Engl J Med.* 2008;359:2135-2142.

10. Ardern CL, Taylor NF, Feller JA, Webster KE. Return-to-sport outcomes at 2 to 7 years after anterior cruciate ligament reconstruction surgery. *Am J Sports Med.* 2012;40:41-48.

11. Ardern CL, Webster KE, Taylor NF, Feller JA. Return to sport following anterior cruciate ligament reconstruction surgery: a systematic review and meta-analysis of the state of play. *Br J Sports Med.* 2011;45:596-606.

12. Ardern CL, Webster KE, Taylor NF, Feller JA. Return to the preinjury level of competitive sport after anterior cruciate ligament reconstruction surgery: two-thirds of patients have not returned by 12 months after surgery. *Am J Sports Med.* 2011;39:538-543.

13. Lohmander LS, Ostenberg A, Englund M, Roos H. High prevalence of knee osteoarthritis, pain, and functional limitations in female soccer players twelve years after anterior cruciate ligament injury. *Arthritis Rheum.* 2004;50:3145-3152.

14. von Porat A, Roos EM, Roos H. High prevalence of osteoarthritis 14 years after an anterior cruciate ligament tear in male soccer players: a study of radiographic and patient relevant outcomes. *Ann Rheum Dis.* 2004;63:269-273.

15. Benjaminse A, Gokeler A, van der Schans CP. Clinical diagnosis of an anterior cruciate ligament rupture: a meta-analysis. *J Orthop Sports Phys Ther.* 2006;36:267-288.

16. Markolf KL, Jackson SR, McAllister DR. Relationship between the pivot shift and Lachman tests: a cadaver study. *J Bone Joint Surg Am.* 2010;92:2067-2075.

17. Kocher MS, Steadman JR, Briggs KK, et al. Relationships between objective assessment of ligament stability and subjective assessment of symptoms and function after anterior cruciate ligament reconstruction. *Am J Sports Med.* 2004;32:629-634.

Anterior Cruciate Ligament Sprain: Nonoperative Management

Mark V. Paterno

A 17-year-old competitive female soccer player presents to physical therapy with a diagnosis of a right acute anterior cruciate ligament (ACL) tear. She reports injuring her knee while participating in a soccer game 1 week ago. At that time, she was running down the field and attempted to execute a cutting maneuver when an opponent collided with her trunk and threw her off balance. She felt a "pop" in her knee and an immediate sensation of her knee "giving way." She was unable to continue playing and sought immediate medical attention. The MRI of her right knee obtained at her medical follow-up demonstrated a complete acute ACL tear with no concomitant meniscal or articular cartilage damage. She is a senior in high school and this injury occurred in the first game of her season.

▶ Based on the patient's diagnosis, what factors would be appropriate to consider before choosing a nonoperative treatment plan?

▶ What are the most appropriate physical therapy interventions if a nonoperative treatment plan is implemented?

▶ What are possible complications that may limit the effectiveness of physical therapy?

KEY DEFINITIONS

COPER: Person with ACL deficiency who is able to resume all preinjury levels of activity without any episodes of the knee giving-way for at least 1 year[1]

NONCOPER: Person with ACL deficiency who experiences knee instability on return to activity[1]

PERTURBATION TRAINING: Nonoperative treatment intervention for ACL-deficient individuals; training includes progressive application of disruptions to the individual's balance on unstable surfaces in an attempt to enhance dynamic neuromuscular stability in the affected knee prior to return to activity[2]

Objectives

1. Describe a decision-making algorithm to determine if an ACL-deficient individual is a candidate to pursue nonsurgical management of ACL injury.

2. Identify appropriate interventions for an individual pursuing nonsurgical management of an ACL injury.

3. Identify appropriate return-to-sport criteria for individuals pursuing conservative management of ACL injury.

Physical Therapy Considerations

Physical therapy considerations during nonoperative management of the individual with a diagnosis of acute anterior cruciate ligament tear:

▶ **General physical therapy plan of care/goals:** Decrease acute pain and effusion; increase strength; increase lower quadrant strength; improve functional stability; prevent or minimize loss of aerobic fitness capacity

▶ **Physical therapy interventions:** Patient education regarding functional anatomy and injury pathomechanics; modalities and manual therapy to decrease pain and effusion; flexibility exercises; resistance exercises to increase strength, activation, and endurance capacity with a focus on the lower extremity and core musculature; balance and proprioceptive interventions; perturbation training

▶ **Precautions during physical therapy:** Monitor all activity to ensure no episodes of knee giving-way; address precautions or contraindications for exercise, based on patient's mechanical instability (e.g., limit open kinetic chain knee extension in the range from 30° to full extension to decrease anterior shear forces at tibiofemoral joint)

▶ **Complications interfering with physical therapy:** Residual knee instability with activities of daily living (ADLs) or exercise

Understanding the Health Condition

Rupture of the ACL is a devastating injury. The primary role of the ACL is to create stability in the knee joint. The ACL is positioned obliquely in the knee joint attaching the anterior tibial plateau to the posterior portion of the inner wall of the lateral femoral condyle (Fig. 24-1).[3] In this position, the ACL provides a primary restraint to anterior tibial translation and assists in rotatory stability in the knee.[4] Therefore, injury to the ACL results in excessive anterior translation of the tibia on the femur, with subsequent mechanical instability. The sensation of the knee "giving way" is often the product of a collection of impairments, including mechanical instability, altered neuromuscular control, and altered proprioception, and is referred to as functional instability. Typical management of ACL injury in the United States is surgical reconstruction—90% of patients who sustain an ACL tear pursue this course of care.[5] Despite the preponderance of patients selecting surgical management of ACL insufficiency, some patients may be able to maintain an acceptable functional level without surgical reconstruction.

The athlete attempting to participate in pivoting and cutting sports in the absence of the mechanical stability provided by an intact ACL represents a clinical challenge to rehabilitation professionals. In the early 1980s, Noyes et al.[6] discussed their theory of the "rule of thirds." The authors hypothesized that approximately one-third of ACL-deficient individuals could execute light recreational activities without repeated episodes of the knee giving-way. More recently, researchers from the University of Delaware have developed a decision-making scheme to more objectively identify individuals who may be able to participate

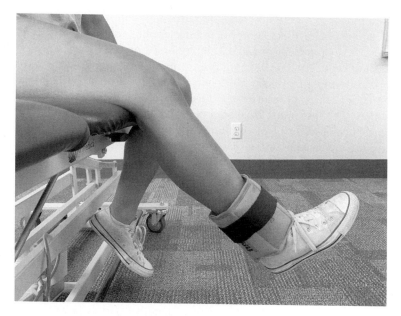

Figure 24-1. Seated knee extension in a range from 90° to 45°.

in pivoting and cutting activity without giving way ("copers") and those who are less likely to be able to accomplish this level of activity without surgical intervention ("noncopers").[2,7] Specific and objective criteria to identify individuals who have the potential to succeed without surgical intervention is critical. The consequences of experiencing repeated giving-way episodes with an ACL-deficient knee can be catastrophic. Repeated knee giving-way episodes due to mechanical and functional instability are often associated with additional meniscus injury, articular cartilage damage, and further joint degeneration.[8,9] Considering current evidence that suggests the incidence of osteoarthritis after ACL injury is between 50% and 100%,[10-12] any activity that has the potential to accelerate this negative joint cascade should be pursued with extreme caution.

Choosing nonoperative management after an ACL injury is a multifactorial decision. Ultimately, all factors under consideration must focus on a scenario that minimizes the potential for repeated giving-way of the knee. First, the patient must present with an absence of any secondary knee pathology.[2] Second, the patient must qualify via an objective algorithm that identifies candidates with the greatest likelihood for success and minimal chance of repeated giving-way. The patient's preference for a treatment plan is often driven by lifestyle choices. Some may choose to limit pivoting or cutting activity post-ACL tear as a means to decrease risk of repeated giving-way. Others may choose to delay surgical ACL reconstruction in an attempt to return to pivoting or cutting activity on a limited basis due to work-related demands or short-term athletic goals, such as in the scenario of the high school senior at the end of her competitive athletic career. Many factors including long-term joint health and short-term goals must be considered prior to selecting a treatment plan.

Physical Therapy Patient/Client Management

There may be one or more appropriate interventions for a patient who chooses nonoperative management of an ACL injury based on the patient's presentation. Once identified as a potential candidate for nonoperative management, physical therapy interventions may include resolving typical impairments such as acute effusion, limitations in range of motion (ROM) and mobility, and decreased strength. In addition, emphasis must be placed on maximizing lower extremity proprioception as a component of establishing dynamic stability prior to attempting to return to functional activities, such as sports. One specific intervention which has proven to increase success with the ability to return to sport in a targeted population is perturbation training as described by Fitzgerald et al.[2] The primary goal for most injured athletes/individuals is to return to pain-free sport or activity as quickly and as safely as possible in a manner that optimizes functional stability in the knee and limits the potential for giving-way episodes.

Examination, Evaluation, and Diagnosis

A clinical diagnosis of an acute ACL injury is outlined in Case 23. This injury often presents with hallmark impairments. Acute hemarthrosis within the knee joint[13] with potential reflex inhibition of the quadriceps musculature is common after ACL rupture.[14] These patients may also present with a limitation in full ROM[15] and residual deficits in lower extremity muscle activation with functional weakness.[16] Collectively, these impairments may contribute to an altered gait pattern.[17] Coinciding with damage to the native ACL is a loss of proprioceptive input to the knee joint.[18] The intact ACL possesses robust mechanoreceptor innervation that allows the ACL to provide proprioceptive input to the knee joint.[14,19] Hence, injury to this structure disrupts this feedback and decreases joint position sense of the extremity. These impairments must be objectively assessed and adequately addressed prior to return to activity. Evidence suggests that factors such as preinjury level of function and amount of antero-posterior translation (mechanical stability) do *not* predict successful functional outcome after ACL injury.[1,20] Rather, assessments of functional movements may be a more accurate predictor of successful outcome in this population.

The ultimate selection of individuals appropriate for a nonoperative course of treatment should be the product of an objective, algorithmic assessment that can identify those with the best potential to succeed with minimal risk of repeated giving-way episodes. For individuals with acute unilateral ACL tear, Fitzgerald et al.[2,7] outlined a selection **algorithm to identify potential "copers," or those who had the potential to successfully return to high-level functional activity without giving-way.** Those who failed the selection algorithm were described as "noncopers" and were candidates for surgical reconstruction. The selection algorithm begins with a determination of the extent of knee damage. If there is evidence of multiligamentous injuries, repairable meniscus pathology or chondral defects, the individual is already excluded as a candidate for nonoperative management. The screening assessment for nonoperative candidates consists of 4 single-leg hop tests,[21] self-reported number of giving-way episodes, the Knee Outcome Survey of Activities of Daily Living (ADLs) Scale,[22] and a global rating of knee function.[2] Those who demonstrate an 80% limb symmetry score on all hop tests, report no more than one episode of giving-way since initial injury, score ≥80% on the Knee Outcome Survey of ADLs, and have a global rating score of ≥60% are candidates for nonoperative rehabilitation.[2] In a 10-year follow-up of over 800 patients with an ACL injury, 17.5% were initially identified as potential copers. Approximately 10% of the patients chose to pursue conservative management. Within this group, 75% were able to return to sports without an ACL reconstruction. However, this represents less than 8% of the initial cohort of patients who suffered an ACL injury.[1,20]

Plan of Care and Interventions

Physical therapy interventions must address findings from the musculoskeletal examination. Acute impairments including effusion, pain, loss of motion, and altered gait patterns should be initially addressed in the early phases of rehabilitation to develop an appropriate foundation. Modalities may help reduce acute signs and symptoms. **Moderate to strong evidence supports the use of supervised targeted progressive resistance exercises, neuromuscular electrical stimulation, and neuromuscular re-education for individuals with altered knee stability.**[23] Targeted balance training and perturbation training should be utilized to address impaired proprioceptive function.[24,25] A return-to-sport progression should be used to ensure the individual's ability to successfully resume prior levels of function.

The development of sufficient muscle performance is critical for success on higher-level performance tests as well as for the ultimate transition to function and sport. Marked deficits in quadriceps strength and timing of quadriceps activation are common due to reflex muscle inhibition[14] as well as disuse atrophy after injury. Current evidence has shown improved quadriceps strength with the use of neuromuscular electrical stimulation in patients with an ACL injury.[26] Targeted progressive resistive exercises are also critical to increase lower extremity strength and should include a mixture of both open and closed kinetic chain interventions. However, the physical therapist must carefully choose ranges to strengthen the quadriceps that *minimize* the anterior shear forces at the ACL-deficient tibiofemoral joint. Open kinetic chain (OKC) interventions provide an opportunity to train a specific muscle in relative isolation to target specific strength deficits that may exist. Quadriceps strengthening in an OKC (*e.g.*, seated leg extension with foot non-weightbearing) is an effective way to increase strength. Leg extension exercises performed in a limited range (between 45° and 90° of flexion [Fig. 24-1]) results in minimal anterior shear at the tibiofemoral joint. In contrast, extending the knee from 45° to full extension can result in excessive anterior shear forces.[27,28] Resisted knee flexion in an OKC also improves the strength of the hamstrings, which helps in the development of functional knee stability. A complement of closed kinetic chain (CKC) interventions is appropriate to train impaired muscle groups in functional positions. Exercises such as leg presses, squatting, "wall sitting" (Fig. 24-2)

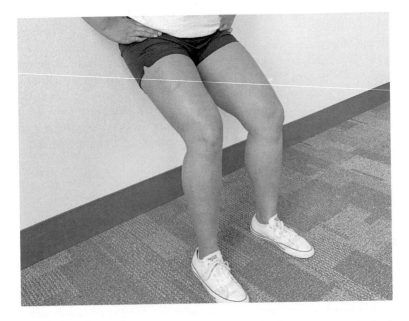

Figure 24-2. Wall sitting exercise.

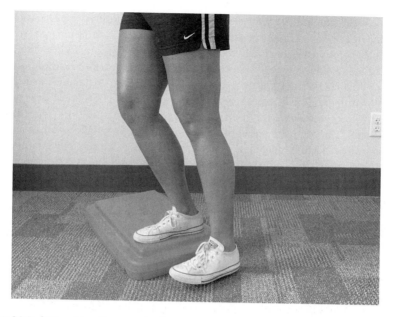

Figure 24-3. Step up/step down exercise. Patient stands on ACL-deficient limb at the edge of an elevated surface, lowers the contralateral limb toward the floor to only lightly touch the heel, then returns to starting position.

and step-ups/step-downs (Fig. 24-3) through a knee range of motion that limits excessive shear and stress on the tibiofemoral joint (0°-60°) can progressively strengthen the lower extremity in the presence of ACL deficiency.[28] Thus, the ideal knee ranges in which to perform strengthening exercises with minimal anterior shear forces at the tibiofemoral joint are between 45° and 90° for OKC exercises and between 0° and 60° for CKC exercises.

Balance and proprioception impairments are common after ACL injury[29-31] and these deficits are thought to contribute to functional instability.[32] Methods currently used to assess proprioceptive deficits may not provide sufficient information related to the clinical correlates of this deficit.[33] Despite limitations with assessment, consensus exists in the literature that an attempt to restore proprioceptive function in the ACL-deficient knee is necessary to enhance dynamic stability.[34] Interventions such as single-limb standing on stable and unstable surfaces are sufficient to initiate balance and proprioceptive training on the ACL-deficient limb. These interventions can be advanced from single-plane movement to more dynamic interventions that can challenge the joint in three planes of movement. A very structured proprioceptive intervention used in a population of patients with ACL deficiency is perturbation training.[2] Perturbation training is a progression of balance exercises in which the patient stands on unstable surfaces such as roller boards and tilt boards. The patient is progressively challenged to maintain single-limb balance on unstable surfaces as various perturbations are applied to the unstable surface. The challenge of the perturbation task advances as the patient becomes more skilled in controlling the movement and demonstrates increased stability. In theory, these interventions help improve reactive stability of the joint by developing appropriate neuromuscular responses to external stress in the absence of mechanical stability. Based on results of clinical studies with physically active individuals with ACL injuries who are appropriately selected for non-operative management, Fitzgerald et al.[2] have suggested including perturbation training within a rehabilitation program for 2 to 3 sessions per week for a total of 10 visits to promote successful return to prior level of function.

Progression beyond the initial phases of nonoperative management of an ACL injury requires the individual to demonstrate an ability to successfully attain certain criteria directed toward return to sport. To participate in a dynamic functional progression (and before returning to sport), an individual must be able to demonstrate normal knee ROM and sufficient strength (>90% limb symmetry index), balance, proprioception, and neuromuscular control.[35] Failure to meet these goals prior to functional reintegration can result in the development of compensations and abnormal movement patterns.[25,36] Once these goals are met, a functional progression back to activity and/or sports is recommended prior to initiation of desired sports-specific activities.[35,37] **Prior to return to sport, a functional reintegration program should be developed to meet the unique, activity-specific goals of each patient.** Emphasis should be on the development of progressive reintegration with initial interventions occurring at reduced speed and/or intensity. With the current young female soccer player, after resolution of her impairments (i.e., attainment of normal knee ROM and strength), successful completion of perturbation training, and an absence of any giving-way with activity, a functional progression should begin with light pivoting and cutting activities that simulate maneuvers experienced on the soccer field. These may include soccer-specific drills, dribbling drills, and light plyometric activities. Typically, these should be initiated in a single plane and at a submaximal (50%) speed. As she demonstrates success with these maneuvers, the intensity of the drills can be increased by adding multiplanar movements, focusing more on single-limb activities, and increasing the speed to 75% and eventually to 100%. If she is able to successfully execute these drills, a final progression to "live-game" activity should be executed during a simulated game or during a scrimmage situation. If she successfully completes this phase of rehabilitation without episodes of giving-way, consideration can be made to return to sport. Objective criteria to evaluate readiness to return to sport may include patient-reported outcomes such as the International Knee Documentation Committee (IKDC) self-report measure,[22] single-limb hop testing,[21] and functional movement tools such as a drop vertical jump maneuver.[38]

Evidence-Based Clinical Recommendations

SORT: Strength of Recommendation Taxonomy

A: Consistent, good-quality patient-oriented evidence
B: Inconsistent or limited-quality patient-oriented evidence
C: Consensus, disease-oriented evidence, usual practice, expert opinion, or case series

1. An objective algorithmic assessment can be used to identify "copers"—those ACL-deficient individuals who may be able to return to high-level functional activity without surgical ACL reconstruction and without repeated giving-way episodes. **Grade A**

2. Participation in interventions that incorporate neuromuscular re-education and improve lower extremity strength, balance, and proprioception increases the likelihood that ACL-deficient individuals can successfully return to pivoting and cutting activity without undergoing ACL reconstruction. **Grade B**

3. ACL-deficient individuals who choose nonoperative management should participate in a structured, functional reintegration program before returning to sport. **Grade C**

COMPREHENSION QUESTIONS

24.1 Which of the following is NOT a criterion for a patient with an anterior cruciate ligament tear to be classified as a potential "coper"?

A. 80% limb symmetry score or greater on all single-limb hop testing

B. Knee Outcome Survey of ADLs of $\geq 80\%$

C. Reports of no more than one episode of giving way since injury

D. No asymmetries with movement patterns on a drop vertical jump assessment

24.2 Open kinetic chain (OKC) knee extension exercises should be performed in which of the following ranges of motion to minimize anterior shear forces within the ACL-deficient knee joint?

A. 90° flexion to full extension

B. 90° flexion to 10° flexion

C. 90° flexion to 45° flexion

D. 90° flexion to 60° flexion

ANSWERS

24.1 **D.** The drop vertical jump assessment is not a criterion to be considered a coper. All other answers were included in the algorithm defined by Fitzgerald et al.[2,7]

24.2 **C.** A safe range to perform OKC knee extension with ACL deficiency is 90° to 45° because it minimizes the anterior shear forces at the tibiofemoral joint.

REFERENCES

1. Hurd WJ, Axe MJ, Snyder-Mackler L. A 10-year prospective trial of a patient management algorithm and screening examination for highly active individuals with anterior cruciate ligament injury: part 1, outcomes. *Am J Sports Med.* 2008;36:40-47.

2. Fitzgerald GK, Axe MJ, Snyder-Mackler L. Proposed practice guidelines for nonoperative anterior cruciate ligament rehabilitation of physically active individuals. *J Orthop Sports Phys Ther.* 2000;30:194-203.

3. Duthon VB, Barea C, Abrassart S, et al. Anatomy of the anterior cruciate ligament. *Knee Surg Sports Traumatol Arthrosc.* 2006;14:204-213.

4. Butler DL, Noyes FR, Grood ES. Ligamentous restraints to anterior-posterior drawer in the human knee. A biomechanical study. *J Bone Joint Surg Am.* 1980;62:259-270.

5. Linko E, Harilainen A, Malmivaara A, Seitsalo S. Surgical versus conservative interventions for anterior cruciate ligament ruptures in adults. *Cochrane Database Syst Rev.* 2005(2):CD001356.

6. Noyes FR, Matthews DS, Mooar PA, Grood ES. The symptomatic anterior cruciate-deficient knee. Part II: the results of rehabilitation, activity modification, and counseling on functional disability. *J Bone Joint Surg Am.* 1983;65:163-174.

7. Fitzgerald GK, Axe MJ, Snyder-Mackler L. A decision-making scheme for returning patients to high-level activity with nonoperative treatment after anterior cruciate ligament rupture. *Knee Surg Sports Traumatol Arthrosc.* 2000;8:76-82.

8. Levy AS, Wetzler MJ, Lewars M, Laughlin W. Knee injuries in women collegiate rugby players. *Am J Sports Med.* 1997;25:360-362.

9. Beynnon BD, Johnson RJ, Abate JA, et al. Treatment of anterior cruciate ligament injuries, part I. *Am J Sports Med.* 2005;33:1579-1602.

10. Lohmander LS, Ostenberg A, Englund M, Roos H. High prevalence of knee osteoarthritis, pain, and functional limitations in female soccer players twelve years after anterior cruciate ligament injury. *Arthritis Rheum.* 2004;50:3145-3152.

11. von Porat A, Roos EM, Roos H. High prevalence of osteoarthritis 14 years after an anterior cruciate ligament tear in male soccer players: a study of radiographic and patient relevant outcomes. *Ann Rheum Dis.* 2004;63:269-273.

12. Spindler KP, Wright RW. Clinical practice. Anterior cruciate ligament tear. *N Engl J Med.* 2008;359:2135-2142.

13. Daniel DM, Stone ML, Dobson BE, et al. Fate of the ACL-injured patient. A prospective outcome study. *Am J Sports Med.* 1994;22:632-644.

14. Kennedy JC, Alexander IJ, Hayes KC. Nerve supply of the human knee and its functional importance. *Am J Sports Med.* 1982;10:329-335.

15. McHugh MP, Tyler TF, Gleim GW, Nicholas SJ. Preoperative indicators of motion loss and weakness following anterior cruciate ligament reconstruction. *J Orthop Sports Phys Ther.* 1998;27:407-411.

16. Ageberg E, Pettersson A, Friden T. 15-year follow-up of neuromuscular function in patients with unilateral nonreconstructed anterior cruciate ligament injury initially treated with rehabilitation and activity modification: a longitudinal prospective study. *Am J Sports Med.* 2007;35:2109-2117.

17. Berchuck M, Andriacchi TP, Bach BR, Reider B. Gait adaptations by patients who have a deficient anterior cruciate ligament. *J Bone Joint Surg Am.* 1990;72:871-877.

18. Friden T, Roberts D, Zatterstrom R, et al. Proprioceptive defects after an anterior cruciate ligament rupture-the relation to associated anatomical lesions and subjective knee function. *Knee Surg Sports Traumatol Arthrosc.* 1999;7:226-231.

19. Haus J, Halata Z. Innervation of the anterior cruciate ligament. *Int Orthop.* 1990;14:293-296.

20. Hurd WJ, Axe MJ, Snyder-Mackler L. A 10-year prospective trial of a patient management algorithm and screening examination for highly active individuals with anterior cruciate ligament injury: part 2, determinants of dynamic knee stability. *Am J Sports Med.* 2008;36:48-56.

21. Noyes FR, Barber SD, Mangine RE. Abnormal lower limb symmetry determined by function hop tests after anterior cruciate ligament rupture. *Am J Sports Med.* 1991;19:513-518.

22. Irrgang JJ, Snyder-Mackler L, Wainner RS, et al. Development of a patient-reported measure of function of the knee. *J Bone Joint Surg Am.* 1998;80:1132-1145.

23. Logerstedt DS, Snyder-Mackler L, Ritter RC, et al. Orthopaedic Section of the American Physical Therapy Association. Knee stability and movement coordination impairments: knee ligament sprain. *J Orthop Sports Phys Ther.* 2010;40:A1-A37.

24. Chmielewski TL, Hurd WJ, Rudolph KS, et al. Perturbation training improves knee kinematics and reduces muscle co-contraction after complete unilateral anterior cruciate ligament rupture. *Phys Ther.* 2005;85:740-749.

25. Chmielewski TL, Rudolph KS, Snyder-Mackler L. Development of dynamic knee stability after acute ACL injury. *J Electromyogr Kinesiol.* 2002;12:267-274.

26. Snyder-Mackler L, Delitto A, Bailey SL, Stralka SW. Strength of the quadriceps femoris muscle and functional recovery after reconstruction of the anterior cruciate ligament. A prospective, randomized clinical trial of electrical stimulation. *J Bone Joint Surg Am.* 1995;77:1166-1173.

27. Beynnon BD, Johnson RJ, Fleming BC. The science of anterior cruciate ligament rehabilitation. *Clin Orthop Relat Res.* 2002(402):9-20.

28. Beynnon BD, Fleming BC, Johnson RJ, et al. Anterior cruciate ligament strain behavior during rehabilitation exercises in vivo. *Am J Sports Med.* 1995;23:24-34.

29. Hewett TE, Paterno MV, Myer GD. Strategies for enhancing proprioception and neuromuscular control of the knee. *Clin Orthop Relat Res.* 2002(402):76-94.

30. Paterno MV, Hewett TE, Noyes FR. The return of neuromuscular coordination after anterior cruciate ligament reconstruction. *J Orthop Sports Phys Ther.* 1998;27:94.

31. Paterno MV, Hewett TE, Noyes FR. Gender differences in neuromuscular coordination of controls, ACL-deficient knees and ACL-reconstructed knees. *J Orthop Sports Phys Ther.* 1999;29:A-45.

32. Friden T, Roberts D, Ageberg E, et al. Review of knee proprioception and the relation to extremity function after an anterior cruciate ligament rupture. *J Orthop Sports Phys Ther.* 2001;31:567-576.

33. Gokeler A, Benjaminse A, Hewett TE, et al. Proprioceptive deficits after ACL injury: are they clinically relevant? *Br J Sports Med.* 2012;46:180-192.

34. Irrgang JJ, Neri R. The rationale for open and closed kinetic chain activities for restoration of proprioception and neuromuscular control following injury? In Lephart SM, Fu FH, eds. *Proprioception and Neuromuscular Control in Joint Stability.* Champaign, IL: Human Kinetics; 2000.

35. Schmitt L, Byrnes R, Cherny C, et al. Cincinnati Children's Hospital Medical Center: Evidence-based clinical care guideline for return to activity after lower extremity injury. Available at: http://www.cincinnatichildrens.org/svc/alpha/h/health-policy/otpt.htm, Guideline 38, pages 1-13, May 24, 2010. Accessed January 16, 2012.

36. Chmielewski TL, Hurd WJ, Snyder-Mackler L. Elucidation of a potentially destabilizing control strategy in ACL deficient non-copers. *J Electromyogr Kinesiol.* 2005;15:83-92.

37. Myer GD, Paterno MV, Ford KR, et al. Rehabilitation after anterior cruciate ligament reconstruction: criteria-based progression through the return to sport phase. *J Orthop Sports Phys Ther.* 2006;36:385-402.

38. Paterno MV, Schmitt LC, Ford KR, et al. Biomechanical measures during landing and postural stability predict second anterior cruciate ligament injury after anterior cruciate ligament reconstruction and return to sport. *Am J Sports Med.* 2010;38:1968-1978.

ACL Reconstruction: Rehabilitation and Return to Play

Pedro Zavala
Michael R. Conway
Charles Nathan Vannatta
Sadie J. Zebell
George J. Davies

CASE 25

A 20-year-old female presents to an outpatient physical therapy clinic 3 months after anterior cruciate ligament (ACL) reconstruction with a bone-tendon (patella)-bone graft. The tear occurred in her right nondominant lower extremity when she fell while skiing. She reports that her knee "bent and pivoted," and she felt a "popping" sensation in her knee. Although she was able to ski down the hill, when she attempted to ski the following day, her knee felt "unstable" and she stopped. Due to persistent swelling and instability in the knee, she sought medical care. She was evaluated by a sports medicine orthopedic surgeon. An ACL tear without concomitant injuries was confirmed via MRI scan. The surgeon advised the patient to participate in a prehabilitation program prior to surgical repair. Prehabilitation consisted of outpatient visits with a board-certified sports physical therapist and the prescription of a comprehensive home exercise program. The patient was managed by the same physical therapist for the first 3 months post-ACL reconstruction. Due to unforeseen circumstances, the patient was transferred to another board-certified sports physical therapist. The patient's goals are to resolve any remaining impairments and learn whether she can start a return-to-running program.

- ▶ What are the examination priorities?
- ▶ Aside from biomechanical constraints, what are adverse neuroplastic effects following ACL injury?
- ▶ What domains of function should be included as part of return-to-sport criteria?

KEY DEFINITIONS

ARTHROGENIC MUSCLE INHIBITION: Inability to volitionally contract a muscle due to reflex inhibition of the muscle/s surrounding a joint following damage[1]

CYCLOPS LESION: Development of fibrotic tissue in the anterior aspect of the intercondylar notch that results in loss of knee extension[2]

KINESIOPHOBIA: Unrealistic, disproportionate, and irrational fear of physical movement secondary to a traumatic injury[3]

PERIODIZATION: Planned manipulation of training variables (*e.g.*, load, sets, and repetitions) to maximize training adaptations and prevent the onset of overtraining syndrome[4]

POST-TRAUMATIC OSTEOARTHRITIS (PTOA): Onset of osteoarthritis within a joint secondary to an intra-articular injury[5]

RETURN TO PARTICIPATION: Training to participate in the desired sport to *some* degree, but at a lower level than desired and with some degree of restriction[6]

RETURN TO PERFORMANCE: Resumption of prior level of performance in the athlete's preferred sport[6]

RETURN TO SPORT: Participation in sport without restriction, but *not* at the desired level of performance[6]

RETURN-TO-SPORT CONTINUUM: Concept that allows clinicians to parallel recovery and rehabilitation as part of the process of returning athletes to sport[6]

Objectives

1. Understand the epidemiology and impact of ACL injuries.

2. Identify pertinent aspects of a patient's history that may influence re-injury risk and subsequent rehabilitation strategies.

3. Describe a staged progression to structure rehabilitation interventions to return athletes to their desired level of sport participation.

4. Provide recommended reference values to guide decisions in progressing athletes through stages of rehabilitation.

5. Implement a shared decision-making process for guiding athletes in returning to athletic participation.

Physical Therapy Considerations

Physical therapy considerations during management of the individual after ACL reconstruction:

▶ **General physical therapy plan of care/goals:** Protect knee during early phases of healing; decrease pain; treat impairments; normalize gait; increase strength of core and lower extremity; improve functional movements and progress into sport-specific activities using a criterion-based approach

▶ **Physical therapy interventions:** Patient education and establishment of realistic expectations at start of rehabilitation program; appropriate and progressive therapeutic exercises (*e.g.*, basic exercises in early stages with progression to weightbearing functional exercises); biofeedback and blood flow restriction in early stages to enhance muscle function; open- and closed-kinetic chain resistance exercises for the core and lower extremity, with progression from muscle activation and motor control, to load tolerance, strengthening, power, rate of force development, and finally to functional specificity to meet demands required for the athlete's performance in a given sport

▶ **Precautions during physical therapy:** Recognition and reinforcement of early weightbearing precautions to protect healing graft during early rehabilitation; decrease pain and effusion to allow knee movement (which may prevent a cyclops lesion); respect the lengthy rehabilitation program and avoid rushing because patient "feels good"; ensure thorough assessment in multiple domains to help establish readiness for return to sport and reduce risk of reinjury

▶ **Complications interfering with physical therapy:** Postsurgical complications such as deep vein thrombosis, infection, and arthrofibrosis; patient nonadherence with rehabilitation program may lead to difficulties restoring range of motion (ROM), strength, and/or function; apprehension or kinesiophobia, which may warrant referral to a sport psychologist.

Understanding the Health Condition

Safe and successful resumption of activity is the ultimate goal for patients and their providers following an ACL injury or reconstruction. How well this goal is realized has been the center of much discussion within the sports medicine community.[7] Approximately 81% of athletes return to some participation with sport. However, only 65% return to their preinjury level of sport and of those who participate at a competitive level, only 55% return to competition.[8] These statistics have led many healthcare professionals to adopt a "continuum" approach beginning with a "return to participation" when athletes just begin to reintegrate into sport activities.[6] Following this stage, the athlete may "return to sport" by resuming practice or competition to some degree. The final part of the continuum is "return to performance" when athletes have restored their prior level of function.[6,9] Participation in elite sport increases the likelihood of returning to sport (OR = 2.5).[8] Perhaps due to additional motivation and drive to "return to performance," 83% of elite athletes have been able to return to their prior level of sport.[10]

Many other factors besides motivation are associated with successful return to sport. These include symmetrical hop test performance, younger age, male sex, psychological readiness, earlier surgery after injury, graft type, time from surgery, and absence of cartilage injury.[8,11,12] Each of these factors should be considered when considering an individual athlete's readiness to return to sport.[6]

The decision to return to sport must also take into consideration the risk for reinjury. Second ACL injury is a very real concern for any athlete choosing to return to sport. Although over 90% of children and adolescents return to *some* level of sport following ACL reconstruction, 13% experience a graft rupture and 14% injure the contralateral ACL.[13] The overall incidence of second ACL injury has been estimated to be as high as 15%,[14] with younger athletes experiencing higher rates ranging from 23% to 35%.[14,15] The majority of second ACL injuries appear to occur in the contralateral limb.[14,16] The relatively high incidence of second ACL injury has caused some to question the prognostic validity of current return-to-sport testing.[17,18] **While passing a battery of return-to-sport tests reduces the risk of graft rupture,[18,19] athletes that have met return-to-sport testing criteria are still at increased risk for *contralateral ACL injury*.[18]** Therefore, **careful attention to sport reintegration and other qualitative[17] and psychosocial variables[20] during the return-to-sport continuum is of paramount importance.**

In addition to reducing the risk for a second ACL injury, the physical therapist must talk with the patient about long-term knee health following ACL injury or reconstruction. After a joint injury, post-traumatic osteoarthritis (PTOA) often develops. Specifically, 50% to 90% of ACL injuries progress to PTOA.[5] A number of factors increase the risk of PTOA, including female sex, older age, high body mass index, lower physical activity level, smoking, low education level, increased time interval between injury and surgery, and varus alignment of the uninjured knee.[5]

Physical Therapy Patient/Client Management

ACL tears are initially diagnosed based on the mechanism of injury, the patient's subjective history, and clinical examination. Imaging is often performed to confirm the diagnosis and to examine the joint for any additional pathology. On confirmation of an ACL tear, the **primary goals for prehabilitation (*before* surgery) are to decrease pain, minimize knee effusion, increase ROM, improve quadriceps function, reduce postoperative complications, and to educate the patient on the plan of care and long-term prognosis after surgery.[2]** In both athletic and highly active populations, ACL reconstruction is the gold standard treatment following an acute ACL injury. Surgical intervention is primarily performed arthroscopically. Selection of graft type depends on several factors and is a shared decision between surgeon and patient. **Regardless of graft type, postoperative rehabilitation is progressed through criterion-based phases over a 9- to 15-month period.** Returning to sport after ACL reconstruction is a long and extensive process that aims to restore preinjury knee function.

Examination, Evaluation, and Diagnosis

A thorough patient history is a crucial component of the clinical examination. It provides the clinician with important information regarding mechanism of injury, location, and nature of symptoms (*e.g.*, presence of knee locking or buckling), alleviating and aggravating factors, review of other systems, and helps frame the plan of care.

The postoperative physical examination starts with observation of the patient's limb for presence of global knee effusion, knee discoloration, and quadriceps muscle atrophy. Tests and measures consist of general palpation, anthropometric measurements, ROM (*i.e.*, goniometry), flexibility, joint play, strength, special tests, postural control, and functional movement (if able). Anthropometric measurements, such as a circumferential girth measurement at the tibiofemoral joint line and 10 cm proximal, allow objective tracking of both knee effusion and quadriceps atrophy. A 1.0 to 1.63 cm change has been reported as the minimal detectable change in another knee surgical population (total knee arthroplasty).[21]

ROM, joint play assessment, and flexibility are assessed to quantify motion restriction, joint laxity, and overall soft tissue mobility. During ROM assessment, quantity and quality of motion, and end-feel should be assessed on both the involved and uninvolved limb. ROM symmetry is an important element in the initial phases of rehabilitation both pre- and postoperatively.[2] A cyclops lesion is the development of fibrotic tissue in the anterior aspect of the intercondylar notch that results in loss of knee extension, which may require surgical intervention to resolve. The possibility of a cyclops lesion should be considered if difficulty in restoring ROM is encountered.[2] Assessment of hamstring, gastrocnemius, and quadriceps (when tolerable) flexibility should be assessed and restored to be symmetrical compared to the uninvolved limb.

Assessment of strength, especially the involved quadriceps, is a critical component of the evaluation. Hart and colleagues[22] reported that within the first 8 weeks following ACL injury, individuals exhibit only 85% and 82% of quadriceps activation for the uninvolved and involved limbs respectively, which has been attributed to arthrogenic muscle inhibition. This phenomenon affects both afferent and efferent pathways, making it difficult to activate the quadriceps and avoid atrophy. Following ACL injury, cross-sectional area of the quadriceps also decreases.[23] Both impaired neural pathways and reduced cross-sectional area of the quadriceps contribute to the quadriceps weakness. We recommend formal strength assessment of the quadriceps using isokinetic or isometric dynamometry at 12 weeks postsurgical repair, when the extent of biologic healing may afford safe opportunity to do so. Following assessment of strength, tests to evaluate higher level functional activities including dynamic balance, jumping, hopping, agility tests, and sport-specific movements are recommended in the late stages of ACL rehabilitation.

Early after ACL reconstruction, it is important that clinicians assess ligament laxity, static and dynamic postural stability, and perform a functional movement analysis. Performing a Lachman test provides information regarding the integrity of the surgical repair to ensure no further surgical intervention is warranted prior to partaking in a rehabilitation program.[24] A common early postural control assessment is bipedal static balance with eyes open and eyes closed. Four to six weeks later, single-leg balance should be assessed.[25] A double-leg squat can be performed within the first 4 weeks following ACL reconstruction. This functional assessment can illustrate altered movement patterns such as unequal weight distribution or presence of apprehension in placing weight on the surgical limb. A single-leg squat

Table 25-1 ADVANTAGES AND DISADVANTAGES OF GRAFT SOURCES FOR ANTERIOR CRUCIATE LIGAMENT RECONSTRUCTION

Graft Type	Advantages	Disadvantages
Bone-patellar tendon-bone	• Strong graft[28,29] • Presence of bony fixation on each end[30,31]	• Quadricep weakness • Higher risk of development of anterior knee pain[28]
Hamstring (semimembranosus or gracilis)	• Less risk of development of anterior knee pain[28,29] • Strong graft choice with multiple strands[28]	• Lacks bony fixation[28] • Presence of hamstring weakness[30]
Quadriceps tendon	• Strong graft choice[28] • Less pain at donor site[28]	• Lacks bony fixation[32]

test has been used clinically to assess the dynamic strength of proximal hip muscles and knee extensors, as well as neuromuscular control and coordination.[26,27]

In developing a management strategy, it is important to know what type of graft was used. Table 25-1 outlines the advantages and disadvantages of graft sources for ACL reconstruction that may impact the plan of care.[28-32]

Plan of Care and Interventions

Postoperative rehabilitation following ACL reconstruction should follow a periodized and progressive rehabilitation through several phases that gradually increase demands on the patient to adequately prepare for resumption of prior level of activity. Currently, there is no consensus on the optimal progression through rehabilitation.[6,7] Following principles of periodization (progressive overload and specific adaptations to imposed demands), the rehabilitation plan can be divided into several phases. This case describes a combination of criterion- and time-based milestones to guide progression through 5 phases: (1) protection and restoration (Weeks ~0-6); (2) foundational strengthening, neuromuscular control, and load tolerance (Weeks ~6-16); (3) advanced strengthening, plyometric training, and running progression (Weeks 16-24); (4) power development and sport-specific training (6-9 months); and (5) sport integration and return to competition (9+ months).[6,7] The expected timeframe for each phase and the implementation of certain interventions depend on the presence of comorbidities, expected healing time of the graft, and the ability of the patient to achieve objective milestones during rehabilitation. This case focuses on Phases 2 through 4, but Phase 1 will be briefly summarized.

The goals of Phase 1 (protection and restoration) are to protect the surgical fixation and graft integrity, reduce pain and joint effusion, increase ROM, improve quadriceps activation, and normalize gait. During the initial postoperative visit, education regarding the prognosis and plan of care helps guide patient expectations and ease concerns. The following criteria should be used to assess the patient's readiness to progress to Phase 2: circumferential girth measurements at the joint line within 1.0 cm compared to uninvolved knee; achievement of full knee extension (0°) or if relevant, hyperextension, comparable to the uninvolved knee; knee flexion >120°; volitional quadriceps setting contraction (visible superior patellar glide into femoral trochlear groove) without the presence of muscle fasciculations; ability to complete a straight leg raise without an extensor lag; and, a normalized gait pattern. Typically, these milestones are achieved within the first 4 to 6 postoperative weeks.[7]

The goals of Phase 2 (weeks 6-16) are to improve neuromuscular control, progress lower extremity and core strengthening intensity, and increase the patient's ability to tolerate loads imparted to the knee.

Following ACL injury, individuals tend to rely more on visual input than proprioception to maintain postural control.[33] This *sensory reweighting* occurs due to disruption of the mechanoreceptors within the tibiofemoral joint and changes in higher brain centers including the cerebellum and frontal, parietal, and occipital lobes.[33] The observed neuromuscular deficits throughout rehabilitation following ACL reconstruction have been attributed to multiple adverse neuroplastic alterations associated with the injury.

The use of motor learning principles to enhance automaticity with movement control patterns may be beneficial to address the sensory-visual motor control and motor cortex alterations that occur after ACL reconstruction.[33,34] Interventions such as proprioceptive neuromuscular facilitation (PNF), incorporation of external cues, and dual tasks may improve motor control and motor learning.[33,34] For example, one way to effectively stimulate the mechanoreceptors is by joint approximation in combination with alternating isometrics.[35-37] The purpose behind these interventions is to minimize *conscious* focus on proper quadriceps activation and neuromuscular stability to determine whether the patient is able to maintain proper neuromuscular control while completing dual tasks. Because competitive environments are often unpredictable and require the athlete's focus to be task-oriented, this trained automaticity may assist in protecting athletes from re-injury.

For successful rehabilitation, progressive resistance training—especially for the quadriceps and hamstrings—is imperative throughout each phase. As goals shift from focusing on hypertrophy, strength, or endurance, it is vital for the physical therapist to apply the principles of resistance training and periodization appropriately. The reader is referred to the American College of Sports Medicine (ACSM)'s guidelines for more details.[38]

If the patient plans to return to jumping, cutting, and/or pivoting sports, plyometric training (exercises that require various loads to be moved at higher velocities with different movements to promote muscular power) should be initiated when sufficient strength has been restored. There is no consensus on a specific minimum strength necessary to indicate readiness to initiate plyometric training. Several authors have reported biomechanical changes in jumping tasks with a quadriceps strength leg symmetry index (LSI) of less than 80% to 85%, which may suggest a *minimum* strength symmetry of 80% prior to initiating plyometric training.[39,40] However, consideration of absolute strength (*e.g.*, peak torque to body weight ratio) and the intensity of the plyometric task are also important considerations.[41] Plyometric training is typically introduced when patients achieve a LSI >70% to

80% and demonstrate the ability to control eccentric loading during double-leg and single-leg squats.

Appropriately timed inclusion of plyometric training is recommended because this type of training improves athletic performance by stimulating fast-twitch muscle fibers, which results in improved strength, power, agility, speed, and coordination.[42,43] Plyometric training also enhances eccentric force production, develops an efficient stretch-shortening cycle, and improves neuromuscular performance and movement quality.[42-44] Last, plyometric training has been theorized to result in increased confidence levels for athletes, a psychological factor noted to influence return-to-sport rates.[45]

By 3 to 4 months post-ACL reconstruction, the degree of biologic healing may afford the opportunity to initiate a return-to-running program.[46] In addition to surgeon clearance for running, additional criteria are recommended to help inform this decision. A thorough strength assessment of proximal hip musculature, quadriceps, hamstrings, gastrocnemius, and soleus should be performed. Strength of the proximal hip musculature (abductors, extensors, external and internal rotators) can be assessed via hand-held dynamometry (HHD), which has demonstrated good validity and reliability.[47] Deficits in proximal hip strength should be addressed with open- and closed-chain exercises, as proximal hip weakness has been associated with an increased risk of non-contact ACL injury.[48] Evaluation of gastrocnemius and soleus strength can be assessed using a heel raise test.[49] For evaluation of quadriceps and hamstrings strength, isokinetic dynamometry is preferred. However, if this is not available, HHD should be used. Hirano and colleagues[50] found a positive correlation between HHD and isokinetic measurements of isometric knee extension strength in males. If strength assessment can be performed via isokinetic dynamometry, variables of interest are extensor peak torque, extensor peak torque to body weight ratio, and hamstring to quadriceps ratio. The athlete should achieve an LSI of 70% to 75% for knee extension before initiating a return-to-running program.[51] LSI should be interpreted along with peak torque to body weight ratio and functional assessment of strength such as single-leg squats.

Prior to returning to running, the athlete must also demonstrate adequate dynamic balance. The Y-Balance test and Star Excursion Balance Test (SEBT) are reliable and easy tools that provide qualitative and quantitative information regarding dynamic postural control.[52] In the SEBT, the goal is for the athlete to perform an anterior reach *within* 4 cm relative to the contralateral limb because an anterior reach of less than 4 cm relative to contralateral limb has been shown to be associated with certain lower extremity injuries in athletes[52,53] Additional assessments to consider are qualitative evaluations of submaximal jumping and hopping.

If the athlete demonstrates adequate strength, neuromuscular control, and minimal signs of apprehension following a running trial, the patient may be safe to initiate a running program. De Fontenay and colleagues[54] determined that individuals with hamstring grafts that had higher subjective International Knee Document Committee scores (≥ 64) were 3 times more likely to successfully complete a return-to-running program with minimal presence of knee swelling and no pain during and after a running session. Completing a running assessment using a treadmill and high-speed camera is a feasible way to assess running kinematics and identify compensations early. Knurr et al.[55] found that gait kinematics and kinetics may not return to preinjury level even one year following ACL reconstruction. Therefore, focused gait training may be necessary to attempt to normalize running kinematics. If the athlete tolerates the initial running trial well, a return-to-running program may begin with close monitoring of symptoms and attention to whether the patient's running gait normalizes or may benefit from additional intervention.

The primary goal of Phase 2 is to attain adequate strength of the involved extremity to ensure the tissues have the capacity to tolerate the demands of plyometric movements. Initiation of submaximal plyometrics has been shown to be safe and can improve strength, power, agility, speed, and coordination.[44,45] Focusing on restoring neuromuscular control and integrating training of different sensory systems may overcome the neuromuscular deficits and sensory reweighting that occurs secondary to ACL injury. Although timelines following ACL reconstruction are fluid, progression through each phase should be criterion-based. To progress to Phase 3, knee effusion must remain within 1.0 cm of the uninvolved side; ROM must be symmetric (within 5° of the uninvolved side); quadriceps and hamstring LSI must be near 70% to 80%; and, the athlete must not demonstrate abnormal kinematics during double- and single-leg tasks (e.g., weight shift away from involved limb during a squat or stiff knee landing on completion of submaximal plyometrics). It is important that a team approach involving the orthopedic surgeon, physical therapist, coaches, and the patient is implemented when determining the future plan of care.

Phase 3 of rehabilitation (weeks 16-24) includes the exercises and activities previously performed with progression of advanced strengthening, plyometric training and running. The goal of this phase is to continue challenging the athlete by progressing toward the demands of the sport she will be returning to. As the athlete is participating in more advanced dynamic movements, it is imperative that she continues independent strength training because treatment sessions may focus on neuromuscular control and other aspects of rehabilitation.

Balance and proprioceptive training should consist of single-leg balance activities (Fig. 25-1) and reactive postural stability training with the addition of perturbations (Fig. 25-2). Single-leg balance activities can be performed using the Star Excursion Balance Test grid (Fig. 25-1). Perturbation training enhances neuromuscular control, increases the readiness of muscles to respond to disruptive forces, and improves joint stability by stimulating afferent pathways.[56] Advancing plyometric training can aid in neuromuscular control as the athlete improves both double-leg and single-leg control during dynamic movements. Neuromuscular control training with double- and single-leg movements progressing from hops in place to anterior and lateral hops, and finally adding a rotatory component with dual tasks improves knee biomechanical and neuromuscular deficits during single-leg landing tasks.[57,58]

During each of these activities, dual-task training should continue to be used because the goal is to transition each skill toward automaticity with adequate performance even in the presence of distractions. Dual tasks can consist of both cognitive and motor tasks and should be used during the progression of neuromuscular training. Multidirectional movements (beyond jumping activities) are encouraged here since these activities are crucial for athletic participation.

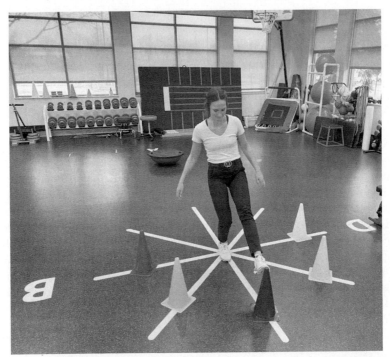

A

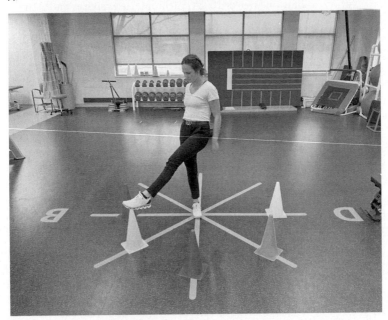

B

Figure 25-1. Single-limb balance and proprioceptive training using the Star Excursion Balance grid. **A.** Single-leg stance on ACL-reconstructed limb with contralateral limb reaching in an anterior direction and **B**, reaching in anterolateral direction.

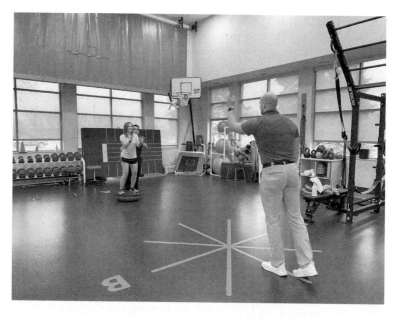

Figure 25-2. Reactive postural stability training on a BOSU® ball in double-limb stance while preparing to catch a weighted object (with therapist guarding the patient for safety). Perturbations can also be performed by standing on a foam surface or tilt board, or can be directly applied by the physical therapist.

Phase 3 is when the athlete is introduced to agility training as a progression of the running program and training moves from low-intensity to high-intensity drills. Between 4 and 6 months post-ACL reconstruction, Souissi and colleagues[59] found that more aggressive and complex exercises designed to increase neuromuscular control, muscle strength and power, proprioception, speed, and agility significantly improved performance in functional tests compared to a standardized rehabilitation program.[59] The speed and agility training implemented in this group progressed as follows: moderate speed forward and backward running; forward running into single-leg forward and backward hops; high-speed running; backward running into single-leg forward hopping; high-speed running around cones slalom style; sprinting into a lateral shuffle, and figure-8 running.[59] Clinicians can use this framework to guide the progression through multidirectional running, cutting, and pivoting according to the patient's tolerance level.

As patients demonstrate the ability to complete agility and plyometric training at higher intensities, strength gains should be monitored. Prior to initiating maximum effort agility and plyometrics, it is recommended that patients achieve a quadriceps LSI near 90%[39,40,60] and demonstrate good tolerance and qualitative control of agility and plyometric tasks. Once these criteria are met, it may be appropriate to advance to more sport-specific training in Phase 4.

Phase 4 (months 6-9) emphasizes developing explosive power in preparation for sport-specific tasks. While strength deficits may still be present, the foundation of progressive overload through strengthening, running, plyometrics, and agility drills has been established. Strengthening exercises should be increased to develop power and the intensity of agility and plyometric tasks may be completed at maximal efforts. As the athlete develops qualitative control during these tasks, the therapist can add elements of challenge to prepare the athlete for the more open environment encountered outside the clinic.

For strength and functional hop testing, the passing criterion is typically set at ≥90% LSI.[7] To ensure reliable and accurate measurement, strength should be evaluated using the same tests administered in Phase 2. Four hop tests that are valid and reliable measures of function for this population[61] should be used: single-leg hop test for distance (SLHT), 6-meter timed test, triple-hop test for distance, and crossover hop test for distance. Although hop tests provide a quantitative assessment, their use to make return-to-sport determinations is less clear.[62] It is becoming increasingly recognized that the clinician should note the presence of any altered kinematics during performance. However, there is no consensus on what kind of kinematic criteria should be implemented in making return-to-sport decisions.

It appears that achieving a 90% LSI may not indicate restoration of knee function, nor does achieving this benchmark eliminate increased risk of further injury. Wellsandt and colleagues[63] compared strength and functional hop testing in individuals following ACL injury. They tested the *uninvolved* limb prior to ACL reconstruction and both the uninvolved and involved limb at the 6-month follow-up. They found that using the *baseline* measurement of the *uninvolved* limb prior to ACL reconstruction may serve as a better reference point to determine return to sport and risk of further injury, compared to measurement of the uninvolved limb at 6-month follow-up. A recent investigation examined power output using various methods including isokinetic dynamometry and hop testing in individuals 8 months post-ACL reconstruction.[64] They found that LSIs from isokinetic testing at 60°/sec and 180°/sec (72.8% and 84.8%, respectively) were significantly lower than LSIs for the single-hop test and triple-hop test (92.7% and 94.0%, respectively). These findings indicate that measures of LSI may *overestimate* knee function and may also be task dependent. Therefore, LSIs should be interpreted in the context with other measures such as jump distance relative to body height or peak torque to body weight ratios.

The last functional assessments to assist in determining return to sport are agility tests and/or sport-specific movements.[6,7] Figure 25-3 shows the Lower Extremity Functional Test (LEFT), a valid and reliable test that incorporates 8 multidirectional skills consisting of acceleration and deceleration maneuvers and progressive cutting and pivoting motions to the knee. Normative values for the LEFT are ≤120 seconds for females and ≤100 seconds for males.[65] Other agility tests include the modified pro-shuffle, modified agility T-test, shuttle run, and 505 test.[6,66,67] None of these tests has been validated for return-to-sport determinations and no consensus exists for which test is preferred. It may also be appropriate to incorporate sport-specific drills in a controlled environment prior to determining return-to-sport decision.

Patient-reported outcomes also serve as tools to measure progress throughout the postoperative rehabilitation journey. Some patient-reported outcomes may provide additional information regarding lack of psychological readiness

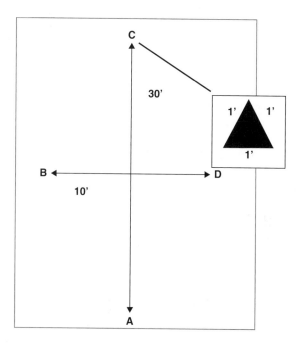

Figure 25-3. Diagram of the Lower Extremity Functional Test (LEFT). The LEFT course measures 9.14 m (30 feet) in the north-south direction and 3.05 m (10 feet) in the east-west direction (A = south, B = east, C = north, D = west). Triangles consisting of 0.305 m (1 ft) strips of athletic tape are positioned at the end of each axis. The test is initiated with the patient starting at the southernmost (A) triangle. Sequence of multidirectional skills: (1) forward run, (2) backward run, (3) side shuffle, (4) carioca, (5) Figure 8's, (6) 45° cuts, (7) 90° cuts, (8) crossover 90° cuts, (9) forward run, (10) backward run. The forward and backward runs start at the southern triangle (A) with the patient running to the northern triangle (C) and returning back to the start (A). The other drills are performed counterclockwise (A-D-C-B-A) then clockwise (A-B-C-D-A).

that may delay return to sport: Anterior Cruciate Ligament-Return to Sport after Injury Scale (ACL-RSI), International Knee Documentation Committee (IKDC), Knee Injury and Osteoarthritis Outcome Scores (KOOS), Tegner Activity Scale, Lysholm Scale, and Tampa Kinesiophobia Index.

Returning an athlete back to her respective sport is a long journey following ACL reconstruction. The goal of the entire rehabilitation process is to restore knee function, return to preinjury status, and ultimately minimize further risk of injury. Despite using criterion-based assessments, there are limitations and minimal consensus on what should constitute return-to-sport criteria.[68] Unfortunately, individuals passing return-to-sport benchmarks are still at increased risk of sustaining a subsequent ACL rupture and at an increased risk (235%) of a contralateral ACL injury.[18] Therefore, it may be worthwhile to include an additional phase once all of the above clinical criteria are met.

Phase 5 (9+ months) consists of gradually reintroducing the athlete into the team environment through a staged approach.[7] Because the risk for second ACL injury is substantially lower when waiting at least 9 months following ACL reconstruction, it is recommended that this phase should begin no sooner than 9 months *and* not before the aforementioned clinical criteria have been met.[69] Athletes can begin with a period of team participation through non-contact drills and then move toward contact drills in controlled settings under close supervision of coaching and athletic training staff to observe for any athlete apprehension or knee symptoms.

Once the athlete demonstrates adequate qualitative performance (*e.g.*, minimal presence of apprehension with sport-specific movements) during drills in an open team environment, the athlete may participate in scrimmages to progress into more sport-specific type environments. Close supervision for apprehension, kinesiophobia, or development of symptoms should continue. When an athlete has demonstrated the ability to participate in scrimmages within team practices, introduction of "friendly" matches could follow prior to participation with competition. Moving through the continuum of return to participation, return to sport, and then return to prior level of performance is advocated by the International Olympic Committee.[6] While there are no set guidelines for how to *precisely* navigate this process, with close supervision of the athlete by the coaching staff and medical team, a shared decision on readiness to return to competition can be made.

Evidence-Based Clinical Recommendations

SORT: Strength of Recommendation Taxonomy

A: Consistent, good-quality patient-oriented evidence
B: Inconsistent or limited-quality patient-oriented evidence
C: Consensus, disease-oriented evidence, usual practice, expert opinion, or case series

1. Passing a battery of return-to-sport tests reduces the risk of ACL graft rupture and determines the patient's readiness to return to practice, return to competition, and return to performance. **Grade B**

2. Patients who participate in a prehabilitation program prior to ACL reconstruction may experience fewer postoperative complications. **Grade C**

3. Regardless of graft type for ACL reconstruction, postoperative rehabilitation is progressed through criterion-based phases over 9 to 15 months. **Grade C**

COMPREHENSION QUESTIONS

25.1 Which of the following criteria does NOT need to be achieved prior to the patient initiating a return to running program?

    A. 16 weeks postsurgery

    B. Quadriceps strength limb symmetry index (LSI) at least 70%

    C. Star Excursion Balance Test anterior asymmetry scores >4 cm side-to-side difference

    D. Subjective International Knee Document Committee score of ≥64

25.2 What are *adverse* neuroplastic effects that have been documented in individuals following an ACL reconstruction?

A. Increase in sensory proprioception information

B. Increase reliance on visual cues for both static and dynamic postural control

C. Unilateral deficits with spinal reflex and corticospinal pathway excitability

D. Increased ability to dual task

ANSWERS

25.1 **A.** At around 3 to 4 months following ACL reconstruction, the degree of biologic healing may afford the opportunity for patients to initiate a return-to-running program. In addition to this timeframe and surgeon clearance for running, certain criteria are recommended to help inform this decision. A thorough strength assessment consists of evaluating proximal hip musculature, quadriceps, hamstrings, gastrocnemius, and soleus. A common goal to initiate a return-to-running program is a leg symmetry index (LSI) of 70% to 75% for knee extension.[51] Adequate dynamic balance also needs to be present. On the Star Excursion Balance Test (SEBT), the quantitative goal is for the athlete to perform an anterior reach *within* 4 cm relative to the contralateral limb. De Fontenay and colleagues[54] determined that individuals with higher subjective International Knee Document Committee scores (≥64) were 3 times more likely to successfully complete a return-to-running program with minimal presence of knee swelling and no pain both during and post-running session in individuals with hamstring graft.

25.2 **B.** After ACL reconstruction, individuals tend to rely more on visual input to maintain postural control, and less on proprioception.[33,34] In addition, changes in spinal reflex and corticospinal pathway excitability results in *more* neural input needed to reach motor threshold, and postural control and gait deficits occur during dual-task performance.

REFERENCES

1. Snyder-Mackler L, De Luca PF, Williams PR, et al. Reflex inhibition of the quadriceps femoris muscle after injury or reconstruction of the anterior cruciate ligament. *J Bone Jt Surg Am.* 1994;76:555-560.

2. Kambhampati SBS, Gollamudi S, Shanmugasundaram S, Josyula VVS. Cyclops lesions of the knee: a narrative review of the literature. *Orthop J Sport Med.* 2020;8:2325967120945671.

3. Huang H, Nagao M, Arita H, et al. Reproducibility, responsiveness and validation of the Tampa Scale for Kinesiophobia in patients with ACL injuries. *Health Qual Life Outcomes.* 2019;17:150.

4. Lorenz D, Morrison S. Current concepts in periodization of strength and conditioning for the sports physical therapist. *Int J Sports Phys Ther.* 2015;10:734-747.

5. Wang LJ, Zeng N, Yan ZP, et al. Post-traumatic osteoarthritis following ACL injury. *Arthritis Res Ther.* 2020;22:57.

6. Ardern CL, Glasgow P, Schneiders A, et al. 2016 Consensus statement on return to sport from the First World Congress in Sports Physical Therapy, Bern. *Br J Sports Med*. 2016;50:853-864.

7. Meredith SJ, Rauer T, Chmielewski TL, et al. Panther Symposium ACL Injury Return to Sport Consensus Group. Return to sport after anterior cruciate ligament injury: Panther Symposium ACL injury return to sport consensus group. *Knee Surg Sport Traumatol Arthrosc*. 2020;28:2403-2414.

8. Ardern CL, Taylor NF, Feller JA, Webster KE. Fifty-five per cent return to competitive sport following anterior cruciate ligament reconstruction surgery: an updated systematic review and meta-analysis including aspects of physical functioning and contextual factors. *Br J Sports Med*. 2014;48:1543-1552.

9. Buckthorpe M. Optimising the late-stage rehabilitation and return-to-sport training and testing process after ACL reconstruction. *Sport Med*. 2019;49:1043-1058.

10. Lai CCH, Ardern CL, Feller JA, Webster KE. Eighty-three per cent of elite athletes return to preinjury sport after anterior cruciate ligament reconstruction: a systematic review with meta-analysis of return to sport rates, graft rupture rates and performance outcomes. *Br J Sports Med*. 2018;52:128-138.

11. Ithurburn MP, Longfellow MA, Thomas S, et al. Knee function, strength, and resumption of preinjury sports participation in young athletes following anterior cruciate ligament reconstruction. *J Orthop Sports Phys Ther*. 2019;49:145-153.

12. Muller B, Yabroudi MA, Lynch A, et al. Return to preinjury sports after anterior cruciate ligament reconstruction is predicted by five independent factors. *Knee Surge Sport Traumatol Arthrosc*. 2021;30:84-92.

13. Kay J, Memon M, Marx RG, et al. Over 90% of children and adolescents return to sport after anterior cruciate ligament reconstruction: a systematic review and meta-analysis. *Knee Surg Sport Traumatol Arthrosc*. 2018;26:1019-1036.

14. Wiggins AJ, Grandhi RK, Schneider DK, et al. Risk of secondary injury in younger athletes after anterior cruciate ligament reconstruction: a systematic review and meta-analysis. *Am J Sports Med*. 2016;44:1861-1876.

15. Webster KE, Feller JA. Exploring the high reinjury rate in younger patients undergoing anterior cruciate ligament reconstruction. *Am J Sports Med*. 2016;44:2827-2832.

16. Paterno MV, Rauh MJ, Schmitt LC, et al. Incidence of second ACL injuries 2 years after primary ACL reconstruction and return to sport. *Am J Sports Med*. 2014;42:1567-1573.

17. Kotsifaki A, Whiteley R, Van Rossom S, et al. Single leg hop for distance symmetry masks lower limb biomechanics: Time to discuss hop distance as decision criterion for return to sport after ACL reconstruction? *Br J Sports Med*. 2022;56:249-256.

18. Webster KE, Hewett TE. What is the evidence for and validity of return-to-sport testing after anterior cruciate ligament reconstruction surgery? A systematic review and meta-analysis. *Sport Med*. 2019;49:917-929.

19. Ashigbi EYK, Banzer W, Niederer D. Return to sport tests' prognostic value for reinjury risk after anterior cruciate ligament reconstruction: a systematic review. *Med Sci Sports Exerc*. 2020;52:1263-1271.

20. Ardern CL, Taylor NF, Feller JA, et al. Psychological responses matter in returning to preinjury level of sport after anterior cruciate ligament reconstruction surgery. *Am J Sports Med*. 2013;41:1549-1558.

21. Jakobsen TL, Christensen M, Christensen SS, et al. Reliability of knee joint range of motion and circumference measurements after total knee arthroplasty: does tester experience matter? *Physiother Res Int*. 2010;15:126-134.

22. Hart JM, Pietrosimone B, Hertel J, Ingersoll CD. Quadriceps activation following knee injuries: a systematic review. *J Athl Train*. 2010;45:87-97.

23. Birchmeier T, Lisee C, Kane K, et al. Quadriceps muscle size following ACL injury and reconstruction: a systematic review. *J Orthop Res*. 2020;38:598-608.

24. Cooperman JM, Riddle DL, Rothstein JM. Reliability and validity of judgments of the integrity of the anterior cruciate ligament of the knee using the Lachman's test. *Phys Ther*. 1990;70:225-233.

25. Kouvelioti V, Kellis E, Kofotolis N, Amiridis I. Reliability of single-leg and double-leg balance tests in subjects with anterior cruciate ligament reconstruction and controls. *Res Sport Med*. 2015;23:151-166.

26. Crossley KM, Zhang WJ, Schache AG, et al. Performance on a single-leg squat task indicates hip abductor muscle function. *Am J Sports Med*. 2011;39:866-873.

27. Batty LM, Feller JA, Hartwig T, et al. Single-leg squat performance and its relationship to extensor mechanism strength after anterior cruciate ligament reconstruction. *Am J Sports Med*. 2019;47:3423-3428.

28. Mouarbes D, Menetrey J, Marot V, et al. Anterior cruciate ligament reconstruction: a systematic review and meta-analysis of outcomes for quadriceps tendon autograft versus bone–patellar tendon–bone and hamstring-tendon autografts. *Am J Sports Med*. 2019;47:3531-3540.

29. Hurley ET, Calvo-Gurry M, Withers D, et al. Quadriceps tendon autograft in anterior cruciate ligament reconstruction: a systematic review. *Arthroscopy*. 2018;34:1690-1698.

30. Huber R, Viecelli C, Bizzini M, et al. Knee extensor and flexor strength before and after anterior cruciate ligament reconstruction in a large sample of patients: influence of graft type. *Phys Sportsmed*. 2019;47:85-90.

31. Thaunat M, Fayard JM, Sonnery-Cottet B. Hamstring tendons or bone-patellar tendon-bone graft for anterior cruciate ligament reconstruction? *Orthop Traumatol Surg Res*. 2019;105:S89-S94.

32. Lu H, Chen C, Xie S, et al. Tendon healing in bone tunnel after human anterior cruciate ligament reconstruction: a systematic review of histological results. *J Knee Surg*. 2019;32:454-462.

33. Baez S, Andersen A, Andreatta R, et al. Neuroplasticity in corticolimbic brain regions in patients after anterior cruciate ligament reconstruction. *J Athl Train*. 2021;56:418-426.

34. Grooms DR, Page SJ, Nichols-Larsen DS, et al. Neuroplasticity associated with anterior cruciate ligament reconstruction. *J Orthop Sports Phys Ther*. 2017;47:180-189.

35. Voss DE. Proprioceptive neuromuscular facilitation. *Am J Phys Med*. 1967;46:838-899.

36. Riemann BL, Lephart SM. The sensorimotor system, part II: the role of proprioception in motor control and functional joint stability. *J Athl Train*. 2002;37:80-84.

37. Riemann BL, Lephart SM. The sensorimotor system, part I: the physiologic basis of functional joint stability. *J Athl Train*. 2002;37:71-79.

38. Pescatello LS. *ACSM's Guidelines for Exercise Testing and Prescription*. 9th ed. Wolters Kluwer/Lippincott Williams & Wilkins Health; 2014.

39. Ithurburn MP, Paterno MV, Ford KR, et al. Young athletes with quadriceps femoris strength asymmetry at return to sport after anterior cruciate ligament reconstruction demonstrate asymmetric single-leg drop-landing mechanics. *Am J Sports Med*. 2015;43:2727-2737.

40. Palmieri-Smith RM, Lepley LK. Quadriceps strength asymmetry after anterior cruciate ligament reconstruction alters knee joint biomechanics and functional performance at time of return to activity. *Am J Sports Med*. 2015;43:1662-1669.

41. Pietrosimone B, Davis-Wilson HC, Seeley MK, et al. Gait biomechanics in individuals meeting sufficient quadriceps strength cutoffs after anterior cruciate ligament reconstruction. *J Athl Train*. 2021;56:960-966.

42. Fischetti F, Vilardi A, Cataldi S, Greco G. Effects of plyometric training program on speed and explosive strength of lower limbs in young athletes. *J Phys Educ Sport*. 2018;18:2476-2482.

43. Booth MA, Orr R. Effects of plyometric training on sports performance. *Strength Cond J*. 2016;38:30-37.

44. Buckthorpe M, Della Villa F. Recommendations for plyometric training after ACL reconstruction—a clinical commentary. *Int J Sports Phys Ther*. 2021;16:879-895.

45. Kasmi S, Zouhal H, Hammami R, et al. The effects of eccentric and plyometric training programs and their combination on stability and the functional performance in the post-ACL-surgical rehabilitation period of elite female athletes. *Front Physiol.* 2021;12:688385.

46. Scheffler SU, Unterhauser FN, Weiler A. Graft remodeling and ligamentization after cruciate ligament reconstruction. *Knee Surg Sport Traumatol Arthrosc.* 2008;16:834-842.

47. Mentiplay BF, Perraton LG, Bower KJ, et al. Assessment of lower limb muscle strength and power using hand-held and fixed dynamometry: a reliability and validity study. *PLoS One.* 2015;10:e0140822.

48. Khayambashi K, Ghoddosi N, Straub RK, Powers CM. Hip muscle strength predicts noncontact anterior cruciate ligament injury in male and female athletes: a prospective study. *Am J Sports Med.* 2016;44:355-361.

49. Brown M, Avers D. *Daniels and Worthingham's Muscle Testing. Techniques of Manual Examination and Performance Testing.* 10th ed. Elsevier Health Sciences; 2018.

50. Hirano M, Katoh M, Gomi M, Arai S. Validity and reliability of isometric knee extension muscle strength measurements using a belt-stabilized hand-held dynamometer: a comparison with the measurement using an isokinetic dynamometer in a sitting posture. *J Phys Ther Sci.* 2020;32:120-124.

51. Rambaud AJM, Ardern CL, Thoreux P, et al. Criteria for return to running after anterior cruciate ligament reconstruction: a scoping review. *Br J Sports Med.* 2018;52:1437-1444.

52. Powden CJ, Dodds TK, Gabriel EH. The reliability of the star excursion balance test and lower quarter y-balance test in healthy adults: a systematic review. *Int J Sports Phys Ther.* 2019;14:683-694.

53. Plisky PJ, Rauh MJ, Kaminski TW, Underwood FB. Star excursion balance test as a predictor of lower extremity injury in high school basketball players. *J Orthop Sports Phys Ther.* 2006;36:911-919.

54. de Fontenay B, van Cant J, Gokeler A, Roy JS. Reintroduction of running after ACL reconstruction with a hamstring autograft: can we predict short-term success? *J Athl Train.* 2021;Oct 8. Epub ahead of print.

55. Knurr KA, Kliethermes SA, Stiffler-Joachim MR, et al. Running biomechanics before injury and 1 year after anterior cruciate ligament reconstruction in division I collegiate athletes. *Am J Sports Med.* 2021;49:2607-2614.

56. Hurd WJ, Chmielewski TL, Snyder-Mackler L. Perturbation-enhanced neuromuscular training alters muscle activity in female athletes. *Knee Surg Sport Traumatol Arthrosc.* 2006;14:60-69.

57. Nagelli C, Wordeman S, Di Stasi S, et al. Biomechanical deficits at the hip in athletes with ACL reconstruction are ameliorated with neuromuscular training. *Am J Sports Med.* 2018;46:2772-2779.

58. Nagelli CV, Di Stasi S, Wordeman SC, et al. Knee biomechanical deficits during a single-leg landing task are addressed with neuromuscular training in anterior cruciate ligament–reconstructed athletes. *Clin J Sport Med.* 2019;31:e347-e353.

59. Souissi S, Wong del P, Dellal A, et al. Improving functional performance and muscle power 4 to 6 months after anterior cruciate ligament reconstruction. *J Sport Sci Med.* 2011;10:655-664.

60. Schmitt LC, Paterno MV, Ford KR, et al. Strength asymmetry and landing mechanics at return to sport after anterior cruciate ligament reconstruction. *Med Sci Sports Exerc.* 2015;47:1426-1434.

61. Reid A, Birmingham TB, Stratford PW, et al. Hop testing provides a reliable and valid outcome measure during rehabilitation after anterior cruciate ligament reconstruction. *Phys Ther.* 2007;87:337-349.

62. Hegedus EJ, McDonough S, Bleakley C, et al. Clinician-friendly lower extremity physical performance measures in athletes: a systematic review of measurement properties and correlation with injury, part 1. The tests for knee function including the hop tests. *Br J Sports Med.* 2015;49:642-648.

63. Wellsandt E, Failla MJ, Snyder-Mackler L. Limb symmetry indexes can overestimate knee function after anterior cruciate ligament injury. *J Orthop Sports Phys Ther.* 2017;47:334-338.

64. Nagai T, Schilaty ND, Laskowski ER, Hewett TE. Hop tests can result in higher limb symmetry index values than isokinetic strength and leg press tests in patients following ACL reconstruction. *Knee Surg Sport Traumatol Arthrosc.* 2020;28:816-822.

65. Brumitt J, Heiderscheit BC, Manske RC, et al. Lower extremity functional tests and risk of injury in division III collegiate athletes. *Int J Sports Phys Ther.* 2013:8:216-227.

66. Myer GD, Schmitt LC, Brent JL, et al. Utilization of modified NFL combine testing to identify functional deficits in athletes following ACL reconstruction. *J Orthop Sports Phys Ther.* 2011;41:377-387.

67. Stewart PF, Turner AN, Miller SC. Reliability, factorial validity, and interrelationships of five commonly used change of direction speed tests. *Scand J Med Sci Sport.* 2014;24:500-506.

68. Flagg KY, Karavatas SG, Thompson S Jr, Bennett C. Current criteria for return to play after anterior cruciate ligament reconstruction: an evidence-based literature review. *Ann Transl Med.* 2019;7:S252.

69. Grindem H, Snyder-Mackler L, Moksnes H, et al. Simple decision rules can reduce reinjury risk by 84% after ACL reconstruction: the Delaware-Oslo ACL cohort study. *Br J Sports Med.* 2016;50:804-808.

Medial Collateral Ligament Sprain

Janice K. Loudon

A 16-year-old high school football player was injured when he was hit on the lateral side of the right knee while running with the football. He immediately fell to the turf and was unable to bear weight on his right leg. He did not return to play. After a sideline examination, the team doctor diagnosed him with a grade II medial collateral ligament sprain. The football player's goal is to return to play as soon as possible.

▶ What examination signs may be associated with this diagnosis?
▶ What are the most appropriate examination tests?
▶ Based on his diagnosis, what do you anticipate will be the contributors to activity limitations?
▶ What are the most appropriate physical therapy interventions?
▶ What are the most appropriate physical therapy outcome measures for return to sport?
▶ What is his rehabilitation prognosis?

KEY DEFINITIONS

GRADE II LIGAMENT SPRAIN: Ligament injury that involves tearing of 25% to 75% of the ligament; signs and symptoms include pain, swelling, loss of motion, and possible joint instability

MEDIAL COLLATERAL LIGAMENT (MCL): Major ligament of the knee that maintains medial stability

VALGUS STRESS: Force applied to the lateral side of a joint that creates tensile stress to the medial joint

Objectives

1. Describe the anatomy of the medial collateral ligament of the knee.
2. Identify the most accurate clinical tests for assessing an MCL sprain.
3. Differentiate between the three grades of MCL sprains.
4. Prescribe appropriate therapeutic exercises for an individual with a grade II MCL sprain.
5. Determine the most appropriate functional tests needed for return to sport after an MCL sprain.

Physical Therapy Considerations

Physical therapy considerations during management of the individual with a diagnosis of a grade II medial collateral ligament sprain:

▶ **General physical therapy plan of care/goals:** Decrease pain; increase joint range of motion (ROM); increase lower quadrant strength; prevent or minimize loss of aerobic fitness capacity

▶ **Physical therapy interventions:** Patient education regarding functional anatomy and injury pathomechanics; modalities and manual therapy to decrease pain; muscular flexibility exercises; resistance exercises to increase muscular endurance capacity of the core and to increase strength of lower extremity muscles; aerobic exercise program; knee brace

▶ **Precautions during physical therapy:** Monitor vital signs; address precautions or contraindications for exercise, based on the stages of healing

▶ **Complications interfering with physical therapy:** Excessive swelling; excessive scarring that limits normal knee ROM

Understanding the Health Condition

Knee injuries are common in sporting activities, and injury to ligaments of the knee account for close to 40% of these injuries.[1] Of these ligament injuries, the MCL is the most commonly injured.[2,3] Anatomically, the MCL complex contains three

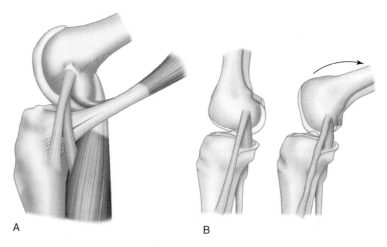

Figure 26-1. A. Medial side of the knee, showing the superficial and deep portions of the medial collateral ligament. **B.** In knee extension, posterior fibers of the MCL are relatively tight. In knee flexion, tension in the posterior fibers decreases. (Reproduced with permission from Cole BJ, Sekiya JK. *Surgical Techniques of the Shoulder, Elbow, and Knee in Sports Medicine.* Philadelphia, PA: Saunders; 2008. Figure 4-55.)

components: the superficial MCL (sMCL), the deep MCL (dMCL), and the posterior oblique ligament (POL). These three components blend and exist as a continuous band of tissue (Fig. 26-1). The sMCL is a flat band that originates on the femur, proximal and posterior to the medial epicondyle and distal to the adductor tubercle.[4] The tibial insertion has two components, one proximal that blends with the anterior part of the semimembranosus tendon and a more distal one that is located anterior to the posteromedial crest of the tibia.[5] The sMCL is barbell shaped and ranges in length from 6 to 12 cm depending on the size of the individual.[4,6] The sMCL is extracapsular and is separated from the dMCL by a bursa. The dMCL is also termed the medial capsular ligament and can be further divided into the meniscofemoral and meniscotibial portions. The deep fibers of the MCL originate slightly anterior and distal to the femoral attachment of the sMCL. The dMCL is composed of short vertically oriented bands that directly attach to the medial meniscus and the knee capsule. This anatomical relationship accounts for the high association of medial meniscal tears with MCL sprains. The third component of the MCL complex is a fibrous bundle that is located posterior to the sMCL and is termed the POL.[7] The POL blends with the posterior medial joint capsule, medial meniscus, and semimembranosus tendon sheath. Some authors refer to this anatomical area as the posteromedial corner.[5,7] The detailed anatomy of the MCL complex is described in Table 26-1.

The MCL complex is the primary stabilizer of the medial knee to direct valgus stress.[6] Grood *et al.*[8] determined that the MCL is the primary restraint for valgus at 5° of knee flexion (57% of anatomical restraint) and 25° (78% of anatomical restraint) of knee flexion. Portions of the MCL complex are taut throughout knee ROM Fig. 26-1B). The anterior fibers of the sMCL are taut in flexion and the posterior fibers are taut in extension. The MCL is dynamically reinforced by the pes anserine and semimembranosus muscles when the knee is extended.[9]

Table 26-1 ANATOMY OF THE MCL COMPLEX	
Structure	Anatomical Attachments
Superficial MCL (sMCL)	Originates on the distal femur, proximal and posterior to the medial epicondyle and distal to the adductor tubercle
	Courses distally attaching to medial tibia, eventually blending with the periosteum and semimembranosus
Deep MCL (dMCL)	Broader, shorter, and deeper to the sMCL
	Attaches to the joint capsule and medial meniscus
Posterior oblique ligament (POL)	Originates posterior to the sMCL
	Blends with posterior medial joint capsule, medial meniscus, and semimembranosus tendon sheath

The meniscofemoral ligament of the dMCL is a secondary stabilizer to valgus stress at all angles of knee motion.[6] In addition to protecting against valgus stress, the MCL complex contributes to restraining rotatory motion (tibial external rotation) and anterior-posterior translation.[10]

Modes for which the MCL is injured include contact and noncontact incidents in which valgus stress is directed at a flexed knee. An isolated injury to the MCL often occurs from a direct blow to the lateral aspect of the thigh while the foot is planted, which produces a direct valgus moment. This type of injury is common in football and rugby. The dMCL fibers are shorter and experience a greater percentage of stretch when subject to valgus strain.[6] Therefore, the dMCL is ruptured more frequently than the sMCL. In addition, most MCL injuries occur at the femoral origin or in the mid-substance directly over the joint line.

A second mechanism of injury to the MCL is a valgus stress coupled with tibial external rotation. This pivoting maneuver occurs commonly in sports such as skiing, basketball, and soccer. With this type of injury, the POL is injured first, followed by the deep and superficial fibers of the MCL.[7] Frequently, other structures such as the anterior cruciate ligament (ACL) and medial meniscus are also injured.[11]

Ligament sprains are commonly graded based on signs and symptoms gathered from the clinical examination. The physical therapist needs to be cognizant of the fact that an individual may have laxity at the knee joint, but still be functional and without instability. The grade of ligament injury is based on the amount of laxity (in millimeters) as compared to the stable extremity. A grade I sprain involves microscopic tears of the superficial and dMCL with no resultant instability or laxity detected with an applied valgus stress. A grade II MCL sprain is an incomplete tear with microscopic and gross disruption of fibers of the superficial and dMCL. With this grade, there are 5° to 15° of valgus instability at 30° of knee flexion with a definite end point. At full knee extension, there is no straight plane valgus or rotational instability. A grade III MCL sprain is a complete tear of the MCL complex with more than 15 mm of instability to valgus stress at 30° knee flexion and possibly at full knee extension. Rotational instability is often present. Of individuals that sustain a Grade III MCL injury, 78% sustain associated injuries to structures such as the ACL.[5] Table 26-2 outlines the grades of MCL ligament sprains.[9]

Table 26-2   GRADES OF MEDIAL COLLATERAL LIGAMENT SPRAIN

Grade	Damage	Clinical Exam	Laxity (mm)	MRI Findings
I	Microscopic tear of superficial and deep MCL	No increase in medial joint line opening at 30° knee flexion Tenderness with palpation over ligament Stiffness	0-5	Grossly intact ligament with periligamentous edema
II	Microscopic and gross disruption of superficial and deep fibers of MCL	Increased laxity at 30° knee flexion, but firm end feel Swelling Pain with palpation Limited knee ROM, especially extension Antalgic gait	6-10	Partial tear of the sMCL with surrounding edema
III	Complete tear of MCL complex	Instability at 30° knee flexion and full extension Empty end feel Loss of full knee ROM Pain and swelling Limited weightbearing tolerance	>10	Full-thickness tear of the sMCL and varying degrees of dMCL tear, periligamentous edema

Physical Therapy Patient/Client Management

Most MCL sprains can be managed nonoperatively. Because Grades I and II sprains generally heal spontaneously and sufficiently, nonsurgical management has become the treatment of choice.[12] However, remodeling of the collagen fibers takes years and the mechanical properties of the healed MCL remain inferior to those of the normal MCL.[13] The intact, normal MCL has strain rates that are 30 times higher along its longitudinal direction compared to its transverse direction.[14] Physical therapy interventions include therapeutic exercise and potentially ultrasound.[15] The primary goal for most injured athletes/individuals is to return to pain-free sport or activity as quickly and safely as possible in a manner that does not overload the healing tissues.

Examination, Evaluation, and Diagnosis

A comprehensive musculoskeletal examination is conducted to rule out other potential sources of knee pain including injuries to the ACL or meniscus, adolescent epiphyseal fracture, and/or patellofemoral pain. During the subjective examination, the physical therapist identifies the mechanism of injury, location of pain, if tearing or popping occurred on the medial side of the knee, and the athlete's functional limitations.

The objective examination includes palpation, performance of special tests and assessment of ROM, swelling, muscle strength, and function. In the acute phase after injury, knee ROM is usually limited in flexion and extension primarily due to swelling. Swelling localized to the medial aspect of the knee is consistent with isolated MCL complex injury because the MCL is extra-articular and rarely results in intra-articular swelling. Significant traumatic effusion is a sign of ACL rupture.[10] Muscle strength, especially the quadriceps, may be deficient due to pain and swelling. Palpation should include the entire course of the MCL complex. Tenderness, specifically at one attachment site, indicates the injury likely occurred at that location. A mid-substance tear can cause tenderness near the medial joint line. The combination of pain, swelling, and muscle inhibition may result in an antalgic gait.

Special tests for the MCL complex include the two-part **valgus stress test** and the Swain test (Table 26-3). The valgus stress test is performed with the knee at 30° of flexion (Fig. 26-2A) and with the knee in full extension (Fig. 26-2B). At 30° of knee flexion, medial laxity of 0 to 5 mm compared to the uninvolved limb indicates tearing of the sMCL (grade I sprain).[16] Greater than 5 mm of laxity is a grade II sprain and suggests further injury to the dMCL, POL, and posteromedial corner.[17] With the knee in full extension, a valgus stress test will be negative if the injury is an isolated superficial grade I or II MCL sprain.[17] If the valgus stress test is positive at full knee extension, then the entire MCL complex and posterior cruciate ligament

Table 26-3	SPECIAL TESTS ASSOCIATED WITH THE MEDIAL COLLATERAL LIGAMENT COMPLEX			
Tests	**Patient Position**	**Findings**	**Sensitivity**	**Specificity**
Valgus stress test with knee at 30° flexion (Fig. 26-2)	Patient is supine with the test leg slightly over the side of the table. The therapist lifts the test leg using the table to support the femur. The therapist bends the knee to 30° and then applies a valgus stress to the limb at the knee.	Increased laxity as compared to the uninvolved side	91%[20]	49%[20]
Valgus stress test with knee in full extension (Fig. 26-3)	Patient is supine with the test leg slightly over the side of the table. The therapist lifts the test leg using the table to support the femur. The therapist keeps the knee in full extension and then applies a valgus stress to the limb at the knee.	Increased laxity as compared to the uninvolved side	NA	NA
Swain test (Fig. 26-4)	The patient is sitting on the side of the table. Therapist passively rotates the tibia into external rotation.	Pain along the medial side of joint indicates injury to MCL complex	NA	NA

Abbreviation: NA, not available.

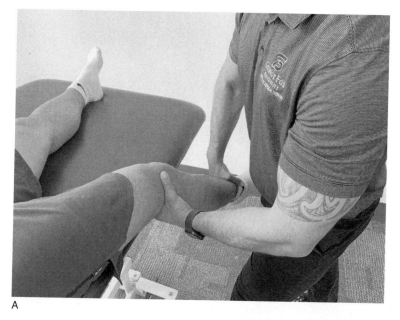

A

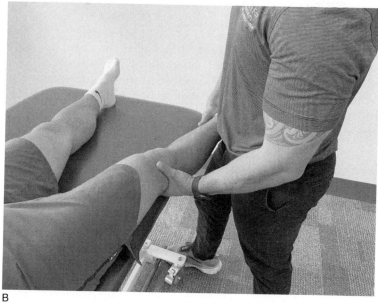

B

Figure 26-2. Valgus stress test at **A**, 30° knee flexion and **B**, full knee extension.

are compromised. The sensitivity of the valgus stress test at 30° flexion is excellent (91%).[18,19]

The Swain test is an examination for testing the presence of chronic MCL injury and rotatory instability.[20] This test is performed with the knee flexed to 90° and the

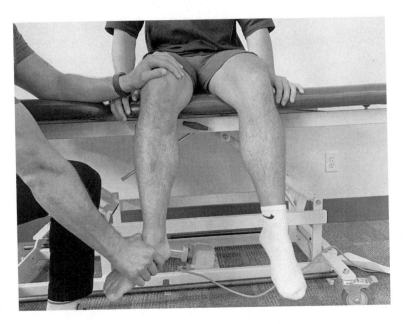

Figure 26-3. Swain test.

tibia passively externally rotated (Fig. 26-3). Pain along the medial side of the joint and excessive tibial rotation indicates injury to the MCL complex.

In adolescents, a stress radiograph should be performed to exclude a physeal injury. Although magnetic resonance imaging (MRI) is the gold standard for identifying ligamentous injury, diagnostic ultrasound is a less expensive alternative that has a 94% accuracy of identifying injury location and severity.[5]

Plan of Care and Interventions

Treatment of grade I and grade II MCL sprains is similar, with the exception that individuals with grade I injuries are progressed at a faster rate with regard to weight-bearing, ROM, and strengthening. Grade III sprains may be treated conservatively or surgically. **Prognosis for nonoperative isolated grade III MCL sprains is good.**[7]

When individuals present with loss of function and chronic valgus instability, or do not respond to conservative measures, surgical intervention is often considered.[21,22] Other indications for operative treatment of an MCL injury include: a large bony avulsion; concomitant tibial plateau fracture; and/or associated cruciate ligament injury. Approximately 80% of grade III MCL injuries have associated ACL or meniscal damage, so surgery for this grade is not uncommon.[23] Surgical fixation can be achieved by the orthopedist performing a primary repair or a reconstruction with an autograft or allograft. The most common procedure is the Slocum procedure which involves a semimembranosus tendon reconstruction. **A systematic review by Varelas et al. concluded that patient outcomes following reconstruction of the MCL were significantly improved from baseline.**[24] Specifically, patients had improved subjective and objective International Knee Documentation Committee (IKDC) scores and improved Lysholm knee activity scores. In addition, following surgery, patients had significantly reduced valgus laxity.[24]

The nonsurgical rehabilitation program following an MCL sprain can be divided into four phases (Table 26-4). The duration of each phase depends on the grade of injury. For example, an individual with a grade I MCL sprain may be able to return to sport in 10 to 14 days, whereas an individual with a grade II sprain can expect rehabilitation to last for up to 6 weeks.[25]

Phase I begins postinjury and lasts up to 1 week. MCL injuries are best treated with early mobilization and strengthening. Active motion significantly reduces laxity and increases the tensile strength of the healing sMCL compared to immobilization of the limb.[26,27] That being said, there may be a brief period of knee immobilization and symptomatic management with ice, elevation, and compression. A grade II/III sprain requires a longer immobilization period with limited ROM. In these circumstances, the individual wears a long-legged rehabilitation brace that limits knee ROM in the extremes of extension and flexion. **During phase I of the rehabilitation, low-intensity ultrasound may be beneficial.** In animal studies, ultrasound improved the proportion of type I collagen (the primary component of mature scar tissue) after MCL transection.[15] The athlete may need

Table 26-4	REHABILITATION FOR MCL SPRAIN[26,28]
Phase I (1 wk)*	Rehabilitation brace (limited motion)
	Partial weightbearing with crutches
	Low-intensity ultrasound over MCL
	Exercise in brace (3 times per day)
	• Straight leg raise (limit hip adduction)
	• Active ankle ROM
	• Active knee flexion to 90°
	• Active hip flexion and extension
	• Upper extremity active exercise
	• Ice, compression on knee
	Stationary cycling without resistance
Phase II (2 wk)*	Progress to full weightbearing
	Aerobic exercise
	Knee ROM without pain
	Ultrasound over MCL
	Partial squats
	Step-up and step-down exercises
	Stationary cycling
Phase III (3 wk)*	Closed-chain exercises with good form (no valgus loading)
	Progress knee flexion and extension (pain-free)
	If no effusion and full motion,
	• Functional exercises including straight ahead level running
	• Balance exercises
Phase IV (after 3 wk)*	Agility exercises

*Timeframe varies depending on grade of MCL injury

crutches and be allowed to bear weight as tolerated. For more severe sprains, crutches may be needed for longer (up to 3 months for grade III).[28] Active knee flexion should begin during this phase, but needs to be pain-free and limited to 90° of knee flexion. Basic straight leg raises should be prescribed, though hip adduction should be initially limited. Stationary cycling can be performed pain-free and resistance-free.

Phase II begins at approximately 2 weeks postinjury. Individuals with grade II or III injuries start later. During this phase, the athlete is progressed to full weight-bearing. ROM should be advanced working toward full motion. Lower extremity strengthening is continued and weightbearing exercises are introduced. Examples of these exercises are partial motion squats and step-up and step-down exercises. Aerobic cross training should be emphasized and may include cycling, upper extremity ergometer, or swimming.

Phase III is characterized by functional training and begins around 3 weeks. Closed-chain exercises are continued with an emphasis on controlling valgus loading. A lunge may be used for this purpose (Fig. 26-4). The athlete must be able to lunge without allowing the knee to collapse toward the midline. Balance training is also incorporated. A running program can be initiated when the athlete has good leg control, full ROM, and no knee effusion.

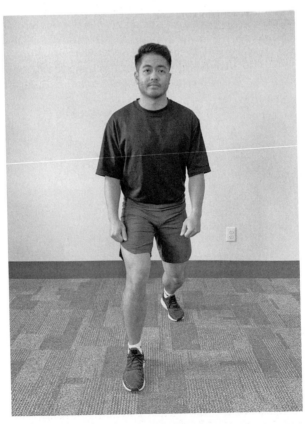

Figure 26-4. A lunge performed to assess the patient's ability to avoid right knee valgus.

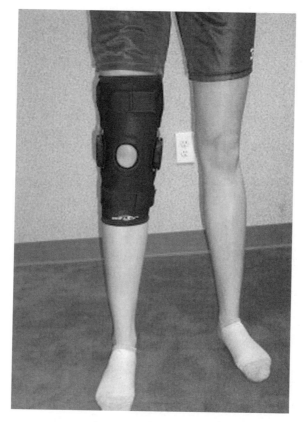

Figure 26-5. Functional brace. (Reproduced with permission from De Carlo M, Armstrong B. Rehabilitation of the knee following sports injury. *Clin Sports Med.* 2010 Jan;29(1):81-106.)

Phase IV is the phase in which the athlete is working to return to sport. Agility exercises and sport-specific skills are emphasized. A functional brace is worn for return to sport, especially for contact sports (Fig. 26-5). The brace may be worn up to 6 months. The brace should be a lightweight hinged knee brace with medial and lateral upright supports to control frontal plane stresses.[27] **Most athletes with MCL sprains can return to sport within 8 weeks.** The return-to-sport criteria are listed in Table 26-5.

Table 26-5   FULL RETURN-TO-SPORT CRITERIA[26]
No swelling
Minimal to no pain that is localized over the superficial MCL
Full knee ROM
Knee stable when tested in full extension
Minimal valgus opening at 30° knee flexion with definite end point
Strength of quadriceps and hamstrings equal to 90% of that of the contralateral limb
Good movement performance with functional tests (*e.g.,* no valgus knee moment with cutting, landing from jump)

Evidence-Based Clinical Recommendations

SORT: Strength of Recommendation Taxonomy

A: Consistent, good-quality patient-oriented evidence
B: Inconsistent or limited-quality patient-oriented evidence
C: Consensus, disease-oriented evidence, usual practice, expert opinion, or case series

1. Valgus stress testing is sensitive for diagnosing a medial collateral ligament (MCL) sprain. **Grade A**

2. The functional outcome for an individual with an isolated nonoperative grade III MCL injury is good. **Grade B**

3. MCL reconstruction results in good patient functional outcomes such as improved IKDC and Lysholm outcome scores and reduced valgus laxity. **Grade A**

4. Low-intensity ultrasound improves collagen synthesis and strength of the injured MCL. **Grade B**

5. Most athletes are able to return to sport 8 weeks following MCL sprain. **Grade C**

COMPREHENSION QUESTIONS

26.1 Valgus stress to the knee in weightbearing is the most common mechanism of injury to a medial collateral ligament. The second most common mechanism of injury is

   A. Tibial external rotation

   B. Tibial internal rotation

   C. Knee hyperextension

   D. Deceleration

26.2 The medial collateral ligament complex has three components that include the superficial band, deep band, and the _____.

   A. Medial meniscus

   B. Posterior cruciate ligament

   C. Posterior oblique ligament

   D. Meniscofemoral ligament

26.3 Which of the following statements is correct with regard to rehabilitation following an MCL injury?

   A. Complications and re-ruptures are common.

   B. Individuals that sustain a Grade I or II MCL sprain are treated conservatively.

   C. Return to sport occurs in approximately 50% of athletes.

   D. Conservative measures are usually unsuccessful, and surgery is required.

ANSWERS

26.1 **A.** Based on the origin and insertion of the MCL, tibial external rotation will cause the MCL to become taut, putting it at higher risk of injury.

26.2 **C.** The fibrous bundle that is located posterior to the sMCL is termed the posterior oblique ligament (POL).[6] The POL blends with the posterior medial joint capsule, medial meniscus, and semimembranosus tendon sheath. Some authors refer to this anatomical area as the posteromedial corner.[5,7]

26.3 **B.** Grades I and II MCL sprains respond well to conservative treatment that includes early range of motion and progressive thigh strengthening. The fibers of the MCL tend to heal if gradual and progressive stress is placed to the ligament.[5,12,21,26]

REFERENCES

1. Mack CD, Kent RW, Coughlin MJ, et al. Incidence of lower extremity injury in the National Football League: 2015 to 2018. *Am J Sports Med*. 2020;48(9):2287-2294.

2. Phisitkul P, James SL, Wolf BR, Amendola A. MCL injuries of the knee: current concepts review. *Iowa Orthop J*. 2006;26:77-90.

3. Rothenberg P, Grau L, Kaplan L, Baraga MG. Knee injuries in American football: an epidemiological review. *Am J Orthop (Belle Mead NJ)*. 2016;45(6):368-373.

4. LaPrade RF, Engebretsen AH, Ly TV, et al. The anatomy of the medial part of the knee. *J Bone Joint Surg Am*. 2007;89(9):2000-2010.

5. Encinas-Ullán CA, Rodríguez-Merchán EC. Isolated medial collateral ligament tears: An update on management. *EFORT Open Rev*. 2018;3(7):398-407.

6. Robinson JR, Bull AMJ, Thomas RRD, Amis AA. The role of the medial collateral ligament and posteromedial capsule in controlling knee laxity. *Am J Sports Med*. 2006;34(11):1815-1823.

7. Marchant MH, Tibor LM, Sekiya JK, et al. Management of medial-sided knee injuries, part 1: medial collateral ligament. *Am J Sports Med*. 2011;39(5):1102-1113.

8. Grood ES, Noyes FR, Butler DL, Suntay WJ. Ligamentous and capsular restraints preventing straight medial and lateral laxity in intact human cadaver knees. *J Bone Joint Surg Am*. 1981;63(8):1257-1269.

9. Hughston JC, Andrews JR, Cross MJ, Moschi A. Classification of knee ligament instabilities. Part I. The medial compartment and cruciate ligaments. *J Bone Joint Surg Am*. 1976;58(2):159-172.

10. Griffith CJ, LaPrade RF, Johansen S, et al. Medial knee injury: Part 1, static function of the individual components of the main medial knee structures. *Am J Sports Med*. 2009;37(9):1762-1770.

11. Elkin JL, Zamora E, Gallo RA. Combined anterior cruciate ligament and medial collateral ligament knee injuries: anatomy, diagnosis, management recommendations, and return to sport. *Curr Rev Musculoskelet Med*. 2019;12(2):239-244.

12. Frank C, Woo SL, Amiel D, et al. Medial collateral ligament healing. A multidisciplinary assessment in rabbits. *Am J Sports Med*. 1983;11(6):379-389.

13. Woo SL, Gomez MA, Inoue M, Akeson WH. New experimental procedures to evaluate the biomechanical properties of healing canine medial collateral ligaments. *J Orthop Res*. 1987;5(3):425-432.

14. Quapp KM, Weiss JA. Material characterization of human medial collateral ligament. *J Biomech Eng*. 1998;120(6):757-763.

15. Sparrow KJ, Finucane SD, Owen JR, Wayne JS. The effects of low-intensity ultrasound on medial collateral ligament healing in the rabbit model. *Am J Sports Med.* 2005;33(7):1048-1056.

16. Grood ES, Noyes FR, Butler DL, Suntay WJ. Ligamentous and capsular restraints preventing straight medial and lateral laxity in intact human cadaver knees. *J Bone Joint Surg Am.* 1981;63(8):1257-1269.

17. Haimes JL, Wroble RR, Grood ES, Noyes FR. Role of the medial structures in the intact and anterior cruciate ligament-deficient knee. Limits of motion in the human knee. *Am J Sports Med.* 1994;22(3):402-409.

18. Kastelein M, Wagemakers HPA, Luijsterburg PAJ, et al. Assessing medial collateral ligament knee lesions in general practice. *Am J Med.* 2008;121(11):982-988.e2.

19. Simonsen O, Jensen J, Mouritsen P, Lauritzen J. The accuracy of clinical examination of injury of the knee joint. *Injury.* 1984;16(2):96-101.

20. Lonergan KT, Taylor DC. Medial collateral ligament injuries of the knee: an evolution of surgical reconstruction: *Techniques in Knee Surgery.* 2002;1(2):137-145.

21. Duffy PS, Miyamoto RG. Management of medial collateral ligament injuries in the knee: an update and review. *Phys Sportsmed.* 2010;38(2):48-54.

22. Indelicato PA. Isolated medial collateral ligament injuries in the knee. *J Am Acad Orthop Surg.* 1995;3(1):9-14.

23. Hastings DE. The non-operative management of collateral ligament injuries of the knee joint. *Clin Orthop Relat Res.* 1980;(147):22-28.

24. Varelas AN, Erickson BJ, Cvetanovich GL, Bach BR. Medial collateral ligament reconstruction in patients with medial knee instability: a systematic review. *Orthop J Sports Med.* 2017;5(5):2325967117703920.

25. Holden DL, Eggert AW, Butler JE. The nonoperative treatment of grade I and II medial collateral ligament injuries to the knee. *Am J Sports Med.* 1983;11(5):340-344.

26. Giannotti BF, Rudy T, Graziano J. The non-surgical management of isolated medial collateral ligament injuries of the knee. *Sports Med Arthrosc Rev.* 2006;14(2):74-77.

27. Hart DP, Dahners LE. Healing of the medial collateral ligament in rats. The effects of repair, motion, and secondary stabilizing ligaments. *J Bone Joint Surg Am.* 1987;69(8):1194-1199.

28. Brotzman SB, Wilk K. *Handbook of Orthopaedic Rehabilitation.* 2nd ed. Elsevier; 2006.

Posterior Collateral Ligament (PCL) Sprain

Matt Mymern
Laurie Griffin

A 24-year-old male is referred to a physical therapy clinic after sustaining a right knee injury playing soccer 6 days ago. The patient reports that the injury occurred when another player tackled him. He describes the impact as a posterior and laterally directed force to the medial tibia. Since the incident, he reports pain with prolonged walking and difficulty descending stairs. The patient reports minimal to no knee instability. Anti-inflammatory medication decreases the pain and allows him to descend stairs without difficulty. The patient reports a history of right patellar tendinitis. The patient's medical history is unremarkable.

► What examination signs may be associated with this suspected diagnosis?
► What are the most appropriate examination tests?
► What are the most appropriate physical therapy interventions?
► What objective criteria may be used to determine appropriateness for return-to-sport participation?

KEY DEFINITIONS

POSTERIOR CRUCIATE LIGAMENT (PCL): Intracapsular ligament of the knee that limits posterior translation of the tibia

POSTEROLATERAL CORNER (PLC): Region of the knee composed of the popliteofibular ligament, fibular collateral ligament, and the popliteus muscle

VARUS FORCE: Force applied to a limb that results in the distal aspect of the limb moving toward the midline of the body

Objectives

1. Describe pathomechanics for a posterior cruciate ligament injury.

2. Identify appropriate clinical special tests to evaluate a patient with potential injury to the posterior cruciate ligament.

3. Implement evidence-based rehabilitation treatments for posterior cruciate ligament injuries.

Physical Therapy Considerations

Physical therapy considerations during management of the individual with a diagnosis of PCL injury:

▶ **General physical therapy plan of care/goals:** Decrease pain and swelling; prevent muscular inhibition; normalize gait abnormalities; restore range of motion (ROM); maintain cardiovascular fitness

▶ **Physical therapy interventions:** Patient education; prescription of home exercise program (HEP); modalities; manual therapy to decrease pain, swelling, and increase ROM; patellar mobilization; gait training

▶ **Precautions during physical therapy:** Assess vital signs, monitor neurovascular status (e.g., distal pulses, sensory and motor function); decrease posterior tibial shear forces

▶ **Complications interfering with physical therapy:** Fibular nerve dysfunction with possible progression into foot drop, which may require an ankle-foot orthosis

Understanding the Health Condition

The PCL is approximately twice as thick and strong as the anterior cruciate ligament (ACL).[1,2] Roughly 13 millimeters (mm) wide and 38 mm long,[1,2] the PCL originates from the anterolateral aspect of the medial femoral condyle near the intercondylar notch. The PCL inserts on the posterior tibial plateau, approximately 1 cm distal to the joint line. Although the PCL is intracapsular, it is isolated with the ACL from the synovial cavity. The PCL can be further divided into an anterolateral bundle and posteromedial bundle. The anterolateral bundle is larger and represents 65% of the substance. In knee flexion, the anterolateral bundle is taut and the posteromedial bundle is lax. The posteromedial bundle, comprising the remaining 35% of the PCL substance, is taut in knee extension, while the anteromedial bundle is lax.[1-3]

Several PCL injury mechanisms have been described in the literature. A common mechanism is a posteriorly directed force to the tibia, which creates a supraphysiologic load to the PCL. The classic example is a football player's shoulder pad or helmet coming into direct contact with a player's tibia during a tackle. Another example is the enormous posteriorly directed force that occurs during a motor vehicle accident when the passenger's tibia strikes the dashboard. Traumatic hyperextension of the knee may also cause a PCL injury (e.g., slide tackle in soccer when the player's foot is securely planted on the turf). If the mechanism of injury also involves forceful twisting, other structures may be compromised, resulting in a multiligamentous injury.[3-5]

PCL injuries are categorized into three grades by the extent of the damage.[5] In grade I injuries, the ligament is stretched and only mildly damaged (up to 25% of the ligament substance is torn). Posterior translation of the tibia on the femur may be up to 5 mm greater than the uninvolved side. In a grade II injury, the ligament is considered moderately damaged (25%-50% of the ligament substance is torn). A posterior translation difference of 6 to 10 mm compared to the uninvolved side is expected. A grade III injury is a completely torn ligament that may occur in any part of the PCL. Translation difference of >10 mm is expected in the grade III tear.[6] PCL injuries may occur in isolation or in combination with other soft tissue damage. An isolated PCL injury means that only the PCL is damaged. Combined ligament injuries of the PCL may involve several structures, most often the posterolateral structures of the knee[3-5] including the popliteofibular ligament, fibular collateral ligament, and popliteus muscle.[7]

Physical Therapy Patient/Client Management

Many approaches can be utilized in the management of both nonoperative and surgically indicated knee injuries. Good outcomes have been reported with conservative management for Grades I and II isolated PCL injuries.[8] Surgical management may be recommended for acute Grade III injury or for individuals with persistent pain and impairments after a trial of conservative management.[9] Published protocols for postoperative management vary in regard to bracing, weightbearing, ROM restrictions, timing of the initiation of hamstring exercises, and return-to-sport participation. Due to the traumatic nature of this injury, interventions and the plan of care are individualized and depend on the mechanism of injury to the PCL and any associated ligamentous damage. Surgical consultation should be considered for individuals who are unable to fulfill their daily, occupational, or athletic demands.

Examination, Evaluation, and Diagnosis

Isolated injury to the PCL, or combined ligamentous injury, occurs less frequently than injuries to other areas of the knee. Hence, less research has been directed to the posterolateral aspect of the knee. PCL injuries have been reported in 1% to

40% of acute injuries[10,11] and up to 40% of knee injuries in the traumatic setting.[12] Acute injuries to the PCL are typically the result of a noncontact mechanism (*e.g.*, work-related injuries, sports injuries, and low-energy or low-velocity falls). The most common cause of traumatic PCL injury is motor vehicle collision, followed by high-energy or high-velocity sporting injuries.[13]

To enable a comprehensive examination, both lower extremities should be exposed to compare alignment of the limbs, joint effusion, and previous scars. Gait should be specifically examined for a varus thrust pattern or hyperextension thrust pattern, both of which indicate chronic injury of the PCL and posterolateral corner.[14-16] A varus thrust gait is common with chronic posterolateral deficiency and indicates lateral compartment opening as the knee shifts into varus on foot strike.[16] If not addressed in the plan of care, an abnormal gait pattern secondary to chronic posterolateral deficiency of the knee may result in degenerative changes.

The neurovascular screen should specifically determine whether the common fibular nerve has been affected, which is not uncommon because of the location of the fibular nerve and popliteal artery in relation to the lateral compartment and the varus stress that occurs with PCL injuries. Sensation or strength changes reflective of the function of the common fibular nerve and its branches should be assessed. Damage should be suspected if the patient presents with numbness or altered sensation on the dorsum of the foot (excluding the first dorsal web space) or weakness in ankle dorsiflexion or eversion or great toe extension.[16] Injury to the popliteal artery can be evaluated by the ankle-brachial index (ABI). An ABI <0.9 has been reported to be 95% to 100% sensitive and 80% to 100% specific in detecting arterial injuries that require surgical intervention.[17]

Palpation and special tests provide additional objective data to further refine or refute a hypothesis during the examination process. The anterior joint line can be palpated with the patient supine, knees flexed to 90°, and feet flat on the table. With an intact PCL, the anterior border of the medial tibial plateau is approximately 1 cm anterior to the medial femoral condyle. An injury to the PCL can be suspected by the degree of posterior subluxation of the tibial plateau in comparison to the femoral condyle.[16] Table 27-1 describes special tests that can be performed to further rule in or rule out injury to the PCL and/or associated ligamentous injury.

To determine the extent of damage to the PCL, imaging is generally performed after the injury and before a patient is referred for physical therapy. If available, the physical therapist should thoroughly review the radiographs. Anteroposterior, lateral, and oblique images can determine the presence of a fracture to the tibial plateau, femoral condyles, or patella.[14] In individuals with chronic PCL injury, the standing anteroposterior view and sunrise view (supine or prone with the knee flexed) may show joint space narrowing.[19] If gross instability is present, a lateral view may identify significant posterior tibial subluxation.[15] A kneeling stress radiograph may be performed to quantify posterior instability. For this technique, the patient kneels in 90° flexion on a radiopaque pad that supports the legs up to the tibial tubercle, leaving the femoral condyles unsupported.[20] Schulz *et al.*[13] have reported that a 5 to 12 mm side-to-side difference in posterior tibial displacement on the kneeling stress radiographs indicates an isolated PCL sprain, whereas a displacement greater than 12 mm indicates a combined posterior instability. However, the ability to differentiate between a complete and partial PCL tear is not reliable with stress radiographs. Magnetic resonance imaging (MRI) has become the gold standard to examine PCL integrity.[21] Because MRI allows for the examination of intra-articular structures and any osteochondral injury, an MRI scan may be performed to further examine a knee when the diagnosis is uncertain or when a complex injury to the knee has occurred.

Table 27-1   SPECIAL TESTS TO RULE IN OR RULE OUT PCL AND/OR CONCOMITANT LIGAMENTOUS INJURY

Special Test	Test Performance	Findings
Godfrey test	Patient is supine. Therapist lifts patient's lower legs, holding them parallel to the table, with hips and knees flexed to 90°. Therapist views patient's knees from the side.	Using the tibial tuberosity as a landmark, the therapist observes the patient's knees from the lateral aspect. If the PCL is lax (or torn), gravity allows the tibia to rest in a posteriorly subluxed position, which can be seen as a posterior sag.[14]
Quadriceps Active test	Patient is supine with involved hip and knee flexed to 90°. Therapist stabilizes foot on the treatment table and asks patient to contract the quadriceps.	If the PCL is torn, the therapist will observe a reduction of the posteriorly subluxed tibia as quadriceps contract.[16] For PCL injuries[18]: 54% sensitivity and 97% specificity
Posterior drawer test	Patient is supine with hips flexed to 45° and involved knee flexed to 90°. Therapist pushes proximal tibia posteriorly.	Therapist feels the movement to assess posterior tibial plateau translation. Grade I injury: 0-5 mm translation Grade II injury: 6-10 mm translation Grade III injury: ≥11 mm[6]

(Continued)

Table 27-1 SPECIAL TESTS TO RULE IN OR RULE OUT PCL AND/OR CONCOMITANT LIGAMENTOUS INJURY (CONTINUED)

Special Test	Test Performance	Findings
Reverse pivot shift	Patient is supine with hip flexed 90°, tibia externally rotated at the foot, and knee flexed to 70°-80°. Therapist applies valgus stress to the knee while extending the knee.	If the PCL is not intact, the patient and therapist perceive an audible "clunk" when the posteriorly subluxed tibia suddenly reduces as the knee approaches full extension.[11] For posterolateral corner injuries[15]: positive predictive value 68%; negative predictive value 89%
External rotation recurvatum	Patient is supine with legs extended. Therapist lifts the patient's great toe off the plinth and compares bilaterally.	A positive test is defined as an increase in knee recurvatum, varus, or external rotation of the tibia, likely due to posterolateral opening of the joint.[14] Positive test may detect both an ACL and PCL injury has occurred.[7]

(Continued)

Table 27-1   SPECIAL TESTS TO RULE IN OR RULE OUT PCL AND/OR CONCOMITANT LIGAMENTOUS INJURY (CONTINUED)

Special Test	Test Performance	Findings
Dial test	Patient is supine (or prone). Therapist externally rotates the tibia at the foot and examines for differences in external rotation with the knee flexed at 30° and 90°. Therapist compares the difference in tibial external rotation bilaterally at 30° and 90° of knee flexion.	If a difference of 10°-15° is noted between the injured and contralateral leg, injury of the PCL and posterolateral corner may be suspected. If a difference is noted at *only* 30° of knee flexion, injury to the posterolateral corner may be likely.[15] If tibial external rotation is increased at *both* 30° and 90° compared to the uninvolved side, both posterolateral corner and the PCL may be involved.[15,16,18]

Plan of Care and Interventions

To formulate a treatment plan, the physical therapist must take into consideration the patient's primary complaints, activity level, occupational demands, comorbidities, and whether the PCL injury is acute or chronic.

For the acute PCL injury like the one sustained by the patient in this case, the efficacy of conservative management has not been well studied. Grade I or II isolated PCL injuries may be managed without surgical intervention. One of the main goals is to maintain the knee in the best possible anatomical position. To limit gravitational pull on the anterolateral bundle of the PCL, Cosgarea and Jay[22] and LaPrade[16] recommend immobilizing the patient's knee in extension with a knee immobilizer brace for 2 to 4 weeks. These authors also recommend decreasing inflammation, maintaining knee ROM through passive ROM, and **avoiding hamstring over-activation (*i.e.*, isolated hamstring resistance exercises) early in the rehabilitation**.[16,22-24] Recommended interventions also include knee passive ROM in the prone position (to minimize posterior-directed forces), patellar mobilization, **isometric quadriceps muscle activation (*i.e.*, quad sets)**, and ice. Table 27-2 describes the exercises that should be the primary focus from injury onset to approximately 6 weeks post-injury. Bracing a PCL-injured knee may help keep the posteriorly subluxed tibia in a more neutral position which may reduce stress on the healing structures and allow for healing in a more anatomical position. However, evidence to support the effectiveness of PCL-specific bracing to improve long-term stability is lacking.

Table 27-2 KNEE EXERCISES TO MAINTAIN ROM AND DECREASE INFLAMMATION IN ACUTE PHASE AFTER PCL INJURY

Therapeutic Exercise	Position	Exercise Technique
Prone passive ROM 	Patient prone on table to decrease the force of gravity and posterior tibial positioning.	Therapist or caregiver flexes patient's knee to end range, as tolerated by the patient. Instruct patient to avoid hamstring activation and to remain passive during ROM.
Patellar mobilizations Superior-inferior Medial-lateral	Patient in long sitting with legs extended and quadriceps relaxed.	Instruct patient to mobilize the patella in superior-inferior and medial-lateral directions.

(Continued)

Table 27-2 KNEE EXERCISES TO MAINTAIN ROM AND DECREASE INFLAMMATION IN ACUTE PHASE AFTER PCL INJURY (CONTINUED)		
Therapeutic Exercise	**Position**	**Exercise Technique**
Quadriceps muscle sets	Patient supine or in long sitting.	Instruct patient to actively draw the patella superiorly while contracting the quadriceps. Hold 5 seconds, repeat 20 times.

Operative management is considered for individuals with grade III PCL injuries, as well as for those with grade II PCL injuries who have failed conservative treatment. Although many PCL reconstruction techniques have been used, newer methods that reconstruct both bundles with allograft should, in theory, result in improved stability.[3,25] However, evidence is inconclusive regarding the precise surgical technique that results in the best outcomes.

One of the concerns after surgical intervention is how to maintain proper positioning of the PCL to avoid stretching of the graft over time due to the posterior tibial sag from the effects of gravity. Due to the infrequency of isolated PCL injury and differing surgical techniques, there is no standard postsurgical rehabilitation protocol. Recommendations for weightbearing after isolated PCL reconstruction vary from nonweightbearing for 2 to 8 weeks to full weightbearing immediately.[9,25-27] Similarly, **bracing protocols vary from having the knee immobilized in full extension or in a PCL-specific brace, with timeframes ranging from 8 weeks to 6 months after surgery.**[26,27]

There are also different protocols for postoperative ROM restrictions, with a few authors recommending that patients perform ROM exercises initially in the prone position. Some authors recommend achieving 90° knee flexion by 2 weeks, with long-term goals of 120° to 130° by 2 to 3 months.[28,29] It should be kept in mind that unnecessarily restricting ROM can lead to difficulties obtaining full mobility later, as well as an increased risk of arthrofibrosis.

Quadricep and hamstring strength deficits have been identified up to 2 years after PCL reconstruction.[30] Some sources recommend avoiding hamstring activation early in the rehabilitation program (ranging from 6 weeks to 3-4 months postsurgery[30,31]) because contraction of this muscle group increases posterior shear forces within the tibiofemoral joint that may compromise healing of the PCL graft. However, failure to incorporate knee flexion exercises may explain why strength deficits are still observed 2 years after surgery. To achieve the balance between protecting the graft and minimizing atrophy, it has been recommended that patients perform co-contraction in both open- and closed kinetic chain exercises for the quadriceps and hamstrings within protective ranges: 0° to 50° minimally stresses PCL grafts.[32]

Despite the variability among PCL reconstruction rehabilitation protocols, each protocol shares a focus on restoring function, minimizing disability, reducing pain and swelling, improving mobility, and increasing strength and proprioception. Because of the low-level evidence guiding postsurgical PCL rehabilitation, the standard for activity progression continues to be based on time since surgery. Initially, progressive ROM should be performed with prevention of hyperextension and posterior tibial translation. Progressive weightbearing with appropriate exercise should be administered through the rehabilitation to increase muscular endurance and strength. For example, a patient can perform step-ups/step-downs as an exercise to support the functional task of reciprocal stair ambulation. Quelard et al.[33] recommended a **postoperative rehabilitation program** allowing for progressive weightbearing at the tenth week after surgery, avoiding open kinetic chain hamstring exercise for 5 months with a plan to return to training at 8 months. With their protocol, Quelard et al.[33] found **significant improvement in differential laxity, International Knee Documentation Committee (IKDC) scores, and Tegner Lysholm Knee Scale scores after an average of 5 years follow-up.** The majority of patients can expect to return to sports and heavy labor 9 months after surgical repair of the PCL.[12,25]

Consensus for return-to-sport participation for the PCL continues to be limited and undefined within the literature. For guidance, we recommend a criterion-based progression for return-to-sport participation. Table 27-3 identifies sample criteria that may be used for different functional aspects of knee control. The administration of tests in Table 27-3 should be based on the surgeon's postoperative rehabilitation protocol. A battery of validated tests including subjective questionnaires and objective measures should be administered at multiple timeframes throughout the recovery.

Functional tasks such as single-leg squatting and Y-Balance Test—Lower Quarter have been used to assess compensatory strategies, neuromuscular control, and dynamic balance.[34-36] The single-leg squat test is performed with the patient standing on a 20-cm height box. The patient is instructed to squat to 60° of knee flexion

Table 27-3 RETURN-TO-PARTICIPATION CRITERIA	
Test	**Sample Passing Criteria**
ROM	Symmetrical active knee extension Passive flexion >125°
Neuromuscular control and dynamic balance	Single-leg squat: test performance rated as "good"[34,35] Y-Balance Test—Lower Quarter: • Side-to-side symmetry • Anterior reach ≤4 cm compared to contralateral limb[37]
Strength (measured using hand-held dynamometer or isokinetic machine)	Limb symmetry index ≥90% for the quadriceps and for the hamstring compared to contralateral limb[38]
Power (examples of hop tests: single-leg for distance, triple-hop for distance, cross-over hop for distance)	Hop testing series >90% compared to contralateral limb[39]
Agility	T-test <11 seconds[40]

at a rate of 1 squat per 2 seconds, while holding arms in front, keeping the trunk upright, and holding the opposite leg in a slightly extended position. After 3 practice trials, the patient performs three test trials. Poor performance (*i.e.*, technique errors) include ipsilateral trunk lean, pelvic tilt, adduction or internal rotation of the hip, loss of balance, and/or dynamic knee valgus (medial collapse of the knee).[34,35] The patient receives a "good" score if he/she can perform the squat 2 out of 3 times without any of the five aforementioned technique errors.[34,35]

Dynamic balance can be assessed using the Y-Balance Test—Lower Quarter (YBT-LQ). The YBT-LQ is a commercial device with a central weightbearing platform with three extensions that form the "Y."[36] To assess dynamic balance with the YBT-LQ, the patient balances on one lower extremity while using the opposite lower extremity to slide a moveable platform along one of the three axes. The distance that the patient is able to slide the moveable platform along an axis is used to track progress during rehabilitation and to compare performance to the uninvolved extremity. Addressing side-to-side asymmetries with balance exercises may help reduce the risk of subsequent injury. For example, an asymmetry ≥4 cm in the anterior direction when performing the star excursion balance test (a precursor to the YBT-LQ) has been reported to be associated with lower extremity injury in a population of healthy, high school basketball players.[37]

Strength testing using hand-held dynamometry or isokinetic testing should be incorporated to determine the *symmetry* of limb strength. A goal of >90% limb symmetry for the quadriceps and hamstrings is recommended for return-to-sport participation.[38] Lower extremity power and performance can be assessed through hop testing and execution of the T-test.[39,40] Hop tests are frequently administered to track progress during rehabilitation to evaluate one's readiness to return to activity.[39] Examples of hop tests include the single-leg hop for distance, the triple-hop for distance, and the cross-over hop for distance. Hop tests should be administered bilaterally with a goal of the patient demonstrating a limb symmetry index >90%. The T-Test is an agility drill performed on a "T"-shaped course. Four cones are positioned to form the "T": two cones are positioned 10 yards apart in a north (B)-south (A) direction and the other two cones (west cone = C and east cone = D) are positioned five yards to each side of cone B. The patient starts at cone A, sprints to cone B and touches its base with the right hand. Next, the athlete side shuffles first to cone C and touches the base with the left hand followed by shuffling to cone D and touches the base with the right hand. The patient side shuffles back to B, touches the base with the left hand, and runs backward to cone A. For most populations, passing criteria score on the T-Test is less than 11 seconds.[40] Before initiating either running, sport-specific drills, or power development, it may be beneficial to repeat PCL kneeling stress radiographs to demonstrate whether sufficient graft healing has occurred to withstand training advancement. Common subjective outcome measures used for long-term postoperative knee ligament management include the International Knee Documentation Committee (IKDC), Tegner, and Lysholm scales.[41] In addition, the ACL-RSI (return to sport after injury) has gained popularity as an outcome measure to address mental readiness for returning to sport participation. This tool has only been validated for individuals with ACL injuries, but clinicians may consider this tool as an option to identify readiness in patients with other knee ligament injuries.

Evidence-Based Clinical Recommendations

SORT: Strength of Recommendation Taxonomy

A: Consistent, good-quality patient-oriented evidence
B: Inconsistent or limited-quality patient-oriented evidence
C: Consensus, disease-oriented evidence, usual practice, expert opinion, or case series

1. Limiting isolated hamstring strengthening and promoting strengthening of the quadriceps improve the stability and decrease the tibial sag of the knee with a PCL injury. **Grade B**

2. Bracing that prevents further posterior tibial sag (*e.g.*, knee extension immobilizer or brace that provides anteriorly directed force on tibia) is beneficial for individuals with PCL-deficient knees. **Grade C**

3. After PCL reconstruction and rehabilitation, individuals experience statistically significant improvements in differential laxity, IKDC scores, and Tegner and Lysholm scores at 5 years follow-up. **Grade B**

COMPREHENSION QUESTIONS

27.1 A patient is referred to a physical therapy clinic with a diagnosis of a PCL tear. He expresses concern about surgical repair and states that he would rather conservatively rehabilitate his knee. Which of the following sets of interventions would be the MOST appropriate plan to assist the patient in the acute stage of rehabilitation?

A. Supine ROM, towel under the knee with quad sets, patellar mobilization, ice

B. Prone passive knee ROM, towel under proximal tibia during gastrocnemius-soleus towel stretching in long sitting position, quad sets, patellar mobilization, ice

C. Prone active knee ROM, hamstring sets, patellar mobilization, ice

D. Supine passive ROM, hamstring sets, patellar mobilization, ice

27.2 A patient complains of knee instability. In the physical therapy examination, he has positive posterior drawer and quadriceps active tests. Which additional special test should the physical therapist perform to help *rule in* a posterior lateral corner injury versus an isolated PCL tear?

A. Godfrey

B. Anterior drawer

C. Dial

D. McMurray

27.3 With respect to the anatomy of the PCL, which of the following is a true statement?

    A. The anteromedial bundle is larger of the two bundles and is taut in extension.

    B. The anteromedial bundle is smaller of the two bundles and is lax in flexion.

    C. The posteromedial bundle is larger of the two bundles and is taut in extension.

    D. The posteromedial bundle is smaller of the two bundles and is lax in flexion.

27.4 When considering objective criteria to assess your patient's ability to return-to-sport participation, which of the following provides the most complete results for safe participation?

    A. Symmetrical knee flexion active range of motion

    B. Limb Symmetry Index >90%; YBT-LQ <4 cm; hop test scores >90% of contralateral side; T-Test <11 seconds

    C. Normalized gait; vertical hop >90% of the contralateral limb

    D. T-Test >30 seconds

ANSWERS

27.1 **B.** Prone ROM decreases the effect of gravity and any posterior tibial translation with ROM. Support under the proximal tibia also assists in preventing posterior tibial sag and reduces hamstring involvement with gastrocnemius-soleus stretching in the long sitting position. Hamstring activation will be limited because the prone position promotes further posterior tibial translation, decreasing stress to the healing posterolateral structures.[12,23,26]

27.2 **C.** If a difference is noted from the contralateral side of 10° to 15° on the dial test, injury of the PCL and posterolateral corner may be suspected. If a difference is noted at *only* 30° of flexion, injury to the posterolateral corner may be likely.[19] If tibial external rotation is increased at 30° and 90° compared to the contralateral side, both posterolateral corner and the PCL may be involved.[15] The posterior tibial sag noted on the Godfrey test indicates that the PCL is lax (option A). The anterior drawer test is commonly used to assess for anterior cruciate ligament laxity (option B). The McMurray test is performed to diagnose a meniscal tear (option D).

27.3 **D.**

27.4 **B.** Criteria for suggested for return to participation include the following: limb symmetry index >90%, YBT-LQ anterior asymmetry <4 cm, hop tests >90% of contralateral side, T-Test <11 seconds.[37-40]

REFERENCES

1. Lopes OV Jr, Ferretti M, Shen W, et al. Topography of the femoral attachment of the posterior cruciate ligament. *J Bone Joint Surg Am.* 2008;90:249-255.

2. Tajima G, Nozaki M, Iriuchishima T, et al. Morphology of the tibial insertion of the posterior cruciate ligament. *J Bone Joint Surg Am.* 2009;91:859-866.

3. Moorman CT III, Murphy Zane MS, Bansai S, et al. Tibial insertion of the posterior cruciate ligament: a sagittal plane analysis using gross, histologic, and radiographic methods. *Arthroscopy.* 2008;24:269-275.

4. Matava MJ, Ellis E, Gruber B. Surgical treatment of posterior cruciate ligament tears: an evolving technique. *J Am Acad Orthop Surg.* 2009;17:435-446.

5. Wind WM Jr, Bergfeld JA, Parker RD. Evaluation and treatment of posterior cruciate ligament injuries: revisited. *Am J Sports Med.* 2004;32:1765-1775.

6. American Medical Association. Committee on the medical aspects of sports. *Standard Nomenclature of Athletic Injuries.* Chicago, IL: American Medical Association;1968:92-101.

7. Lunden JB, Bzdusek PJ, Monson JK, et al. Current concepts in the recognition and treatment of posterolateral corner injuries of the knee. *J Orthop Sports Phys Ther.* 2010;40:502-516.

8. Bedi A, Musahl V, Cowan JB. Management of posterior cruciate ligament injuries: An evidence-based review. *J Am Acad Orthop Surg.* 2016;24:277-289.

9. Chahla J, Nitri M, Civitarese D, et al. Anatomic double-bundle posterior cruciate ligament reconstruction. *Arthroscopy.* 2016;5:149-156.

10. Gray H. *Anatomy of the Human Body.* 20th ed. Philadelphia, PA: Lea and Febiger; 1918.

11. LaPrade RF, Terry GC. Injuries to the posterolateral aspect of the knee. Association of anatomic injury patterns with clinical instability. *Am J Sports Med.* 1997;25:433-438.

12. Fanelli GC, Edson CJ. Posterior cruciate ligament injuries in trauma patients: Part II. *Arthroscopy.* 1995;11:526-529.

13. Schulz MS, Russe K, Weiler A, et al. Epidemiology of posterior cruciate ligament injuries. *Arch Orthop Trauma Surg.* 2003;123:186-191.

14. Lopez-Vidriero E, Simon DA, Johnson DH. Initial evaluation of posterior cruciate ligament injuries: history, physical examination, imaging studies, surgical and nonsurgical indications. *Sports Med Arthrosc.* 2010;18:230-237.

15. Miller MD, Cooper DE, Fanelli GC, et al. Posterior cruciate ligament: current concepts. *Instr Course Lect.* 2002;51:347-351.

16. LaPrade RF. *Posterolateral Knee Injuries: Anatomy, Evaluation, and Treatment.* New York, NY: Thieme; 2006.

17. Johnson ME, Foster L, DeLee JC. Neurologic and vascular injuries associated with knee ligament injuries. *Am J Sports Med.* 2008;36:2448-2462.

18. Rubinstein RA Jr., Shelbourne KD, McCarroll JR, et al. The accuracy of the clinical examination in the setting of posterior cruciate ligament injuries. *Am J Sports Med.* 1994;22:550-557.

19. Rigby JM, Porter KM. Posterior cruciate ligament injuries. *Trauma.* 2010;12:175-181.

20. Schulz MS, Russe K, Lampakis G, Strobel MJ. Reliability of stress radiography for evaluation of posterior knee laxity. *Am J Sports Med.* 2005;33:502-506.

21. Feltham GT, Albright JP. The diagnosis of PCL injury: literature review and introduction of two novel tests. *Iowa Orthop J.* 2001;21:36-42.

22. Cosgarea AJ, Jay PR. Posterior cruciate ligament injuries: evaluation and management. *J Am Acad Orthop Surg.* 2001;9:297-307.

23. Fanelli GC, Edson CJ. Combined posterior cruciate ligament-posterolateral reconstructions with Achilles tendon allograft and biceps femoris tendon tenodesis: 2- to 10-year follow-up. *Arthroscopy.* 2004;20:339-345.

24. Montgomery SR, Johnson JS, McAllister DR, Petrigliano FA. Surgical management of posterior cruciate ligament injuries: indications, techniques, and outcomes. *Current Rev Musculoskeletal Medicine*. 2013;6:115-123.

25. Harner CD, Janaushek MA, Kanamori A, et al. Biomechanical analysis of a double-bundle posterior cruciate ligament reconstruction. *Am J Sports Med*. 2000;28:144-151.

26. Fanelli GC, Beck JD, Edson CJ. Double bundle posterior cruciate ligament reconstruction: surgical technique and results. *Sports Med Arthrosc Rev*. 2010;18:242-248.

27. Lee YS, Jung YB. Posterior cruciate ligament: Focus on conflicting issues. *Clin Orthop Surg*. 2013;5:256-262.

28. Wu CH, Chen AC, Yuan LJ. Arthroscopic reconstruction of posterior cruciate ligament by using a quadriceps tendon autograft. A minimum 5-year follow-up. *Arthroscopy*. 2007;23:420-427.

29. Adler GG. All-inside posterior cruciate ligament reconstruction with a graftlink. *Arthrosc Techn*. 2013;2:e111-e115.

30. Cavanaugh JT, Saldivar A, Marx RG. Postoperative rehabilitation after posterior cruciate ligament reconstruction and combined posterior cruciate ligament-posterolateral corner reconstruction. *Operative Tech Sports Med*. 2015;23:372-384.

31. Li B, Shen P, Wang JS, et al. Therapeutic effects of tibial support braces on posterior stability after posterior cruciate ligament reconstruction with autogenous hamstring tendon graft. *European J Phys Rehab Med*. 2015;51:163-170.

32. Escamilla RF, Macleod TD, Wilk KE, et al. Cruciate ligament loading during common knee rehabilitation exercise. *Proc Inst Mech Eng H*. 2012;226:670-680.

33. Quelard B, Sonnery-Cottet B, Zayni R, et al. Isolated posterior cruciate ligament reconstruction: is non-aggressive rehabilitation the right protocol? *Orthop Traumatol Surg Res*. 2010;96:256-262.

34. Hall MP, Raik RS, Ware AJ, et al. Neuromuscular evaluation with single leg squat test at 6 months after anterior cruciate ligament reconstruction. *Orthop J Sports Med*. 2015;3:1-8.

35. Crossley KM, Zhang WJ, Schache AG, et al. Performance on the single-leg squat task indicates hip abductor muscle function. *Am J Sports Med*. 2011;39:866-873.

36. Plisky PJ, Gorman PP, Butler RJ, et al. The reliability of an instrumented device for measuring components of the star excursion balance test. *N Am J Sports Phys Ther*. 2009;4:92-99.

37. Plisky, PJ, Rauh MJ, Kamisniski TW, Underwood FB. Star excursion balance test as a predictor of lower extremity injury in high school basketball players. *J Orthop Sports Phys Ther*. 2006;36:911-919.

38. Welling W, Benjaminse A, Seil R, et al. Low rates of patients meeting return to sport criteria 9 months after anterior cruciate ligament reconstruction: a prospective longitudinal study. *Knee Surg Sports Traumatol Arthrosc*. 2018;26:3636-3644.

39. Noyes FR, Barber SD, Mangine RE. Abnormal lower limb symmetry determined by function hop tests after anterior cruciate ligament rupture. *Am J Sports Med*. 1991;19:513-518.

40. Haff GC, Triplett NT. 4th ed. *Essentials of Strength Training and Conditioning*. Human Kinetics; 2015.

41. Shelbourne KD, Benner RW, Ringenberg JD, Gray T. Optimal management of posterior cruciate ligament injuries: current perspectives. *Orthop Res Rev*. 2017;9:13-22.

Meniscus Sprain

Jason Brumitt

A 24-year-old female injured her right knee 2 days ago during a city-league basketball game. She was unable to continue playing and required "a little" assistance from a teammate to get to her car. She was evaluated by her primary care provider (PCP) the next day. The PCP recommended the use of over-the-counter nonsteroidal anti-inflammatory medication and referred the patient to physical therapy. Five days postinjury, the patient reports to the physical therapist that the injury occurred when she planted her right leg and cut toward the left to evade a defender. She denies hearing a pop, but the immediate pain was severe (8 out of 10 on a visual analog scale). Her current pain level is 5 out of 10. The patient's pain and mechanism of injury are consistent with a meniscus injury.

▸ What examination signs may be associated with this suspected diagnosis?
▸ What are the most appropriate examination tests?

KEY DEFINITIONS

SENSITIVITY: Ability of a diagnostic test to correctly identify individuals who have the target disease or health condition (Table 28-1). Sensitivity is calculated by dividing the number of true positive test results by the sum of true positive test results and false negative test results. SnNout is a helpful mnemonic for a highly sensitive test (high sensitivity, negative, rules out).[1]

SPECIFICITY: Ability of a diagnostic test to correctly identify individuals who do *not* have the target disease or health condition (Table 28-1). Specificity is calculated by dividing the number of true negative test results by the sum of true negative test results and false positive test results. SpPin is a helpful mnemonic for a highly specific test (high specificity, positive, rules in).[1]

Table 28-1 2 × 2 TABLE FOR DIAGNOSTIC TESTS		
	Disease/Health Condition Present	**Disease/Health Condition Absent**
Test positive	True positive (A)	False positive (B)
Test negative	False negative (C)	True negative (D)

Sensitivity = A/(A + C); Specificity = D/(B + D)

Objectives

1. Describe the anatomy and function of the menisci.
2. Describe the pathomechanics associated with a meniscal injury.
3. Recognize symptoms associated with a meniscal injury.
4. Describe clinical examination tests that may help rule in a diagnosis of meniscus sprain.

Physical Therapy Considerations

Physical therapy considerations during management of the individual with a suspected meniscus sprain:

► **General physical therapy plan of care/goals:** Rule out other knee injuries; decrease pain; increase flexibility; increase (or prevent loss of) knee range of motion; increase lower quadrant strength; prevent or minimize loss of aerobic fitness capacity

► **Physical therapy interventions:** Modalities to reduce pain; interventions to restore range of motion deficits; therapeutic exercises to restore strength and aerobic fitness

► **Precautions during physical therapy:** Monitor vital signs; avoid exercises that place a rotatory force on the knee during acute and subacute phases of healing

▶ **Complications interfering with physical therapy:** Damage to additional knee structures such as anterior cruciate or medial collateral ligaments; articular cartilage pathology; osteochondritis dissecans, fracture, tumor,[2] cysts[3]

Understanding the Health Condition

The menisci are wedge-shaped fibrocartilage structures located on the proximal (articular) portion of the tibia. Each knee has a lateral and medial meniscus: the lateral meniscus (circular shaped) is smaller than the medial meniscus (C-shaped; Fig. 28-1). The menisci have several attachments on the tibia: the anterior and posterior horns via insertional ligaments, the joint capsule, the anterior intermeniscal ligament, and the coronary ligaments. The lateral meniscus has additional attachments to the meniscofemoral ligaments and a portion of the popliteal tendon.[4,5] The medial meniscus attaches to the deep portion of the medial collateral ligament of the knee.[5]

The menisci provide several functions at the knee. Their primary function is to protect the joint by serving as shock absorbers to transmit loads across the joint.[4,6] The menisci also help improve joint congruence and overall stability.[4,6-9] Additional roles include joint lubrication and nutrition provision to the cartilage.[6,10]

Meniscus injuries can result from an acute injury or from normal age-related degenerative changes.[11] Acute meniscal tears are typically the result of a violent twisting motion. An example of a meniscal injury mechanism is a basketball player attempting to evade a defender by planting the leg then quickly rotating the body to move in another direction. The rotational stress that is created through the loaded knee may sprain or tear a portion of the meniscus. The meniscus is also at risk for injury during valgus forces at the knee. It is common for the meniscus to

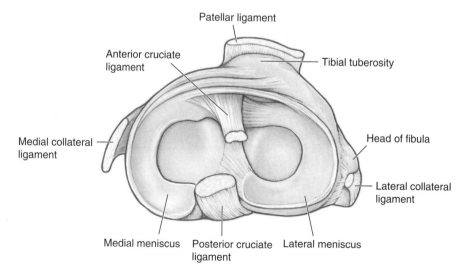

Figure 28-1. The menisci of the right knee. (Reproduced with permission from Morton DA, Foreman KB, Albertine KH, eds. *The Big Picture: Gross Anatomy.* New York: McGraw-Hill; 2011.)

be sprained in conjunction with a sprain of either the anterior cruciate ligament (ACL) or medial collateral ligament (MCL). Indeed, 82% to 96% of knees with an ACL sprain have an associated meniscal injury.[12] Isolated sprains of the meniscus are also common. In some orthopedic surgery practice settings, more than 20% of all surgical procedures on the knee are for the meniscus.[10]

Examination, Evaluation, and Diagnosis

Diagnosis is based on patient history and clinical examination. Table 28-2 presents key questions that should be asked during the subjective (patient history) portion of the examination. A patient may describe that the injury occurred when rotating or twisting. The date of injury provides information regarding the stage of healing and may aid prognosis. An audible popping sound is frequently associated with a ligament tear (*e.g.*, ACL). However, a "pop" is *not* usually associated with an isolated meniscus injury. Swelling is common and may impair range of motion and contribute to pain (secondary to stimulation of mechanoreceptors). A patient with a meniscal injury may report pain "in the knee" and/or pain along the joint line. The patient may also describe that her knee "catches" or "locks." In contrast, a patient with a degenerative meniscal injury may lack recall of a mechanism of injury and report a gradual onset of symptoms (*e.g.*, pain, locking, giving way).[11]

Table 28-2   INTERVIEW QUESTIONS THAT SHOULD BE ASKED IF A MENISCAL INJURY IS SUSPECTED
When and how did you injure your knee? (*i.e.*, mechanism of injury)
How long have you been experiencing this pain?
Did you hear a "pop"?
Was there any swelling (immediately postinjury or residual)?
Where is your pain located?
Does the knee "lock" or does it "catch"?

Table 28-3 presents a sample physical examination for a patient with suspected knee pathology. Information from the subjective portion of the examination helps guide decision-making as to which tests to administer. Special tests for meniscal pathology may be performed in standing, supine, and prone positions (Table 28-4).

If the patient is able to bear weight through the involved extremity and ambulate with assistance, the Thessaly test may be performed at this time. Other special tests reported to assess meniscus integrity are performed in supine (McMurray test, joint line tenderness), in prone (Apley's compression test), or standing (*e.g.*, Ege's test).[13-16] However, the diagnostic utility of one special test to identify a meniscus injury is poor.[17-19] A 2007 systematic review and meta-analysis of common special tests for meniscal integrity concluded that no single physical examination test was able to assist the clinician in accurately identifying a meniscal injury.[17] Since that report, additional studies have presented diagnostic accuracy statistics for joint line tenderness, Thessaly, and joint fullness tests in detecting meniscal injury.[13-15,20] In some cases, higher sensitivity and specificity values were reported, especially in situations where the diagnostic utility of performing two tests was assessed.[15,20]

Table 28-3   PHYSICAL EXAMINATION FOR INDIVIDUALS WITH SUSPECTED KNEE PATHOLOGY

Standing
- General observation (view patient anteriorly, posteriorly, and laterally in static and dynamic postures)
- Gait
- Special and functional tests (Table 28-4)

Sitting
- Active and passive range of motion (goniometry)
- Muscle flexibility testing
- Resisted testing (*i.e.*, manual muscle testing)
- Neurovascular testing

Supine
- Observation
- Active and passive range of motion (goniometry)
- Muscle flexibility testing
- Resisted testing (*i.e.*, manual muscle testing)
- Special tests (Table 28-4)
- Joint play
- Palpation

Sidelying
- Resisted testing

Prone
- Muscle flexibility testing
- Resisted testing
- Special tests (Table 28-4)

Table 28-4   SPECIAL TESTS REPORTED TO IDENTIFY MENISCAL INJURY

Test	Patient Position	Test Performance	Positive Test
McMurray test	Supine	Therapist grasps patient's heel with one hand and knee with the other hand. While palpating the tibio-femoral joint line with one finger and thumb, the thera-pist flexes the knee fully and then rotates the leg either internally or externally. Next, the therapist extends the knee. Repeat again, extend-ing the knee from the flexed position and with the leg rotated in the opposite direction.	Audible or palpable click

(Continued)

Table 28-4   SPECIAL TESTS REPORTED TO IDENTIFY MENISCAL INJURY (CONTINUED)

Test	Patient Position	Test Performance	Positive Test
Thessaly test[13,14] at A, 5° knee flexion B, 20° knee flexion A B	Standing in single-limb stance on involved leg, placing hands on therapist's hands to assist with balance	Patient flexes involved leg to either 5° (Fig. A) or 20° (Fig. B). Patient is instructed to rotate body to the left and then to the right, while maintaining the desired degree of knee flexion. This movement is repeated 3 times.	Reproduction of pain or other symptoms
Bounce home test	Supine	Therapist supports involved lower extremity with one hand on posterior side of knee and the other hand supporting the foot. The hip is passively flexed to ~45° and the knee is passively flexed to ~25°-30°. Without informing the patient, the therapist quickly removes the hand from behind the patient's knee, allowing the knee to passively extend.	Reproduction of pain Inability to achieve full extension

(Continued)

Table 28-4   SPECIAL TESTS REPORTED TO IDENTIFY MENISCAL INJURY (CONTINUED)

Test	Patient Position	Test Performance	Positive Test
Test for joint line tenderness 	Supine with hips flexed to 45° and knees flexed ~90°	Therapist palpates the tibiofemoral joint line on each side.	Reproduction of pain
Joint line fullness	Supine with hips flexed to 45° and involved knee flexed 70°-90° to assess medial compartment and 30°-45° to assess lateral compartment	Therapist palpates the tibiofemoral joint line for "palpable fullness."[20]	Fullness that limits "normal joint compression"[20]
Apley's test 	Prone, with involved knee flexed to 90°	Distraction component (not pictured): Therapist grasps the foot and ankle of the involved lower extremity with both hands. The therapist stabilizes the posterior thigh with a knee. Next, therapist distracts the tibia and rotates the leg. Compression component (pictured):	Reproduction of pain or other symptoms

(Continued)

Table 28-4	SPECIAL TESTS REPORTED TO IDENTIFY MENISCAL INJURY (CONTINUED)		
Test	Patient Position	Test Performance	Positive Test
		Therapist grasps foot and ankle of involved lower extremity with one hand. The therapist's other hand is used to apply gentle stabilizing pressure to patient's posterior thigh (therapist may also use the same hand and knee posture described in distraction component). Therapist applies compressive force through the foot directed toward the knee, while internally and externally rotating the leg.	

Table 28-5 presents **sensitivity and specificity for special tests reported to identify meniscal pathology.**[13-15,20,21-25] **The diagnostic utility of these special tests is compared to arthroscopy—the gold standard for determining the presence or absence of a meniscus injury.**[26] The higher the sensitivity and specificity of a test, the greater the confidence the clinician has in the results. Early studies showed that a positive Thessaly test at 20° knee flexion (sensitivity: 89%-92%; specificity: 96%-97%) can help rule *in* a meniscal injury because of its high specificity (SpPin), whereas a negative Thessaly test can help rule *out* a meniscal injury

Table 28-5	SENSITIVITY AND SPECIFICITY ASSOCIATED WITH SELECT SPECIAL TESTS FOR MENISCAL PATHOLOGY			
Author (Year)	Population	Test	Sensitivity (%)	Specificity (%)
Kocher et al.[21] (2001)	113 patients (64 girls; mean age: 11.9 y)	1. Clinical exam 2. MRI	1. 62.1,[a] 50.0[b] 2. 79.3,[a] 66.7[b]	1. 80.7,[a] 89.2[b] 2. 92.0,[a] 82.8[b]
Kocabey et al.[22] (2004)	50 patients (mean age: 22 y; range: 12-42 y)	1. Clinical exam consisting of four tests: McMurray Joint line tenderness Steinmann Modified Apley's test 2. MRI	1. 87[a], 75[b] 2. 80[a], 85[b]	1. 68[a], 95[b] 2. 79[a], 97[b]

(Continued)

Table 28-5 SENSITIVITY AND SPECIFICITY ASSOCIATED WITH SELECT SPECIAL TESTS FOR MENISCAL PATHOLOGY (CONTINUED)

Author (Year)	Population	Test	Sensitivity (%)	Specificity (%)
Karachalios et al.[14] (2005)	213 patients (56 females; mean age: 29.4 y) and 197 volunteers (53 females; mean age: 31.1 y)	1. McMurray test 2. Apley's test 3. Joint line tenderness 4. Thessaly test 5° 5. Thessaly test at 20°	1. 48,[a] 65[b] 2. 41,[a] 41[b] 3. 71,[a] 78[b] 4. 66,[a] 81[b] 5. 89,[a] 92[b]	1. 94,[a] 86[b] 2. 93,[a] 86[b] 3. 87,[a] 90[b] 4. 96,[a] 91[b] 5. 97,[a] 96[b]
Harrison et al.[13] (2009)	116 patients (57 females) with suspected meniscal injury	1. Thessaly test	1. 90.3	1. 97.7
Konan et al.[15] (2009)	109 patients (29 females; mean age: 39 y)	1. McMurray test 2. Joint line tenderness 3. Thessaly test at 20° 4. McMurray test and joint line tenderness 5. Thessaly test at 20° and joint line tenderness	1. 50,[a] 21[b] 2. 83,[a] 68[b] 3. 59,[a] 32[b] 4. 91,[a] 75[b] 5. 93,[a] 78[b]	1. 77,[a] 94[b] 2. 76,[a] 97[b] 3. 67,[a] 95[b] 4. 91,[a] 99[b] 5. 92,[a] 99[b]
Couture et al.[20] (2011)	100 patients (43 females; mean age: 46.1 y) to have knee arthroscopic surgery	1. Joint line tenderness 2. McMurray test 3. Joint line fullness	1. 90,[a] 87[c] 2. 28,[a] 32[c] 3. 73,[a] 70[c]	1. 0,[a] 30[c] 2. 87,[a] 78[c] 3. 73,[a] 82[c]
Gobbo et al.[23] (2015)	117 male and 45 female patients (mean age: 39 y) scheduled for video arthroscopy	Clinical examination consisting of five tests: 1. McMurray 2. Apley's test 3. Childress 4. Steinmann I 5. Steinmann II	89.02[a] 85.71[b]	31.25[a] 24.17[b]
Goossens et al.[24] (2015)	593 patients (252 females) with suspected meniscal injury; mean age: 49.4 y	1. Thessaly test at 20° 2. McMurray test 3. Combined analysis	1. 1.64,[a] 64[b], 64[c] 2. 2.69,[a] 72[b], 70[c] 3. 3.52,[a] 55[b], 53[c]	1. 45[a], 40[b], 53[c] 2. 37[a], 34[b], 45[c] 3. 54[a], 52[b], 62[c]

(Continued)

Table 28-5 SENSITIVITY AND SPECIFICITY ASSOCIATED WITH SELECT SPECIAL TESTS FOR MENISCAL PATHOLOGY (CONTINUED)

Author (Year)	Population	Test	Sensitivity (%)	Specificity (%)
Hashemi et al.[25] (2020)	86 patients (mean age: 27 y; range: 15 to 45 y) who were candidates for arthroscopic surgery	1. Thessaly test at 20° 2. McMurray 3. Apley's compression test	1. 90.7 2. 72.2 3. 70.4	1. 90.6 2. 71.9 3. 68.7

[a]Medial meniscus
[b]Lateral meniscus
[c]Combined results for medial and lateral meniscus

because of its high sensitivity (SnNout).[1,14] However, it is important for physical therapists to stay current with research evaluating the diagnostic accuracy of special tests. For example, subsequent studies have questioned the ability of the Thessaly test at 20° knee flexion performed in isolation to accurately diagnose a meniscal injury. In 2015, Goossens et al.[24] reported significantly lower sensitivity (64% for both medial and lateral meniscus) and specificity (45% for medial meniscus, 40% for lateral meniscus) than earlier reports.[13,14] Konan et al.[15] also reported low sensitivity (59%) and specificity (31%) for the Thessaly test at 20° for the medial meniscus and low sensitivity (67%) and high specificity (95%) for the lateral meniscus. However, when Konan et al.[15] combined the Thessaly test at 20° knee flexion with joint line tenderness, they found both high sensitivity (93% for medial meniscus and 78% for lateral meniscus) and specificity (92% for medial meniscus and 99% for lateral meniscus). As evolving evidence shows that the ability of a single test to accurately diagnose a meniscus injury is not strong, many authors recommend that one's "diagnostic certainty" may be increased by performing several tests.[15,20,22,23]

Plan of Care and Interventions

The physical therapy plan of care depends on the severity of the meniscal sprain and the patient's point of entry into the healthcare system. Physical therapy treatment may include modalities to reduce pain (e.g., electrical stimulation, cryotherapy, low-level laser therapy), interventions to restore range of motion (therapeutic exercises, joint mobilization, manual therapy), and therapeutic exercises to restore strength and aerobic fitness.[27-29] The ability to progress the patient may be limited by the location of the tear (less vascularization to the inner 2/3 of the meniscus), the extent of the tear, and the presence of comorbid conditions. Regardless of whether a patient has been referred by a PCP or self-referred, the physical therapist may initiate treatment for a patient with a suspected meniscal sprain. If the patient fails to improve with treatment, referral for a knee arthroscopy is indicated to confirm the presence and extent of a meniscus injury.

Evidence-Based Clinical Recommendations

SORT: Strength of Recommendation Taxonomy

A: Consistent, good-quality patient-oriented evidence
B: Inconsistent or limited-quality patient-oriented evidence
C: Consensus, disease-oriented evidence, usual practice, expert opinion, or case series

1. Special clinical examination tests performed to identify meniscal pathology have moderate to high sensitivity and specificity, especially when the results of more than one test are combined. **Grade B**

2. The gold standard test to confirm or rule out a meniscus injury is arthroscopy. **Grade A**

COMPREHENSION QUESTIONS

28.1 The Thessaly test is performed with the patient's knee in ___ ° and ___ ° of knee flexion.

    A. 5, 10

    B. 10, 20

    C. 5, 20

    D. 20, 30

28.2 According to Couture et al.,[20] the McMurray test has poor sensitivity (28%) for detecting medial meniscus pathology; however, the test is associated with a high specificity (87%). If a patient with a suspected meniscus injury has a positive McMurray test, which of the following is true?

    A. The patient does not have a medial meniscus injury.

    B. A positive McMurray test will help to rule in a meniscal injury.

    C. A positive McMurray test will help to rule out a meniscal injury.

    D. The patient has a medial meniscus injury.

ANSWERS

28.1 **C.**

28.2 **B.** If a test with high specificity is positive, then the test may help to rule *in* the target disorder (SpPin). In this case, a positive McMurray test helps to rule in medial meniscus injury, because the test has high specificity (87%). Option D is incorrect because, although one can suspect that there is a meniscus injury based on the test's high specificity, it would be incorrect to state that the patient *does* have this injury. It is only accurate to state that the post-test *probability* of a meniscal tear is higher in the presence of a positive test with high specificity because arthroscopy is the gold standard test to *confirm* the presence or absence of a meniscus injury.

REFERENCES

1. Sackett DL. *Evidence-Based Medicine: How to Practice and Teach EBM.* Edinburgh: Churchill Livingstone;2000.

2. Muscolo DL, Ayerza MA, Makino A, et al. Tumors about the knee misdiagnosed as athletic injuries. *J Bone Joint Surg Am.* 2003;85A:1209-1214.

3. Pinar H, Boya H, Satoglu IS, Oztekin HH. A contribution to Pisani's sign for diagnosing lateral meniscal cysts: a technical report. *Knee Surg Sports Traumatol Arthrosc.* 2009;17:402-404.

4. Masouros SD, McDermott ID, et al. Biomechanics of the meniscus-meniscal ligament construct of the knee. *Knee Surg Sports Traumatol Arthrosc.* 2008;16:1121-1132.

5. Kohn D, Moreno B. Meniscus insertion anatomy as a basis for meniscus replacement: a morphologic cadaveric study. *Arthroscopy.* 1995;11:96-103.

6. Gee SM, Posner M. Meniscus anatomy and basic science. *Sports Med Arthrosc Rev.* 2021; 29:e18-e23.

7. Levy IM, Torzilli PA, Warren RF. The effect of medial meniscectomy on anterior-posterior motion of the knee. *J Bone Joint Surg Am.* 1982;64:883-888.

8. Levy IM, Torzilli PA, Gould JD, Warren RF. The effect of lateral meniscectomy on motion of the knee. *J Bone Joint Surg Am.* 1989;71:401-406.

9. Allen CR, Wong EK, Livesay GA, et al. Importance of the medial meniscus in the anterior cruciate ligament-deficient knee. *J Orthop Res.* 2000;18:09-115.

10. Renstrom P, Johnson RJ. Anatomy and biomechanics of the menisci. *Clin Sports Med.* 1990;9:523-538.

11. Howell R, Kumar NS, Patel N, Tom J. Degenerative meniscus: pathogenesis, diagnosis, and treatment options. *World J Orthop.* 2014;5:597-602.

12. Bellabarba C, Bush-Joseph CA, Bach BR Jr. Patterns of meniscal injury in the anterior-cruciate deficient knee: a review of the literature. *Am J Orthop.* 1997;26:18-23.

13. Harrison BK, Abell BE, Gibson TW. The Thessaly test for detection of meniscal tears: validation of a new physical examination technique for primary care medicine. *Clin J Sport Med.* 2009;19:9-12.

14. Karachalios T, Hantes M, Zibis AH, et al. Diagnostic accuracy of a new clinical test (the Thessaly test) for early detection of meniscal tears. *J Bone Joint Surg Am.* 2005;87:955-962.

15. Konan S, Rayan F, Haddad FS. Do physical diagnostic tests accurately detect meniscal tears? *Knee Surg Sports Traumatol Arthrosc.* 2009;17:806-811.

16. Solomon DH, Simel DL, Bates DW, et al. The rational clinical examination. Does this patient have a torn meniscus or ligament of the knee? Value of the physical examination. *JAMA.* 2001;286:1610-1620.

17. Hegedus EJ, Cook C, Hasselblad V, et al. Physical examination tests for assessing a torn meniscus in the knee: a systematic review with meta-analysis. *J Orthop Sports Phys Ther.* 2007;37:541-550.

18. Malanga GA, Andrus S, Nadler SF, McLean J. Physical examination of the knee: a review of the original test description and scientific validity of common orthopedic tests. *Arch Phys Med Rehabil.* 2003;84:592-603.

19. Stratford PW, Binkley J. A review of the McMurray test: definition, interpretation, and clinical usefulness. *J Orthop Sports Phys Ther.* 1995;22:116-120.

20. Couture JF, Al-Juhani W, Forsythe ME, et al. Joint line fullness and meniscal pathology. *Sports Health.* 2012;4:47-50.

21. Kocher MS, DiCanzio J, Zurakowski D, Micheli LJ. Diagnostic performance of clinical examination and selective magnetic resonance imaging in the evaluation of intraarticular knee disorders in children and adolescents. *Am J Sports Med.* 2001;29:292-296.

22. Kocabey Y, Tetik O, Isbell WM, et al. The value of clinical examination versus magnetic resonance imaging in the diagnosis of meniscal tears and anterior cruciate ligament rupture. *Arthroscopy.* 2004;20:696-700.

23. Gobbo Rda R, Rangel Vde O, Karam FC, Pires LA. Physical examinations for diagnosing meniscal injuries: correlation with surgical findings. *Rev Bras Ortop.* 2015;46:726-729.

24. Goossens P, Keijsers E, Van Geenen RJC, et al. Validity of the Thessaly test in evaluating meniscal tears compared with arthroscopy: a diagnostic accuracy study. *J Orthop Sports Phys Ther.* 2015;45:18-24.

25. Hashemi SA, Ranjbar MR, Tahami M, et al. Comparison of accuracy in expert clinical examination versus magnetic resonance imaging and arthroscopic exam in diagnosis of meniscal tear. *Adv Orthop.* 2020;2020:1895852.

26. Jackson JL, O'Malley PG, Kroenke K. Evaluation of acute knee pain in primary care. *Ann Intern Med.* 2003;139:575-588.

27. Lim HC, Bae JH, Wang JH, et al. Non-operative treatment of degenerative posterior root tear of the medial meniscus. *Knee Surg Sports Traumatol Arthrosc.* 2010;18:535-539.

28. Malliaropoulos N, Kiritsi O, Tsitas K, et al. Low-level laser therapy in meniscal pathology: a double-blind placebo-controlled trial. *Lasers Med Sci.* 2013;28:1183-1188.

29. Thorlund JB, Juhl CB, Ingelsrud LH, Skou ST. Risk factors, diagnosis and non-surgical treatment for meniscal tears: evidence and recommendations: a statement paper commissioned by the Danish Society of Sports Physical Therapy (DSSF). *Br J Sports Med.* 2018;52:557-565.

Tibial Stress Fracture

Michael D. Rosenthal
Shane A. Vath

A local fireman who has no significant prior running experience plans to enter a marathon in 7 months. He had 28 weeks to train and started running 1 mile every other day, and then added an additional mile weekly to meet the goal of 26 miles in time for the race. After 3 weeks of running, the patient noted medial shin pain that occurred near the end of the run or during the cool-down walking period. The leg pain dissipated after sitting and resting for a few hours and was not present on awakening or throughout the next day. The fireman continued training, which resulted in a gradual increase and earlier onset of pain. The fireman experienced leg pain at the beginning of runs that would ease with continued running. After 6 weeks of training, the leg pain occurred at the beginning and throughout the entire run and no longer resolved with cessation of running. The pain intensity increased, and the patient was unable to continue running. He started taking nonsteroidal anti-inflammatory drugs (NSAIDs), which allowed completion of one more week of painful training. Now, the patient has shin pain at rest that increases with standing and walking activities. On wakening, he experiences moderate discomfort and the pain increases during and following prolonged standing and walking. After prolonged sitting, symptoms ease, but remain present. The patient is frustrated and concerned about the potential inability to run the local marathon, so he self-referred to an outpatient physical therapy clinic. At the time of evaluation, the patient had not run for 2 days. As he walked through the therapy office, his gait was notably antalgic, with an exaggerated trunk lean toward the more involved side. Strength testing, range of motion (ROM), and visual inspection were all normal. Diffuse medial shin pain was reproduced with ROM and strength testing. The most significant finding on examination was localized tenderness to palpation about 2 cm in length along the medial tibia (right leg greater than left), at the junction of the mid to distal one-third of the tibias. There was also mild bilateral tenderness over the central third of the medial tibias. Other than the recent increase in training, the patient's past medical history was unremarkable.

Signs, symptoms, and history are consistent with tibial stress fractures. The fireman's main goal is to return pain-free to his training program to be able to complete the local marathon.

▶ Based on the patient's suspected diagnosis, what do you anticipate may be the contributing factors to the condition?
▶ What physical examination signs may be associated with this diagnosis?
▶ What ancillary tests (*e.g.*, imaging) are most sensitive and specific for diagnosing a tibial stress fracture?

KEY DEFINITIONS

BONE STRESS INJURY (BSI): Overuse injury resulting in the bone's inability to withstand repeated mechanical loading which results in micro- or macro-structural failure, increased intracortical porosity, and reduction in local mechanical properties; condition presents with progressive localized pain and tenderness[1]

EXTRINSIC RISK FACTORS: Characteristics of an individual's training or competition schedule that may influence the likelihood of sustaining a stress fracture (*e.g.*, training regimen, shoe selection, training surface or terrain, type of sport)

INTRINSIC RISK FACTORS: Characteristics of the individual that may influence the likelihood of sustaining a stress fracture (*e.g.*, sex, knee alignment, leg length discrepancy nutritional factors, hormonal factors)

OSTEOBLASTS: Cells that produce bone matrix, ultimately resulting in increased bone strength and healing of a (stress) fracture

OSTEOCLASTS: Cells that resorb bone, which can ultimately produce a resorption cavity and decrease in bone strength

TIBIAL STRESS FRACTURE: Overuse injury that primarily occurs in response to a significant increase in training intensity and or volume (usually running); marked by localized tenderness of 2 to 3 cm along the medial tibia; pain at rest and at night are common

Objectives

1. Describe tibial stress fracture symptoms and potential intrinsic and extrinsic risk factors associated with this diagnosis.

2. Identify rationale for referral for further evaluation and imaging.

3. Identify commonly used clinical tests for diagnosing tibial stress fractures.

4. Distinguish between high- and low-risk stress fractures and provide appropriate protection to allow stress fracture healing.

5. Design a rehabilitation program to ensure healing while aiding in rapid return to daily activities and sports including running.

Physical Therapy Considerations

Physical therapy considerations during management of the individual with a suspected diagnosis of medial tibial stress fracture:

▶ **General physical therapy plan of care/goals:** Differential diagnosis; consultation with an orthopedic/musculoskeletal specialist; decrease pain; protect from further injury with immobilization and/or appropriate assistive devices to normalize gait and reduce tibial load; address any underlying medical conditions; provide education regarding diagnosis and prognosis; minimize lower extremity deconditioning without interrupting healing; aid in managing progression back to running by educating patient on training variables (frequency, intensity, type, duration); assess pain and function with gradual increase in activity to reduce likelihood of further injury

▶ **Physical therapy interventions:** Patient education regarding functional anatomy and injury pathomechanics; modalities; musculotendinous flexibility and joint mobility exercises; resistance exercises to promote maintenance and recovery of muscular endurance and strength; alternate low-impact aerobic conditioning to allow fitness training; gradual progression of impact-loading exercises; orthotic fabrication; continue discussion with patient to minimize likelihood that frustration with injury will alter psychological wellbeing

▶ **Precautions during physical therapy:** Differentiate low-risk versus high-risk stress fractures; avoid compressive, tensile, or torsional strains to the lower extremity that may result in non-union, malunion or fracture completion; monitor response of leg pain to prescribed exercise program and reduce tissue loads if patient experiences increased symptoms during training or the following day; address precautions or contraindications for exercise based on patient's pre-existing condition(s); monitor response to reduced activity and impact on individual's career, sport, or leisure activities; monitor patient's use of NSAIDs

▶ **Complications interfering with physical therapy:** Patient/client who is unwilling or unable to alter training regimen; work schedule; comorbidities (*e.g.,* hormonal status, nutritional status, osteopenia, osteoporosis, radiation therapy, and other cancer treatments)

Understanding the Health Condition

The tibia is the major weightbearing bone in the leg and the second largest bone in the human body next to the femur. Ninety percent of the lower extremity load is carried by the tibia with the fibula taking the remaining 10%.[2] The tibia is prismoid in shape, having a broadened flat trabecular bone epiphyseal plateau proximally which articulates with the femoral condyles. Below the tibial plateau, the bone transitions to a cortical bone diaphysis. The diameter is smallest between the middle third and distal third of the length of the bone. Near the ankle, the tibia expands again into an epiphysis forming the tibial plafond, a concave dense trabecular bony region that articulates with the talar dome. The cortical bone shaft of the tibia is made up of three surfaces: the medial, posterior, and lateral. Multiple muscles attach to the tibia and are contained within four compartments: anterior, lateral, superficial posterior, and deep posterior. The borders of each compartment are defined by varying proportions of tough fascia, soft tissue, and bone. Variability in borders makes some compartments more or less compliant and able to tolerate increases in size whether due to muscle hypertrophy, bony callus, edema or other space occupying lesion(s), which may result in increased intra-compartmental pressures. The fascia of the anterior compartment attaches to the anterior margin of the tibia. The fibula attaches to the tibia by a tough interosseous membrane, proximal and distal bony articulations, and associated ligaments. The tibia undergoes varied loading throughout the gait cycle, the magnitude of which is influenced by several factors (*e.g.*, bony anatomy, muscular endurance, running style). The anterior cortex experiences tensile strain while the posterior cortex has a compressive strain during impact loading.[3] With running, the tibia is cyclically loaded with vertical forces measuring 2.5 to 2.8 times body weight.[4] Microdamage formation depends on the interaction between the number of bone strain cycles, strain magnitude, and the speed at which strain is introduced (*i.e.*, strain rate). Once the threshold for microdamage has been surpassed, further increases in bone strain cycles are likely to result in additional structural damage.[1] To slow the progression of bone stress injury (BSI), decreased bone loading is required to slow osteoclastic activity and enable remodeling to "catch up" without further damage accumulating. Osteoclast activation and resorption in cortical bone take approximately 4 weeks, and replacement with new bone takes 3 months, with up to a year required for full mineralization.[5]

Medial tibial pain accounts for 13% to 17% of all running injuries.[6] Stress fractures are typically one of the top 5 most common running injuries and account for 5% to 50% of all musculoskeletal running injuries.[7,8] While the site of the stress fracture varies by sport and activity, over 80% of stress fractures occur in the lower body.[9-11] BSI are common in distance runners impacting between one-third to two-thirds of competitive cross-country and long-distance runners, while track and field athletes have incidence rates ranging from 4.9% to 21.1%.[11,12] Recurrence rates are high, up to 50% in track-and-field athletes and 10.3% to 12.6% for cross-country athletes, and a history of previous stress fracture is most predictive of a future stress fracture.[13] The tibia is the most common location of stress fracture,[14-15] accounting for 24% to 55% of all stress fractures.[9,10,16] Fibular bone stress injuries (7%-12% of all stress fractures[10,12]) should also be considered in the differential diagnosis due to proximity to tibia and similar clinical history and symptom presentation. The majority of tibial stress fractures are "low risk"—occurring in the posteromedial aspect at the junction of the mid to distal third of its length.[17] This area has been deemed a low-risk stress fracture because healing typically occurs with protection and activity modification.[18] Tibial stress fractures can also occur in the region of the medial tibial condyle (Fig. 29-1) and the anterior mid-diaphyseal cortex of the tibia, with the specific location determined by the combination of stresses incurred by the tibia.[1,17] For individuals with anterior tibial cortex stress fractures (known as "the dreaded black line"; Fig. 29-2), the combination of poor blood supply and tension, vice compression, and forces to the injured region make this a high-risk stress fracture.[17] These high-risk stress fractures are associated with delayed union, nonunion progression to complete fracture, and problematic return to sports.[19]

Stress fractures are an overuse injury experienced primarily by individuals who rapidly increase running or other high-impact activities. Stress fractures often occur during the second and third weeks following an increase in training volume, but have also been reported at later stages of training.[20] Development of a stress fracture is the result of an accumulation of microtrauma from repetitive loading, continuation of loading, and loss of bone homeostasis due to inadequate rest and repair.[1,21] Following a disturbance in homeostasis, the time required to reach a new equilibrium is 3 to 4 months in cortical bone.[1] If insufficient time is given to adapt to new mechanical stimulus, then more bone damage occurs. Responses to bone

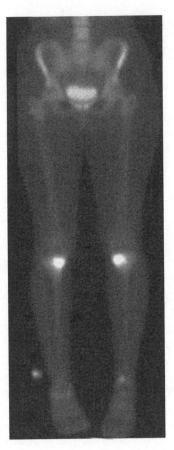

Figure 29-1. Technetium bone scan image of patient with bilateral medial tibial condyle stress fractures. The brighter regions indicate an increased rate of bone turnover (more radioactive technetium is taken up by osteoblast cells).

loading occur along a continuum—beginning with normal remodeling and then advancing to accelerated remodeling, stress reaction, stress injury, stress fracture, and complete fracture when excessive loading without adequate rest is continued.[1,19] There are two types of stress fractures: fatigue fractures and insufficiency fractures.[22] Fatigue fractures occur due to repetitive submaximal stress to normal bone, which creates a region of accelerated bone remodeling. Insufficiency fractures occur when bones deficient in microstructure and/or mineralization (*i.e.*, osteopenia or osteoporosis) undergo normal loading.[23]

Effective training programs that include well-planned loading and rest periods promote bony adaptation and subsequent increases in bone mass (*i.e.*, strength). Bone is a dynamic tissue that continually undergoes remodeling with osteoclasts that resorb bone and osteoblasts that form new bone. Osteoclastic activity creates tunnels within the bone that weaken its architecture and can result in pain with repeated loading. If loading continues and interrupts healing, the activity of osteoclasts outpaces that of osteoblasts, which can result in microtrabecular disruption (stress injury). Continued loading can lead to a cortical break (stress fracture).[1]

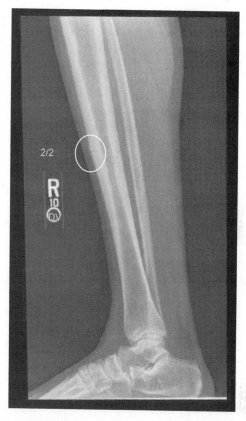

Figure 29-2. Lateral radiograph of the tibia showing an anterior cortex stress fracture and the "dreaded black line" (within circle).

Regardless of the etiology of fatigue stress fractures, relative rest and appropriate nutrition allow the body to restore balance in bone remodeling and heal appropriately. However, continued training, cyclic impact loading, and inadequate recovery periods may perpetuate shin pain and allow a stress fracture to progress to a complete fracture.[24,25]

Muscular strength, endurance, and power are thought to mitigate ground reaction forces and protect against the development of stress fractures.[19,25] As muscle fatigue develops, muscular shock absorption decreases, and the bone experiences a significantly greater load, with reports indicating ground reaction and shear strain forces increasing by 10% to 35%.[26,27] Runners that experience abnormal loading with high ground reaction force and rates, and accelerations or torsion during running may be at increased risk of BSI.[28,29]

Stress fractures may be the result of extrinsic and/or intrinsic factors. **Extrinsic factors** proposed to contribute to the onset of stress fracture include: rapid increase in training (intensity, frequency, and duration), old or inappropriate footwear, recent change in running surface (*e.g.*, hills), and recent change in running technique.[30] Proposed **intrinsic risk factors** include: prior history of BSI, sex, race, bone size, anatomic factors (*e.g.*, foot shape, leg length discrepancy, knee alignment), decreased muscular strength, suboptimal lower extremity biomechanics, and nutritional factors.[19,30-32] Female adolescent runners with a history of BSI are 6 times more likely of having a future BSI. Female runners without a history of BSI, but with other risk factors such as body mass index <19.0 kg/m^2, delayed menarche, ≥15 years of age, or absence or irregular menses have a 2-fold greater risk of a BSI compared to peers without these intrinsic factors.[25,33,34] The presence of female athlete triad components: decreased bone mineral density, low energy availability (*i.e.*, disordered eating), and hormonal factors (*i.e.*, menstrual cycle irregularity) also increase the risk of stress fracture.[19,34] If any concerns for the female athlete triad are identified during rehabilitation, the therapist should refer the patient to a primary care provider for further evaluation and treatment. In contrast, having a higher level of physical fitness and a history of previous impact-loading sports activity seem to be protective of overuse injuries.[35] Untrained individuals are 10 times more likely to develop overuse injuries compared to individuals who have a higher level of physical fitness.[36]

Examination, Evaluation, and Diagnosis

A thorough patient history helps the physical therapist develop potential differential diagnoses prior to initiating the physical examination. The therapist should gather information regarding: history of trauma, mechanism of injury, past medical history, history of similar symptoms, previous medical attention sought for the condition and type of medical providers seen, whether a diagnosis had been established, past imaging studies and results, easing and aggravating factors, and current status of symptoms (improving, worsening, or static). In addition, the physical therapist should inquire about the patient's specific training routine, including frequency, intensity, type of training (sprints, hills), distance, types of running surfaces, type and age of running shoes, and positions or activities that reproduce symptoms. The therapist should also explore what is motivating the individual to perform their current exercise program (*e.g.*, job qualification or training, sport, leisure, health).

Patients presenting with suspicion of tibial stress fracture are most likely to report atraumatic shin pain with weightbearing activity that began as a result of a recent increase in running intensity and/or volume. However, given the spectrum of BSI, it may be difficult to base the diagnosis purely on a clinical examination. Furthermore, the physical therapist must remember that it is possible to have a concomitant condition (*e.g.*, periostitis). Early symptoms of a tibial stress fracture may be like those of medial tibial stress syndrome (MTSS). Differential diagnoses for tibial stress fracture include: MTSS, chronic periostalgia secondary to tension between fascial attachments to the periosteum, chronic exertional compartment syndrome, tendinitis, periostitis, fibular stress fracture, muscle hernia, intermittent claudication, venous insufficiency, osteoid osteoma, ligamentous injuries, cartilage pathologies, meniscal tears, osteomyelitis (in younger patients), and metastases (in older patients).[37] While less common, bone stress injuries of the medial tibial condyle or medial malleolus can present like meniscal tears, ligamentous injuries, or cartilage pathologies.[38]

The primary symptoms associated with tibial stress fracture are atraumatic local tenderness, swelling, and occasionally warmth and pain that increases with exercise.[38-40] Initial symptoms are typically mild and resolve with prolonged sitting or sleep. If the aggravating activity is continued, the symptoms tend to worsen, and pain limits the patient's ability to perform the desired activity. If the individual is not involved in an organized sport or lacks a specific training goal, they will typically refrain from further training due to pain and the symptoms will resolve over time. With continued training, the condition typically worsens. Symptoms become more frequent, have an earlier onset, interrupt the ability to train, and are present for longer durations after cessation of activity. In many cases, patients experience pain at rest that increases after prolonged standing and eases somewhat after prolonged sitting. Pain at rest, especially at night, is also common with stress fractures.[41]

Pain may initially be diffuse. However, after a period of relative rest from pain-producing activities, the pain becomes more localized. A key physical examination finding is localized tenderness within a 2- to 3-cm region, often accompanied by palpable thickening of the bone.[1,38] This contrasts with the diffuse pain over an area >5 cm, which is more indicative of MTSS.[42] **Numerous special tests may assist in the clinical diagnosis of tibial stress fracture** (Table 29-1). However, none has consistently demonstrated high diagnostic value.[43,44]

Table 29-1 SPECIAL TESTS ASSOCIATED WITH TIBIAL STRESS FRACTURES

Test	Patient Position	Findings
Fulcrum test[43,44]	Sitting at edge of treatment table. Therapist grasps ankle with one hand and provides a medial/lateral stress to the tibia in the symptomatic region.	Reproduction or increase in patient's pain is a positive sign for potential tibial stress fracture.
Percussion test	Supine on treatment table. Therapist passively elevates the straight leg off examination table and provides a rapid percussive force through the heel along the long axis of the leg/tibia.	Reproduction or increase in patient's pain is a positive sign for potential tibial stress fracture.
Tuning fork test[43,44]	Supine on treatment table with knee flexed ~ 90° to relax posterior leg musculature. Therapist strikes a 128-Hz tuning fork and applies it to the tibia at the region of tenderness. The tuning fork may be held stationary or slowly moved across the region of tenderness.	Reproduction or increase in patient's pain is a positive sign for potential tibial stress fracture.
Ultrasound test[43]	Supine on treatment table with knee flexed ~ 90° to relax posterior leg musculature. Continuous therapeutic ultrasound of 1 MHz for 3-5 min is applied to the region of greatest tenderness to palpation. The ultrasound head is moved over an area ~3 times the size of the sound head at an intensity of 0.5-3.0 W/cm^2.	Reproduction or increase in patient's pain is a positive sign for potential tibial stress fracture.
Single-leg hop[44]	Standing on one leg, patient performs vertical jump. This more provocative test should only be performed if previous tests do not reproduce symptoms, or to aid in determining ability to return to impact activities.	Reproduction of the patient's pain is a positive sign for potential tibial stress fracture.

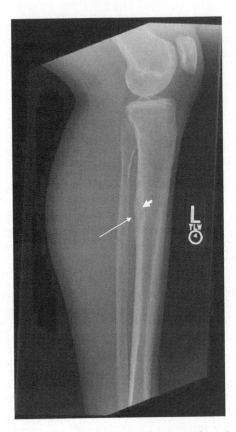

Figure 29-3. Lateral radiograph of the tibia demonstrating periosteal reaction (long arrow) and linear lucency (short arrow) through the proximal posterior tibial cortex, consistent with a healing stress fracture.

Because radiographic examination is the least expensive and the most widely available imaging modality, x-rays are recommended as the first imaging study when a stress fracture is suspected.[45] At early stages of BSI, the sensitivity of radiographs is only 15% to 35%. If initial radiographs of the leg are negative, they should be repeated in 10 to 14 days, which increases sensitivity, but is less sensitive than magnetic resonance imaging (MRI). Changes on plain radiographs are usually not evident for at least 2 to 3 weeks after symptom onset, are often normal for up to 3 months, and in some cases may remain normal.[46,47] Findings on radiographs indicating stress fracture are often nonspecific and may include periosteal thickening, subtle periosteal reaction "gray cortex" sign, or distinct lucency (Figs. 29-3 and 29-4).[47] Periosteal thickening is the most common finding. However, this nonsensitive finding is often present in individuals with an extensive physical training background.

The **gold standard for diagnosis of tibial stress fractures is MRI.**[39,40,41] The American College of Radiology Appropriateness Criteria® recommends the use of MRI in most cases of suspected stress fracture following negative radiographs.[45]

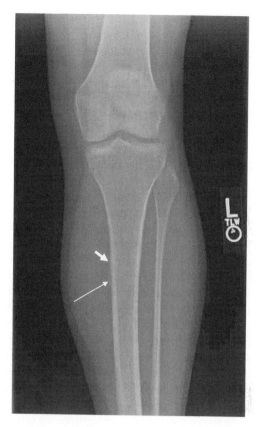

Figure 29-4. Anteroposterior radiograph of the tibia demonstrating a thickening, or periosteal reaction (long arrow) and a fracture line (short arrow) at the medial tibial cortex.

Bone scans and computed tomography (CT) scans are recommended in lieu of MRI for select reasons, though these imaging modalities expose the individual to higher levels of ionizing radiation.[45] MRI grading scales for BSI may be helpful in determining injury severity and potential time for return to running.[40,48] Low-risk/low-grade BSI have a more favorable outcome and more rapid return to sport (averaging 9 weeks). Low-risk/high-grade BSIs and all high-risk BSIs are associated with a more prolonged recovery with return to sport around 20 weeks.[1,48] The time to return to activity after BSI is highly variable and rehabilitation must be progressed based on each individual's healing response, using pain as a guide.[25]

Plan of Care and Interventions

Physical therapy interventions should address findings from the history and musculoskeletal examination. If the physical therapist suspects a stress fracture, the individual should be advised to decrease weightbearing on the involved extremity(ies) using crutches and referred to an orthopedic or musculoskeletal specialist for further evaluation and management. If diagnosis of a tibial stress fracture is confirmed via imaging, the therapist can develop a comprehensive rehabilitation program to minimize deconditioning, optimize return to preinjury activity levels, and address intrinsic and extrinsic factors to mitigate the potential for reinjury while ensuring that the BSI does not progress, especially in high-risk anterior cortex stress fractures.

Once an individual with a high-risk anterior tibial stress fracture is cleared to initiate rehabilitation by the physician, return to activity can be progressed the same as for individuals with low-risk stress fractures.[1] NSAIDs should only be used for a short duration because they may mask the symptoms of excessive loading (pain) and may reduce bone formation during bone healing.[24] The goal of rehabilitation is to return the individual to preinjury level of function and fitness in the shortest time possible without interrupting or delaying bone healing. This begins with intentionally reduced activity to decrease loads to allow healing. Pain is used as the key indicator of healing and the patient is allowed to return only to pain-free activities of daily living (ADLs).[25] The presence of pain during, after, or the day after activity indicates that the injured bone needs to have a further reduced load. Individuals with a rearfoot or leg BSI may use cushioned shoes and/or insoles to dissipate impact forces during ADLs. If individuals are unable to demonstrate a normal gait pattern or have pain with required daily walking, then assistive devices should be used to offset weightbearing. A pneumatic leg brace or a controlled ankle motion (CAM) boot may also reduce loads, though CAM boots should be used with caution as they may alter gait mechanics and cause secondary musculoskeletal overuse injuries. Individuals with low-risk stress fractures should be returned to unassisted ambulation as soon as they are able to demonstrate a normal pain-free gait. The patient should be progressed back to normal activity slowly while monitoring for any return of pain at rest, at night, or an increase in pain during, after, or the following day after an increase in activity/loads. Close monitoring and education on pain are vital. If pain increases, this indicates that the bone has been mechanically or chemically irritated and loading must be reduced to avoid delayed healing or reinjury. For individuals with a history of repeated BSI, especially in the same region, the physical therapist must perform a thorough re-examination to identify and address any previously overlooked intrinsic or extrinsic risk factors that may be leading to deleterious loading of the bone.

Progressive resistance exercises, guided by pain response, can be safely initiated for low-risk posteromedial tibial BSI, but should be delayed for high-risk anterior tibial cortex BSI.[25] As long as there is no increase in pain, low-impact activities (e.g., stationary cycling, swimming, deep water running, elliptical, and anti-gravity treadmill training) should be implemented and progressed to maintain cardiovascular fitness. Once an individual has progressed to pain-free unassisted daily activities for 5 to 7 consecutive days, a progressive walk-run program can be initiated at a low pace and intensity.[1,25] If pain returns, the athlete rests until the pain resolves. Progressive running is designed to incrementally load bone, not to improve aerobic conditioning. Safe progression of bone loading is supported by increasing only one training variable—frequency, intensity, type, or time—by 5% to 10% per week while continuing to closely monitor pain.[25] As the individual returns to running, the therapist continues to identify and address any faulty mechanics that may increase bone loading. Techniques to help the patient maintain running velocity with reduced bone strain and reduce recurrence of BSI include increasing step rate (cadence), reducing stride length, and modifying foot strike pattern.[49,50] The physical therapist must be aware that disuse impacts all lower extremity bones and peaks at around 12 weeks—the likely timeframe corresponding to the individual's return-to-running program.[51] Thus, cross-training and jump training to load the bone in multiple directions with planned periods of rest should be encouraged to support continued musculoskeletal health.[35]

Evidence-Based Clinical Recommendations

SORT: Strength of Recommendation Taxonomy

A: Consistent, good-quality patient-oriented evidence
B: Inconsistent or limited-quality patient-oriented evidence
C: Consensus, disease-oriented evidence, usual practice, expert opinion, or case series

1. Extrinsic risk factors are associated with development of tibial stress fractures. **Grade A**

2. Intrinsic risk factors are associated with development of tibial stress fractures. **Grade B**

3. Special clinical tests can assist in the diagnosis of tibial stress fractures. **Grade B**

4. Magnetic resonance imaging (MRI) is the most specific and sensitive tool for diagnosis of tibial stress fractures. **Grade A**

COMPREHENSION QUESTIONS

29.1 What is the MOST common cause of tibial stress fracture?

    A. Training errors (extrinsic risk factor)
    B. Pes planus (intrinsic risk factor)
    C. Incorrect shoe selection (extrinsic risk factor)
    D. High body mass index (intrinsic risk factor)

29.2 What is the MOST sensitive and specific imaging modality for diagnosis of tibial stress fracture?

    A. Bone densitometry
    B. Magnetic resonance imaging (MRI)
    C. Technetium bone scan
    D. Standard (plain) radiographs

29.3 What are the current American College of Radiology recommendations for imaging of suspected tibial stress fracture?

A. Bone scan; if abnormal, then MRI

B. Radiographs; if normal, then MRI within 7 days

C. Radiographs; if normal, then repeat in 10 to 14 days and consider MRI to rule out high-risk stress fractures and/or make return to sport/work decisions

D. Radiographs; if normal, then repeat in 21 days and if still normal, 95% probability there is no stress fracture

29.4 What intrinsic risk factor is MOST highly associated with development of a bone stress injury?

A. Leg length discrepancy

B. Old, worn-out shoes

C. Pes planus

D. Prior history of bone stress injury

29.5 What are the components of the female athlete triad?

A. Caucasian, low energy availability, regular menstruation

B. Decreased bone mineral density, low energy availability, irregular menstruation

C. Mileage greater than 20 miles/week, high running cadence, worn-out shoes

D. Under 22 years of age, competitive athlete, well-nourished

ANSWERS

29.1 **A.** The most prevalent cause of tibial stress fracture is training errors.[1,13,21]

29.2 **B.** MRI is considered the gold standard for diagnosing tibial stress fractures. It provides the most sensitive and specific information when evaluating bone stress injuries.[40,41] While the technetium bone scan provides a high level of sensitivity, the specificity is not as high as MRI.

29.3 **C.** According to American College of Radiology Appropriateness Criteria®, stress fractures of the tibia should initially be imaged using radiography, although radiographic imaging lacks sensitivity. If the initial radiographs of the leg (tibia and fibula) are negative, radiographs should be repeated in 10 to 14 days, which increases sensitivity, but is less sensitive than MRI. MRI without contrast may be considered if there is concern for high-risk anterior tibial diaphysis stress fracture, or there is an immediate need to know for return to sports for high-level athletes or resumption of work for military and manual laborers.[44]

29.4 **D.** The intrinsic risk factor most highly associated with development of a bone stress injury is a prior history of bone stress injury.[1,33]

29.5 **B.** Components of female athlete triad are decreased bone mineral density (osteopenia or osteoporosis), low energy availability (disordered eating), and hormonal factors (menstrual cycle irregularity).[34]

REFERENCES

1. Warden SJ, Davis IS, Fredericson M. Management and prevention of bone stress injuries in long-distance runners. *J Orthop Sports Phys Ther*. 2014;44(10):749-765.

2. Takebe K, Nakagawa A, Minami H, et al. Role of the fibula in weight-bearing. *Clin Orthop Relat Res*. 1984;184:289-292.

3. Meardon SA, Willson JD, Gries SR, et al. Bone stress in runners with tibial stress fracture. *Clin Biomech*. 2015;30:895-902.

4. Miller DI. Ground reaction forces in distance running. In: Cavanagh PR, ed. *The Biomechanics of Distance Running*. Champaign, IL: Human Kinetics; 1990:203-224.

5. Eriksen EF. Cellular mechanisms of bone remodeling. *Rev Endocri Metab Disord*. 2010;11:219-227.

6. Taunton JE, Clement DB, Webber D. Lower extremity stress fractures in athletes. *Phys Sportsmed*. 1981;9:77-86.

7. Bennell KL, Malcolm SA, Brukner PD, et al. A 12-month prospective study of the relationship between stress fractures and bone turnover in athletes. *Calcif Tissue Int*. 1998;63:80-85.

8. Losito JM, Laird RC, Alexis MR, Mora J. Tibial and proximal fibular stress fracture in a rower. *J Am Pod Med Assoc*. 2003;9:340-343.

9. Brukner P, Bradshaw C, Khan KM, et al. Stress fractures: a review of 180 cases. *Clin J Sport Med*. 1996;6:85-89.

10. Matheson GO, Clement DB, McKenzie DC, et al. Stress fractures in athletes. A study of 320 cases. *Am J Sports Med*. 1987;15:46-58.

11. Changstrom BG, Brou L, Khodaee M, et al. Epidemiology of stress fracture injuries among US high school athletes, 2005-2006 through 2012-2013. *Am J Sports Med*. 2014;43:26-33.

12. Bennell KL, Malcolm SA, Thomas SA, et al. The incidence and distribution of stress fractures in competitive track and field athletes. A twelve-month prospective study. *Am J Sports Med*. 1996;24:211-217.

13. Kelsey JL, Bachrach LK, Procert-Gray E, et al. Risk factors for stress fracture among young female cross-country runners. *Med Sci Sports Exerc*. 2007;39:1457-1463.

14. James SL, Bates BT, Osternig LR. Injuries to runners. *Am J Sports Med*. 1978;6:40-50.

15. McBryde AM Jr. Stress fractures in runners. *Clin Sports Med*. 1985;4:737-752.

16. Giladi M, Milgrom C, Simkin A. Stress fractures and tibial bone width: a risk factor. *J Bone Joint Surg*. 1987;69:326-329.

17. Fredericson M, Jennings F, Beaulieu C, Matheson GO. Stress fractures in athletes. *Top Magn Reson Imaging*. 2006;17:309-325.

18. McCormick F, Nwachukwu BU, Provencher MT. Stress fractures in runners. *Clin Sports Med*. 2012;31:291-306.

19. Brukner P, Bennell K, Matheson G. *Stress Fractures*. Victoria, Australia: Human Kinetics;1999.

20. Burr DB. Bone, exercise, and stress fractures. *Exerc Sport Sci Rev*. 1997;25:171-194.

21. Pepper M, Akuthota V, McCarty EC. The pathophysiology of stress fractures. *Clin Sports Med*. 2006;25:1-16.

22. Matcuk GR, Mahanty SR, Skalski MR, et al. Stress fractures: pathophysiology, clinical presentation, imaging features, and treatment options. *Emerg Radiol.* 2016;23:365-375.

23. Li ZC, Dai LY, Jiang LS, Qiu S. Difference in subchondral cancellous bone between postmenopausal women with hip osteoarthritis and osteoporotic fracture: implication for fatigue microdamage, bone microarchitecture, and biomechanical properties. *Arthritis Rheum.* 2012;64:3955-3962.

24. Warden SJ, Thompson WR. Becoming one with the force: optimising mechanotherapy through an understanding of mechanobiology. *Br J Sports Med.* 2017;51:989-990.

25. Warden SJ, Edwards WB, Willy RW. Optimal load for managing low-risk tibial and metatarsal bone stress injuries in runners: the science behind the clinical reasoning. *J Orthop Sports Phys Ther.* 2021;51:322-330.

26. Beck BR. Tibial stress injuries. An aetiological review for the purposes of guiding management. *Sports Med.* 1998;26:265-79.

27. Milgrom C, Radeva-Petrova DR, Finestone A, et al. The effect of muscle fatigue on in vivo tibial strains. *J Biomech.* 2007;40:845-850.

28. Pohl MB, Mullineaux DR, Milner CE, et al. Biomechanical predictors of retrospective tibial stress fractures in runners. *J Biomech.* 2008;41:1160-1165.

29. Van der Worp H, Vrielink JW, Bredeweg SW. Do runners who suffer injuries have higher vertical ground reaction forces than those who remain injury-free? A systematic review and meta-analysis. *Br J Sports Med.* 2016;50:450-457.

30. Kasitinon D, Ramey Argo L. Risk Factors for Developing Stress Fractures. In: Miller T.L., Kaeding C.C. (eds). *Stress Fractures in Athletes.* 2nd ed. Springer, Cham, Switzerland; 2020.

31. Arendt E, Agel J, Heikes C, Griffiths H. Stress injuries to bone in college athletes: a retrospective review of experience at a single institution. *Am J Sports Med.* 2003;31:959-968.

32. Armstrong DW III, Rue JP, Wilckens JH, Frassica FJ. Stress fracture injury in young military men and women. *Bone.* 2004;35:806-816.

33. Wright AA, Taylor JB, Ford KR, et al. Risk factors associated with lower extremity stress fractures in runners: a systematic review with meta-analysis. *Br J Sports Med.* 2015;49:1517-1523.

34. Abbott A, Bird ML, Wild E, et al. Part I: epidemiology and risk factors for stress fractures in female athletes. *The Physician and Sportsmedicine* 2020;48:17-24.

35. Milgrom C, Simkin A, Eldad A, et al. Using bone's adaptation ability to lower the incidence of stress fractures. *Am J Sports Med.* 2000;28:245-251.

36. Rosendal L, Langberg H, Skov-Jensen A, Kjaer M. Incidence of injury and physical performance adaptations during military training. *Clin J Sport Med.* 2003;13:157-163.

37. Lohrer H, Malliaropoulos N, Korakakis V, Padhiar N. Exercise-induced leg pain in athletes: diagnostic, assessment, and management strategies. *Phys Sportsmed.* 2019;47:47-59.

38. Kahanov L, Eberman LE, Games KE, Wasik M. Diagnosis, treatment, and rehabilitation of stress fractures in the lower extremity in runners. *Open Access J Sports Med.* 2015;6:87-95.

39. Young AJ, McAllister DR. Evaluation and treatment of tibial stress fractures. *Clin Sports Med.* 2006;25:117-128.

40. Fredericson M, Bergman AG, Hoffman KL, Dillingham MS. Tibial stress reaction in runners. Correlation of clinical symptoms and scintigraphy with a new magnetic resonance imaging grading system. *Am J Sports Med.* 1995;23:472-481.

41. Batt ME, Ugalde V, Anderson MW, Shelton DK. A prospective controlled study of diagnostic imaging for acute shin splints. *Med Sci Sports Exerc.* 1998;20:1564-1571.

42. Schneiders AG, Sullivan SJ, Hendrick PA, et al. The ability of clinical tests to diagnose stress fractures: a systematic review and meta-analysis. *J Orthop Sports Phys Ther.* 2012;42:760-771.

43. Nussbaum ED, Gatt CJ, Bjornarra J, Yang C. Evaluating the clinical tests for adolescent tibial bone stress injuries. *Sports Health.* 2021;13;502-510.

44. Bencardino JT, Stone TJ, Roberts CC, et al. ACR Appropriateness Criteria Stress (Fatigue/Insufficiency) Fracture, Including Sacrum, Excluding Other Vertebrae. *J Am Coll Radiol.* 2017;14:S293-S306.

45. Savoca CJ. Stress fractures. A classification of the earliest radiographic signs. *Radiol.* 1971; 100:519-524.

46. Deutsch AL, Coel MN, Mink JH. Imaging of stress injuries to bone. Radiography, scintigraphy and MR imaging. *Clin Sports Med.* 1997;16:275-290.

47. Wright AA, Hegedus EJ, Lenchik L, et al. Diagnostic accuracy of various imaging modalities for suspected lower extremity stress fractures: a systematic review with evidence-based recommendations for clinical practice. *Am J Sports Med.* 206;45:255-263.

48. Dobrindt O, Hoffmeyer B, Ruf J, et al. Estimation of return-to-sports-time for athletes with stress fracture—an approach combining risk level of fracture site with severity based on imaging. *BMC Musculoskeletal Disorders.* 2012;13:139

49. Huang Y, Xia H, Chen G, et al. Foot strike pattern, step rate, and trunk posture combined gait modifications to reduce impact loading during running. *J Biomech.* 2019;86:102-109.

50. Kliethermes KA, Stiffler-Joachim MR, Wille CM, et al. Lower step rate is associated with a higher risk of bone stress injury: a prospective study of collegiate cross country runners. *Br J Sports Med.* 2021;55:851-856.

51. Popp KL, Ackerman KE, Rudolph SE, et al. Changes in volumetric bone mineral density over 12 months after a tibial bone stress injury diagnosis. *Am J Sports Med.* 2021;49:226-235.

DISCLAIMER

The views expressed in this article are those of the authors and do not necessarily reflect the official policy or position of the Department of the Navy, Department of Defense, or the U.S. Government.

Medial Tibial Stress Syndrome

Michael D. Rosenthal
Shane A. Vath

CASE 30

A 25-year-old businessman initiated a running program with a goal to get into shape and lose weight. The program consisted of running 2 miles 4 to 5 times per week and he continued this regimen for 4 weeks. He initially noted medial shin pain after 2 weeks of running that occurred near the end of his run or with cool-down walking. When the pain started to interfere with his exercise program, he self-referred to an outpatient physical therapy clinic for evaluation and treatment. Signs, symptoms, and history are consistent with medial tibial stress syndrome (MTSS). The individual's main goal is to return to pain-free running and improve his fitness.

- ▶ Based on the patient's suspected diagnosis, what do you anticipate may be the contributing factors to the condition?
- ▶ What examination signs may be associated with this diagnosis?
- ▶ What are the most appropriate physical therapy interventions?
- ▶ What are possible complications that may limit the effectiveness of physical therapy?

KEY DEFINITIONS

EXTRINSIC RISK FACTORS: Characteristics of an individual's training or competition schedule that may influence the likelihood of developing MTSS (*e.g.,* training regimen, shoe selection, training surface or terrain, type of sport)

INTRINSIC RISK FACTORS: Characteristics of the individual that may influence the likelihood of developing MTSS (*e.g.,* sex, lower extremity strength deficits, excessive hip rotation mobility, high body mass index, navicular drop)

MEDIAL TIBIAL STRESS SYNDROME: Overuse injury that primarily occurs with a rapid increase in frequency, intensity, and/or duration of impact activities (usually running); marked by diffuse tenderness >5 cm in length along the posteromedial border of the tibia of one or both legs, and most commonly affects the middle to distal thirds of the tibia

Objectives

1. Describe medial tibial stress syndrome and identify potential risk factors that may result in this condition.
2. Provide appropriate patient education regarding MTSS.
3. Design and prescribe appropriate resistance exercises to treat MTSS.
4. Prescribe alternate aerobic activities aimed to improve fitness that minimize lower extremity loads and reduce the risk for further injury.
5. Discuss an appropriate plan for increasing activity and returning to impact activities while preventing a recurrence of the condition.

Physical Therapy Considerations

Physical therapy considerations during management of the individual with a diagnosis of medial tibial stress syndrome:

▶ **General physical therapy plan of care/goals:** Decrease pain; protect from injury progression; provide education regarding diagnosis and prognosis; increase muscular flexibility and lower extremity strength; minimize lower extremity deconditioning without interrupting healing; encourage low-impact aerobic conditioning to maintain or increase aerobic fitness; educate patient on training variables (frequency, intensity, type, duration) and recommended progression of exercise volume to reduce likelihood of further injury

▶ **Physical therapy interventions:** Patient education regarding functional anatomy and injury pathomechanics; modalities and manual therapy to decrease pain; musculotendinous and joint mobility/flexibility exercises; resistance exercises to increase lower extremity and core strength and muscular endurance; low-impact aerobic exercise program; gait retraining and biomechanical analysis; trial use of foot orthoses

▶ **Precautions during physical therapy:** Monitor shin pain in response to prescribed exercise program and reduce tissue loads if the patient experiences increased pain; address precautions or contraindications for exercise based on patient's pre-existing condition(s); monitor impact on individual's career, sport, or leisure activities in response to reduced activity; continue open line of communication with patient during period of care to ensure physical and psychological well-being

▶ **Complications interfering with physical therapy:** Unwillingness or inability of patient/client to alter training regimen; work schedule; comorbidities (e.g., connective tissue disorders, nutritional status, overall health status)

Understanding the Health Condition

Medial tibial pain accounts for 13% to 19% of all running injuries[1-4] and stress injuries account for 15% to 20% of all musculoskeletal running injuries.[5,6] The term "shin splints" is often used in the literature and by patients and medical professionals to describe exercise-related leg pain. Although frequently used in reference to MTSS, shin splints is a nonspecific diagnosis and physical therapists should utilize more appropriate terminology in the differential diagnosis of patients with leg pain. While a diagnosis of MTSS can be reliably made based on a sound clinical examination, concurrent lower leg pathology has been reported in up to a third of cases.[6-8] In 15% of cases, MTSS has been reported to occur in conjunction with posterior exertional compartment syndrome. Differential diagnoses for medial tibial pain includes: tibial bone stress injury (including tibial stress fracture, covered in Case 29), chronic periostalgia secondary to tension between muscle and fascia attachments to the periosteum, exertional compartment syndrome, tendinopathy, periostitis, muscle hernia, intermittent claudication, venous insufficiency, chronic deep posterior compartment syndrome, infection, peripheral neuropathy, lumbosacral radiculopathy, and neoplasm.[9-11]

Pertinent anatomy associated with MTSS includes muscles, vasculature, and nerves within the leg that are contained within four compartments (Fig. 30-1): anterior (tibialis anterior, extensor digitorum longus, extensor hallucis longus, fibularis tertius, anterior tibial artery and vein, deep fibular nerve), lateral (fibularis longus, fibularis brevis, perforating branches of the anterior tibial artery and fibular artery and vein, superficial fibular nerve), superficial posterior (gastrocnemius, soleus, plantaris, popliteal and sural arteries, popliteal, soleal and gastrocnemial veins, tibial nerve), and deep posterior (popliteus, tibialis posterior, flexor digitorum longus, flexor hallucis longus, posterior tibial artery and vein, tibial nerve). The borders of each compartment are defined by varying proportions of fascia, soft tissue, and bone. Some compartments are less compliant and unable to tolerate an increase in size (whether due to muscle hypertrophy or edema), which may result in increased intra-compartmental pressures.

The etiology of MTSS is most often attributed to bone stress injury, although there is some evidence that the condition may result from fascial traction—but not inflammation—of the periosteum.[12-15] MTSS represents the early stages in the continuum of bone stress injury.[16] Normally, when the tibia is exposed to higher

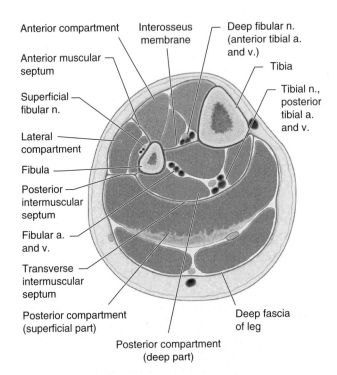

Anterior compartment   Interosseus membrane   Deep fibular n. (anterior tibial a. and v.)

Anterior muscular septum

Tibia

Superficial fibular n.

Tibial n., posterior tibial a. and v.

Lateral compartment

Fibula

Posterior intermuscular septum

Fibular a. and v.

Transverse intermuscular septum

Posterior compartment (superficial part)

Deep fascia of leg

Posterior compartment (deep part)

Figure 30-1. Cross-section of the right leg. (Reproduced with permission from Morton DA, Foreman KB, Albertine KH, eds. *The Big Picture: Gross Anatomy.* 2nd Ed. New York: McGraw-Hill; 2019.)

loads, osteoclastic activity (bone resorption) produces channeling within the tibia that can be more pronounced on the concave (compressive) side of the postero-medial aspect of the tibia. Next, osteoblastic activity (bone formation) produces periosteal thickening, which results in stronger bone that is able to tolerate the increased loads. However, if the activity of osteoclasts outpaces that of osteoblasts during bone remodeling, tunnels are produced within the bone, causing structural weakness that may result in pain with repeated loading. If repetitive high-impact loading is continued, the healing process is further interrupted and microfracture lines can propagate across the bone—resulting in a stress fracture. Bone biopsies have shown osseous metabolic changes with inflammatory changes at periosteal attachments (tendinous and deep crural fascia connections to the bone).[17]

Individuals with MTSS have reduced bone mineral density and altered tibial bone structure.[18] In individuals without MTSS, plain radiographs demonstrate clear, consistent tibial cortical thickness (Fig. 30-2A). In contrast, radiographs from patients with nonacute MTSS may show thickening of the posteromedial tibial cortex in response to osteoblastic activity (Fig. 30-2B).[19] In 18 adult male athletes with longstanding MTSS, Magnusson *et al.*[20] noted that the posteromedial tibial border was 15% more porous than nonathletic control subjects and 23% more porous than athletic controls. These results indicate that despite thickening of the cortex, MTSS is associated with areas of low bone mineral density. A technetium bone scan in a patient with MTSS demonstrates vertically oriented *diffuse* uptake along the posteromedial tibia (Fig. 30-3), indicating increased bone metabolism in this region. This pattern is distinct from the *localized* uptake in the patient with a tibial stress fracture (Fig. 29-1).

While the pathoanatomy underlying MTSS remains a source of discussion, there is growing agreement regarding the pathomechanics. One plausible cause is tibial bending resulting from recurrent impact loading that causes compression of the tibia posteromedially and tension anteriorly. Another potential cause is traction produced by muscular and fascial insertions along the posteromedial tibia. Stickley et al.[15] proposed that a traction-induced injury results from the pull of the deep crural fascia, and not from the muscles of the deep and superficial posterior compartments. In contrast, Bouche and Johnson[21] reported that tension produced by the deep posterior compartment muscles on the distal tibial fascia increases the tension on the medial tibia crest. Additional authors attribute MTSS symptoms to a short tibialis posterior tendon or traction from the soleus and/or flexor digitorum longus on the tibia, which corresponds to the typical area of tenderness.[22-25] Stress

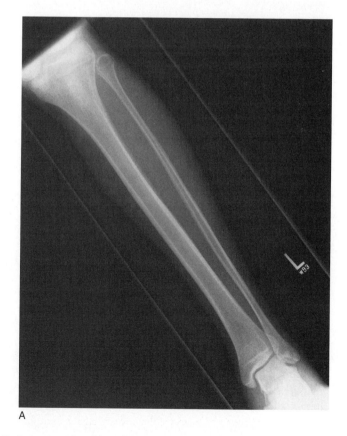

A

Figure 30-2. Anteroposterior plain radiographs of: **A**, leg of a patient without a history of MTSS. Note the clear, consistent periosteal thickness in the medial tibial metaphysis.

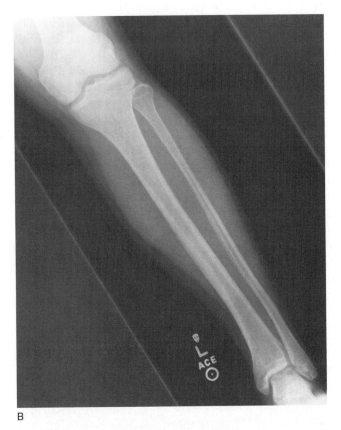

B

Figure 30-2. *(Continued)* **B**, leg of a patient with MTSS. Note region of periosteal thickening in the mid-distal third of the medial tibia.

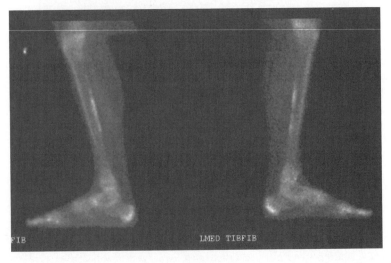

Figure 30-3. Bone scan showing vertically oriented, nonfocal, radioisotope uptake consistent with the diagnosis of MTSS.

to the tibia may also increase when muscles fatigue with running, which reduces muscular shock absorption and produces faulty biomechanics that increase load to the tibia.[4,20,26-29] Regardless of the cause or causes of MTSS, relative rest allows the body to restore balance and heal appropriately.

The primary symptom associated with MTSS is diffuse pain along the postero-medial border of the tibia, most commonly affecting the mid to distal thirds of the tibia.[30-32] Diffuse pain over an area greater than 5 cm is indicative of MTSS, while a smaller region of 2 to 3 cm of localized tenderness potentially accompanied by swelling is more indicative of tibial stress fracture.[32,33] Initial symptoms are typically mild and resolve with periods of nonweightbearing (*e.g.*, sitting or sleep). If the aggravating activity is continued, the symptoms tend to worsen and activity limitations develop due to pain. If the individual is not involved in an organized sport or lacks a specific training goal, they will typically refrain from further training, which allows the pain to resolve over time. With continued training, the condition typically worsens with pain that becomes more frequent, with earlier onset, interrupts the ability to train, and remains for longer durations after cessation of activity. In many cases, patients experience pain with prolonged standing. Less commonly, pain occurs in prolonged nonweightbearing positions.

Numerous intrinsic and extrinsic risk factors have been proposed to contribute to the development of MTSS. Although much of the available research is retrospective in nature, MTSS is likely the result of a combination of these factors. **Extrinsic factors** reported to increase the likelihood of developing MTSS include: rapid increase in weekly training (increasing intensity appears more important than increasing frequency and distance), insufficient footwear, running history of <5 years, previous history of MTSS or stress fracture, and use of orthotics.[16,34-37] Proposed intrinsic risk factors include: sex (greater risk in women), high body mass index, increased dynamic foot pronation and medial loading duration, female athlete triad, nutritional deficiencies, increased hip internal and external rotation range of motion, muscle strength and endurance deficits at the hip and lower leg, and decreased step rate while running.[16,25-31,34-40]

Physical Therapy Patient/Client Management

The physical therapist may be the first medical professional sought out by a patient for evaluation and treatment of exertional leg pain. Patients may also be referred by other healthcare professionals who commonly evaluate patients with musculoskeletal conditions. If referred to the physical therapist, it is not uncommon for the patient to present with a nonspecific diagnosis of "leg pain" or "shin splints." Patients may have had imaging studies such as radiographs, magnetic resonance imaging (MRI), and/or bone scans prior to referral, but the therapist may not have available resources for reviewing the images or have access to the radiology report. When presenting to physical therapy, the athlete is often seeking immediate relief of symptoms with the ability to continue pain-free high-impact activities. The physical therapist must perform a thorough subjective and objective examination and must have a clear understanding of the athlete's training regimen to provide appropriate education on training variables and progressive return to high-impact activities. The primary goal for most injured individuals is to maintain the greatest level of fitness possible while returning to pain-free sport or activity as quickly and as safely as possible. A systematic loading program should be utilized to provide appropriate stress to systems (*e.g.*, cardiovascular) and tissues (*e.g.*, musculoskeletal) throughout the healing process.

Examination, Evaluation, and Diagnosis

Individuals presenting with symptoms consistent with MTSS are likely involved in high-impact activities and have had a recent and rapid increase in training. Individuals frequently report diffuse posteromedial shin pain in one or both legs after performing high-impact activities. Typically, pain progresses in the following manner: pain after exercise that resolves with rest; pain during exercise that is reduced with continued training but returns after activity and resolves slowly with rest; pain that continues during and interrupts daily activities and curtails training.

A thorough history often enables the physical therapist to develop a reasonable differential diagnosis prior to initiating the physical examination. If the patient reports a prior history of similar symptoms, it is imperative that the physical therapist learn whether they sought out medical attention, what type of medical providers were seen, whether there was an established diagnosis, and the results of any previous imaging studies. Patient questioning includes easing/aggravating factors and status of symptoms (improving, worsening, or static). In particular, the physical therapist should ask specific questions about the patient's training routine including frequency, intensity, distance, type of training (sprints, hills), types of running surfaces, running shoe type (including any recent change), age of running shoes, and which positions or activities reproduce pain during daily activity. Additional questions should include information related to dietary intake and habits and frequency of menstrual cycle (for women). The therapist should explore what is motivating the individual to perform the exercise program (*e.g.*, training required for job qualification or training, sport, or leisure/health).

Patients presenting with suspicion of MTSS are likely to report a recent history of increased running volume. However, given the spectrum of bone stress injury, it may be difficult to base the diagnosis purely on a clinical examination. Furthermore, the physical therapist must remember that it is possible to have a concomitant condition. Early symptoms of MTSS may be similar to that of tibial stress fracture (Case 29). A key physical examination finding that helps distinguish MTSS from tibial stress fracture is *diffuse* tenderness of 5 cm or greater.[25,32] Although many special tests have been reported to assist in the clinical diagnosis of MTSS and tibial stress fracture, none has consistently shown high diagnostic value.

If the individual is adherent to the prescribed conservative management program but is not experiencing decreased tibial pain after 3 to 4 weeks, radiographic examination should be considered. If the patient experiences an *increase* in pain despite treatment adherence, the therapist should consider referral for radiographs even earlier. However, radiographs are typically of minimal benefit because they usually do not begin to demonstrate abnormalities for 14 to 21 days. In some cases, x-rays remain normal.[19,41] Although the most common abnormal finding on radiographs consistent with MTSS is periosteal thickening,[20] this is a nonspecific finding often present in individuals with an extensive physical training background. As a result, technetium bone scan, computed tomography, and MRI are used to improve sensitivity and specificity in diagnosing the etiology of tibial pain.[42-44] Findings on MRI may yield prognostic information to help inform return to high-level activities.[45]

Plan of Care and Interventions

Few intervention studies are available to guide therapists in evidence-based choices to accelerate recovery from MTSS. There have been only four randomized controlled trials (three conducted in military populations) for the treatment of MTSS.[14,46] Physical therapy interventions must be directed at the etiology of the painful overuse syndrome, which most commonly involves an overly aggressive training progression. Relative rest is agreed upon as equal to, if not better than, other treatment options for MTSS. Relative rest means reducing cyclic loading of the tibias and soft tissues especially during weightbearing. Aquatic therapy, cycling, rowing, gravity-reduced walking/jogging (*e.g.*, harness supported treadmill activity or anti-gravity treadmills), and elliptical trainers may be incorporated to promote physical conditioning during this period of relative rest as long as the patient adheres to *pain-free* activity. Occasionally, assistive devices (*e.g.*, axillary crutches) may be required to reduce the load sufficiently to ensure ambulation is pain-free. Before returning to running, the patient should be able to walk during daily activities pain-free and with full weightbearing.[47] Without appropriate rest, the condition typically progresses in severity.

Ice is helpful in reducing MTSS-related pain.[48,49] Nonsteroidal anti-inflammatory drugs (NSAIDs) may also be taken to provide pain relief.[50] However, taking NSAIDs to decrease pain and allow increased tolerance for excessive daily activity or exercise may delay restoration of tissue homeostasis, result in injury progression, and extend symptom duration.[47,51] During the period of relative rest, the individual should experience a gradual reduction in pain in conjunction with some increase in functional ability. The presence of pain during, after, or the day after activity indicates that the injured bone needs to have a reduced load. If the individual is unable to demonstrate a normal gait pattern or has pain with daily walking, the therapist should prescribe an assistive device to employ appropriate partial weightbearing to relieve pain. Once the individual has progressed to pain-free unassisted daily activities for 5 to 7 consecutive days, a progressive walk-run program at a low pace and intensity can be initiated.[47,52] If pain increases, function decreases, or the patient experiences a lack of improvement, the therapist should re-assess daily activity and adjust appropriately.

Although there is a documented association between the use of orthotics and an increased risk of MTSS, orthotics have been shown to help reduce symptoms associated with MTSS.[53-55] The response to orthotics is dependent on the individual patient, ranging from immediate relief to improvement over days to weeks. While shoe selection based on foot type has been long advocated, evidence suggests no significant effect of shoe selection on preventing leg injuries in military populations.[56] Stretching of the posterior leg muscles (*e.g.*, gastrocnemius-soleus, posterior tibialis) has been advocated primarily based on the fact that the muscular insertions are in the region of pain associated with MTSS.[15,21,24] In a prospective study of 23 adults with symptoms of MTSS, Loudon and Dolphino[57] found that 65% of the subjects had a 50% reduction in pain at the end of a 3-week intervention of calf stretches and use of off-the-shelf shoe inserts. Because the study design did not isolate stretching as an independent intervention and did not include a comparison or control group, these results only support calf stretching as a component of the treatment of MTSS. This should be noted especially because limited passive ankle dorsiflexion has not consistently been found to be a risk factor for MTSS.[35-37] Of interest, runners with a higher step rate (cadence) have a reduced incidence of MTSS compared to those with a lower step rate.[4,28] Thus, the therapist may consider running re-training with an emphasis on increasing the step rate (i.e., shortening step length) as another intervention that may facilitate return to pain-free running. Last, the therapist must be aware of interventions that are not well supported to treat MTSS. Ultrasound, phonophoresis, cortisone injections, bone electrical stimulators, extracorporeal shock wave therapy, and acupuncture have not demonstrated consistent benefit in treating exercise-induced leg pain, including MTSS.[58-61]

If the condition fails to improve after 4 weeks of physical therapy interventions, we recommend that the patient be referred to another healthcare provider that specializes in musculoskeletal injuries (such as an orthopedic surgeon) for additional evaluation and to ensure that no other condition is responsible for the patient's symptoms. In recalcitrant cases of MTSS, patients have reported up to 78% improvement after fasciotomy of the superficial and deep posterior compartments.[61-63] Surgery involving cauterization of the periosteum of the tibia had a 90% success rate at 6-month follow-up.[9] Surgical intervention may act to denervate the periosteum.[64] Although significant improvement in pain has been reported following these types of surgery, the rate of return to presymptomatic levels of activity has been reported at <50%.[65]

Evidence-Based Clinical Recommendations

SORT: Strength of Recommendation Taxonomy

A: Consistent, good-quality patient-oriented evidence
B: Inconsistent or limited-quality patient-oriented evidence
C: Consensus, disease-oriented evidence, usual practice, expert opinion, or case series

1. Extrinsic risk factors are associated with development of MTSS. **Grade C**

2. Intrinsic risk factors are associated with development of MTSS. **Grade B**

3. Interventions such as ice and stretching are associated with better patient outcomes than relative rest in the management of MTSS. **Grade C**

COMPREHENSION QUESTIONS

30.1 What intrinsic risk factor for medial tibial stress syndrome (MTSS) is MOST consistently supported in the literature?

A. Higher BMI

B. Increased Q-angle

C. Limited ankle dorsiflexion range of motion

D. Limited hip internal rotation range of motion

30.2 What treatment approach has been demonstrated to be MOST effective in the management of MTSS?

A. Acupuncture

B. Laser treatment

C. Relative rest

D. Phonophoresis

30.3 What is the key clinical examination finding that suggests the presence of MTSS?

A. Diffuse tenderness to palpation of ≥5 cm along the posteromedial border of the tibia

B. Focal tenderness to palpation of approximately 2.5 cm along the posteromedial border of the tibia.

C. Symptom reproduction with repeated single-leg heel raises

D. Symptom reproduction with single-leg vertical jump

ANSWERS

30.1 **A.** From the options provided, higher BMI is the most agreed upon intrinsic risk factor for the development of MTSS.[35,36]

30.2 **C.** There is a lack of intervention studies to guide the management of MTSS. There have been four randomized controlled trials on the treatment of MTSS. Relative rest is agreed upon as equal to, if not better than, other treatment options.[46,48]

30.3 **A.** Diffuse tenderness to palpation is the key finding which differentiates the likelihood of an individual having MTSS versus a stress fracture which would be likely to have more focal (2.5 cm region) of tenderness.[31]

REFERENCES

1. Taunton JE, Clement DB, Webber D. Lower extremity stress fractures in athletes. *Phys Sportsmed.* 1981;9:77-86.

2. Clement DB, Taunton JE, Smart GW, McNicol KL. Survey of overuse running injuries. *Phys Sportsmed.* 1981;9:47-58.

3. Epperly T, Fields K. Epidemiology of running injuries. In: O'Conner FG, Wilder R, Nirschl R, eds. *Textbook of Running Medicine.* New York, NY:McGraw-Hill; 2001:1-11.

4. Luedke LE, Heiderscheit BC, Williams DSB, Rauh MJ. Influence of step rate on shin injury and anterior knee pain in high school runners. *Med Sci Sports Exerc.* 2016;48:1244-1250.

5. Bennell KL, Malcolm SA, Thomas SA, et al. The incidence and distribution of stress fractures in competitive track and field athletes. A twelve-month prospective study. *Am J Sports Med.* 1996; 24:211-217.

6. Brubaker CE, James SL. Injuries to runners. *J Sports Med.* 1974;2:189-198.

7. Styf J. Diagnosis of exercise-induced pain in the anterior aspect of the lower leg. *Am J Sports Med.* 1988;16:165-169.

8. Winters M, Bakker EWP, Moen MH, et al. Medial tibial stress syndrome can be diagnosed reliably using history and physical examination. *Br J Sports Med.* 2018;52:1-6.

9. Detmer DE. Chronic shin splints: classification and management of medial tibial stress syndrome. *Sports Med.* 1986;3:436-446.

10. Chambers HG. Medial tibial stress syndrome: evaluation and management. *Oper Techniq Sports Med.* 1995;3:274-277.

11. Edwards PH Jr, Wright ML, Hartman JF. A practical approach for the differential diagnosis of chronic leg pain in the athlete. *Am J Sports Med.* 2005;33:1241-1249.

12. Tweed JL, Avil SJ, Campbell JA, Barnes MR. Etiologic factors in the development of medial tibial stress syndrome: a review of the literature. *J Am Podiatr Med Assoc.* 2008;98:107-111.

13. Craig DI. Current developments concerning medial tibial stress syndrome. *Phys Sportsmed.* 2009;37:39-44.

14. Moen MH, Tol JL, Weir A, et al. Medial tibial stress syndrome: a critical review. *Sports Med.* 2009;39:523-546.

15. Stickley CD, Hetzler RK, Kimura IF, Lozanoff S. Crural fascia and muscle origins related to medial tibial stress syndrome symptom location. *Med Sci Sports Exec.* 2009;41:1991-1996.

16. Brukner P, Bennell K, Matheson G. *Stress Fractures.* Victoria, Australia: Blackwell Science Asia;1999.

17. Johnell O, Rausing A, Wendeberg M, Westlin N. Morphological bone changes in shin splints. *Clin Orthop Relat Res.* 1982;167:180-184.

18. Franklyn M, Oakes B. Aetiology and mechanisms of injury in medial tibial stress syndrome: Current and future developments. *World J Orthop.* 2015;6:577-589.

19. Deutsch AL, Coel MN, Mink JH. Imaging of stress injuries to bone. Radiography, scintigraphy and MR imaging. *Clin Sports Med.* 1997;16:275-290.

20. Magnusson HI, Westlin NE, Nyqvist F, et al. Abnormally decreased regional bone density in athletes with medial tibial stress syndrome. *Am J Sports Med.* 2001;29:712-715.

21. Bouche RT, Johnson CH. Medial tibial stress syndrome (tibial fasciitis): a proposed pathomechanical model involving fascial traction. *J Am Podiatr Med Assoc.* 2007;97:31-36.

22. Saxena A, O'Brien T, Bunce D. Anatomic dissection of the tibialis posterior muscle and its correlation to medial tibial stress syndrome. *J Foot Surg.* 1990;29:105-108.

23. Michael RH, Holder LE. The soleus syndrome. A cause of medial tibial stress (shin splints). *Am J Sports Med.* 1985;13:87-94.

24. Beck BR, Osternig LR. Medial tibial stress syndrome. The location of muscles in the leg and relation to symptoms. *J Bone Joint Surg Am.* 1994;76:1057-1061.

25. Naderi A, Moen MH, Degens H. Is high soleus muscle activity during the stance phase of the running cycle a potential risk factor for the development of medial tibial stress syndrome? A prospective study. *J Sport Sci.* 2020;38:2350-2358.

26. Huang Y, Xia H, Chen G, et al. Foot strike pattern, step rate, and trunk posture combined gait modification to reduce impact loading during running. *J Biomech.* 2019;86:102-109.

27. Becker J, James S, Wayner R, et al. Biomechanical factors associated with Achilles tendinopathy and medial tibial stress syndrome in runners. *Am J Sports Med.* 2017;45:2614-2621.

28. Kliethermes KA, Stiffler-Joachim MR, Wille CM, et al. Lower step rate is associated with a higher risk of bone stress injury: a prospective study of collegiate cross country runners. *Br J Sports Med.* 2021;55:851-856.

29. Hollander K, Johnson CD, Outerleys J, Davis IS. Multifactorial determinants of running injury locations in 550 injured recreational runners. *Med Sci Sports Exerc.* 2021;53:102-107.

30. Yates B, White S. The incidence and risk factors in the development of medial tibial stress syndrome among naval recruits. *Am J Sports Med.* 2004;32:772-780.

31. Bennett JE, Reinking MF, Pluemer B, et al. Factors contributing to the development of medial tibial stress syndrome in high school runners. *J Orthop Sports Phys Ther.* 2001;31:504-510.

32. Batt ME, Ugalde V, Anderson MW, Shelton DK. A prospective controlled study of diagnostic imaging for acute shin splints. *Med Sci Sports Exerc.* 1998;30:1564-1571.

33. Anderson MW, Ugalde V, Batt M, Gacayan J. Shin splints: MR appearance in a preliminary study. *Radiology.* 1997;204:177-180.

34. Burne SG, Khan KM, Boudville PB, et al. Risk factors associated with exertional medial tibial pain: a 12-month prospective clinical study. *Br J Sports Med.* 2004;38:441-445.

35. Moen MH. Bongers T, Bakker EW, et al. Risk factors and prognostic indicators for medial tibial stress syndrome. *Scan J Med Sci Sports.* 2012;22:34-39.

36. Hamstra-Wright KL, Huxel Bliven KC, Bay C. Risk factors for medial tibial stress syndrome in physically active individuals such as runners and military personnel: a systematic review and meta-analysis. *Br J Sports Med.* 2015;49:362-369.

37. Winkelmann ZK, Anderson D, Games KE, Eberman L. Risk factors for medial tibial stress syndrome in active individuals: an evidence-based review. *J Athl Train.* 2016;51:1049-1052.

38. Lauder TD, Williams MV, Campbell CS, et al. The female athlete triad: prevalence in military women. *Mil Med.* 1999;164:630-635.

39. Yagi S, Muneta T, Sekiya I. Incidence and risk factors for medial tibial stress syndrome and tibial stress fracture in high school runners. *Knee Surg Sports Traumatol Arthrosc.* 2013;21:556-563.

40. Mattock J, Steele JR, Mickle K. Lower leg muscle structure and function are altered in long-distance runners with medial tibial stress syndrome: a case control study. *J Foot Ankle Res.* 2021;14:47.

41. Savoca CJ. Stress fractures. A classification of the earliest radiographic signs. *Radiol.* 1971;100:519-524.

42. Fredericson M, Bergman AG, Hoffman KL, Dillingham MS. Tibial stress reactions in runners. Correlation of clinical symptoms and scintigraphy with a new magnetic resonance imaging grading system. *Am J Sports Med.* 1995;23:472-481.

43. Gaeta M, Minutoli F, Vinci S, et al. High-resolution CT grading of tibial stress reactions in distance runners. *AJR Am J Roentgenol.* 2006;187:789-793.

44. Bencardino JT, Stone TJ, Roberts CC, et al. ACR Appropriateness Criteria Stress (Fatigue/Insufficiency) Fracture, Including Sacrum, Excluding Other Vertebrae. *J Am Coll Radiol.* 2017;14:S293-S306.

45. Moen MH, Schmikli SL, Weir A, et al. A prospective study on MRI findings and prognostic factors in athletes with MTSS. *Scand J Med Sci Sports.* 2014;24:204-210.

46. Moen MH, Holtslag L, Bakker E, et al. The treatment of medial tibial stress syndrome in athletes; a randomized clinical trial. *Sports Med Arthrosc Rehabil Ther Technol.* 2012;4:12.

47. Warden SJ, Edwards WB, Willy RW. Optimal load for managing low-risk tibial and metatarsal bone stress injuries in runners: the science behind the clinical reasoning. *J Orthop Sports Phys Ther*. 2021;51:322-330.

48. Andrish JT, Bergfeld JA, Walheim J. A prospective study of the management of shin splints. *J Bone Joint Surg Am*. 1974;56:1697-1700.

49. Winters M, Eskes M, Weir A, et al. Treatment of medial tibial stress syndrome: a systematic review. *Sports Med*. 2013;43:1315-1333.

50. Couture CJ, Karlson KA. Tibial stress injuries; decisive diagnosis and treatment of 'shin splints'. *Phys Sportsmed*. 2002;30:29-36.

51. Warden SJ, Thompson WR. Becoming one with the force: optimising mechanotherapy through an understanding of mechanobiology. *Br J Sports Med*. 2017;51:989-990.

52. Warden SJ, Davis IS, Fredericson M. Management and prevention of bone stress injuries in long-distance runners. *J Orthop Sports Phys Ther*. 2014;44(10):749-765.

53. Schwellnus MP, Jordaan G, Noakes TD. Prevention of common overuse injuries by the use of shock absorbing insoles. A prospective study. *Am J Sports Med*. 1990;18:636-641.

54. Hubbard TJ, Carpenter EM, Cordova ML. Contributing factors to medial tibial stress syndrome: a prospective investigation. *Med Sci Sports Exerc*. 2009;41:490-496.

55. Eickhoff CA, Hossain SA, Slawski DP. From the field. Effects of prescribed foot orthoses on medial tibial stress syndrome in collegiate cross-country runners. *Clin Kinesiol*. 2000;54:76-80.

56. Knapik JJ, Trone DW, Swedler DI, et al. Injury reduction effectiveness of assigning running shoes based on plantar shape in marine corps basic training. *Am J Sports Med*. 2010;38:1759-1767.

57. Loudon JK. Dolphino MR. Use of foot orthoses and calf stretching for individuals with medial tibial stress syndrome. *Foot Ankle Spec*. 2010;3:15-20.

58. Beck BR. Tibial stress injuries. An aetiological review for the purposes of guiding management. *Sports Med*. 1998;26:265-279.

59. Morris RH. Medial tibial syndrome: a treatment protocol using electric current. *Chiropractic Sports Med*. 1991;5:5-8.

60. Schulman RA. Tibial shin splints treated with a single acupuncture session: case report and review of the literature. *J Am Med Acupuncture*. 2002;13:7-9.

61. Korakakis V, Whiteley R, Tzavara A, Malliaropoulos N. The effectiveness of extracorporeal shock-wave therapy in common lower limb conditions: a systematic review including quantification of patient rated pain reduction. *Br J Sports Med*. 2018;52:387-407.

62. Clanton TO, Solcher BW. Chronic leg pain in the athlete. *Clin Sports Med*. 1994;13:743-759.

63. Holen KJ, Engebretsen L, Grontvedt T, et al. Surgical treatment of medial tibial stress syndrome (shin splint) by fasciotomy of the superficial posterior compartment of the leg. *Scand J Med Sci Sports*. 1995;5:40-43.

64. Wallensten R. Results of fasciotomy in patients with medial tibial syndrome or chronic anterior-compartment syndrome. *J Bone Joint Surg Am*. 1983;65:1252-1255.

65. Yates B, Allen MJ, Barnes MR. Outcome of surgical treatment of medial tibial stress syndrome. *J Bone Joint Surg Am*. 2003;85-A:1974-1980.

DISCLAIMER

The views expressed in this chapter are those of the authors and do not necessarily reflect the official policy or position of the Department of the Navy, Department of Defense, or the U.S. Government.

Achilles Tendinosis

Tyler Cuddeford
Lyndsay Stutzenberger

CASE 31

A 30-year-old male was referred to an outpatient physical therapy clinic with a diagnosis of midportion Achilles tendinopathy on his right side. He has experienced a gradual increase in pain for 5 years. His worsening symptoms have limited his ability to run recreationally or play basketball or volleyball without pain. Previous therapies (nonsteroidal anti-inflammatory drugs eccentric exercises, manual therapy) have failed to improve symptoms. His orthopedist has recommended surgery. However, the patient would like to try physical therapy again.

▶ Based on the patient's diagnosis, what do you anticipate may be the contributing factors to his condition?
▶ What are the most appropriate physical therapy interventions?

KEY DEFINITIONS

ECCENTRIC EXERCISE: Form of exercise in which the muscle(s) are allowed to lengthen gradually in the presence of an applied load

MICRODIALYSIS: Laboratory technique in which a catheter is inserted into a tendon at the site of suspected degenerative changes to study metabolism within the tendon

NEOVASCULARIZATION: Growth of new blood vessels

TENDINOPATHY: General term for a diseased state of a tendon; tendinosis may be referred to as a chronic tendinopathy

TENDINOSIS: Chronic, painful degenerative condition of a tendon marked by *absence* of inflammation, a loss of function, and the presence of a thickened region (*i.e.*, a painful nodule)

Objectives

1. Describe the differences between tendinitis and tendinosis.
2. Describe the pathophysiology associated with midportion Achilles tendinopathy.
3. Prescribe an evidence-based resistance training program for an individual with midportion Achilles tendinopathy.

Physical Therapy Considerations

Physical therapy considerations during management of the individual with a diagnosis of Achilles tendinosis:

▶ **General physical therapy plan of care/goals:** Increase lower quadrant strength; decrease pain; increase muscular flexibility

▶ **Physical therapy interventions:** Resistance exercises to increase strength of the gastrocnemius and soleus; patient education regarding activity level; stretching exercises; aerobic exercise program

▶ **Precautions during physical therapy:** Monitor vital signs; presence of intrinsic risk factors (decreased ankle range of motion, decreased plantarflexion strength, increased foot pronation, abnormal tendon structure); presence of extrinsic risk factors (obesity, hypertension, hyperlipidemia, diabetes mellitus)

▶ **Complications interfering with physical therapy:** Nonadherence with exercise program

Understanding the Health Condition

The Achilles tendon is the distal extension of the gastrocnemius and soleus muscles and inserts into the calcaneus. The tendon is the strongest tendon in the human body. The capacity of the Achilles tendon to tolerate high loads during eccentric contractions is significant. Cuddeford et al.[1] demonstrated that normal subjects were able to perform a single-leg eccentric load of well over 200% of their body weight, highlighting the fact that rehabilitation programs may not adequately load the tendon for collagen remodeling to occur.

The Achilles tendon is at risk for acute injury (tendinitis), degeneration (tendinosis), and/or rupture.[2-4] Tendinosis is thought to be the result of overuse and age-related changes with a failure of proper tissue remodeling.[3,5] de Mos et al.[6] confirmed findings of increased water content, matrix degeneration, increased collagen turnover rate, high concentrations of denatured or damaged collagen, and increased enzymatic activity in a study of 10 adults undergoing surgery for Achilles tendinopathy. The pathogenesis of Achilles tendinopathy is multifactorial and related to the body's inability to adapt to increased stress. The condition affects novice, recreational, and elite runners, soccer players, rock climbers, badminton players, adventure racers, as well as many other moderately active and sedentary individuals.[4,7-14]

Tendinosis is distinct from acute tendon injury (tendinitis) because it is *not* associated with local chemically mediated inflammation.[15,16] Intratendinous microdialysis studies have investigated the metabolism within the tendonitic Achilles. Prostaglandins associated with chemical inflammation are *absent*, suggesting that if any swelling is present, it may be the result of neurogenic inflammation.[15,16] In fact, neuropeptides (substance P and calcitonin gene-related peptide) that may contribute to neurogenic inflammation have been identified in individuals with Achilles tendinosis.[16-18] In patients with Achilles tendinosis, neovascularization has been visualized (utilizing gray-scale ultrasonography and color Doppler techniques) primarily on the ventral side of the Achilles at the tendon's midportion (the region of the thickened painful nodule). Importantly, these blood vessels are *not* present in individuals without Achilles tendinosis.[19] The neovascularization in the region of the Achilles may occur in response to a hypoxic environment and/or increased glutamate concentrations. Accompanying the neovascularization are sensory and sympathetic nerves.[19-22]

Physical Therapy Patient/Client Management

The mainstay of conservative treatment continues to be eccentric exercises consisting of relatively low load and high repetitions.[5,16,23-24] Slow, heavy-load concentric exercise programs are also effective in decreasing pain and improving function.[25] The efficacy of interventions such as modalities, soft tissue mobilization, footwear evaluation and/or orthotics, taping, dry needling, and manual therapy are not sufficiently supported by evidence.[24] In the most recent clinical practice guidelines for Achilles tendinopathy, **evidence supports the efficacy of patient education directed toward active rest (*e.g.*, swimming, deep water running, or cycling) and activity modification.**[24] Sclerosing injections or surgery are invasive treatments performed by orthopedic physicians for patients who fail to improve with conservative management.[5,16]

Examination, Evaluation, and Diagnosis

A diagnosis of tendinosis is based on clinical examination findings and may be confirmed with imaging studies.[5,24] Diagnostic imaging techniques (ultrasonography, magnetic resonance imaging) or biopsy are used by physicians to confirm the diagnosis.[5] The patient with suspected or confirmed Achilles tendinosis typically reports pain, an inability to participate in sports without pain, and/or a loss of function. The Victorian Institute of Sport Assessment-Achilles (VISA-A) can be used to evaluate the clinical severity of the condition. Administration of this questionnaire can be used before and after treatment to assess changes in pain and stiffness and with time and treatment.[24] The patient may present with decreased strength and/or pain during manual muscle testing; therefore, a functional movement such as a heel raise on the involved side is also recommended.[24] An elite athlete may need to perform a single-legged vertical jump or hop to reproduce symptoms. Palpation of the tendon may reveal tenderness and a nodule usually at the mid-portion of the tendon (2-6 cm proximal to the insertion site). To help rule out an Achilles tendon rupture, the physical therapist should confirm that the patient has a negative Thompson test (*i.e.*, with an intact Achilles tendon, the non-weightbearing, involved ankle should passively plantarflex when the therapist squeezes the calf).

Plan of Care and Interventions

The **primary intervention for Achilles tendinosis is heavy loading with eccentric or concentric exercises.** The majority of research has focused on exercise for *midportion* Achilles tendinopathy. Modalities, orthotics, low level laser therapy, and manual therapy techniques are not recommended interventions.[24]

Several investigators have found that 10- to 12-week eccentric exercise programs for the gastrocnemius and the soleus significantly decreased pain and increased calf strength in recreational adult runners with Achilles tendinosis.[1,23,24,26] In the study by Alfredson *et al.*[26], 30 recreational athletes who had failed to improve with prior bouts of physical therapy and other conservative treatments were either in the experimental group (mean age 44.3 ± 7.0 years) or the control group (mean age 39.6 ± 7.9 years). Only two exercises were prescribed for the experimental group; each was performed twice daily with 3 sets of 15 repetitions. To perform each exercise, the patient first assumes an upright posture with forefeet supported on a step or stair. Next, the patient elevates his body by plantarflexing *both* ankles (Fig. 31-1A). Next, the patient shifts his weight to load the injured lower extremity. Finally, the patient performs the eccentric component of the exercise by lowering the heel of his *symptomatic* limb below the plane of the step (Fig. 31-1B). Subjects were instructed to complete all repetitions even in the presence of pain. Once each subject was able to perform the exercises without pain, they were instructed to perform the exercises with a weighted backpack or to perform the exercises with a standing calf machine or weighted sled. At the end of the 12-week training period, all individuals in the experimental group were able to return to preinjury training levels, whereas those in the control group (who did not receive any treatment) elected to have surgery and took an average of 24 weeks to return to running after surgery.[26]

In a randomized controlled trial comparing traditional loaded and unloaded eccentric exercises with slow and heavy concentric resistance exercises, Beyer *et al.*[25] demonstrated that there was no difference between the two modes of exercises at the end of the 12-week program or at the 52-week follow-up assessment. Figure 31-2 demonstrates the use of a leg-press machine to load the Achilles tendon.

Eccentric training programs appear to decrease (*i.e.*, normalize) tendon size.[27,28] The observed destruction of new blood vessels and associated nerves after an eccentric program may account for the decrease in pain experienced by patients. It is thought that the forces generated during the eccentric exercises destroy those structures.[5,29] Tendon adaptation also appears to require a precise load to change its properties.[30-33] Performing low load and high repetitions of ankle dorsiflexion

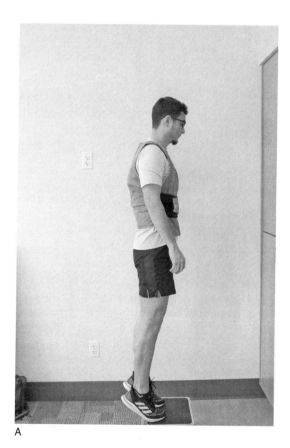

A

Figure 31-1. Loaded eccentric exercise (with use of weighted vest) emphasizing the gastrocnemius. **A.** Patient plantarflexes both ankles while standing on a stair or stool.

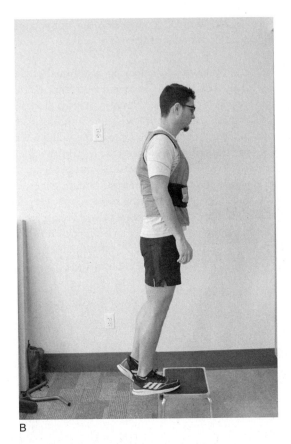

B

Figure 31-1. *(Continued)* **B.** Patient shifts weight to the involved right lower extremity and lowers his body by allowing dorsiflexion at the ankle, keeping the right knee in full extension.

and plantarflexion may not load the tendon *enough* to generate collagen synthesis for tendon remodeling. Similarly, collagen synthesis may be closely related to the nature of how the load is applied.[33-34] In a comparison study of high- and low-strain isometric plantarflexion exercise programs, Arampatzis *et al.*[33] found a strain threshold that triggers tendon adaptation. The heavier load exercises provided the necessary collagen adaptation to the plantarflexor group, whereas lower loads were insufficient to produce adequate tendon change.[33] Further, lower-load exercises used in this study were equivalent to daily activities, suggesting exercises that equate to body weight are *not* adequate for tendon remodeling. Tendons require extreme loads (80%-90% of maximum voluntary contraction) followed by rest to create positive changes in tendon thickness and stiffness.

Silbernagel *et al.*[35] used a four-phase exercise program for patients with Achilles tendinopathy. The first phase starts with concentric heel raises (single- and double-legged standing and sitting toe raises) and standing eccentric toe raises (eccentric loading of the involved ankle; similar to that described by Alfredson *et al.*[26]). Later stages include eccentric calf muscle training (with added weight) as described by

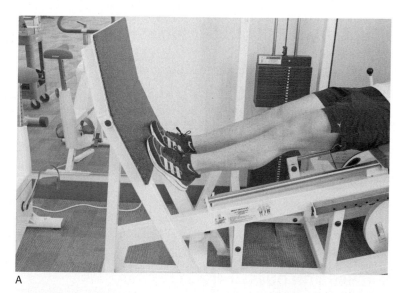

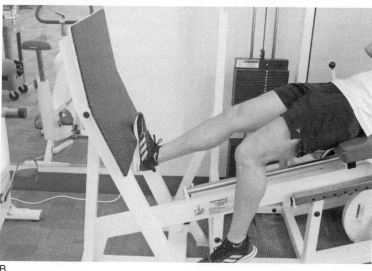

Figure 31-2. On a weighted sled or calf press, **A.** patient elevates body by plantarflexing both ankles. **B.** At the top of the motion (full plantarflexion), the patient shifts all his weight to the involved right leg, eccentrically lowering the weight by slowly dorsiflexing the ankle.

Alfredson *et al.*[26], double- and single-legged heel raises at the edge of a stair, quick-rebounding toe raises, and plyometrics.[35] Subjects experienced significant improvements in pain, power, and muscular endurance compared to baseline measures. At the 5-year follow-up, a majority of subjects had made a full recovery.[36] Future investigations are warranted to determine which of the aforementioned programs lead to the best patient outcomes.

Evidence-Based Clinical Recommendations

SORT: Strength of Recommendation Taxonomy

A: Consistent, good-quality patient-oriented evidence
B: Inconsistent or limited-quality patient-oriented evidence
C: Consensus, disease-oriented evidence, usual practice, expert opinion, or case series

1. Rehabilitation for individuals with Achilles tendinosis should include education that includes activity modification and advice for active rest (swimming, deep water running, and biking). **Grade A**

2. Exercise programs consisting of eccentric and/or concentric exercises for the gastrocnemius and soleus muscles help reduce pain and restore function in patients with *midportion* Achilles tendinosis. **Grade A**

COMPREHENSION QUESTIONS

31.1 The reduction of pain experienced by patients after completing a 12-week eccentric exercise program for midportion Achilles tendinosis is thought to be due to destruction of which of the following structures?

　　A. New blood vessels and associated nerves

　　B. Tendon sheath

　　C. Collagen fibers

　　D. Scar tissue

31.2 Which of the following statements is accurate when performing exercise interventions for midportion Achilles tendinosis?

　　A. The ankle should be allowed to dorsiflex to 10°.

　　B. The patient should not experience pain during exercise.

　　C. The exercises can either be concentric or eccentric.

　　D. The patient should only include eccentric exercises.

ANSWERS

31.1 **A.** Imaging studies performed after the completion of a training program have revealed a normalized tendon structure with a decrease in new blood vessels and associated nerves.

31.2 **C.** Alfredson et al.[5,26], Silbernagel et al.[23], and Beyer et al.[25] all demonstrated significant benefits from the various forms of eccentric and/or concentric exercise. Pain is allowed during the performance of these exercises.

REFERENCES

1. Cuddeford T, Houck J, Palmer D, et al. What maximum ankle torque is appropriate for training patients with non-insertional Achilles tendinopathy? *Orthop Phys Ther Pract.* 2018;30:543-547.

2. Mann RA, Chou L. Effective intervention for Achilles tendinitis and tendinosis: toe rise helps differentiate tendinitis from tendinosis. *J Musculoskeletal Med.* 1998;15:57-62.

3. Heckman DS, Gluck GS, Parekh SG. Tendon disorders of the foot and ankle, part 2: Achilles tendon disorders. *Am J Sports Med.* 2009;37:1223-1234.

4. Schepsis AA, Jones H, Haas AL. Achilles tendon disorders in athletes. *Am J Sports Med.* 2002;30:287-305.

5. Alfredson H. The chronic painful Achilles and patellar tendon: research on basic biology and treatment. *Scand J Med Sci Sports.* 2005;15:252-259.

6. de Mos M, van El B, DeGroot J, et al. Achilles tendinosis: changes in biochemical composition and collagen turnover rate. *Am J Sports Med.* 2007;35:1549-1556.

7. Magnussen RA, Dunn WR, Thomson AB. Nonoperative treatment of midportion Achilles tendinopathy: a systematic review. *Clin J Sport Med.* 2009;19:54-64.

8. Kujala UM, Sarna S, Kaprio J. Cumulative incidence of Achilles tendon rupture and tendinopathy in male former elite athletes. *Clin J Sport Med.* 2005;15:133-135.

9. Gajhede-Knudsen M, Ekstrand J, Magnusson H, Maffulli N. Recurrence of Achilles tendon injuries in elite male football players is more common after early return to play: an 11-year follow-up of the UEFA Champions League injury study. *Br J Sports Med.* 2013;47:763-768.

10. Nielsenx RO, Rønnow L, Rasmussen S, Lind M. A prospective study on time to recovery in 254 injured novice runners. *PLoS One.* 2014;9:e99877.

11. Buda R, Di Caprio F, Bedetti L, et al. Foot overuse diseases in rock climbing: an epidemiologic study. *J Am Podiatr Med Assoc.* 2013;103:113-120.

12. Paavola M, Kannus P, Paakkala T, et al. Long-term prognosis of patients with Achilles tendinopathy. An observational 8-year follow-up study. *Am J Sports Med.* 2000;28:634-642.

13. Sobhani S, Dekker R, Postema K, Dijkstra PU. Epidemiology of ankle and foot overuse injuries in sports: a systematic review. *Scand J Med Sci Sports.* 2013;23:669-686.

14. Astrom M. Partial rupture in chronic Achilles tendinopathy. A retrospective analysis of 342 cases. *Acta Orthop Scand.* 1998;69:404-407.

15. Alfredson H, Lorentzon M, Backman S, et al. cDNA-arrays and real-time quantitative PCR techniques in the investigation of chronic Achilles tendinosis. *J Orthop Res.* 2003;21:970-975.

16. Alfredson H, Cook J. A treatment algorithm for managing Achilles tendinopathy: new treatment options. *Br J Sports Med.* 2007;41:211-216.

17. Scott A, Khan KM, Roberts CR, et al. What do we mean by the term "inflammation"? A contemporary basic science update for sports medicine. *Br J Sports Med.* 2004;38:372-380.

18. Andersson G, Danielson P, Alfredson H, Forsgren S. Presence of substance P and the neurokinin-1 receptor in tenocytes of the human Achilles tendon. *Regul Pept.* 2008;150:81-87.

19. Ohberg L, Lorentzon R, Alfredson H. Neovascularization in Achilles tendons with painful tendinosis but not in normal tendons: an ultrasonographic investigation. *Knee Surg Sports Traumatol Arthrosc.* 2001;9:233-238.

20. Alfredson H, Ohberg L, Forsgren S. Is vasculo-neural ingrowth the cause of pain in chronic Achilles tendinosis? An investigation using ultrasonography and colour Doppler, immunohistochemistry, and diagnostic injections. *Knee Surg Sports Traumatol Arthrosc.* 2003;11:334-338.

21. Andersson G, Danielson P, Alfredson H, Forsgren S. Nerve-related characteristics of ventral paratendinous tissue in chronic Achilles tendinosis. *Knee Surg Sports Traumatol Arthrosc.* 2007;15:1272-1279.

22. Bjur D, Alfredson H, Forsgren S. The innervation pattern of the human Achilles tendon: studies of the normal and tendinosis tendon with markers for general and sensory innervation. *Cell Tissue Res.* 2005;320:201-206.

23. Silbernagel KG, Brorsson A, Lundberg M. The majority of patients with Achilles tendinopathy recover fully when treated with exercise alone: a 5-year follow-up. *Am J Sports Med.* 2011;39:607-613.

24. Martin R, Chimenti R, Cuddeford T, et al. Achilles pain, stiffness, and muscle power deficits: mid-portion Achilles tendinopathy revision 2018. *J Orthop Sports Phys Ther.* 2018;48:A1-A38.

25. Beyer R, Kongsgaard M, Hougs Kjaer B, et al. Heavy slow resistance versus eccentric training as treatment for Achilles tendinopathy: a randomized controlled trial. *Am J Sports Med.* 2015;43:1704-1711.

26. Alfredson H, Pietila T, Jonsson P, Lorentzon R. Heavy-load eccentric calf muscle training for the treatment of chronic Achilles tendinosis. *Am J Sports Med.* 1998;26:360-366.

27. Gardin A, Movin T, Svensson L, Shalabi A. The long-term clinical and MRI results following eccentric calf muscle training in chronic Achilles tendinosis. *Skeletal Radiol.* 2010;39:435-442.

28. Shalabi A, Kristoffersen-Wilberg M, Svensson L, et al. Eccentric training of the gastrocnemius-soleus complex in chronic Achilles tendinopathy results in decreased tendon volume and intratendinous signal as evaluated by MRI. *Am J Sports Med.* 2004;32:1286-1296.

29. Ohberg L, Alfredson H. Effects of neovascularization behind the good results with eccentric training in chronic mid-portion Achilles tendinosis? *Knee Surg Sports Traumatol Arthrosc.* 2004;12:465-470.

30. Kjaer M. Role of extracellular matrix in adaptation of tendon and skeletal muscle to mechanical loading. *Physiol Rev.* 2004;84:649-698.

31. Kjaer M, Langberg H, Miller BF, et al. Metabolic activity and collagen turnover in human tendon in response to physical activity. *J Musculoskelet Neuronal Interact.* 2005;5:41-52.

32. Kjær M, Langberg H, Heinemeier K, et al. From mechanical loading to collagen synthesis, structural changes and function in human tendon. *Scand J Med Sci Sports.* 2009;19:500-510.

33. Arampatzis A, Albracht K, Karamanidis K. Adaptations responses of the human Achilles tendon by modulation of the applied cyclic strain magnitude. *J Exp Bio.* 2007;210:2743-2753.

34. Chaudhry S, Morrissey D, Woledge R, et al. Eccentric and concentric exercise of the triceps surae: an in vivo study of dynamic muscle and tendon biomechanical parameters. *J Appl Biomech.* 2015;31:69-78.

35. Silbernagel KG, Thomee R, Eriksson BI, Karlsson J. Continued sports activity, using a pain-monitoring model, during rehabilitation in patients with Achilles tendinopathy: a randomized controlled study. *Am J Sports Med.* 2007;35:897-906.

36. Silbernagel KG, Brorsson A, Lundberg M. The majority of patients with Achilles tendinopathy recover fully when treated with exercise alone: a 5-year follow-up. *Am J Sports Med.* 2011;39:607-613.

Lateral Ankle Sprain

Charles Greene

A 17-year-old female high school soccer player sustained a noncontact injury to her right ankle during a game. The injury occurred while she was cutting with the soccer ball. She reported that she immediately fell to the pitch, could not bear weight on her right ankle, and could not return to the game. After the sideline evaluation, the player was sent to the team physician, who immediately ordered x-rays. After re-evaluating the athlete and reviewing the x-rays the following day, the team physician diagnosed the athlete with a lateral ankle sprain and referred her to physical therapy for evaluation and treatment. The athlete's goal is to return to play as soon as possible to finish her senior season.

▶ What signs and symptoms may be associated with this diagnosis?
▶ What are the most appropriate examination tests?
▶ What are the most appropriate physical therapy interventions?
▶ What objective criteria should the athlete meet prior to returning to play?

KEY DEFINITIONS

ANTERIOR TALOFIBULAR LIGAMENT (ATFL): One of three ligaments forming the lateral collateral ligament (LCL) complex of the ankle; the ATFL originates on the lateral malleolus of the fibula and inserts on the talus.

CALCANEOFIBULAR LIGAMENT (CFL): Middle portion of the LCL complex of the ankle that forms a narrow band originating from the lateral malleolus of the fibula and inserts on the calcaneal tubercle

LATERAL ANKLE SPRAIN (LAS): "Roll in" sprain injury of the ATFL that occurs when an inversion force is applied to the lateral ankle with the foot in plantarflexion; if the inversion force extends posteriorly, the CFL and posterior talofibular ligament may also be injured.

POSTERIOR TALOFIBULAR LIGAMENT (PTFL): Posterior portion of the LCL complex of the ankle that originates on the lateral malleolus of the fibula and inserts on the posterior surface of the talus

Objectives

1. Describe the anatomy of the LCL complex of the ankle.
2. Describe the risk factors associated with LAS.
3. Identify the most accurate clinical tests for assessing a LCL complex sprain.
4. Compare and contrast the signs and symptoms associated with the different grades of ankle sprain.
5. Implement evidence-based rehabilitation treatments for LCL complex of the ankle.

Physical Therapy Considerations

Physical therapy considerations during the management of the individual with a diagnosis of LCL sprain:

▶ **General physical therapy plan of care/goals:** Decrease pain; increase flexibility and/or joint range of motion; increase lower quadrant strength; restore balance; prevent or minimize loss of aerobic fitness capacity

▶ **Physical therapy interventions:** Patient education regarding functional anatomy and injury pathomechanics; modalities and manual therapy to decrease pain and increase range of motion (ROM); flexibility exercises; resistance exercises to increase endurance capacity of the core muscles and strength of lower extremity muscles; balance exercises; aerobic exercise program; prophylactic taping/bracing

▶ **Precautions during physical therapy**: Monitor vital signs; address precautions or contraindications for exercise based on stages of healing; address precautions or contraindications for the use of modalities

▶ **Complications interfering with physical therapy**: Excessive edema; excessive scarring that limits normal ankle ROM

Understanding the Health Condition

Since the National Federation of State High School Associations started keeping records, participation in high school athletics has increased annually.[1] From 2005 to 2016, high school sports participation increased from 7.1 to 11.1 million, with female participation approximately doubling during that time.[1] Increased sports participation has resulted in an increased frequency of injuries. Each year, there are an estimated 807,222 lower extremity sports-related injuries (LESRIs) in American high school athletes.[2] Sports with the highest LESRI rate were football and girls' soccer.[2] The most frequently injured lower extremity regions were ankles (40%), knees (25%), and thighs (14%), with the most common diagnoses of sprains (50%), strains (17%), contusions (12%), and fractures (5%).[2]

In a comprehensive study covering the same 11-year span (2005-2016), researchers evaluated data from High School Reporting Information Online, a national high school sports injury surveillance system for athletes participating in 8 gender-comparable sports (soccer, volleyball, basketball, baseball/softball, swimming and diving, track and field, cross-country, and tennis) to determine rates and patterns of LESRIs.[3] Similar to the aforementioned study, the authors found LESRI rates were highest in girls' soccer followed by basketball.[2,3] In a study from 2005/06 to 2010/11 describing ankle injury rates in 20 sports using the High School Reporting Information Online, the authors also found that ankle sprain rates were higher for girls in gender-comparable sports.[2-4] The ATFL was most frequently injured, involving 85.3% of sprains.[4]

The lateral ankle is stabilized by the LCL complex, which is comprised of three ligaments: the ATFL, the CFL, and the PTFL (Fig. 32-1). The medial ankle is stabilized by the medial collateral ligament (also known as the deltoid ligament).

The ATFL originates from the anterior-inferior border of the lateral malleolus of the fibula and inserts on the neck of the talus. The function of the ATFL is to prevent the talus from being displaced anteriorly and internally rotated when the talocrural joint is plantarflexed.[5] The ATFL is the weakest of the three ligaments comprising the LCL. A load of approximately 138.9 newtons injures the ATFL, which is roughly half the load required to injure the PTFL (261.2 newtons) and one-third of the force required to injure the CFL (345.7 newtons).[6,7] Due to its low-load capability, anatomical position, and the unstable plantarflexed position, the ATFL is the most commonly injured component of the LCL complex.[2-7]

Risk factors for a LAS can be categorized as intrinsic (originating within the body) or extrinsic (originating outside the body).[8-10] Intrinsic risk factors include age, sex, body composition, prior medical history (*e.g.*, previous LCL injury, history of concussion), anatomical variations (*e.g.*, increased foot width or cavovarus deformity), beginner skill level, poor postural control, decreased reaction time, increased ankle

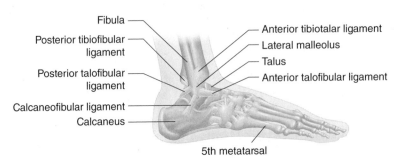

Figure 32-1. Ligaments of the foot, lateral aspect. (Reproduced with permission from Mark H. Hankin, Dennis E. Morse, Carol A. Bennet-Clarke: *Clinical Anatomy: A case-study approach.* NY: McGraw Hill LLC, 2013.)

eversion to inversion strength, decreased ligament tensile strength, limited dorsi-flexion ROM, and psychological factors (*e.g.*, fear of re-injury).[8-14] Extrinsic factors that increase the risk of LAS include participation in sports that involve cutting maneuvers and types of shoes worn (*i.e.*, high-tops compared to low-tops). In addition, failing to use braces or orthoses increases the risk of reinjury.[8-14]

A LAS injury occurs when an athlete is transitioning from nonweightbearing to weightbearing.[15-17] The characteristic biomechanical features of LAS injury are a rapid increase in inversion and internal rotation with or without plantarflexion.[15-17] Therefore, LAS injury results from a sudden inversion and internal rotation loading of the foot-ankle complex regardless of sagittal plane position.[15-17] In addition, kinematic studies demonstrate that peak inversion occurs very rapidly after initial contact, typically between 0.09 and 0.13 seconds.[15-17] Delayed eversion reaction time of peroneal muscles at the lateral aspect of the ankle may contribute to the body's inability to counteract the rapidly occurring inversion force allowing for the LAS.[18]

There are numerous grading systems used to classify LAS injury. The most common is the anatomic system that categorizes injury into three grades (I, II, III) according to the ligaments damaged (Table 32-1).[19-24] An expanded classification system explicitly designed for categorizing LAS injury severity includes clinical tests, active ROM deficits, edema and stress radiograph differences between limbs, and full rehabilitation time/return-to-play timelines.[25] The LAS expanded injury classification consists of 4 injury grades: I, II, IIIA, and IIIB. Grade I is characterized by side-to-side active range of motion (AROM) differences up to 5°, side-to-side edema difference of 0.5 cm, and a return to play in approximately 7 days. Grade II LAS injury is characterized by a positive anterior drawer test, AROM differences >5° but <10°, edema difference >0.5 cm but <2.0 cm, and return to play in approximately 15 days. Grade IIIA is characterized by positive anterior drawer and talar tilt tests, AROM differences >10°, edema difference >2.0 cm, normal stress radiographs, and return to play at approximately 3 weeks. A Grade IIIB LAS injury is characterized by positive anterior drawer and talar tilt tests, AROM differences >10°, edema differences >2.0 cm, >3.00 mm side-to-side difference on stress radiographs, and a return to play of approximately 2 months.[25] Full rehabilitation time refers to the time between the initial injury and the time for the athlete to be able to return to play.

Table 32-1   ANATOMIC SYSTEM FOR CATEGORIZING LAS INJURY SEVERITY[19-24]

Injury Grade	Anatomical Disruption	Pain	Edema	Debilitating	Initiation of Rehabilitation	Time Loss (days)
I	Stretching of ligament only No disruption of fibers, and no ankle instability	Discomfort to mild pain	Absent to mild	Seldom	Can begin immediately	0-7
II	Some tearing of ligament fibers Moderate ankle instability	Moderate to severe pain	Moderate to severe	Mild	7-10 days after immobilization	21-45
III	Complete ligament rupture Gross ankle instability	Severe pain	Severe	Severe	Several weeks, depending on the plan of care (surgery versus conservative intervention)	Major loss of time from sports

Physical Therapy Patient/Client Management

Most LAS injuries (Grades I-III) can be managed with nonsurgical approaches,[26-28] including short-term immobilization with a semi-rigid brace, neuromuscular training, balance training, joint mobilization, therapeutic exercise, nonsteroidal anti-inflammatory drugs, and limited use of modalities.[10,14,26,28-31] However, for individuals with grade III LAS injuries that do not respond to conservative management, surgical repair may be necessary.[28] The primary goal for most athletes with LAS injury is to return to pain-free sport or activity as quickly and as safely as possible in a manner that does not overload the healing tissues, which can lead to chronic ankle instability (CAI).

Examination, Evaluation, and Diagnosis

A comprehensive musculoskeletal examination must be conducted to rule out other potential sources of lower extremity pain. Individuals who present with signs and symptoms of a grade III LAS injury, a syndesmotic sprain (also known as a high ankle sprain), or with tenderness over the physis during the physical examination should be referred to an orthopedic provider for further evaluation and management.[31] An individual with a suspected grade III LAS is referred to an orthopedist because of the risk of developing CAI, which can lead to long-term disability.[31] There is a lack of consensus in the literature regarding whether a person should have surgery for a grade III LAS injury or attempt a course of rehabilitation. The majority of studies have failed to demonstrate that surgery is superior to functional rehabilitation.[10,26,28,32-34] The only exception is that individuals who had surgery reported feeling less unstable than those who did not have surgical stabilization.[32] If the physical therapist suspects that the athlete has a syndesmotic sprain, referral to an orthopedist is indicated for weightbearing radiographs to rule out the presence of a fracture or tibiofibular diastasis, which often accompany grade II, grade III, or syndesmotic ankle sprains.[35] An MRI scan can be useful for assessing the extent of the syndesmotic injury and the presence of nondisplaced fractures or bony edema.[35,36] MRI scans of syndesmotic injuries have revealed that increased injury grade was an important factor in determining prolonged disability. Last, if the physical therapist discovers bony tenderness over the physis in the skeletally immature patient, the patient should be referred for x-rays because of the risk to the growth plate.[31]

During the subjective examination, the physical therapist identifies the mechanism of injury (contact versus noncontact) and location of the pain. Completion of outcome tools, such as the Foot and Ankle Disability Index or the Foot and Ankle Measure, during the initial visit allows the physical therapist to evaluate progress during therapy based on changes in scores at discharge.[29]

The objective examination includes goniometric measurement of ROM, assessment of edema, manual muscle testing, palpation, and special testing. Immediately after the injury, ankle ROM is usually globally limited due to edema. To measure edema surrounding the ankle joint, a tape measure is wrapped around the ankle in the figure-of-eight method. The figure-of-eight (or, figure-of-eight-20) method for assessing edema has excellent inter-rater reliability (intraclass correlation coefficient [ICC] of 0.993 to 0.99) and intra-rater reliability (ICC) of 0.80 to 0.99.[37-39] Since the figure-of-eight method is faster and easier than the water displacement technique and has similar inter-rater reliability (ICC = 0.99), it may be the preferred method for assessing edema.[37-39]

Because of pain and edema, lower leg muscle strength is typically decreased compared to the uninvolved side. The physical therapist should palpate osseous and ligamentous structures including the ATFL, CFL, and PTFL, and the deltoid ligament. The deltoid ligament should be palpated because when the ankle is inverted, supinated, and the lower leg externally rotates, the deltoid ligament can also be injured during a LAS.[9,33,40,41] If the deltoid ligament is tender on palpation, further examination is warranted to rule out an avulsion fracture and/or ligament rupture.[9,33,40,41]

Table 32-2 describes three special tests that can be used to assess the integrity of the lateral ligament complex: anterior drawer test, talar tilt test (also known as inversion stress test), and the squeeze test.[42-54] The anterior drawer test (Fig. 32-2) and talar tilt test (Fig. 32-3) assess the integrity of the ATFL and the CFL. However, adding inversion to the anterior drawer test also evaluates the integrity of the CFL. The talar tilt test primarily assesses the CFL; adding ankle plantarflexion during the test also assesses the ATFL.[41-48,53-56] The squeeze test (Fig. 32-4) assesses the integrity of the interosseous ligament, the interosseus membrane, and the integrity of the tibia and fibula.[42,49-52]

Table 32-2 SPECIAL TESTS ASSOCIATED WITH LATERAL COLLATERAL LIGAMENT COMPLEX[42-54]

Test	Patient Position and Therapist Action	Findings for a Positive Test	Sensitivity	Specificity
Anterior drawer (Fig. 32-2)	Patient is supine or seated with knee flexed 90°, and ankle plantarflexed 10°-20°. Therapist provides gentle anterior translatory force to subtalar joint. Same procedure for testing the CFL, except ankle is placed in neutral position.	Increased laxity compared to the uninvolved side	33%-80%[43-48]	38%-74%[44,45,47]
Talar tilt (also known as inversion stress test) (Fig. 32-3)	Patient seated with ankle in neutral. Therapist stabilizes the distal leg with one hand and uses other hand to grasp the talus and calcaneus and provides an inversion force.	Increased laxity compared to the uninvolved side	50%-52%[43,53]	68%-88%[53,54]
Squeeze (Fig. 32-4)	Using both hands, the therapist compresses the fibula toward the tibia above the midpoint of the calf.	Pain in the interosseous ligament or supporting structures	30%-33%[49-52]	93%[50]

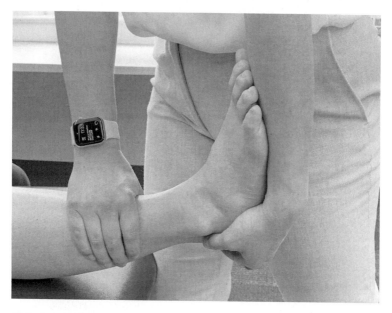

Figure 32-2. Anterior drawer test.

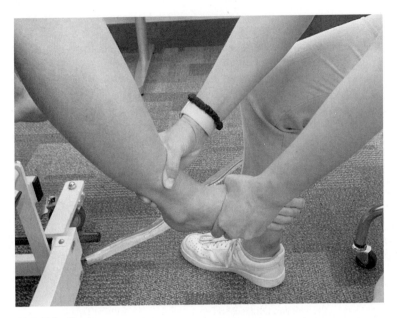

Figure 32-3. Talar tilt test.

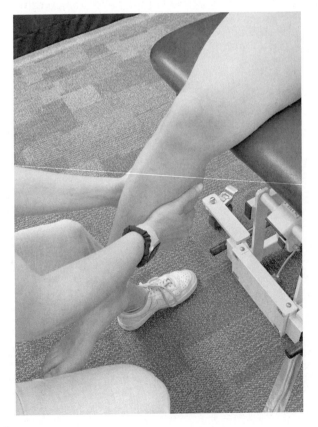

Figure 32-4. Squeeze test.

Plan of Care and Interventions

Grade I and II LAS injuries can be treated with an individualized physical therapy plan of care. The phase of healing (inflammatory, proliferation, or remodeling) and the findings from the examination guide the choice of interventions.[57-59] During the inflammatory phase, the goal is to reduce or control edema and prevent further injury to the ligaments and ankle joint. Treatments include use of ankle braces or stirrups to protect the injured ligament/s by reducing inversion-related movements; cryotherapy and modalities to reduce edema and pain; manual therapy (*e.g.*, joint mobilization or lymphatic drainage techniques) to restore pain-free active ROM and crutches or a walking boot to offset weight from the injured tissue and normalize gait.[10,26,28,33,34,60]

Traditionally, **rest, ice, compression, and elevation (RICE) of the injured lower extremity** have been recommended by physicians and physical therapists as initial interventions for LAS injuries. However, there is weak evidence (anecdotal or case studies) supporting the efficacy of cryotherapy or other modalities to treat pain and edema.[26,28,30,34] The **use of manual therapy compared to rest and immobilization during the acute and post-acute stages to reduce edema, improve ROM, and decrease pain is supported by randomized controlled trials and systematic reviews.**[26,28,30,34] Several systematic reviews also support the use of prescription and over-the-counter anti-inflammatory medication for pain and edema.[26,28,30,34]

During the proliferation phase, healing tissue undergoes vascular ingrowth and proliferation of fibroblasts, leading to new collagen formation.[33] During this stage, the physical therapist continues the strategies employed during the inflammatory phase.[26,28,30,33] Therapeutic activities are progressed to improve ROM and strengthening is initiated. **Joint protection, via the use of ankle braces or stirrups, may be of even greater importance during this phase because overstressing healing tissue may contribute to ligament elongation due to excess formation of weaker type III collagen fibers, which may potentially lead to CAI.**[33,34,61]

During the **remodeling phase (lasting up to 1-year posttrauma), therapeutic interventions are applied to increase strength** (Fig. 32-5), **improve flexibility, aerobic conditioning, and neuromuscular re-education** (Fig. 32-6).[28,30,33,34,62-64] The chosen activities are progressive and simulate the physical demand of the athlete's sport.[32] **To reduce the risk of developing CAI, the athlete must continue protecting the ligament/s with either a lace-up ankle brace or with ankle taping, particularly during physical activity.**[28,30,33,34,62-64]

Knowing when the athlete can return to sport can be complex because several factors go into this decision.[30,32,34,61,65] For an athlete to return to sport, all functional limitations must be fully restored. The athlete should demonstrate: minimal pain (0-2 on a visual analog scale); score of 100% on the Foot Ankle Disability Index for Sport (*i.e.*, demonstrates no dysfunction); ankle passive and active ROM equal to or greater than the noninjured side; minimal ankle edema (*i.e.*, figure-of-eight measurement ≤10% of the noninvolved side); negative stress tests for the LCL complex; strength (*e.g.*, manual muscle tests, isokinetic) and balance/proprioception scores ≥90% compared to noninjured side (*e.g.*, Y Balance Test, Balance Error Scoring System); and sports-specific performance test scores ≥90% (*e.g.*, 1-legged hop test for distance, 6-meter hop for time, hopping agility test, figure-8 agility test).[30,32,34,55,61,65]

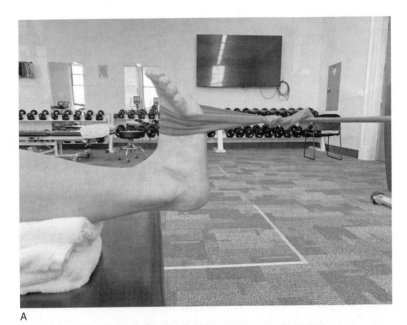

A

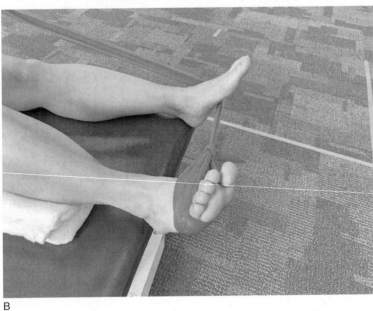

B

Figure 32-5. Resistance band strengthening exercises for ankle. **A.** dorsiflexion, **B.** eversion, **C.** inversion; **D.** plantarflexion

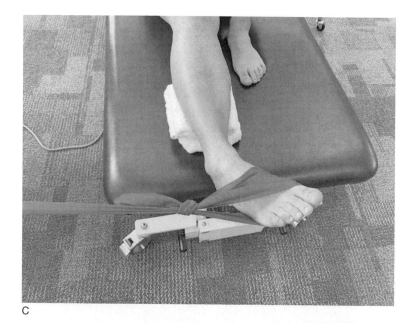

C

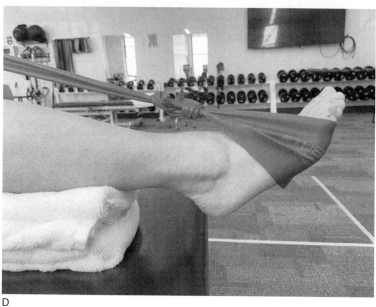

D

Figure 32-5. (*Continued*)

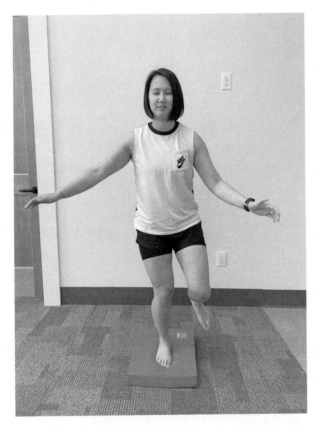

Figure 32-6. Patient performing single-leg balance exercise with eyes closed on unstable surface.

Evidence-Based Clinical Recommendations

SORT: Strength of Recommendation Taxonomy

A: Consistent, good-quality patient-oriented evidence
B: Inconsistent or limited quality patient-oriented evidence
C: Consensus, disease-oriented evidence, usual practice, expert opinion, or case series

1. Rest, cryotherapy (ice), compression, and elevation (RICE) should be used during the first 24 to 48 hours of the initial injury to control pain and edema. **Grade C**

2. Manual therapy such as joint mobilizations can help increase ROM and decrease pain after LAS. **Grade A**

3. Ankle supports (*e.g.*, stirrups, walking boots, ankle braces) should be used during the inflammatory, proliferation, and remodeling phases to reduce the risk of chronic ankle instability injury. **Grade A**

4. Therapeutic exercise is more effective than immobilization and rest alone in managing grade I and II ankle sprains. **Grade A**

COMPREHENSION QUESTIONS

32.1 The most common lateral collateral ligament injured during an inversion mechanism is

A. Deltoid

B. Posterior talofibular

C. Anterior talofibular

D. Calcaneofibular

32.2 To reduce edema, restore ROM, or improve functional performance after a LAS, the MOST effective intervention is:

A. Functional exercise

B. Ankle support post-injury

C. Nonsteroidal anti-inflammatory drugs (NSAIDs)

D. All of the above are correct.

ANSWERS

32.1 **C.** The anterior talofibular ligament is the most common ligament sprained because it is the weakest of the three ligaments and because of its anatomical position (origin and insertion).

32.2 **D.** Convincing evidence has demonstrated that the combination of functional exercise, ankle support, and NSAIDs are recommended for treating LAS injuries.

REFERENCES

1. Federation of State High School Associations. https://members.nfhs.org/participation_statistics. Accessed September 19.2021.

2. Fernandez WG, Yard EE, Comstock RD. Epidemiology of lower extremity injuries among U.S. high school athletes. *Acad Emerg Med.* 2007;14:641-645.

3. Brant JA, Johnson B, Brou L, et al. Rates and patterns of lower extremity sports injuries in all gender-comparable U.S. high school sports. *Orthop J Sports Med.* 2019;7:2325967119873059.

4. Swenson DM, Collins CL, Fields SK, Comstock RD. Epidemiology of U.S. high school sports-related ligamentous ankle injuries, 2005/06-2010/11. *Clin J Sport Med.* 2013;23:190-196.

5. Watanabe K, Kitaoka HB, Berglund LJ, et al. The role of ankle ligaments and articular geometry in stabilizing the ankle. *Clin Biomech.* 2012;27:189-195.

6. Bozkurt M, Doral MN. Anatomic factors and biomechanics in ankle instability. *Foot Ankle Clin.* Sep 2006;11:451-463.

7. Attarian DE, McCrackin HJ, Devito DP, et al. A biomechanical study of human lateral ankle ligaments and autogenous reconstructive grafts. *Am J Sports Med.* 1985;13:377-381.

8. Delahunt E, Remus A. Risk factors for lateral ankle sprains and chronic ankle instability. *J Athl Train.* 2019;54(6):611-616.

9. Fong DT, Chan YY, Mok KM, et al. Understanding acute ankle ligamentous sprain injury in sports. *Sports Med Arthrosc Rehabil Ther Technol.* 2009;1:14.

10. Kerkhoffs GM, van den Bekerom M, Elders LA, et al. Diagnosis, treatment and prevention of ankle sprains: an evidence-based clinical guideline. *Br J Sports Med.* 2012;46:854-860.

11. Doherty C, Delahunt E, Caulfield B, et al. The incidence and prevalence of ankle sprain injury: a systematic review and meta-analysis of prospective epidemiological studies. *Sports Med.* 2014;44: 123-140.

12. Ivarsson A, Johnson U, Andersen MB, et al. Psychosocial factors and sport injuries: meta-analyses for prediction and prevention. *Sports Med.* 2017;47:353-365.

13. Martin RL, Davenport TE, Fraser JJ, et al. Ankle stability and movement coordination impairments: lateral ankle ligament sprains revision 2021. *J Orthop Sports Phys Ther.* 2021;51:CPG1-CPG80.

14. Plisky P, Schwartkopf-Phifer K, Huebner B, et al. Systematic review and meta-analysis of the y-balance test lower quarter: reliability, discriminant validity, and predictive validity. *Int J Sports Phys Ther.* 2021;16:1190-1209.

15. Fong DT, Hong Y, Shima Y, et al. Biomechanics of supination ankle sprain: a case report of an accidental injury event in the laboratory. *Am J Sports Med.* 2009;37:822-827.

16. Kristianslund E, Bahr R, Krosshaug T. Kinematics and kinetics of an accidental lateral ankle sprain. *J Biomech.* 2011;44:2576-2578.

17. Skazalski C, Kruczynski J, Bahr MA, et al. Landing-related ankle injuries do not occur in plantarflexion as once thought: a systematic video analysis of ankle injuries in world-class volleyball. *Br J Sports Med.* 2018;52:74-82.

18. Ashton-Miller JA, Ottaviani RA, Hutchinson C, Wojtys EM. What best protects the inverted weightbearing ankle against further inversion? Evertor muscle strength compares favorably with shoe height, athletic tape, and three orthoses. *Am J Sports Med.* 1996;24:800-809.

19. Mulligan P. Leg, ankle, and foot rehabilitation. In: Andrew JR Harrelson GL, Wilk KE. *Physical Rehabilitation of the Injured Athlete.* 3rd ed. Philadelphia, PA. WB Saunders; 2004:354.

20. Hamilton WG. Ballet. In Reider B. *Sports Medicine: The School-Age Athlete.* Philadelphia, PA. WB Saunders;1991:509.

21. Chinn L, Hertel J. Rehabilitation of ankle and foot injuries in athletes. *Clin Sports Med.* 2010;29:157-167.

22. Thomas J. Ankle sprains classification based on anatomical structures. *Athletic Training.* 1986;21:254,256-257.

23. Balduini FC, Tetzlaff J. Historical perspectives on injuries of the ligaments of the ankle. *Clin Sports Med.* 1982;1:3-12.

24. Jackson DW, Ashley RL, Powell JW. Ankle sprains in young athletes. Relation of severity and disability. *Clin Orthop Relat Res.*1974;101:201-215.

25. Malliaropoulos N, Papacostas E, Papalada A, Maffulli N. Acute lateral ankle sprains in track and field athletes: an expanded classification. *Foot Ankle Clin.* 2006;11:497-507.

26. Doherty C, Bleakley C, Delahunt E, Holden S. Treatment and prevention of acute and recurrent ankle sprain: an overview of systematic reviews with meta-analysis. *Br J Sports Med.* 2017;51:113-125.

27. Dubin JC, Comeau D, McClelland RI, et al. Lateral and syndesmotic ankle sprain injuries: a narrative literature review. *J Chiropr Med.* 2011;10:204-219.

28. Petersen W, Rembitzki IV, Koppenburg AG, et al. Treatment of acute ankle ligament injuries: a systematic review. *Arch Orthop Trauma Surg.* 2013;133:1129-1141.

29. Delahunt E, Bleakley CM, Bossard DS, et al. Clinical assessment of acute lateral ankle sprain injuries (ROAST): 2019 consensus statement and recommendations of the International Ankle Consortium. *Br J Sports Med.* 2018;52:1304-1310.

30. Kaminski TW, Hertel J, Amendola N, et al. National Athletic Trainers' Association. National Athletic Trainers' Association position statement: conservative management and prevention of ankle sprains in athletes. *J Athl Train.* 2013;48:528-545.

31. Myrick KM. Clinical assessment and management of ankle sprains. *Orthop Nurs.* 2014;33:244-248; quiz 249-250.

32. D'Hooghe P, Cruz F, Alkhelaifi K. Return to play after a lateral ligament ankle sprain. *Curr Rev Musculoskelet Med.* 2020;13:281-288.

33. van den Bekerom MP, Kerkhoffs GM, McCollum GA, et al. Management of acute lateral ankle ligament injury in the athlete. *Knee Surg Sports Traumatol Arthrosc.* 2013;21:1390-1395.

34. Vuurberg G, Hoorntje A, Wink LM, et al. Diagnosis, treatment and prevention of ankle sprains: update of an evidence-based clinical guideline. *Br J Sports Med.* 2018;52:956.

35. Hunt KJ, Phisitkul P, Pirolo J, Amendola A. High ankle sprains and syndesmotic injuries in athletes. *J Am Acad Orthop Surg.* 2015;23:661-673.

36. Sikka RS, Fetzer GB, Sugarman E, et al. Correlating MRI findings with disability in syndesmotic sprains of NFL players. *Foot Ankle Int.* 2012;33:371-378.

37. Devoogdt N, Cavaggion C, Van der Gucht E, et al. Reliability, validity, and feasibility of water displacement method, figure-of-eight method, and circumference measurements in determination of ankle and foot edema. *Lymphat Res Biol.* 2019;17:531-536.

38. Rohner-Spengler M, Mannion AF, Babst R. Reliability and minimal detectable change for the figure-of-eight-20 method of measurement of ankle edema. *J Orthop Sports Phys Ther.* 2007;37:199-205.

39. Tatro-Adams D, McGann SF, Carbone W. Reliability of the figure-of-eight method of ankle measurement. *J Orthop Sports Phys Ther.* 1995;22:161-163.

40. Hertel J. Functional anatomy, athomechanics, and pathophysiology of lateral ankle instability. *J Athl Train.* 2002;37:364-375.

41. Lynch SA. Assessment of the injured ankle in the athlete. *J Athl Train.* 2002;37:406-412.

42. Larkins LW, Baker RT, Baker JG. Physical examination of the ankle: a review of the original orthopedic special test description and scientific validity of common tests for ankle examination. *Arch Rehabil Res Clin Transl.* 2020;2:100072.

43. Blanshard KS, Finlay DB, Scott DJ, et al. A radiological analysis of lateral ligament injuries of the ankle. *Clin Radiol.* 1986;37:247-251.

44. Croy T, Koppenhaver S, Saliba S, Hertel J. Anterior talocrural joint laxity: diagnostic accuracy of the anterior drawer test of the ankle. *J Orthop Sports Phys Ther.* 2013;43:911-919.

45. Fujii T, Luo ZP, Kitaoka HB, An KN. The manual stress test may not be sufficient to differentiate ankle ligament injuries. *Clin Biomech.* 2000;15:619-623.

46. Lindstrand A. New aspects in the diagnosis of lateral ankle sprains. *Orthop Clin North Am.* 1976;7:247-249.

47. Phisitkul P, Chaichankul C, Sripongsai R, et al. Accuracy of anterolateral drawer test in lateral ankle instability: a cadaveric study. *Foot Ankle Int.* 2009;30:690-695.

48. van Dijk CN, Lim LS, Bossuyt PM, Marti RK. Physical examination is sufficient for the diagnosis of sprained ankles. *J Bone Joint Surg Br.* 1996;78:958-962.

49. Boytim MJ, Fischer DA, Neumann L. Syndesmotic ankle sprains. *Am J Sports Med.* 1991;19:294-298.

50. de César PC, Avila EM, de Abreu MR. Comparison of magnetic resonance imaging to physical examination for syndesmotic injury after a lateral ankle sprain. *Foot Ankle Int.* 2011;32:1110-1114.

51. Mizel M. Technique tip: a revised method of the Cotton test for intra-operative evaluation of syndesmotic injuries. *Foot Ankle Int.* 2003;24:86-87.

52. Nussbaum ED, Hosea TM, Sieler SD, et al. Prospective evaluation of syndesmotic ankle sprains without diastasis. *Am J Sports Med.* 2001;29:31-35.

53. Hertel J, Denegar CR, Monroe MM, Stokes WL. Talocrural and subtalar joint instability after a lateral ankle sprain. *Med Sci Sports Exerc.* 1999;31:1501-1508.

54. Raatikainen T, Putkonen M, Puranen J. Arthrography, clinical examination, and stress radiograph in the diagnosis of acute injury to the lateral ligaments of the ankle. *Am J Sports Med.* 1992;20:2-6.

55. Gribble PA. Evaluating and differentiating ankle instability. *J Athl Train.* 2019;54:617-627.

56. Magee DJ, Manske RC. *Orthopedic Physical Assessment.* 7th ed. St. Louis, MO. Elsevier; 2020.

57. van den Bekerom MP, Struijs PA, Blankevoort L, et al. What is the evidence for rest, ice, compression, and elevation therapy in the treatment of ankle sprains in adults? *J Athl Train.* 2012;47:435-443.

58. Houglum PA. H. Soft tissue healing and its impact on rehabilitation. *J Sport Rehabil.* 1992;1:19-23.

59. Chamberlain CS, Crowley E, Vanderby R. The spatio-temporal dynamics of ligament healing. *Wound Repair Regen.* 2009;17:206-215.

60. Wells B, Allen C, Deyle G, Croy T. Management of acute grade II lateral ankle sprains with an emphasis on ligament protection: a descriptive case series. *Int J Sports Phys Ther.* 2019;14:445-458.

61. Tassignon B, Verschueren J, Delahunt E, et al. Criteria-based return to sport decision-making following lateral ankle sprain injury: a systematic review and narrative synthesis. *Sports Med.* 2019;49:601-619.

62. Akbari M, Karimi H, Farahini H, Faghihzadeh S. Balance problems after unilateral lateral ankle sprains. *J Rehabil Res Dev.* 2006;43:819-824.

63. McKeon PO, Donovan L. A perceptual framework for conservative treatment and rehabilitation of ankle sprains: an evidence-based paradigm shift. *J Athl Train.* 2019;54:628-638.

64. McKeon PO, Hertel J. Systematic review of postural control and lateral ankle instability, part II: is balance training clinically effective? *J Athl Train.* 2008;43:305-315.64.

65. Hale SA, Hertel J. Reliability and sensitivity of the foot and ankle disability index in subjects with chronic ankle instability. *J Athl Train.* 2005;40:35-40.

Plantar Heel Pain

Casey A. Unverzagt

CASE 33

A 45-year-old male self-referred to an outpatient physical therapy clinic with complaints of left heel pain for the past several months. He denies any specific trauma or pain in the right heel or foot. He reports that ibuprofen temporarily helps his pain, but overall the pain is not improving. The pain is worse in the morning and evening and has forced him to terminate his walking program. His goal is to eliminate his pain and return to walking 1 to 2 miles per day, 4 to 5 times per week.

▶ Based on the patient's subjective report and history of plantar heel pain, what do you anticipate may be contributing factors to his condition?
▶ What examination signs may be associated with this diagnosis?
▶ What are the most appropriate physical therapy outcome measures to assess his functional capacity?
▶ What are the most appropriate physical therapy interventions?

KEY DEFINITIONS

PLANTAR FASCIITIS: Inflammatory condition affecting the plantar fascia and perifascial structures of the foot

PLANTAR HEEL PAIN: Nonspecific term for pain under the heel; historically called plantar fasciitis

WINDLASS MECHANISM: Describes the manner by which the plantar fascia supports the foot during weightbearing; provides a model of the biomechanical stresses placed on the plantar fascia[1]

Objectives

1. Describe differential diagnoses associated with plantar heel pain.
2. Describe plantar heel pain and identify potential risk factors associated with this condition.
3. Describe appropriate joint range of motion and/or flexibility exercises for a person with plantar heel pain.
4. Discuss current evidence supporting the use of modalities, taping, and orthotic fabrications for a person with plantar heel pain.

Physical Therapy Considerations

Physical therapy considerations during management of the individual with a diagnosis of plantar heel pain:

▶ **General physical therapy plan of care/goals:** Decrease pain; increase muscular flexibility; prevent or minimize loss of aerobic fitness capacity

▶ **Physical therapy interventions:** Patient education regarding functional anatomy and injury pathomechanics; modalities to decrease pain and inflammation; manual therapy to decrease pain and increase joint mobility; stretching exercises to address tight triceps surae and plantar fascia; orthotic fabrication

▶ **Precautions during physical therapy:** Address contraindications for exercise based on patient's pre-existing condition(s)

▶ **Complications interfering with physical therapy:** Nonadherence with home exercise program

Understanding the Health Condition

The plantar fascia is a fascial layer investing the plantar aspect of the foot that originates from the calcaneus and, via a complex network, inserts on the plantar aspect of the forefoot.[2] Composed largely of collagen and elastic fibers, the plantar fascia's robust and fibrous structure serves to assist with weightbearing through the feet.[2]

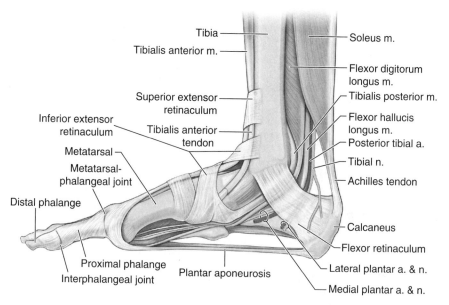

Figure 33-1. Lateral view of the plantar aponeurosis. (Reproduced with permission from Morton DA, Foreman KB, Albertine KH, eds. *The Big Picture: Gross Anatomy.* New York: McGraw-Hill; 2011.)

It is divided into two layers in the transverse plane: the superficial plantar fascia and the deep plantar fascia.[3] The deep plantar fascia is further divided into three layers in the coronal plane (central, lateral, and medial portions).[2] The superficial fascia forms a tough and thick padding over the sole, and has strong *retinacula cutis* (skin ligaments) that tether the skin to the underlying plantar aponeurosis.[3] The deep fascia resembles that within the hand. There is a central plantar aponeurosis that extends forward and divides into digitations for the toes (Fig. 33-1).[3]

Plantar fasciitis is an inflammatory condition affecting the plantar fascia and the perifascial structures of the foot. Historically, physical therapists have attributed plantar fasciitis to faulty biomechanics such as excessive pronation or structural forefoot varus.[1] However, a review of the literature reveals that individuals with either a low-arched or higher-arched foot can experience plantar fasciitis.[1] It has been postulated that individuals with lower arches have impairments resulting from too much motion about the midfoot and rearfoot, whereas individuals with high arches have conditions that result from too little motion.[1,4,5]

The "windlass mechanism" is a model used to provide an explanation of the biomechanical factors and stresses placed upon the foot and plantar fascia.[1] A windlass is a device used to move heavy weights, and it consists of a rope wound around a horizontal cylinder or barrel that is rotated by turning a crank or belt. The windlass effect of the plantar fascia can be illustrated when standing on the ball of the foot (*i.e.*, "tip toes"). The rope is analogous to the plantar fascia and the cylinder is analogous to the metatarsophalangeal joints.[3] During the push-off phase of gait, dorsiflexion causes the plantar fascia to shorten as the winding of the plantar fascia shortens the distance between the calcaneus and metatarsals. This tightening

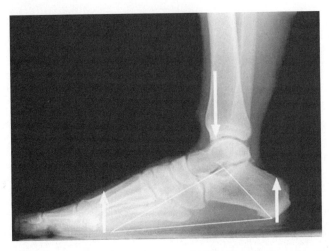

Figure 33-2. Radiograph of foot and ankle. The triangle outlines the truss formed by the calcaneus, midtarsal joint, and metatarsals. The hypotenuse (horizontal line) represents the plantar fascia. Upward arrows depict ground reaction forces. The downward arrow depicts the body's vertical force. The orientation of the vertical and ground reaction forces would cause a collapse of the truss; however, increased plantar fascia tension in response to these forces maintains integrity of the truss. (Reproduced with permission from Bogla LA, Malone TR. Plantar fasciitis and the windlass mechanism: a biomechanical link to clinical practice. *J Athl Train.* 2004;39:77-82.)

of the plantar fascia helps to elevate the medial longitudinal arch. This windlass mechanism can also assist in supinating the foot during the late portion of the stance phase of the gait cycle (Fig. 33-2).

The specific causes of plantar fasciitis are poorly understood, but multiple factors contribute to the condition. Rome *et al.*[6] reported that plantar fasciitis accounts for 15% of all adult foot complaints requiring professional care and the condition is prevalent in both nonathletic and athletic populations. Riddle *et al.*[7] found that the risk of developing plantar fasciitis in a nonathletic population increased with **a decrease in ankle dorsiflexion range of motion. Other independent risk factors include spending the majority of the workday standing and a body mass index (BMI) >30 kg/m^2.**[7] A systematic review examining risk factors associated with chronic plantar heel pain affirmed the independent association between a BMI of 25 and 30 kg/m^2 and the development of plantar fasciitis.[8] This review also identified the presence of a calcaneal spur in a nonathletic population as a significant risk factor. A 2021 case-control study demonstrated that chronic plantar heel pain is not only associated with local foot factors, but also with waist girth, multisite pain, and pain catastrophization.[9]

The term "plantar fasciitis" indicates an inflammatory condition. However, the term has come into question as evidence suggests an absence of inflammatory cells in patients diagnosed with plantar fasciitis.[10] As such, the term "plantar heel pain," which has been used more recently, is likely more appropriate, and will be used hereafter when describing the condition. However, when referring to earlier studies, the term "plantar fasciitis" will be used when the subjects were diagnosed with that condition. In patients with plantar heel pain, other local and regional diagnoses should be considered as either concomitant or independent pathologies. These include plantar heel spurs, bone bruising, fat pad atrophy, tarsal tunnel syndrome, Paget's disease, Sever's disease, plantar fasciopathy (thickening and heterogeneity of the fascia), plantar fascial tearing, calcaneal stress fracture, medial calcaneal nerve entrapment, S1 radiculopathy, and spondyloarthritis. Regardless of the challenges associated with differential diagnosis of plantar heel pain, clinicians must be vigilant to identify and treat the underlying tissue most likely affected (e.g., nerve, tendon, fascia, etc.) and the functional impairments.

Physical Therapy Patient/Client Management

Individuals suffering from plantar heel pain may benefit from several physical therapy interventions including, but not limited to: modalities, manual therapy, taping, night splinting, orthotic devices, and therapeutic exercise.[11] Most patients improve with conservative treatment; however, up to 10% respond poorly and require additional treatment.[12] Cortisone injections, nonsteroidal anti-inflammatory drugs, endoscopic plantar fasciotomy, and extracorporeal shockwave therapy are common interventions available for those who respond poorly to conservative treatment.[11,13-15]

Examination, Evaluation, and Diagnosis

Those at highest risk for developing plantar heel pain, or those who already have the condition, often present with decreased passive ankle dorsiflexion, obesity, and tend to spend the majority of their workday on their feet.[8,11] Individuals will often describe an insidious onset of sharp pain localized to the anteromedial aspect of the heel, or sometimes the center of the plantar aspect of the foot. Pain is most noticeable with initial steps after a period of inactivity (e.g., first steps out of the bed upon wakening), but may worsen following prolonged weightbearing, especially toward the end of the day. During times of increased pain, an antalgic gait may be present.[11] Pain associated with the condition often follows a recent increase in weightbearing activity (e.g., increased walking or running distances). A common clinical presentation also includes immediate pain upon initial steps out of bed in the morning that may gradually decrease with increased activity.

The physical therapist conducts a thorough investigation of the patient's medical history and the current condition. Frequently, a patient reports a recent change in activity level, or employment change that requires more standing or walking. The Foot and Ankle Ability Measure (FAAM) is a reliable and valid self-report questionnaire that assesses impairments, activity limitations, and participation restrictions associated with a patient's heel pain.[11,16] Other validated self-report measures include the Foot Health Status Questionnaire (FHSQ), Foot Function Index (FFI), and the computer-adaptive Lower Extremity Functional Scale (LEFS).[11] The evaluation of a patient with plantar heel pain continues with a comprehensive musculoskeletal examination during which the therapist must be mindful of alternative diagnoses when activity limitations and clinical findings are inconsistent with plantar heel pain.

Table 33-1 CRITERIA USED TO DIAGNOSE PLANTAR FASCIITIS[11]

Plantar medial heel pain, particular after periods of inactivity
Heel pain precipitated by recent increase in weightbearing activity
Pain with palpation of proximal insertion of plantar fascia
Positive windlass test (Table 33-2)
Negative tarsal tunnel test (Table 33-2)
Limited active and passive talocrural joint dorsiflexion range of motion (Table 33-2)
High body mass index in nonathletic individuals

Note the authors from reference 11 used the term plantar fasciitis; however, plantar heel pain is the name of the condition according to the International Classification of Functioning, Disability and Health (ICF).

The examination must also account for possible neurologic, rheumatic, vascular, and central nervous system contributions to the identified impairments.

Table 33-1 presents a list of criteria to use for diagnosis of *plantar fasciitis* according to the International Classification of Diseases (ICD), or *plantar heel pain* according to the International Classification of Functioning, Disability and Health (ICF).[11] Table 33-2 describes how to perform some of the tests used for diagnosis of the condition, as well as their diagnostic accuracy.

Table 33-2 FLEXIBILITY AND SPECIAL TESTS ASSOCIATED WITH PLANTAR HEEL PAIN/PLANTAR FASCIITIS[38]

Test	Patient Position	Positive Findings	Diagnostic Accuracy/ Reliability
Active and passive talocrural joint (ankle) dorsiflexion	Supine on treatment table with feet over edge. Patient actively dorsiflexes ankle and then the therapist passively dorsiflexes ankle. Therapist measures active and passive ROM with goniometer.	≤0° passive dorsiflexion	Intrarater reliability ICC: Passive: 0.64-0.92 Active: 0.74-0.98 Interrater reliability ICC: 0.29-0.81 Odds ratio: 23.3[7] (Those with ≤0° passive dorsiflexion were 23.3 times more likely to have diagnosis compared to those with ≥10° passive dorsiflexion.)
Tarsal tunnel syndrome (dorsiflexion-eversion) test	Seated with foot non-weightbearing, while therapist maximally dorsiflexes ankle, everts foot, and extends all toes for 5-10 second. Then, therapist taps over the region of tarsal tunnel.	Positive Tinel sign or complaint of numbness suggests diagnosis of tarsal tunnel syndrome.	Based on numbness: Sensitivity = 81% Specificity = 99% +LR = 82.73 −LR = 0.19 Based on (+) Tinel sign: Sensitivity = 92% Specificity = 99% +LR = 84.07 −LR = 0.08

(Continued)

Table 33-2   FLEXIBILITY AND SPECIAL TESTS ASSOCIATED WITH PLANTAR HEEL PAIN/PLANTAR FASCIITIS[38] (CONTINUED)

Test	Patient Position	Positive Findings	Diagnostic Accuracy/ Reliability
Windlass test	Test can be performed in two positions: 1. Seated with ankle joint held in neutral by therapist (non-weightbearing), or 2. Standing on step stool with metatarsal heads of foot over edge (weightbearing) Interphalangeal joints are allowed to flex and the first metatarsophalangeal joint is passively extended to end range or until patient's pain is reproduced.	Pain in anteromedial heel or midfoot indicates plantar fasciitis.	Non-weightbearing: Sensitivity = 18% Specificity = 99% +LR = 16.21 −LR = 0.83 Weightbearing: Sensitivity = 33% Specificity = 99% +LR = 28.70 −LR = 0.68
Longitudinal arch angle	Standing with equal weight on both feet. Therapist marks midpoints of medial malleolus, navicular tuberosity, and metatarsal head with a pen, and measures resulting angle of the line with the navicular tuberosity as the fulcrum. (See Fig. 33-3).	Decreased angle (<130°) may correlate to development of plantar fasciitis/ plantar heel pain.	Intrarater reliability ICC: 0.98 Interrater Reliability ICC: 0.67

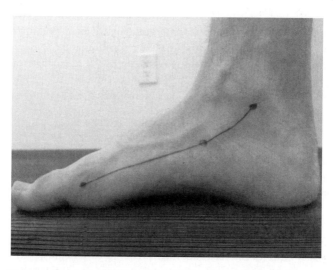

Figure 33-3. Measuring the longitudinal arch angle. Black dots on the midpoints of the medial malleolus, navicular tuberosity, and metatarsal head are connected by a line. Using the navicular tuberosity as the fulcrum, the angle of the line is the longitudinal arch angle.

There is a significant correlation between individuals with plantar heel pain/ plantar fasciitis and decreased passive ankle dorsiflexion with the knee extended (gastrocnemius-soleus complex flexibility).[11,17] While stretching exercises for the gastrocnemius-soleus complex are nearly a universal intervention in a plan of care plantar heel pain/plantar fasciitis, it has been recommended that hamstring length should also be assessed.[18] If the hamstrings demonstrate limited length, stretching of these muscles should be prescribed because increased hamstring tightness may cause prolonged forefoot loading with resultant increased tension on the plantar fascia.[18] Specific stretching of the plantar fascia is beneficial for decreasing pain in individuals with plantar fasciitis, regardless of the initial length of this tissue.[19] After determining that the cause of the patient's pain and dysfunction is due to plantar heel pain, an evidence-based plan of care is implemented and the physical therapist continually monitors the patient's progress through musculoskeletal reassessment and with a self-report questionnaire (*e.g.*, the FAAM).

Plan of Care and Interventions

Physical therapy interventions should address the subjective complaints and objective findings of the initial evaluation. A plan of care to address plantar heel pain includes a combination of anti-inflammatory drugs (NSAIDs), modalities, and taping to provide short-term relief of symptoms (*i.e.*, less than 1 month), while manual therapy, orthotic devices, and night splints may be prescribed to provide more long-term relief of symptoms (*i.e.*, greater than 1 month). Stretching of the gastrocnemius-soleus complex and the plantar fascia provide both short-term and long-term relief, as well as functional improvements.[11]

Prescription and over-the-counter NSAIDs, as well as glucocorticoid injections, are commonly used to decrease pain and inflammation related to plantar heel pain. While the provision of these medications is not within the scope of physical therapy practice, patients often ask the physical therapist for advice regarding their efficacy. Currently, no randomized control trials have been conducted to assess the efficacy of NSAIDs alone. Limited evidence supports the use of glucocorticoid injections for short-term relief (2-4 weeks) of symptoms.[20] Ultimately, the physical therapist should refer patients to their physician or a pharmacist for questions regarding the use, dosage, and efficacy of medications.

Modalities can be used on a short-term basis to treat plantar heel pain. **Ionto-phoresis of either 0.4% dexamethasone or 5% acetic acid**, totaling 6 sessions over 2 to 3 weeks, can provide pain relief and subsequent improvement in function for 2 to 4 weeks after completion of treatment.[11] Low-level laser as well as phonophoresis with ketoprofen gel have also been shown to reduce pain and activity limitations in patients with plantar heel pain/plantar fasciitis.[11]

Several studies, including a recent systematic review support the inclusion of **manual therapy, including mobilization of soft tissue and nerves, to reduce pain, improve range of motion, and facilitate functional improvements in individuals with plantar fasciitis.**[11,21-23] Peripheral joint mobilizations, including posterior glides of the talocrural joint, lateral glides of the subtalar joint, anterior and posterior glides of the first tarsal-metatarsal joint, and distraction of the subtalar joint, appear to be effective at reducing pain and impairments associated with plantar heel pain, though less effective when compared to treatment aimed at soft tissue alone.[22]

Multiple studies have shown that **taping (calcaneal or low-Dye) provides short-term pain relief and functional improvements.**[24-28] However, parameters of taping duration for these benefits have not been specified. The average duration of relief reported by patients was 7 to 10 days.

Orthotics are often prescribed to treat and help prevent recurrences of plantar heel pain. The primary goal of orthotics is to reduce excessive pronation that increases stress on the plantar fascia. Prefabricated and custom orthotics have been shown to provide up to 3 months of pain relief and functional improvement for patients with plantar heel pain.[11,29] There is currently no evidence to support the effectiveness of orthotics for treating plantar heel pain for longer periods of time. In addition, there appears to be no difference in pain intensity or pain interference when comparing soft and hard custom-made orthotics.[30] It is unknown *why* orthotics are effective in treating plantar heel pain because results from studies have been inconclusive.[8]

For individuals who consistently have pain when rising from bed, clinicians should consider recommending a 1 to 3 month trial of night splints.[11] Anterior, posterior, and sock-type night splints have all been shown to provide relief when worn by patients *every* night for 1 to 3 months.[11] Recent evidence suggests that night splints may be less effective at addressing pain and dysfunction associated with chronic plantar heel pain greater than 2 years duration.[31]

There is sufficient evidence to support stretching as a short-term and long-term intervention for pain relief and functional improvement. A number of studies have shown that **calf stretching to increase ankle dorsiflexion correlates with decreased symptoms.**[11] However, authors have not specified whether subjects in the studies had decreased dorsiflexion prior to stretching. Porter *et al.*[32] showed that dorsiflexion stretches improved pain and function in adults with "painful heel syndrome" for up to 4 months. However, there was no difference between groups that performed intermittent stretching (5 sets of 20-second stretches twice per day) versus sustained stretching (3-minute stretches performed 3 times per day). Digiovanni *et al.*[19] showed that **specific stretching of the plantar fascia was also effective at providing long-term (2 years) decreases in pain and improvement in function.** The authors recommended a self-stretch in which the patient dorsiflexes the ankle and extends the toes with one hand while palpating for tension in the fascia with the other hand (Fig. 33-4). Patients were advised to hold the stretch for 10 seconds and repeat 10 times for a single set, with performance of 1 set, 3 times per day, with the first set performed before taking the first step in the morning. There is moderate-quality evidence that self-stretching of the plantar fascia has a larger effect of pain score reduction compared to calf stretching alone.[33] The simultaneous stretching of the Achilles tendon and plantar fascia may be optimal for decreasing pain associated with plantar fasciitis.[34]

Recent meta-analyses and systematic reviews have found that **dry needling of local (Fig. 33-5) and/or regional contributing structures provided statistically significant improvements in pain-related disability and pain intensity** in the short- and long-term in patients experiencing plantar heel pain/plantar fasciitis compared

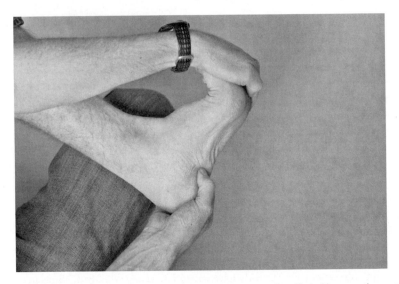

Figure 33-4. Plantar fascia stretching exercise. The patient crosses the affected leg over the contralateral leg. Patient places the fingers across the base of the toes, pulling the toes back toward the shin until a stretch or tautness is felt along the plantar fascia.

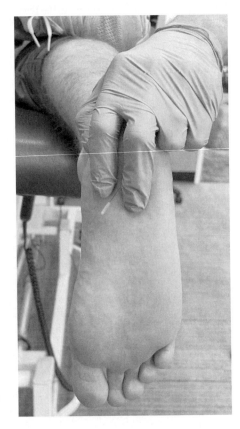

Figure 33-5. Dry needling of the quadratus plantae.

to a control group (placebo or other treatment).[35,36] In a single-blind randomized trial, Rastegar *et al.*[37] compared dry needling to steroid injections in the treatment of plantar fasciitis. The authors found that steroid injections had an immediate analgesic effect, but dry needling produced superior results for patients 12 months after the intervention. More large-scale, adequately powered, placebo-controlled trials should be conducted before recommending dry needling as a stand-alone intervention.

Evidence-Based Clinical Recommendations

SORT: Strength of Recommendation Taxonomy

A: Consistent, good-quality patient-oriented evidence
B: Inconsistent or limited-quality patient-oriented evidence
C: Consensus, disease-oriented evidence, usual practice, expert opinion, or case series

1. Limited ankle dorsiflexion ROM, high BMI (>30 kg/m^2) in nonathletic populations, running, and work-related weightbearing activities are intrinsic risk factors for the development of plantar heel pain/plantar fasciitis. **Grade B**

2. Iontophoresis of 0.4% dexamethasone or 5% acetic acid provides short-term (2-4 weeks) pain relief and improvements in function for individuals with plantar heel pain/plantar fasciitis. **Grade B**

3. Manual therapy consisting of soft tissue, nerve, and joint mobilization should be utilized to decrease pain and improve function in individuals with plantar heel pain/plantar fasciitis. **Grade A**

4. Anti-pronation taping provides short-term (up to 3 weeks) pain relief and improved function in individuals with plantar heel pain. **Grade A**

5. Prefabricated or custom foot orthoses aimed at supporting the arch and reducing abnormal foot pronation provide improvements in function and reduction in pain in patients with plantar heel pain/plantar fasciitis up to 3 months. **Grade A**

6. Night splints should be prescribed for 1 to 3 months as an intervention for patients with plantar heel pain/plantar fasciitis who have pain with the first steps in the morning. **Grade B**

7. Daily stretching, either sustained (1-3 minutes, 3 times per day) or intermittent (5 sets of 20 seconds, 2 times per day) targeting the gastrocnemius-soleus complex provides pain relief and improved calf muscle flexibility in individuals with plantar heel pain/plantar fasciitis for up to 4 months. **Grade B**

8. Stretching of the plantar fascia can decrease pain and improve function in patients with plantar heel pain/plantar fasciitis. **Grade A**

9. When part of a multimodal treatment plan, dry needling of the plantar fascia and/or regional contributing structures can decrease pain-related disability and pain intensity in the short and long term in patients with plantar heel pain/plantar fasciitis. **Grade A**

COMPREHENSION QUESTIONS

33.1 A physical therapist examines a 40-year-old male with complaints of left heel pain for the last 6 months. His pain is worse in the morning when he first steps out of bed. Which intervention would be LEAST effective in providing long-term relief (>1 month) of his symptoms?

 A. Low-Dye taping of the foot

 B. Iontophoresis using 0.4% dexamethasone

 C. Posterior night splint worn for 2 months

 D. Prefabricated orthotics

33.2 A physical therapist examines a 55-year-old female with type 2 diabetes mellitus and recent development of heel pain. She has been diagnosed with plantar heel pain. Which of the following is MOST likely to be a contributing factor to her pain?

 A. Supinated resting foot posture

 B. Pronated resting foot posture

 C. BMI 24 kg/m^2

 D. Decreased active dorsiflexion compared to normal values and her contralateral uninvolved lower extremity

ANSWERS

33.1 **A.** Low-Dye taping has been shown to provide only short-term pain relief, with patients reporting an average of 7 to 10 days of relief. [24-28] All of the other methods listed have been shown to provide months of pain relief to patients who suffer from symptoms of plantar heel pain. [11]

33.2 **D.** According to Riddle et al., [7] decreased dorsiflexion is the greatest risk factor for developing plantar heel pain. While increased BMI has been identified as a risk factor for developing plantar heel pain, a lack of dorsiflexion was shown to be a greater risk factor. A BMI <30 kg/m^2 has not been consistently shown to contribute to plantar heel pain (option C). While historically it was thought that decreased arch height leads to plantar heel pain, this has not been consistently substantiated in the literature. Individuals with high and low arches may develop plantar heel pain/plantar fasciitis (options A and B). [1]

REFERENCES

1. Bolgla LA, Malone TR. Plantar fasciitis and the windlass mechanism: a biomechanical link to clinical practice. *J Athl Train.* 2004;39:77-82.

2. Dutton M. *Orthopaedic Examination, Evaluation, & Intervention.* New York, NY: McGraw-Hill;2004.

3. Rose C, Gaddum-Rosse P, Hollinshead WH. *Hollinshead's Textbook of Anatomy.* 5th ed. Philadelphia, PA:Lippincott-Raven Publishers;1997.

4. Kwong PK, Kay D, Voner RT, White MW. Plantar fasciitis. Mechanics and pathomechanics of treatment. *Clin Sports Med.* 1988;7:119-126.

5. Cornwall MW. Common pathomechanics of the foot. *Athl Ther Today.* 2000;5:10-16.

6. Rome K, Howe T, Haslock I. Risk factors associated with the development of plantar heel pain in athletes. *Foot.* 2001;11:119-125.

7. Riddle DL, Pulisic M, Pidcoe P, Johnson RE. Risk factors for plantar fasciitis: a matched case-control study. *J Bone Joint Surg Am.* 2003;85:872-877.

8. Irving DB, Cook JL, Menz HB. Factors associated with chronic plantar heel pain: a systematic review. *J Sci Med Sport.* 2006;9:11-24.

9. Rogers J, Jones G, Cook JL, et al. Chronic plantar heel pain is principally associated with waist girth (systemic) and pain (central) factors, not foot factors: a case-control study. *J Orthop Sports Phys Ther.* 2021;51:449-458.

10. Lemont H, Ammirati KM, Usen N. Plantar fasciitis: a degenerative process (fasciosis) without inflammation. *J Am Podiatr Med Assoc.* 2003;93:234-237.

11. Martin RL, Davenport TE, Reischl SF, et al. American Physical Therapy Association. Heel Pain—Plantar Fasciitis: Revision 2014. *J Orthop Sports Phys Ther.* 2014;44:A1-A33.

12. Davis PF, Severud E, Baxter DE. Painful heel syndrome: results of nonoperative treatment. *Foot Ankle Int.* 1994;15:531-535.

13. Donley BG, Moore T, Sferra J, et al. The efficacy of oral nonsteroidal anti-inflammatory medication (NSAID) in the treatment of plantar fasciitis: a randomized, prospective, placebo-controlled study. *Foot Ankle Int.* 2007;28:20-23.

14. Urovitz EP, Birk-Urovitz A, Birk-Urovitz E. Endoscopic plantar fasciotomy in the treatment of chronic heel pain. *Can J Surg.* 2008;51:281-283.

15. Malay DS, Pressman MM, Assili A, et al. Extracorporeal shockwave therapy versus placebo for the treatment of chronic proximal plantar fasciitis: results of a randomized, placebo-controlled, double-blinded, multicenter intervention trial. *J Foot Ankle Surg.* 2006;45:196-210.

16. Martin RL, Irrgang JJ, Burdett RG, et al. Evidence of validity for the Foot and Ankle Ability Measure (FAAM). *Foot Ankle Int.* 2005;26:968-983.

17. Drake M, Bittenbender C, Boyles RE. The short-term effects of treating plantar fasciitis with a temporary custom foot orthosis and stretching. *J Orthop Sports Phys Ther.* 2011;41:221-231.

18. Harty J, Soffe K, O'Toole G, Stephens MM. The role of hamstring tightness in plantar fasciitis. *Foot Ankle Int.* 2005;26:1089-1092.

19. Digiovanni BF, Nawoczenski DA, Malay DP, et al. Plantar fascia-specific stretching exercise improves outcomes in patients with chronic plantar fasciitis. A prospective clinical trial with two-year follow-up. *J Bone Joint Surg Am.* 2006;88:1775-81.

20. Crawford F, Thomson C. Interventions for treating plantar heel pain. *Cochrane Database Syst Rev.* 2003:CD000416.

21. Fraser JJ, Corbett R, Donner C, Hertel J. Does manual therapy improve pain and function in patients with plantar fasciitis? A systematic review. *J Man Manip Ther.* 2018;26:55-65.

22. Pollack Y, Shashua A, Kalichman L. Manual therapy for plantar heel pain. *Foot.* 2018;34:11-16.

23. Yelverton C, Rama S, Zipfel B. Manual therapy interventions in the treatment of plantar fasciitis: a comparison of three approaches. *Health SA.* 2019;24(0), a1244.

24. Osborne HR, Allison GT. Treatment of plantar fasciitis by low-Dye taping and iontophoresis: short term results of a double blinded, randomised, placebo-controlled clinical trial of dexamethasone and acetic acid. *Br J Sports Med.* 2006;40:545-549.

25. Hyland MR, Webber-Gaffney A, Cohen L, Lichtman PTSW. Randomized controlled trial of calcaneal taping, sham taping, and plantar fascia stretching for the short-term management of plantar heel pain. *J Orthop Sports Phys Ther.* 2006;36:364-371.

26. Radford JA, Landorf KB, Buchbinder R, Cook C. Effectiveness of low-Dye taping for the short-term treatment of plantar heel pain: a randomised trial. *BMC Musculoskelet Disord.* 2006;7:64.

27. Podolsky R, Kalichman L. Taping for plantar fasciitis. *J Back Musculoskelet Rehabil.* 2015;28:1-6.

28. Verbruggen LA, Thompson MM, Durall CJ. The effectiveness of low-Dye aping in reducing pain associated with plantar fasciitis. *J Sport Rehabil.* 2018;27:94-98.

29. Whittaker GA, Munteanu SE, Menz HB, et al. Effectiveness of Foot Orthoses Versus Corticosteroid Injection for Plantar Heel Pain: The SOOTHE Randomized Clinical Trial. *J Orthop Sports Phys Ther.* 2019;49:491-500.

30. Seligman DAR, Dawson D, Streiner DL, et al. Treating heel pain in adults: a randomized controlled trial of hard vs modified soft custom orthotics and heel pads. *Arch Phys Med Rehabil.* 2021;102:363-370.

31. Wheeler PC. The addition of a tension night splint to a structured home rehabilitation programme in patients with chronic plantar fasciitis does not lead to significant additional benefits in either pain, function or flexibility: a single-blinded randomised controlled trial. *BMJ Open Sport Exerc Med.* 2017;3:e000234.

32. Porter D, Barrill E, Oneacre K, May BD. The effects of duration and frequency of Achilles tendon stretching on dorsiflexion and outcome in painful heel syndrome: a randomized, blinded, control study. *Foot Ankle Int.* 2002;23:619-624.

33. Siriphorn A, Eksakulkla S. Calf stretching and plantar fascia-specific stretching for plantar fasciitis: A systematic review and meta-analysis. *J Bodyw Mov Ther.* 2020;24:222-232.

34. Engkananuwat P, Kanlayanaphotporn R, Purepong N. Effectiveness of the simultaneous stretching of the Achilles tendon and plantar fascia in individuals with plantar fasciitis. *Foot Ankle Intl.* 2018;39:75-82.

35. He C, Ma H. Effectiveness of trigger point dry needling for plantar heel pain: a meta-analysis of seven randomized controlled trials. *J Pain Res.* 2017;10:1933-1942.

36. Llurda-Almuzara L, Labata-Lezaun N, Meca-Rivera T, et al. Is dry needling effective for the management of plantar heel pain or plantar fasciitis? An updated systematic review and meta-analysis. *Pain Med.* 2021;22:1630-1641.

37. Rastegar S, Baradaran Mahdavi S, Hoseinzadeh B, et al. Comparison of dry needling and steroid injection in the treatment of plantar fasciitis: a single-blind randomized clinical trial. *Int Orthop.* 2018;42:109-116.

38. McPoil TG, Martin RL, Cornwall MW, et al. Heel pain-plantar fasciitis: clinical practice guidelines linked to the international classification of function, disability, and health from the orthopaedic section of the American Physical Therapy Association. *J Orthop Sports Phys Ther.* 2008;38:A1-A18.

Note: Page numbers followed by f indicate figures; those followed by t indicate tables.